# INFUSION THERAPY

## TECHNIQUES & MEDICATIONS

**MARILYN FERRERI BOOKER, MS, RN, CRNI**
Regional Director Mid-Atlantic
Premier Medical Services, Inc.
Walnut Creek, California

**DONNA D. IGNATAVICIUS, MS, RN, C**
Instructor, Charles County Community College
Consultant in Gerontological Nursing
La Plata, Maryland

**W.B. SAUNDERS COMPANY**
*A Division of Harcourt, Brace & Company*
Philadelphia London Toronto
Montreal Sydney Tokyo

**W.B. SAUNDERS COMPANY**
*A Division of Harcourt Brace & Company*

The Curtis Center
Independence Square West
Philadelphia, PA 19106

**NOTICE**

Medicine is an ever-changing field. Standard safety precautions must be followed, but as new research and clinical experience broaden our knowledge, changes in treatment and drug therapy become necessary or appropriate. The editors of this work have carefully checked the generic and trade drug names and verified drug dosages to ensure that the dosage information in this work is accurate and in accord with the standards accepted at the time of publication. Readers are advised, however, to check the product information currently provided by the manufacturer of each drug to be administered to be certain that changes have not been made in the recommended dose or in the contraindications for administration. This is of particular importance in regard to new or infrequently used drugs. It is the responsibility of the treating physician, relying on experience and knowledge of the patient, to determine dosages and the best treatment for the patient. The editors cannot be responsible for misuse or misapplication of the material in this work.

THE PUBLISHER

Cover Illustration: Penicillin G

**Library of Congress Cataloging-in-Publication Data**

Booker, Marilyn Ferreri.
Infusion therapy : techniques and medications / Marilyn Ferreri Booker, Donna D. Ignatavicius.
p. cm.
1st ed.
Includes index.
ISBN 0-7216-4923-8
1. Infusion therapy. I. Ignatavicius, Donna D. II. Title.
[DNLM: 1. Home Infusion Therapy. 2. Infusions, Parenteral. 3. Fluid Therapy. WB 354 B7241 1996]
RM170.B66 1996
615'.6—dc20
DNLM/DLC

95-17700

INFUSION THERAPY:
TECHNIQUES AND MEDICATIONS

ISBN 0-7216-4923-8



Printed in the United States of America

Last digit is the print number: 9 8 7 6 5 4 3 2 1

*To Dennis, Reed, and Mary for their love,*
*patience, understanding, and support.*
*To my parents, George and Mary,*
*for their support, love, and encouragement.*

**MFB**

*To Charles and Stephanie for their continuing*
*patience and support.*

**DDI**

*To Elaine Kennedy for her valuable efforts,*
*sense of humor, patience,*
*and above all, her friendship.*

**MFB** and **DDI**

# Reviewers

**Sheila Y. Asbury, MSN, ADN**
School of Nursing, Western Piedmont Community College, Morganton, North Carolina

**Patricia Gauntlett Beare, PhD, MSN, MEd, RN**
College of Nursing, Louisiana State University Medical Center, New Orleans, Louisiana

**Rita F. Bonczek, MS, APRN, CRRN, CS**
Nursing Department, Hospital for Special Care, New Britain, Connecticut

**Elizabeth Carney, MEd, MSN, RN**
College of Nursing, Norwich University, Northfield, Vermont

**Barbara K. Clark, MN, RN, CCRN**
College of Nursing, Washburn University, Topeka, Kansas

**Barbara J. Draude, MSN, RN**
College of Nursing, Middle Tennessee State University, Murfreesboro, Tennessee

**Leonard A. Fahien, MD**
School of Medicine, University of Wisconsin, Madison, Wisconsin

**Barbara E. Gould, MEd, BScPhm**
School of Nursing, Seneca College of Applied Arts and Technology Health Sciences, Toronto, Ontario

**Juanita J. Hoadley, MSN, RN**
Deaconess College of Nursing, St. Louis, Missouri

**Donna M. Morgan, MSN, RN, CCRN**
School of Nursing, Arnot Ogden Medical Center, Elmira, New York

**Linda Morris, BSN, CRNI**
Intravenous Therapy Department, St. Clair Hospital, Pittsburgh, Pennsylvania

**Kathrin Z. Petterelli, MS, RN**
Nursing Department, St. Joseph's Hospital School of Nursing, Syracuse, New York

**Alice Rasmussen, MSN, RN**
School of Nursing, Lake Michigan College, Benton Harbor, Michigan

**Donna Ayers Snelson, MSN, RN**
School of Nursing, Misericordia College, Dallas, Pennsylvania

**Jonathan J. Wolfe, PhD, BS Pharmacy**
Pharmacy Practice, College of Pharmacy, Little Rock, Arkansas

# Acknowledgments

The authors wish to thank the following individuals for their time, assistance, expertise, and encouragement:

From W.B. Saunders, Dan Ruth, Nursing Editor; Susan Bielitsky, Editorial Assistant; Maura Connor, Nursing Editor; Joan Sinclair, Production Manager.

From CRACOM Corporation, Mary Espenschied, Production Editor.

Photography, Monica Ridgely.

Finally, our very special thanks to Elaine Kennedy, EdD, RN, contributor, colleague, and friend, whose assistance in the completion of this project was invaluable.

# Preface

With changes occurring almost daily in the health care delivery system in the United States, clients receiving a variety of infusion therapies are being seen in virtually every clinical setting and in the home. The various types of infusion therapy, the medications administered, and the equipment and infusion systems employed in their delivery contribute to the challenges facing today's nursing students and practitioners. *Infusion Therapy: Techniques and Medications* was written primarily to provide nursing students with in-depth information about the various types of infusion therapy and medications not found in traditional medical-surgical texts. Nurses practicing in hospitals, long-term care facilities, clinics, and home care will find descriptions of the different types of infusion equipment and systems, step-by-step procedures, listings of complications for each type of therapy, and medication monographs helpful in their daily practices. *Infusion Therapy: Techniques and Medications* is a pocket guide that presents the information students and practitioners require in a concise yet thorough manner.

Unlike other pocket guides that address either intravenous therapy techniques or intravenous medications only, *Infusion Therapy: Techniques and Medications* contains the latest information on all types of infusion therapy in addition to complete information on medications and solutions the nurse or student may administer via any infusion route. It is really two books under one cover!

The book is divided into four parts. Part I presents the history and scope of the types of infusion therapy addressed in the book. This part also includes a discussion of the role of each practitioner on the health care team as it relates to infusion therapy, a review of pertinent anatomy and physiology, and infusion systems and equipment.

Part II, Types of Infusion Therapy, includes information on site selection, access devices, administration techniques, and complications for each type of therapy discussed. This part includes peripheral intravenous, central intravenous, subcutaneous, central nervous system, arterial, intraperitoneal, and intraosseous therapies.

Fluids and electrolytes, parenteral nutrition, and transfusion therapies are the topics covered in Part III.

Part IV contains parenteral medication monographs grouped in nine chapters by drug category, rather than merely in alphabetical order. Each chapter in Part IV opens with a general description of the categories of medication found in the chapter and of any subclassifications of medications within the category. Following this there is a discussion of the therapeutic effects, pharmacokinetics (distribution, metabolism/elimination), cautions (side/adverse effects, contraindications, pregnancy and lactation, pediatric, geriatric), and drug/food interactions generally associated with this subclassification. In addition, a table delineating the side/toxic effects the medication subclass may exert on each body system, physical assessment and laboratory indicators of the side/toxic effects the nurse may observe, and general nursing interventions make Part IV valuable as a quick reference. This format affords the learner a general knowledge base about a particular grouping of medications that he or she can apply to other medications that belong to the same classification.

A nursing process framework is used for the medication monographs included in these chapters. The assessment section includes the medication's characteristics (action, indications, cautions, and potential drug/food interaction). The intervention section contains medication administration criteria such as mode/rate of administration, dosing across the life span, types of infusion routes, independent nursing actions, and administration in alternate settings. The evaluation section of each monograph focuses on the client's expected physical assessment and laboratory parameter outcomes. Potential negative outcomes are also listed to help delineate usual side effects from toxicities. Although most medications of a particular classification are listed, only monographs for those medications students and practitioners are most likely to see in their practice settings are included.

**Marilyn Ferreri Booker**
**Donna D. Ignatavicius**

# Contents

## PART IV
## Infusion Medication • 323



## PART V
## Appendixes • 767

PART

# I

# Introduction to Infusion Therapy

CHAPTER 1

# Orientation to Infusion Therapy

*Marilyn Ferreri Booker*



Today's medical and nursing research provides the nurse with exciting innovations for client care. These innovations, while stimulating, are also challenging in that they require the nurse to maintain a knowledge base and skill level that keep step with the rapid changes. Infusion therapy has seen remarkable advances, many of which are because of nursing research. This book integrates findings from nursing research whenever appropriate.

## HISTORY

Unlike other medical treatments, infusion therapy does not have a roster of well-known pioneers. Rather, this evolution, one of the most important aspects of client care as we know it in the twentieth century, is one of technologic advances and chemistry.

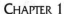

William Harvey described the anatomy of the vascular system in 1628 (*De motre cordis,* 1628). In the mid-1600s Christopher Wren, better known for his accomplishments as an architect, astronomer, meteorologist, and mathematician, observed that access to a dog's entire body could be gained via its foreleg vein. Wren presented his work to his colleagues at Oxford University and later to the Royal Society in London. In *Lancet,* 1832, Dr. Thomas Latta of Scotland outlined a "new" therapy for the treatment of cholera, which was spreading in epidemic proportions throughout the country. His patient was a woman who was near death from the disease. Dr. Latta wrote, "I injected one hundred twenty ounces, when like the effects of magic, instead of the pallid aspect of one whom death had sealed as his own, the vital tide was restored and life and vivacity returned."

During 1898 a number of papers and reports on the topic of infusing saline solution were written. One of the papers was authored by Dr. Thomas Reilly:

> The apparatus commonly employed in the hospitals of New York for this purpose (inEtravenous infusion) consists of a glass funnel connected by a piece of rubber tubing, three feet or more in length, to a cannula, about four inches long by one eighth of an inch in diameter curved for about an inch at its point to facilitate introduction into the vein, and is generally provided with a stopcock.

A problem that plagued intravenous (IV) infusions was pyrogenicity (the infusion of infection-producing agents). Clients receiving IV infusions had a high incidence of fever. Since 1931, terminal sterilization has allowed the commercial manufacturing of IV fluids that are contaminant free, safe, and effective. All IV solutions were in glass containers until the 1970s, when plastic bags were introduced as containers for IV solutions. These bags do not depend on air displacement for infusion and thus eliminate the risk of airborne contamination.

With more research and consequently more knowledge about fluids and electrolytes, solutions other than normal saline solution became available. Today there are hundreds of commercially prepared solutions.

Since the 1970s there have been remarkable advances in infusion therapy. Some of these advances have been in the field of pharmaceuticals, some in equipment, and some in methodologies. Today's nurses may find themselves monitoring drugs or fluid infusions through any of a number of infusion routes.

In 1987 the Centers for Disease Control (CDC) developed and promulgated its system of "universal precautions." These procedures were designed to reduce the risk of transmitting human immunodeficiency virus (HIV), the virus that causes acquired immunodeficiency syndrome (AIDS), and hepatitis B (HBV) to health care workers. In 1992 the Occupational Safety and Health Administration (OSHA) adopted the CDC's approach to infection control and protection of workers and published its "Occupational Exposure to Blood Borne Pathogens; Final Rule" (see Appendix A). These guidelines have been the impetus for the development of new lines of equipment such as "needleless systems" to protect health care workers from exposure.

## SCOPE OF INFUSION THERAPY

Infusion therapy includes the administration of a drug or fluid into the vascular system, subcutaneous tissue, the central nervous system (CNS), a body cavity, or bone. There are many reasons for the physician to prescribe infusion therapy for a particular client. The therapeutic goal may be maintenance, replacement, treatment, diagnosis, monitoring, palliation, or a combination of these. The nurse may administer infusion therapy in short-term-care facilities, outpatient settings, long-term-care facilities, and in clients' homes.

In this book intravascular, subcutaneous, CNS, intraperitoneal (body cavity), and intraosseous infusions are discussed in detail. For a discussion of other body cavity infusions—pleural, pericardial, and bladder—the reader is directed to an oncology text.

## INTRAVASCULAR INFUSIONS

Intravascular administration of medications and fluids results in immediate and complete absorption into the plasma.

### IV Administration

The IV route is the most common method of administering fluids or drugs. IV therapy is the delivery of fluids or drugs into a vein. The vein may be peripheral or central. The peripheral veins used in IV therapy are usually those in the extremities. Central venous therapy is usually designated by the placement of the tip of the access device. For the purpose of this book a catheter whose tip is in the superior or inferior vena cava is considered "central." Both central venous and peripheral IV therapy allow for systemic access via the plasma circulation. The venous system is used for maintenance, replacement, treatment, diagnosis, monitoring, and palliation.

### Arterial Administration

For intraarterial therapy the access device is in an artery. As is true for the IV route, fluids or drugs administered arterially enter the plasma circulation directly. Common uses of arterial therapy are treatment, diagnosis, monitoring, and palliation.

## SUBCUTANEOUS INFUSIONS

Absorption is slower following subcutaneous administration than following intravascular administration. Drugs and fluids enter the plasma through the spaces between the cells of the capillary wall. The most common type of subcutaneous tissue administration the nurse may see is subcutaneous drug administration. Hypodermoclysis (the infusion of an isotonic solution into the subcutaneous tissue) is seldom seen and is not discussed in this book.

In subcutaneous drug administration the nurse administers the drug in small volumes of fluid, usually no more than 1 mL/min, into the space between the cutaneous tissue and the muscle. This method of administering drugs is commonly used for maintenance, treatment, and palliation. Some drugs commonly given subcutaneously include heparin, insulin, morphine, and hydromorphone (Dilaudid).

## CNS INFUSIONS

CNS infusions are seen in the administration of anesthesia, analgesia, chemotherapy, and antibiotics. Unlike intravascular or subcutaneous infusions, in which the plasma acts as the fluid or drug transport agent, drugs administered into the CNS use the cerebrospinal fluid for transport to the site of intended action. Drugs administered via the CNS act in the CNS to provide the desired effects of the treatment. CNS access can also be used for monitoring and palliation.

Two methods are used to gain access to the CNS: epidural and intrathecal.

### Epidural Administration

Epidural administration involves placing an access device into the epidural space. In epidural administration the drug diffuses slowly from the epidural space into the cerebrospinal fluid in the subarachnoid space.

### Intrathecal Administration

Intrathecal administration may be into the spine or the cerebrum. In both cases the drug is administered directly into the cerebrospinal fluid. In spinal intrathecal administration a catheter is placed into the spinal column with the tip of the catheter in the subarachnoid space between the dura and the spinal cord. This area contains the cerebrospinal fluid and the nerve roots. In cerebral intrathecal administration the cerebral port or reservoir (Ommaya reservoir) is placed in the ventricle over the frontal lobe just under the scalp. The catheter attached to this device provides direct access to the cerebrospinal fluid.

## BODY CAVITY INFUSIONS (IRRIGATION)

There are a number of other types of administrations the nurse may see. Most of these are for treatment or palliation in the client with cancer. The desired site of action is local rather than systemic.

### Pleural Administration

Pleural administration involves the placement of a thoracotomy tube or intrapleural needle into the pleural space for the administration of the drug. This therapy is used for intermittent drug administration, not continuous infusion.

### Pericardial Administration

After performing a pericardiocentesis (the insertion of a needle into the space between the pericardial sac and the cardiac muscle tissue for the removal of fluid), the physician administers the drug. The needle is then withdrawn.

### Intraperitoneal Administration

Intraperitoneal therapy involves the administration of a drug or solution into the intraperitoneal cavity via a peritoneal trocar, Tenckhoff catheter, or implanted port. Medication in solution is administered into the peritoneum and is allowed to dwell there for a specified period of time. It is then drained in a manner similar to that in a peritoneal dialysis procedure. This procedure is covered in more detail in Chapter 11.

### Bladder Administration

Bladder administration is similar to intraperitoneal administration. Medication is administered through an indwelling urinary catheter. The nurse permits the medication to dwell for the amount of time ordered by the physician and then drains the fluid from the bladder or has the client void.

## INTRAOSSEOUS INFUSIONS

Entry into the medullary cavity of the long bones of children is the basis of the intraosseous infusions. An intraosseous or bone marrow needle is inserted through the bone into the vascular-rich medullary cavity. Drugs and fluids administered in this manner are rapidly absorbed into the plasma because of the vast circulatory network in the long bones.

## MODE/RATE OF ADMINISTRATION

Unfortunately, there seems to be no convention among health care professionals for the terms used to describe continuous or intermittent administration, IV push, and bolus infusion. For the purposes of this book the following definitions are used.

## Continuous Administration

The physician's order may be to administer the drug or fluid continuously for a certain period of time or until a specified amount of fluid or drug is infused. In this case the nurse administers the infusate (fluid or drug) at a specified rate. The rate may be written in terms of milliliters per hour, as for fluids; units per hour, as seen, for example, in heparin infusion; milligrams per hour, typical of lidocaine (Xylocaine) orders; or micrograms per kilogram per minute, as seen in dopamine (Intropin, 🍁Revimine) infusions.

## Intermittent Administration

An intermittent infusion generally refers to a drug administration regimen given at designated intervals over a period of time. Physician orders for an intermittent infusion may read "Gentamicin 80 mg IV in 50 mL D5W over 30 minutes every 8 hours," meaning that this drug is to infuse for 30 minutes every 8 hours.

## IV Push

IV push administration can be particularly confusing. Usually the drug is administered into a running solution infusion line through a side arm with an intermittent injection cap or heparin lock. Or IV push can be done by encannulating a vein with a needle on the end of the medication syringe and injecting the medication directly into the vein. The nurse must realize that an order for IV push medication does not mean the administration is given as rapidly as possible or "pushed." Certain medications given too rapidly may cause serious complications or even death for the client. Furosemide (Lasix, 🍁Uritrol) given too rapidly may impair the client's hearing. Even when ordered as an IV push, each 20 mg of furosemide is administered over 1 minute. Phenytoin (Dilantin) given too rapidly as an IV push has been known to cause asystole (cessation of cardiac contractions). Even when treating a client having status epilepticus, administration of phenytoin must be no more rapid than 50 mg/min.

## Bolus Infusion

A bolus infusion usually describes the administration of a predetermined amount of drug or solution all at once. The physician may order an amount of IV solution given as a bolus to challenge a client's renal status. A recent use of the term *bolus* is found in pain management therapy. Using a special computerized pump, clients receiving patient-controlled analgesia (PCA) may self-administer a bolus of medication (usually an opioid) when they feel they require it to relieve pain. The nurse programs the pump to administer the medication within parameters set by the physician based on an assessment of the client's pain. In both cases the nurse monitors the client's tolerance of the bolus.

# CHAPTER 2
# Professional Issues

*Donna D. Ignatavicius*



Clients in a variety of health care settings with a diversity of illnesses receive infusion therapy. They range in age from the premature infant to the advanced elderly. The care required for the client receiving infusion therapy is provided by nurses, physicians, pharmacists, dietitians, and family members/significant others.

## ROLE OF INFUSION THERAPY NURSE

The nurse who administers and monitors infusion therapy may be an infusion therapist, a certified specialist, or a nurse generalist (sometimes referred to as a noninfusion therapist), depending on the setting and health care agency policy.

### Infusion Therapist

In some health care settings, particularly hospitals and large nursing homes, one or more registered nurses who specialize in infusion therapy are responsible for administering and monitoring clients receiving various types of therapies. Responsibilities include parenteral nutrition, medications, and blood and blood components. In addition, the infusion therapist is responsible for documentation, client education, and quality improvement relating to therapy.

## Infusion Nursing Team

Some hospitals have a team of personnel managed by a registered nurse and advised by a physician or pharmacist. Since their primary responsibility is intravenous (IV) therapy, many hospitals refer to this group as the IV team (IVT) rather than as an infusion therapy team.

The members of the team may be registered nurses (RNs), licensed practical nurses (LPNs), or IV technicians. Studies have shown that IVTs are cost effective because of their "effective use of equipment and because intravenous nurses practice at high productivity levels. Intravenous nursing teams provide high-quality patient care through more frequent monitoring of intravenous treatment modalities, thereby significantly decreasing the risk of complications related to intavenous therapy" (Intravenous Nurses Society, 1990, p. S11).

A 30-month study at Poudre Valley Hospital showed that the use of an IVT decreased the occurrence and severity of phlebitis after infusions (Scalley et al., 1992). The benefit of the team was consistent on the medical and neuroscience units but not as consistent on the surgical and obstetric/gynecologic units. The IVT also demonstrated a cost savings of about $17,000 per year related to a reduction in IV-related phlebitis.

If infusion therapists are employed by an agency, they are often unable to provide continuous 24-hour monitoring. In most settings, they typically initiate the therapy, check the client once or twice a day (more often in critical care units), and change the infusion dressing and tubing on a regular basis for infection control. The staff nurses, or nurse generalists, provide continuous 24-hour monitoring and notify the infusion therapist when there are changes in the physician's order or problems with the therapy.

## Nurse Generalist

When a health care agency does not employ infusion therapists, or if they are not available on a 24-hour basis, the staff nurse, or nurse generalist, is responsible for therapy. Four out of five clients in a hospital setting require some form of infusion therapy. The average medical-surgical nurse spends about two thirds of his or her time performing tasks and responsibilities related to infusion therapy (Milliam, 1988).

Since infusion therapy is a common treatment modality used in hospitals, many schools of nursing have included this aspect of care in their basic curricula. A study by Kaufman (1992) showed that IV therapy skills are being taught early in the curricula of most associate degree schools. A combination of demonstration and skills laboratory practice helps to prepare the students for caring for clients with IV therapy.

Regardless of formal educational preparation in infusion therapy, most agencies require their staff nurses to complete a continuing education course in which they learn to initiate, administer, and monitor infusions, especially IV infusions. Some states limit the responsibility of infusion therapy to RNs. Other states allow LPNs to perform basic infusion skills such as removing an IV catheter or monitoring the infusion flow rate.

### Intravenous Nurses Society

The Intravenous Nurses Society (INS) is the professional nursing organization for infusion nurses. This group establishes standards and the scope of practice for infusion nurses and offers continuing education and certification in infusion therapy.

The *Intravenous Nursing Standards of Practice* were developed in 1990 by the INS and provide the basis for infusion nursing practice in a variety of health care settings.

## ROLE OF PHYSICIAN

The physician writes the order that specifies the type and amount of infusion therapy that the client is to receive; for example, "IV of 1000 mL D5W to infuse at 125 mL/h." In this case the client should receive 1000 mL of 5% dextrose in water at 125 mL/h via IV in- fusion.

The infusion therapist or nurse generalist makes decisions about the equipment, tubing, and supplies that are needed to provide the prescribed therapy. For example, will an electronic device to monitor the flow be used? Is the client likely to receive medication or additional solution through the IV tubing?

## ROLE OF CLINICAL PHARMACIST

If the physician wants to prescribe a medication, he or she may specify the drug with dosage and frequency of administration or request that the pharmacist calculate the correct drug or dosage based on the client's health condition and laboratory results. For example, the physician may want to start the client on continuous IV heparin for deep vein thrombosis. The physician consults with the pharmacist or asks the pharmacist to calculate the correct heparin dosage based on the client's partial thromboplastin time (PTT).

In most agencies the pharmacist is also involved in calculating parenteral nutrition solutions and mixing medications and solutions under sterile conditions—a procedure known as *admixture*. Although the pharmacist sends the premixed solutions to the nursing unit, the infusion therapist or nurse generalist is responsible for verifying the physician's order and checking the label on the solution for accuracy *before* it is administered.

## ROLE OF DIETITIAN

The dietitian in some agencies is responsible for calculating the caloric, vitamin, and mineral needs for clients receiving parenteral nutrition. The physician orders the base solution and often consults with or requests the dietitian to compute the exact amount of additives that should be administered based on the client's health condition. This task may be done in collaboration with the phar-macist, depending on the specific client or agency policy and procedure.

## PROFESSIONAL RESPONSIBILITIES ASSOCIATED WITH INFUSION THERAPY

### Competence

Health care agencies are responsible for providing competent practitioners who can administer and monitor infusion therapy. A number of malpractice cases have resulted from errors or substandard care associated with this type of therapy.

The INS recommends that infusion nurses become certified in the practice of infusion therapy by achieving certified registered nurse intravenous (CRNI) status. The INS Certification Corporation administers an examination and recertification process to validate the competency of nurses practicing infusion therapy as a specialty.

Another method for validating competence is the agency's continuing education program to certify nurses as competent to practice infusion therapy in that setting. The typical course usually includes classroom and clinical instruction, lasting anywhere from 8 to 60 hours, depending on the agency and the type of clients it serves.

### Transcultural and Age Considerations

Any nurse administering and monitoring infusion therapy must consider differences among individuals. For example, African-Americans tend to have a smaller skinfold thickness in their arms than do Caucasians (Giger et al., 1991). Therefore, the arm veins of African-Americans may be closer to the skin surface.

One of the main considerations related to infusion therapy is age of the client. About two thirds of hospital admissions are clients over 65 years. Caring for these clients can be rewarding yet frustrating and very time consuming. The infusion therapist or nurse generalist must be aware of the physiologic and psychosocial changes of aging that affect the administration of infusion therapy. For example, the small veins of an older adult become more fragile and friable, but the larger veins become sclerotic. Therefore the smallest gauge catheter should be used (Coulter, 1992). A list of implications for IV therapy practice in the elderly is found in Table 6–4 in Chapter 6.

## Documentation

Documentation is one of the standards identified by the INS (1990): "Documentation in the patient's medical record shall contain sufficient information to identify intravenous procedures, prescribed treatments, complications, and nursing interventions" (p. S20).

### PHYSICIAN'S ORDER

The physician initiates infusion therapy by giving the order that specifies the type of therapy and solution or drug to be administered. The infusion therapist or nurse generalist ensures that all necessary components are included in the following order:

- Infusion route
- Type of access device (if not in place)
- Type of base solution (may be determined by pharmacy)
- Specific medication/additives
- Rate of infusion
- Dosage (if medication)
- Frequency of administration

If there are any questions about the physician's order, the nurse notifies the physician for clarification before administering the therapy.

### DRIP RATE/DOSAGE CALCULATION

When the physician gives an order for infusion therapy, the nurse is often responsible for calculating the drip rate. For example, if the order reads "1000 mL D5W to infuse at 125 mL/h," the nurse must calculate the drip rate in drops (gtt) per minute needed to deliver 125 mL/h. Appendix C reviews flow rate (mL/h) and drip rate calculation for IV fluid administration.

If the client's IV is regulated by an electronic controller or pump, the nurse is responsible for knowing how to use the equipment. Even if such a device is used, the nurse must know how to monitor the flow rate. Information about electronic devices is found in Chapter 5.

At times medications are given by infusion therapy. The nurse may need to calculate the dosage of the medication per minute or per hour to comply with the physician's order. In some agencies the pharmacist performs the calculation, but it is still the nurse's responsibility to verify its accuracy before drug administration. For example, the physician's order reads "Give dopamine infusion of 400 mg in 250 mL D5W at 6 mcg/kg/min." In this case the nurse must know the client's current weight to calculate the IV drip rate (gtt/min). Appendix D briefly reviews drug dosage calculation.

### INFUSION/MEDICATION RECORD

The order for infusion therapy is transcribed onto the appropriate infusion, treatment, or medication record. As with any treatment, the nurse records that the infusion was administered. The procedure for this documentation varies from agency to agency. A sample of an infusion Kardex used in short-term care is shown in Figure 2–1.

In the home setting a family member or other caregiver may record the infusions with the guidance of the home health nurse.

### INTAKE AND OUTPUT RECORD

In most health care agencies the infusion is also documented on the intake and output (I&O) record as parenteral intake. The nurse is responsible for documentation in the hospital or nursing home setting, but a family member or other caregiver may document the intake in the home setting.

### CLIENT'S RESPONSE

The nurse observes and records the client's response to infusion therapy. If the client is receiving IV fluids for rehydration, the nurse assesses the client for signs and symptoms that indicate rehydration, such as an improved skin turgor, decreased fever, less dry skin, and improved urinary output. If the client is receiving medication by infusion, such as opioid analgesic, the nurse determines if the drug has been effective in relieving the client's pain.

## Prevention and Assessment of Complications of Therapy

One of the main responsibilities involved in administration of infusion therapy is taking measures to prevent and assess complications that can result from treatment. Most hospitals and nursing homes have flow sheets that list the parameters for which the nurse assesses.

For agencies that do not have flow sheets the nurse generalist is responsible for writing the assessment in the nurses' notes. In addition to assessing the infusion site and

| Date | Time | Type of Solution/Rate | Amount | Route | Initials |
|---|---|---|---|---|---|
| 7/16/94 | 8 15 A | D5/½ NS @ 125 mL/h | 1000 mL | IV | DF |
| 7/16/94 | 4 35 P | D5/¼ NS @ 100 mL/h | 1000 mL | IV | DI |
| 7/17/94 | 2 50 A | D5/¼ NS c̄ 40 mEq K+ @ 100 mL/h | 1000 mL | IV | MB |
| 7/17/94 | 1 30 P | D5/¼ NS c̄ 40 mEq K+ @ 75 mL/h | 1000 mL | IV | KS |
| | | | | | |
| | | | | | |

**FIGURE 2–1.** Example of a Kardex for documenting infusion therapy.

the intake and output, the nurse checks the laboratory test results for indicators of therapeutic and adverse effects of therapy. For example, if the client receives IV potassium for hypokalemia, the nurse checks to determine if the potassium supplement is effective in increasing the serum potassium. If the level rises too high or does not change, the nurse notifies the physician for a possible change in the infusion order.

Later chapters discuss prevention and assessment of complications associated with each of the specific types of infusion.

## CLIENT/FAMILY EDUCATION

When a client receives infusion therapy in any health care setting, the nurse is responsible for providing health teaching. The following areas should be included:

- Purpose of infusion
- Possible complications
- Signs and symptoms (such as burning and redness at the insertion site) that should be reported to the health care provider
- Care of the equipment and solutions (in the home care setting)

Continuous nursing supervision is available in the hospital or nursing home, but the client at home needs in-depth instruction and support. Most often the client receiving infusion therapy at home is discharged directly from the hospital. The nurse discharging the client works with the hospital discharge planner to ensure that the client has access to infusion supplies for home, home health nurse supervision, and a family member or other caregiver available for assistance.

The staff nurse in the hospital is responsible for client/family education regarding infusion therapy and should provide written and verbal instruction (see Appendix B). Written instructions help inform the home health nurse of what has been taught and what information to reinforce with the client and family or other home caregiver.

Before teaching begins, the hospital nurse assesses the client's ability to learn new information and adjusts teaching methods accordingly. For example, if the client is deaf, the nurse uses more written material. If the client cannot read, the nurse relies more on pictures and demonstrations.

The nurse also assesses the client's socioeconomic background and home environment. For instance, if the client does not have running water, the nurse needs to modify the teaching plan to accommodate for this arrangement.

Providing health teaching for a client does not mean that the client has learned the information. For infusion therapy administration it is best for the nurse to demonstrate the procedure and skills involved and then to ask the client or home caregiver to return the demonstration while the nurse evaluates.

## QUALITY IMPROVEMENT

Quality improvement (QI), also known as quality management and quality assurance, is a professional responsibility for any nurse providing client care. QI is one of the INS standards and is defined as a "systematic process to ensure desired patient outcomes. . . . Structure, process, outcome, corrective action, and re-evaluation are the elements of a comprehensive intravenous therapy quality assurance program" (INS, 1990, p. S19).

The purpose of a quality improvement program is to compare the actual care provided against a preset standard, or acceptable level determined by the unit, agency, or institution.

### Outcome Indicators

The best way to evaluate whether quality infusion therapy has been provided is to assess the clients who receive therapy. For example, one indicator of successful infusion therapy is the absence of complications, such as phlebitis and infiltration. The nurse can assess each client for these problems and, if the problems are not present, can conclude that quality care in preventing complications was provided.

Most health care agencies record these data on audit or data collection tools and then analyze the data to make a conclusion about care. In the above example, if complications occur more frequently than the preset standard, the next step is to evaluate process and structure indicators.

### Process Indicators

The term *process* refers to the actual implementation of care. Using the above example, there are many reasons why infusion complications can occur. One reason is poor administration technique. The nurses who initiate therapy can be observed to determine if they are following the agency's procedure for starting therapy. If the technique being used is not acceptable, corrective action is needed to prevent further problems. If, however, the nurses' technique is appropriate, other reasons for the infusion complications must be determined.

## Structure Indicators

The term *structure* refers to the resources and materials available to ensure that quality care is provided. For infusion therapy resources and materials might include adequate nurses for infusion therapy administration and monitoring and adequate and appropriate equipment and supplies. Although unlikely, infusion complications may be the result of poor equipment or contaminated supplies.

## Corrective Action/Reevaluation

Once the cause or causes of a problem have been identified, the nurse can take action to eliminate the cause or correct it. In most health care agencies one or more nurses are designated to coordinate QI studies and provide recommendations for change. These individuals collate data and perform statistical analysis, which is then reported to the agency's QI committee.

All nurses are responsible for identifying problems and collecting the data for analysis. Once a problem has been identified, it is monitored on an ongoing basis to determine if it has been resolved. In any health care agency a successful QI program is dependent on the support of the facility's administration.

# CHAPTER 3
# Anatomy and Physiology

*Marilyn Ferreri Booker*



A knowledge of anatomy and physiology assists the nurse in understanding the way in which the various infusion methods work. This chapter is intended as a review. It assumes the nurse has a working knowledge of anatomy and physiology and thus the clinical significance of the different infusion routes.

## VASCULAR SYSTEM

### Structure

The blood vessels create the vascular system. Arteries carry the blood away from the heart. The artery that emanates from the heart, the aorta, is the largest in the arterial system. This vessel has branches of smaller arteries. These smaller arteries also have artery branches that become smaller as they move away from the heart to the periphery. The smaller arteries become arterioles, which are smaller vessels diverging from the arteries that subdivide into capillaries. The capillaries provide nutrients to and take wastes from the tissues. As the capillaries leave the tissues, this system of decreasing size reverses. The capillaries connect with venules, which are the smallest of the body's veins. The venules in turn connect with small veins that connect with slightly larger veins en route to the heart. This arrangement of increasing size continues as the venous system progresses to the heart. It culminates in the largest vein of the body, the vena cava, which connects directly to the heart.

The vessels of the vascular system not only vary in size according to their location and function but also in vessel wall thickness. With the exception of capillaries, all blood vessels have three discrete layers of tissue: the tunica intima, the tunica media, and the tunica adventitia (Fig. 3–1).

## TUNICA INTIMA

The inner layer of a blood vessel consists of a single layer of endothelial cells lying on a layer of connective tissue. The endothelial cells are flat and smooth, which allows blood cells, platelets, plasma, and intravascularly administered fluid and drugs to run easily along the vessel. Any trauma to these endothelial cells, as in a difficult vein encannulation or cannula removal, may lead to the "roughening" of the endothelial cells, causing cells and platelets to adhere to the vascular lining. This phenomenon is known as thrombosis.

The layer of connective tissue called the internal elastic lamina is most prominent in the large elastic arteries and the medium-caliber muscular arteries. This elastic layer defines the intima from the media. In veins the intima has valves made of the same endothelial cells as the vessel itself. These valves are most common in the smaller, distal veins, but the larger femoral veins also have some. The venous valves provide for unidirectional blood flow to the heart (Solomon, 1992). This arrangement of the valves dictates that the nurse insert venous access devices in the same direction as the blood flow.

## TUNICA MEDIA

The tunica media is the middle layer of tissue and consists of smooth muscle cells. Small amounts of collagen and elastic fibers surround these cells. The collagen, fibers, and muscle cells form a complex pattern of concentric spirals that run along the length of the vessel. A noncontinuous sheet of elastic tissue, the external elastic lamina, separates this layer from the tunica adventitia (Solomon, 1992).

## TUNICA ADVENTITIA

An interwoven pattern of thick bundles of collagen, varying sizes of elastic fibers, and a mixture of smooth muscle cells and fibroblasts compose the outer layer or tunica adventitia. This layer provides the majority of the vessel's strength (Solomon, 1992).

The intima and the inner portion of the media receive nourishment through the lumen by diffusion. However, the

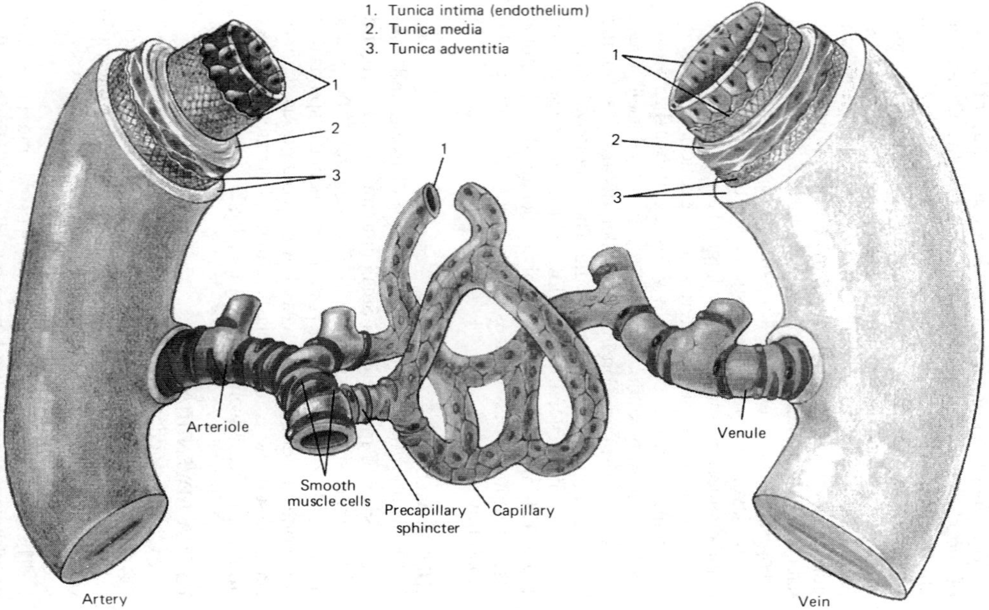


**FIGURE 3–1.** Structure of blood vessel walls. (From Solomon, E. P. [1992]. *Introduction to human anatomy and physiology* [p. 171]. Philadelphia: W. B. Saunders.)

outer portion of the tunica media and the tunica adventitia receive nutrients from the vasa vasorum, small vessels located in the adventitia.

### CAPILLARIES

As mentioned, capillaries connect arteries with veins (Fig. 3–1). These tiny conduits provide for exchanges between the interstitial spaces and the blood. Capillaries consist of a single layer of endothelial cells and connective tissue fibers.

## Function

The arterial and the venous systems have different but complementary functions.

### ARTERIAL SYSTEM

The arterial system delivers blood to the various tissues for nourishment. At the tissues the nutrients, chemicals, and body defense substances are exchanged for cellular wastes, which the arteries take to the excretory organs, the kidneys, liver, and lungs. The arteries also assist with temperature and blood pressure regulation. Blood is directed toward the skin to promote heat loss or away from the skin to conserve heat.

### VENOUS SYSTEM

The venous system's primary function is to provide for the return of blood from the capillaries to the right side of the heart for circulation. It also functions as a reservoir for a large portion of the blood volume.

The differences between veins and arteries are outlined in Table 3–1.

**TABLE 3–1**
**Differences Between Veins and Arteries**

| Veins | Arteries |
|---|---|
| Blood is dark red | Blood is bright red |
| Blood flashback is slow | Blood flashback is pulsating and rapid |
| Has valves for unidirectional blood flow | No valves |
| Takes blood toward the heart | Takes blood away from the heart |
| Peripheral veins have superficial location | Deep location surrounded by muscle |
| An area is supplied by multiple veins | An area is supplied by a single artery |

## Life Span Considerations

### ELDERLY

In the elderly the intima of the veins and arteries increases in thickness. This is a slow, symmetric process, resulting from the gradual accumulation of endothelial cells surrounded by additional connective tissue. The muscular wall becomes less elastic. These changes make the elderly more susceptible to the development of varicosities. These permanently swollen veins, usually seen in the extremities, are prominent and appear tortuous. Varicose veins are not appropriate for intravenous (IV) therapy, as they tend to infiltrate easily. In the arteries these physical alterations cause the larger vessels to become dilated and elongated. These vessels in some elderly clients may become subject to the development of aneurysms, localized sacs in the wall of an artery or vein (Solomon, 1992).

### INFANTS

Scalp veins are often used for IV therapy in infants because scalp veins are prominent and less difficult to locate than an infant's extremity veins. Because veins in the scalp do not have valves, the nurse can insert the needle or catheter in either direction.

# INTEGUMENTARY SYSTEM

Although seemingly simple, the integumentary system is a complex organ with many functions. This, the body's largest organ, is composed of the skin and the subcutaneous tissue.

## Structure

The skin consists of two layers: the epidermis and the dermis. Beneath the dermis is the subcutaneous layer (Fig. 3–2).

The epidermis is the outer layer of the skin. Although less than 1 mm thick in most parts, the epidermis is composed of four separate layers: the stratum corneum, the stratum spinosum, the stratum granulosum, and the stratum germinativum, or basal layer. Most of the cells of the epidermis are keratinocytes. Only the basal layer, however, is capable of mitosis and therefore production of keratinocytes. In the basal layer are also specialized cells called melanocytes. These cells produce melanin, which gives the skin its pigment. There is no difference in the number of melanocytes among races, but there is a difference in the activity of the cells. Because the epidermis has no blood supply or lymph channels of its own, it is totally dependent on the dermis, the underlying layer, for nourishment (Solomon, 1992).

The dermis, or corium, lies just below the basal layer of the epidermis. It varies in thickness from 1 to 4 mm in dif-

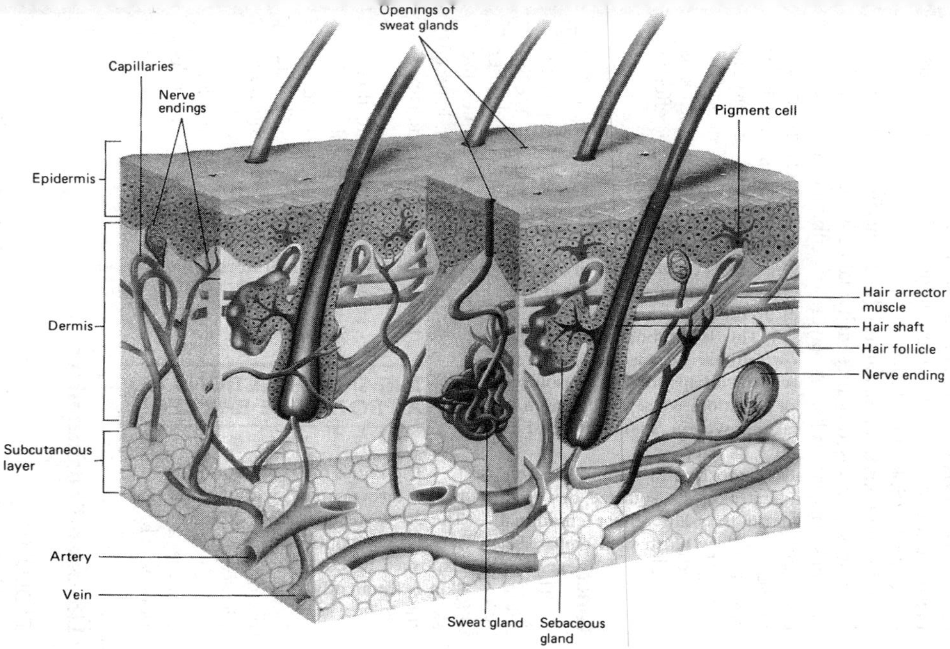


**FIGURE 3–2.** Structure of skin. (From Solomon, E. P. [1992]. *Introduction to human anatomy and physiology* [p. 42]. Philadelphia: W. B. Saunders.)

ferent locations. The dermis is a layer of noncellular connective tissue composed of interwoven collagen and elastic fibers. These give the skin both flexibility and mechanical strength. Collagen is the principal fibrous component of dermal tissue. The fibrous collagen bundles are continually being broken down and resynthesized by dermal cells called fibroblasts. The fibroblasts are also responsible for the production of a gelatinous elastic material called ground substance. The ground substance is thought to have phagocytic properties. Two other cell types make up the dermis: histiocytes and mast cells. The histiocyte is a phagocyte that is part of the reticuloendothelial system. The mast cells are found around blood vessels and synthesize and release heparin. Mast cells also release histamine in the presence of tissue damage (Solomon, 1992).

Subcutaneous tissue separates the dermis from muscle and bone. It is composed of mesenchymal cells that produce the lipocytes or fat cells. A layer of subcutaneous fat is distributed all over the body and varies in thickness based on sex and the various stages of the life cycle. This layer also has a numerous supply of blood vessels of varying sizes. These vessels perforate the fatty tissue and extend into the dermal layer. It is because of these vessels that medications and fluids administered subcutaneously have systemic effects.

## Function

The most important function of the skin is that of providing a barrier between the outside environment and the internal organs. This barrier protects against bacteria and other organisms. When an infusion access device perforates the skin, it causes a breach in the integrity of this barrier, leaving the client at risk for infection. Therefore, strict aseptic care is required for all access device sites.

The skin also functions to prevent loss of body fluids, control body temperature, and manufacture vitamin D. Finally, the skin is a sensory organ conveying impulses to the brain that allow us to discern different sensations. This accounts for the pain the client experiences when the nurse pierces the skin with a vascular access device.

The subcutaneous tissue functions as a heat insulator, provides a protective cushion for the body, and acts as a depot for caloric reserve.

## Life Span Considerations

### ELDERLY

There is no change in the epidermis in the elderly; however, the dermis undergoes major changes as a result of the aging process. There is thinning of the dermis that appears earlier in women than in men. The number of fibrocytes decreases, and the density and amount of collagen are reduced. There are more elastin fibers just beneath the dermis, but they are less effectively organized. The fine elastin fibers in the dermis disappear with age, and this accounts for the laxity of the skin. In addition, the blood vessels in the dermal layer of the skin are less abundant and less well organized in the elderly. This causes problems with heat retention for the elderly client and difficulty with absorption of subcutaneously administered medications and fluids (Hampton, 1991).

The subcutaneous tissue decreases in most areas of the aged body, although total body fat increases until the age of 70 years. The loss of the subcutaneous fat is another factor that impairs heat retention.

#### INFANTS AND YOUNG CHILDREN

Infants and young children have a thin dermis and epidermis with a very small stratum corneum. Absorption of subcutaneously administered drugs is often reduced in the neonate because of the immaturity of blood flow to the various tissues and the decreased amount of subcutaneous tissue (Foster, 1989).

### Transcultural Considerations

African-Americans are susceptible to keloids, an overgrowth of connective tissue in response to a skin cut or puncture (Giger et al., 1991). The nurse providing infusion therapy must be aware of this potential. Using the smallest gauge catheter possible and keeping punctures to a minimum in these clients reduces the formation of these ropelike scars.

African-American clients may have a smaller skinfold thickness in their arms than white clients, but fat distribution over the trunk is the same (Giger et al., 1991). When the nurse or dietician is performing the anthropometric portion of a nutritional assessment on an African-American client, the subscapular skinfold thickness provides a more accurate assessment of nutritional status than the triceps skinfold thickness.

## CENTRAL NERVOUS SYSTEM

A discussion of the support structures of the central nervous system (CNS) is appropriate for the purposes of this book. These support structures include the skull and vertebrae, the three meningeal layers, the ventricular system, and the cerebrospinal fluid (CSF).

## Structure

### SKULL

The calvaria, or roof of the cranial cavity, covers the upper aspects of the brain. The frontal, occipital, two parietal, and two temporal bones fused at suture lines compose this structure. A collection of bony structures with many ridges and grooves makes up the floor of the cranial cavity (Fig. 3–3). The floor mimics the shape of the base of the brain and is divided into three compartments: the anterior, the middle, and the posterior fossae. The anterior fossa houses the frontal lobe; the middle fossa contains parts of the temporal lobes, the upper brain stem, and the pituitary gland. The brain stem and the cerebellar hemispheres are located in the posterior fossa. At the base of the skull a number of small openings, or foramina, permit paired blood vessels and cranial nerves to enter and leave the intracranial cavity. The brain stem connects to the upper cervical spinal cord at a large opening called the foramen magnum. The thickest parts of the skull are the midfrontal and midoccipital bones. The temporal bones are the thinnest parts of the skull (Solomon 1992).

### VERTEBRAL COLUMN

The vertebral column is composed of 7 cervical, 12 thoracic, 5 lumbar, 5 sacral, and 4 fused coccygeal vertebrae (Fig. 3–4). These vertebrae are joined by multiple ligaments and intervening discs, which provide flexibility and stability (Solomon, 1992).

### MENINGES

Three layers of meninges surround the brain and spinal cord (Figs. 3–5 and 3–6). The outer layer, or dura mater, consists of thick, tough connective tissue. The pia mater is the inner vascular membrane, which adheres to the surface of the brain and spinal cord. Folds of pia mater form part of the choroid plexus, support the superficial blood vessels that penetrate the CNS, and provide support for the spinal cord.

Between the dural and pial layers is a spiderweb-like membrane called the arachnoid. The arachnoid surrounds the surface of the brain without following its contour, surrounds the spinal cord, and extends along the roots of the cranial and spinal nerves.

The subdural space is potential space between the dura and the arachnoid (Figs. 3–5 and 3–6). The space between the arachnoid and the pia mater, the subarachnoid space, is filled with CSF. The depth of the subarachnoid space varies. It is narrow over the convexities of the cerebral hemispheres. At the base of the brain and around the brain stem the space widens to form large cisterns. The cisterna magna is the largest cistern and is located between the medulla and the in-

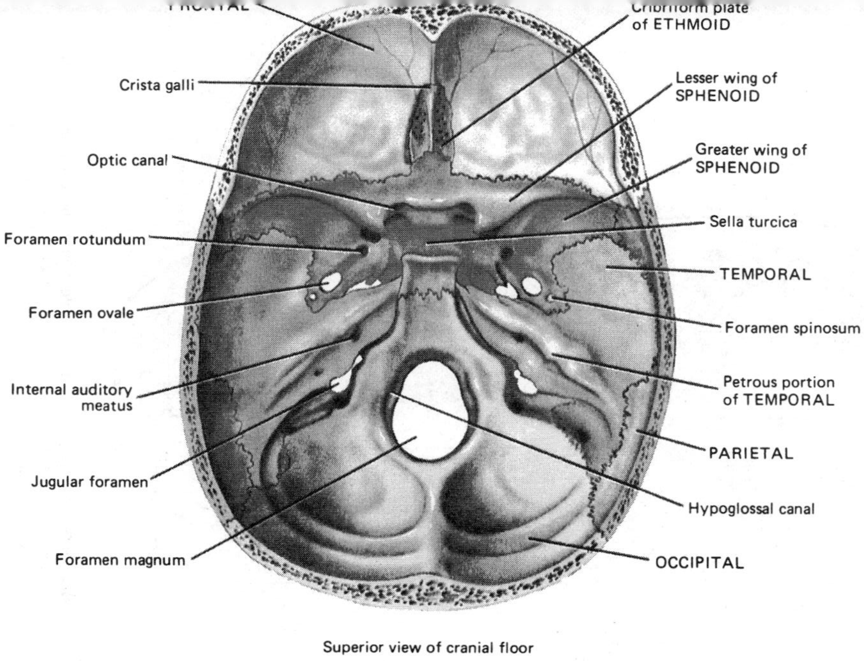


**FIGURE 3–3.** Floor of the cranial cavity. (From Solomon, E. P. [1992]. *Introduction to human anatomy and physiology* [p. 60]. Philadelphia: W. B. Saunders.)

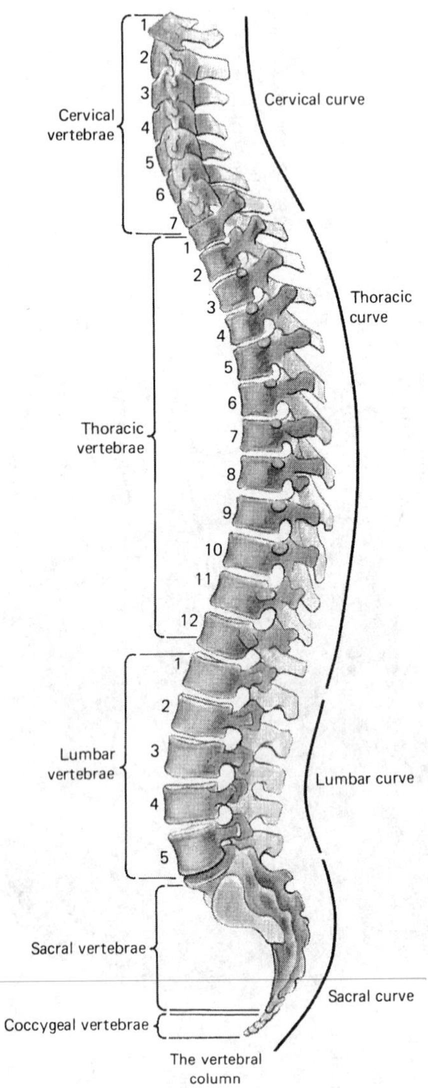


**FIGURE 3–4.** The vertebral column. Note four distinct sections. (From Solomon, E. P. [1992]. *Introduction to human anatomy and physiology* [p. 62]. Philadelphia: W. B. Saunders.)

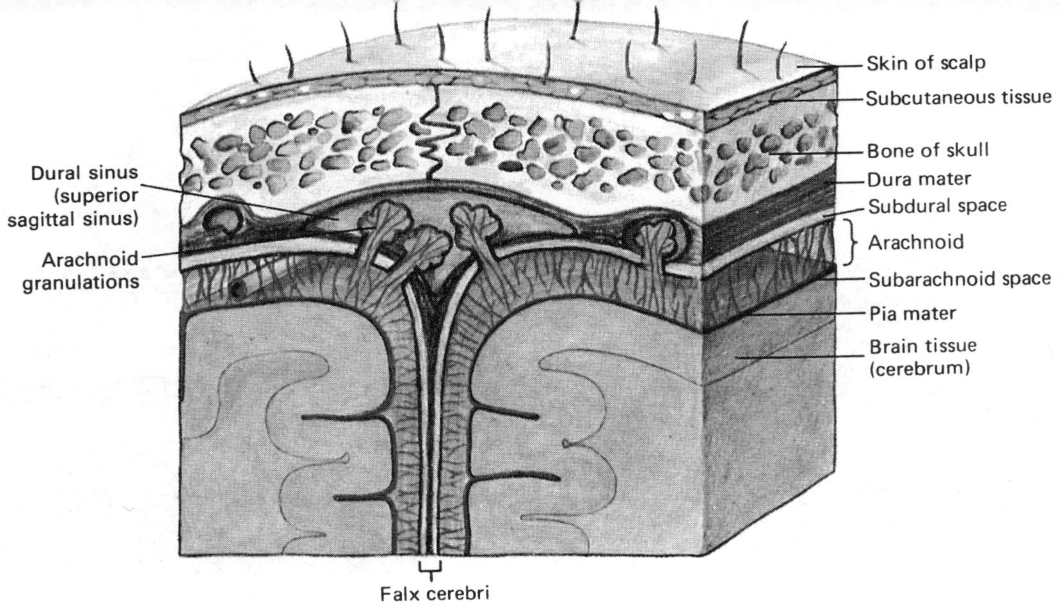


**FIGURE 3–5.** The layers of meninges. (From Solomon, E. P. [1992]. *Introduction to human anatomy and physiology* [p. 102]. Philadelphia: W. B. Saunders.)

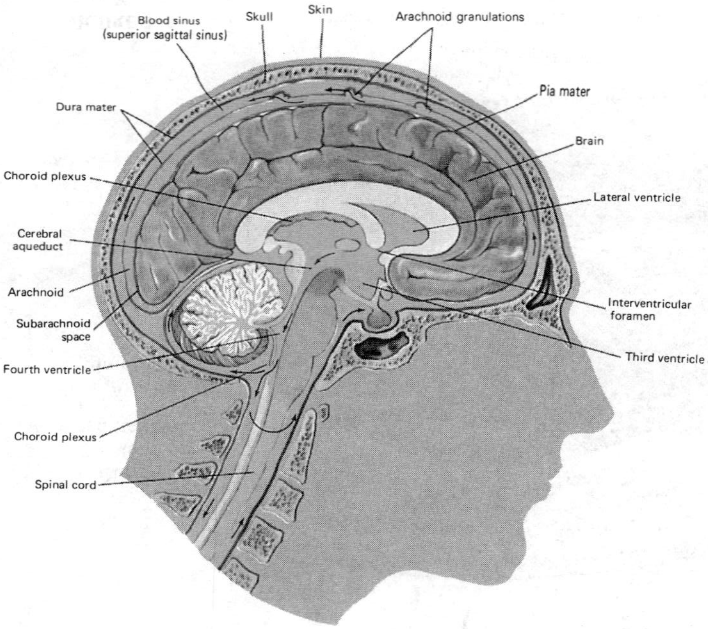


**FIGURE 3–6.** The circulation of the cerebrospinal fluid (CSF) in the brain and spinal cord. (From Solomon, E. P. [1992]. *Introduction to human anatomy and physiology* [p. 103]. Philadelphia: W. B. Saunders.)

ferior surface of the cerebellum. A lumbar cistern is located at the end of the spinal cord and contains sacral nerve roots.

Tiny projections of meninges called arachnoid granulations protrude into the large venous sinuses formed by the dural layers (Fig. 3–6). The CSF in the subarachnoid space is transferred into the venous sinuses as a result of hydrostatic pressure. The arachnoid granulations are permeable and permit one-way flow of CSF, plasma proteins, and serum albumin into the venous blood (Solomon, 1992).

## VENTRICULAR SYSTEM

The ventricular system is located within the brain itself. Four communicating compartments or cavities compose this system (see Fig. 3–6). There are two lateral ventricles and a third and a fourth ventricle. Each of the lateral ventricles is a cavity within the cerebral hemispheres that communicates with the third ventricle by the intraventricular foramen, foramen of Monro. Each lateral ventricle consists of a body and the anterior (frontal), inferior (temporal), and posterior (occipital) horns.

Thalamic structures surround the third ventricle, a thin, centrally located cavity. The third ventricle is con-nected to the fourth ventricle by a narrow channel, the aqueduct of Sylvius. This is located in the midbrain. The fourth ventricle is an angular cavity posterior to the pons and medulla and anterior to the cerebellum that extends to the central canal of the upper cervical cord. Three foramina connect the fourth ventricle with the subarachnoid spaces (Solomon, 1992).

## CEREBROSPINAL FLUID

CSF is a clear, colorless liquid. CSF contains a small amount of protein, glucose, and cells and a large amount of sodium chloride. The CSF is formed principally in the lateral and third ventricles. This is completed by a network of capillaries, the choroid plexus (see Fig. 3–6). CSF is produced as a result of an active transport mechanism, the expenditure of energy and osmotic pressure. The rate of CSF formation is estimated at 500 to 600 mL/d. The CSF circulates from the lateral ventricles through the foramen of Monro into the third ventricle, through the aqueduct of Sylvius into the fourth ventricle and into the cranial and spinal subarachnoid spaces, where it is returned to the venous system. The total volume of CSF in the ventricular system and the subarachnoid spaces at any given time is approximately 140 mL (Solomon, 1992).

## BLOOD-BRAIN BARRIER SYSTEM

The integrity of the CNS is dependent on the physical and chemical environment. A barrier exists between the blood stream and the brain, between the blood stream and CSF, and between CSF and the brain. The barrier system includes the capillary endothelium, the pial-gill membrane, astrocytes, ependymal cells, the choroid plexus, and the arachnoid membrane. It is this system that makes treating cancer and infections of the CNS difficult. These structures attempt to protect the organs of the CNS from any foreign substances including antiinfective and chemotherapeutic agents (Solomon, 1992).

## Function

### SKULL

The skull's function is to protect the brain with its bony structure.

### VERTEBRAL COLUMN

The vertebral column supports the skull and forms a spinal canal that surrounds the spinal cord. This spinal canal protects the spinal cord, the spinal nerves, and the underlying structures.

### MENINGES

The three layers of meninges protect and support the brain and spinal cord.

### CEREBROSPINAL FLUID

CSF provides the CNS with support, a cushion against trauma, and nutrition. The CSF assists in the removal of the waste products of neuronal metabolism and aids in maintaining a consistent intracranial pressure. The pressure of the CSF at the lumbar cistern is normally between 100 and 150 mm of water with the client in the recumbent position.

### BLOOD-BRAIN BARRIER SYSTEM

The complex network of structures called the blood-brain barrier system provides a stable environment for the CNS by regulating the transport of chemical substances between the plasma, the CSF, and the brain.

## Life Span Considerations

### ELDERLY

The permeability of the intervertebral foramina increases with age. Therefore, drugs given epidurally to the elderly client may result in an exaggerated effect because more drug is absorbed than would be in a younger client.

### INFANTS

The myelin sheath decreases the permeability of the blood-brain barrier. In children the myelinization is immature until they reach the age of about 2 years. This immature barrier is associated with drug toxicity in infants, as drugs and bilirubin may enter the CNS (Foster, 1989).

## PLEURA

### Structure

The pleura consists of two serous membranes. The parietal pleural membrane lines the inside walls of the thoracic cavity and the upper surfaces of the diaphragm. The visceral pleura completely encloses both lung surfaces and the fissures between the lobes. The potential cavity between these layers is called the pleural space (Fig. 3–7) (Ignatavicius, Workman, & Mischler, 1995).

### Function

The cells of the pleura produce a thin fluid that lubricates between the two layers. This fluid allows the two pleural surfaces to slide over one another smoothly during respiration.

## PERICARDIUM

### Structure

The pericardium is the protective covering that encapsulates the heart (Fig. 3–8). This protective covering consists of two layers: the visceral pericardium, or inner layer, and the parietal pericardium, or outer layer. The visceral pericardium is

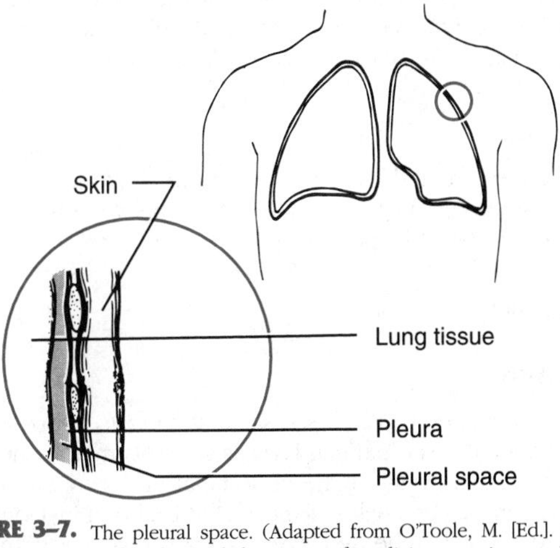


**FIGURE 3–7.** The pleural space. (Adapted from O'Toole, M. [Ed.]. [1992]. *Miller-Keane encyclopedia and dictionary of medicine, nursing, and allied health* [5th ed., p. 1485]. Philadelphia: W. B. Saunders.)

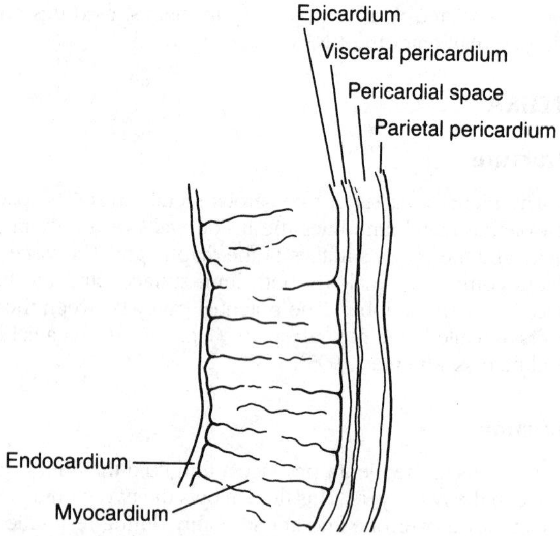


**FIGURE 3–8.** The pericardial space. (From Ignatavicius, D. D., Workman, M. L., & Mishler, M. A. [1995]. *Medical-surgical nursing* [2nd ed., p. 777]. Philadelphia: W. B. Saunders.)

a thin transparent tissue that adheres to the heart muscle itself. The parietal pericardium is a tough, fibrous layer that attaches to the great vessels, the manubrium (the uppermost part of the sternum) and xiphoid process of the sternum (anteriorly), the diaphragm (inferiorly), and the vertebral column (posteriorly). Between the visceral and parietal pericardial layers is the pericardial space, which is filled with 5 to 20 mL of thin pericardial fluid (Ignatavicius, Workman, & Mischler, 1995).

### Function

The pericardial fluid serves two purposes: to lubricate the heart's surfaces and to alleviate friction between the heart's surfaces as the heart pumps.

## PERITONEUM

### Structure

The peritoneum is a closed sac that consists of two layers or membranes. The parietal layer is a serous membrane that lines the inner walls of the abdominal and pelvic cavities. The visceral layer encloses most of the abdominal organs. The area between the two layers is a potential space known as the peritoneal cavity (Fig. 3–9).

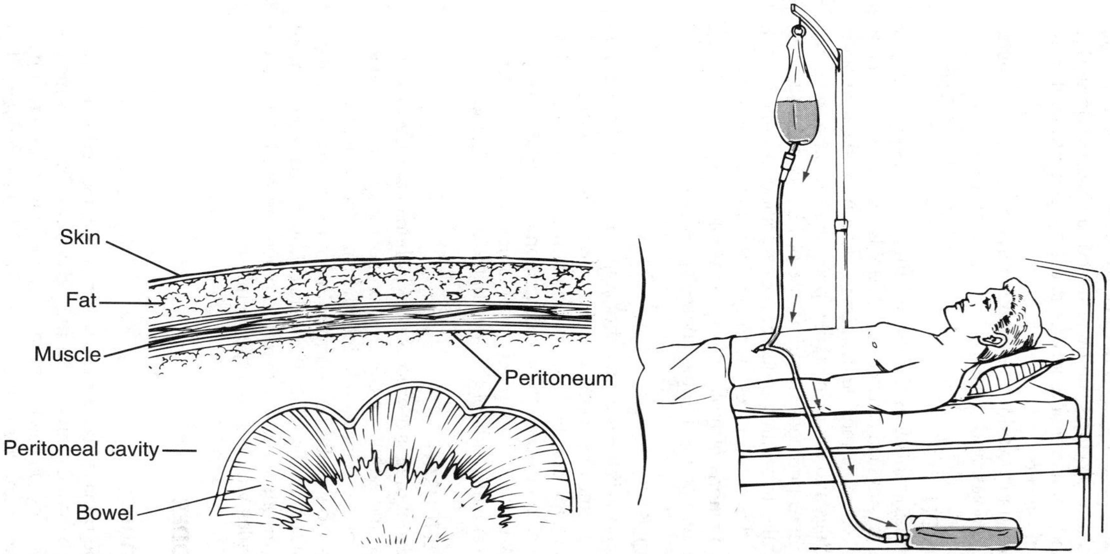


**FIGURE 3–9.** The peritoneal space. (Adapted from Ignatavicius, D. D., Workman, M. L., & Mishler, M. A. *Medical-surgical nursing* [2nd ed., p. 2139]. Philadelphia: W. B. Saunders.)

## Function

The peritoneal membrane functions in the transport of water and electrolytes between the peritoneal cavity and the vascular circulation. It is because of this transport that metabolic waste products can be removed during peritoneal dialysis and chemotherapeutic drugs can be given to treat some ovarian cancers.

This transport involves three physical processes: diffusion, osmosis, and solvent drag.

### DIFFUSION

Diffusion involves the movement of molecules of any of the three physical states (solids, liquids, or gases) in solution across a semipermeable membrane. As long as the size of the molecules and the membrane's pores are of compatible size, movement proceeds from an area of high concentration of molecules to an area of lower concentration of molecules. If this is the only process working, diffusion occurs until the concentrations of molecules of diffusible size on either side of the semipermeable membrane are equal.

### OSMOSIS

Osmosis is the movement of water or other solvent across a semipermeable membrane. This flow moves from the side in which the concentration of nondiffusible molecules is low to the side in which the concentration of nondiffusible molecules is high. This process continues until the concentrations on either side of the membrane are consistent.

### SOLVENT DRAG

Solvent drag is a process by which intermediate-size molecules and solutes move across the semipermeable membrane of the peritoneum. Intermediate-size molecules move across the membrane as a function of the rate of the solvent flow in either direction. If the fluid flow by osmosis is more rapid in one direction than the other, the fluid drags these molecules with it across the membrane.

# BLADDER

## Structure

The urinary bladder is a muscular sac located in the posterior peritoneal cavity near the pelvic floor. In males the urinary bladder is anterior to the rectum. In females the urinary bladder is anterior to the vagina. The bladder is directly behind the pubic symphysis, the point of connection for the pelvic bone structures. The urinary bladder is composed of the fundus, the rounded sac portion, and the bladder neck, a portion of the posterior urethra.

The urinary bladder has an inner lining of epithelial cells known as the urothelium, a middle layer of three types of smooth muscle known as the detrusor muscle, and an outer lining. The trigone is an anatomic landmark on the inner aspect of the posterior urinary bladder formed by the points of ureteral entry on the posterior bladder wall and the urethra. Some bladder cancers are treated by injecting chemotherapeutic drugs directly into the bladder.

## Function

The primary function of the urinary bladder is to provide a site for temporary storage of urine. Thus, the urinary bladder functions to provide continence and enable micturition (voiding).

## Life Span Considerations

### ELDERLY

The aging process may affect the elasticity of the detrusor muscle, causing decreased bladder capacity and urinary retention. This may result in urinary urgency and subsequent incontinence if the client is unable to reach the toilet quickly (Hampton, 1991). Therefore the elderly client may not tolerate drug administration into the bladder, as he or she may not be able to retain the solution long enough for the drug to have its effect on the cancerous cells.

# INTRAOSSEOUS CAVITY

## Structure

Long bones consist of a shaft (diaphysis), two articular ends (epiphyses), and the portion of the bone between them (metaphysis) (Fig. 3–10). The diaphysis is a strong tube of dense or compact bone with a cylindric cavity at its center. The metaphysis is made of cancellous, or spongy, bone that extends a variable distance into the medullary cavity. Long bones are covered almost entirely by a dense fibrous membrane called the periosteum; only the articular surface remains uncovered.

The cavity at the center of the diaphysis, called the medullary cavity, is filled with bone marrow. Bone marrow contains a dense network of sinusoids that drain into large central medullary venous channels. These central venous sinuses drain into veins that retrace the path of the nutrient arteries. These channels exit the bone through both the emissary and nutrient veins, entering the systemic venous circulation. Because of the extensive network of venous sinusoids, absorption into the plasma from the medullary

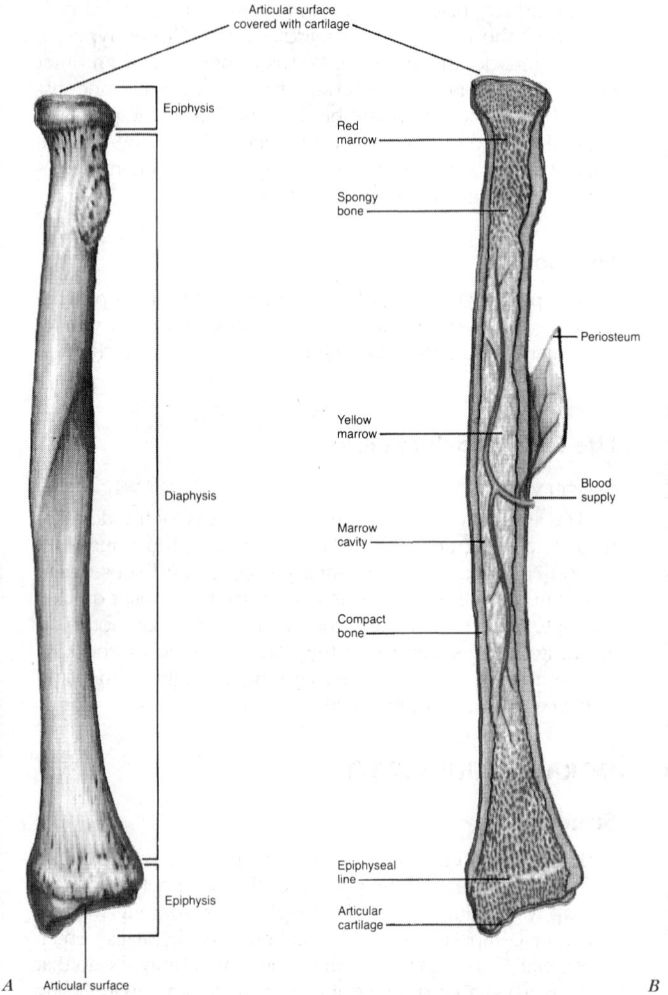


**FIGURE 3–10.** Anatomy of a bone. **A,** Structure of a long bone. **B,** Internal structure of a long bone. (From Solomon, E. P. [1992]. *Introduction to human anatomy and physiology* [p. 48]. Philadelphia: W. B. Saunders.)

cavity is very rapid, mimicking that of direct vascular infusion. This is beneficial in the emergency treatment of young children when vascular access cannot be established.

The periosteum has a rich supply of sensory nerves. There are also vasomotor and sensory nerve fibers associated with the nutrient vessels (Manley, 1988).

## Function

The function of the bones is to (1) provide structure to the body, (2) support surrounding tissues, (3) assist with movement, (4) protect vital organs, (5) manufacture red blood cells, and (6) provide storage for calcium and phosphorus.

## Life Span Considerations

### CHILDREN

Red bone marrow (composed of developing red cells, white cells, and platelets) is abundant at birth. By age 4 years, some fat cells may be found in the child's marrow cavity. At 18 to 20 years the medullary cavity is composed of adipose tissue. From this age on, hematopoietic activity is found only in the vertebrae, ribs, skull, pelvis, and the most proximal portions of the extremities (Spivey, 1987).

CHAPTER 4

# Infusion Systems

*Marilyn Ferreri Booker*



It is important for nurses administering infusions to have a basic understanding of the way in which infusion systems work. This knowledge makes it possible for the nurse to devise methods for use that optimize a particular infusion system's advantages while minimizing the system's risks. Furthermore, the nurse who understands the workings of an infusion system can identify problems readily and troubleshoot or remedy them rapidly.

## CONTAINERS

Two types of containers are available for infusions: glass and plastic.

### Glass

Glass containers have been available for a long time. Early in the manufacturing of infusion solutions glass was chosen because it is essentially inert (unlikely to react with the contents).

#### ADVANTAGES

Glass containers can be manufactured in a variety of designs with walls thick enough to withstand minor trauma and the varying pressures that develop in the sterilization process. Another benefit of glass is its clarity. This attribute allows the nurse to inspect the contents easily for particulate matter (particles floating in the solution). Its rigid sides allow the accurate determination of the container's volume.

## DISADVANTAGES

Glass containers have some disadvantages as well. The integrity of glass is easily impaired but difficult to discern. When dropped or bumped hard, glass containers can shatter. Their rigid sides make storage and disposal bulky. Furthermore, for fluid to drip from glass, air must be available from outside the container to displace it. Therefore, glass infusion systems are "open" systems.

## GLASS INFUSION SYSTEMS

Two types of glass infusion systems are commonly seen: the separate airway design and the integral airway design.

**Separate Airway Design.** The separate airway design has a plastic tube or "straw" attached to the inside of the thick hard cork-type stopper. This tube extends almost the entire length of the bottle to above the fluid level of a full bottle (Fig. 4–1). For the bottle to empty through the administration set, air must come in through the "straw." This air comes unfiltered from the environment into the sterile container. The air exerts pressure on the surface of the fluid, allowing the solution to move through the administration set. The chances of bacterial growth are surprisingly small in this system because (1) most solutions do not support the growth of bacteria nor-

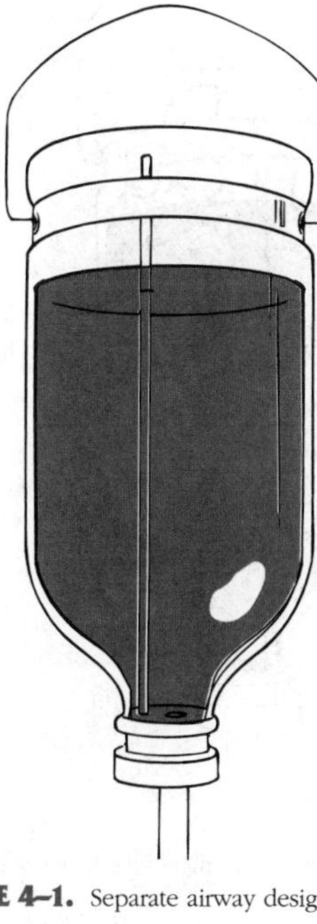

**FIGURE 4–1.** Separate airway design system.

mally found in the environment and (2) particles in the air admitted into the container do not mix with the solution because they meet with surface tension at the fluid level (Fig. 4–2).

The safe use of this system dictates that the nurse consider the following:

1. Because the surface of the fluid level provides a barrier to dust and microbes, the nurse must avoid shaking these containers after they have been hung. Also, the nurse should change containers of this design when about 50 mL remains in the container. The last few drops could carry the environmental contaminants through the administration set and into the client.
2. When opening a new bottle of this design, the nurse carefully removes the metal disk and attached ring. On the top of the bottle stopper, the nurse notices a latex diaphragm. This must be removed before attempting to insert the administration set spike. Usually an edge of the disk can be grasped and pulled straight up. As this diaphragm disk is removed, the nurse should listen for a "whooshing" sound as the vacuum is broken. If this sound is absent, discard this container. The integrity of the contents in any bottle of this design without a discernible vacuum is questionable.

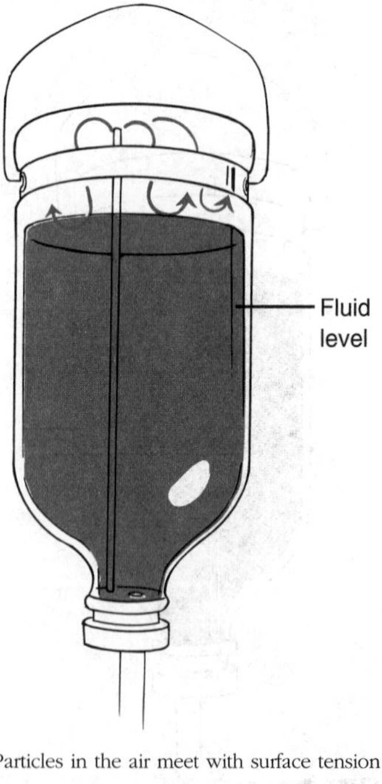


**FIGURE 4–2.** Particles in the air meet with surface tension and cannot mix with the fluid.

3. Sometimes when the bottle is hanging, fluid drips from the plastic air tube hole in the stopper. To remedy this problem the nurse need only create a small amount of negative pressure in the tube by squeezing and releasing the drip chamber of the administration set. This creates negative pressure in the "straw" and stops the dripping.

**Integral Airway Design.** The integral airway design glass system is also "open." In this system, instead of air entering through a "straw," it enters through a side port filter on the administration set. The nurse may find that this tubing is sometimes called "vented tubing." This filter sits above the drip chamber and below the administration set spike (Fig. 4–3). Proponents of this system feel that even though air enters the system from the outside and bubbles through the solution, this air is sterile because it is filtered. This may be so if the filter remains intact. This is not necessarily the case, however, because the filter is removable. To make additions to the solution in this system after it is hanging, man-

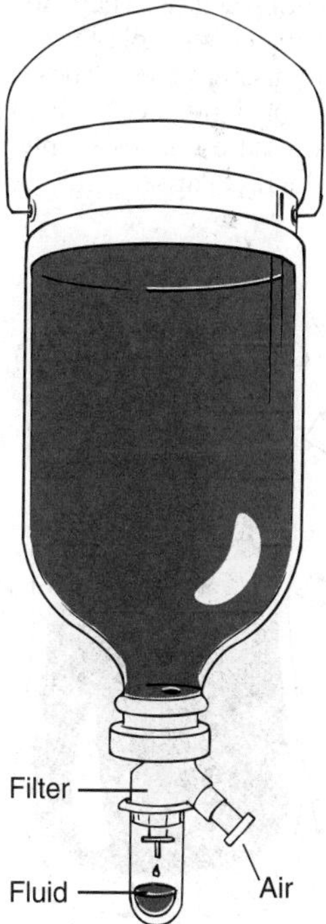


**FIGURE 4–3.** Integral airway design system.

ufacturers' directions include removing the filter, attaching the syringe tip to the airway, and injecting the additive. In doing this the nurse injects any organisms deposited along the airway into the solution and eventually the client.

Another disadvantage of this system occurs when the filter becomes wet. Wet cellulose filters admit air very poorly. Without a steady source of air it is not possible to maintain the infusion rate. Removing the filter cap remedies the problem but allows unfiltered air directly into the solution. Any airborne bacteria are ultimately infused into the client.

## Plastic

In 1971, plastic containers for "large-volume parenterals" (LVPs) became available for hospital use. As with any "new" product, the plastic containers were met with a great deal of skepticism. Actually these containers were well tried during the Vietnam conflict. It was under these severe conditions that plastic became the container of choice.

Plastic containers do not require that air be admitted into the system for the fluid to flow. They are truly a "closed" system. Unlike glass containers, plastic containers do not require "vented" administration sets. These containers run well using "nonvented" or "unvented" administration sets. Outside atmospheric pressure pushes evenly against the flexible container sides, which collapse evenly as the fluid flows by gravity (Fig. 4–4).

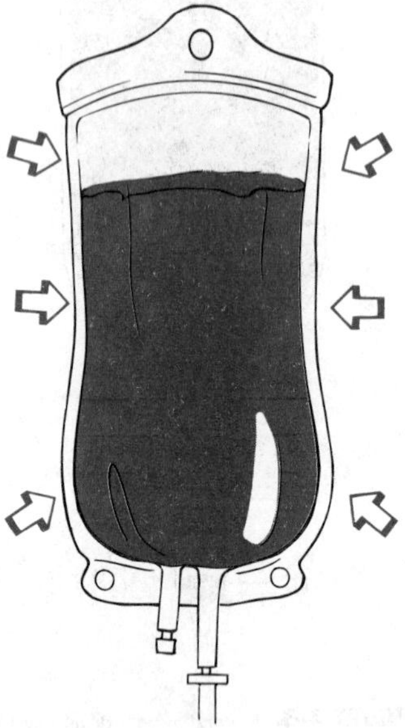

**FIGURE 4–4.** Outside atmospheric pressure collapses the plastic container.

An important feature of the plastic container is the presence of a membrane within the access tube to the fluid. This membrane is far enough up the tube so that the tube is completely sealed by the administration set spike before the spike pierces the membrane (Fig. 4–5).

## ADVANTAGES

Plastic containers do not break under normal conditions. Some designs may be stored on top of one another. Because they collapse when empty, plastic containers are not bulky in disposal. Plastic containers can be manufactured to hold any volume. It is not unusual to see 3-L bags for parenteral nutrition. (Filled glass containers of this volume would be very difficult for most nurses to lift and hang.)

## DISADVANTAGES

The plastic in the container is not clear. It is difficult for the nurse to see particulate matter in the solution. When making additions to the bag, the nurse must take special care not to puncture the side of the bag with the needle. Using a 1-inch (2.5-cm) needle usually alleviates this problem. Measuring the volume left in plastic containers is also more difficult than in glass containers (Fig. 4–6).

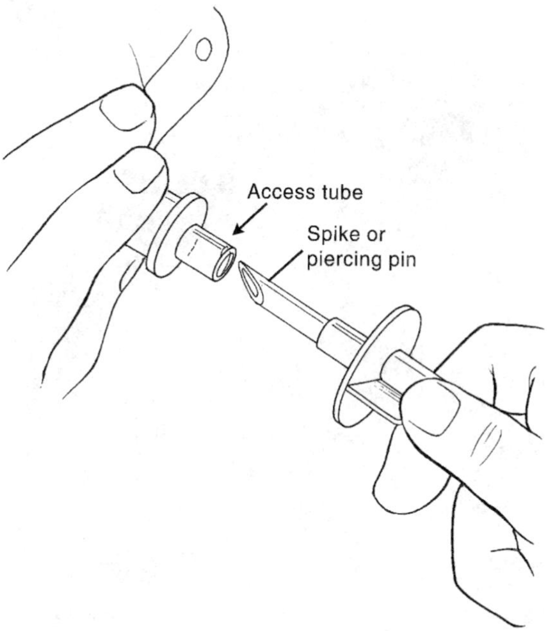


**FIGURE 4–5.** The administration set spike must pierce the membrane.

## ADMINISTRATION SET COMPONENTS

The administration set is the connection between the solution and the client's access device. As infusion therapies have become more complex, manufacturers have adapted these sets to provide the nurse with a variety of products to fit the various therapies. The designs of these sets are limited only by the manufacturers' imaginations. For this reason it is impossible to describe every available administration set. This discussion is limited to the parts that are likely to be found on administration sets. The nurse should keep in mind that these parts can be configured in a variety of ways. Also, electronic pump and controller manufacturers frequently design tubing that can only be used on their devices. These dedicated sets may have cassettes or flow regulation pieces, which are not discussed here (see Chapter 5). Generally, directions appear on the administration set packaging that provide the nurse with the information needed to use the sets properly.

### SPIKE

Administration sets begin with a hard plastic tube with a sharp point. This is called the "spike." The spike penetrates

**FIGURE 4–6.** To read the volume remaining in a plastic IV bag, grasp the bag on either side about 2 inches (5 cm) above the fluid level. Holding the bag taut, read the fluid level. (Photograph courtesy Monica Ridgely.)

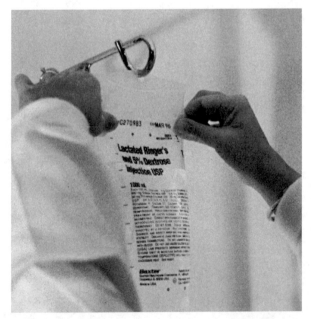

the solution container. When removed from the packaging, the spike has a plastic sheath over it to maintain the spike's sterility (Fig. 4–7).

## SHIELD

Below the spike, most sets have a disk called a shield. The shield acts to prevent the nurse's hands from slipping onto the spike as it is inserted into the container (Fig. 4–7).

## DRIP CHAMBER

Below the shield is usually the drip chamber (Fig. 4–7). This plastic tube is used for priming the set (filling the set with fluid) and verifying flow. Inside the top of the drip chamber is the bottom piece of the spike. Different manufacturers design the size of this piece to control the volume of each drop of fluid. Although there is no standard among the products of most manufacturers, fortunately the size of the drops (called the "drip factor") of a particular set is written on the packaging (Table 4–1). To regulate a gravity flow the nurse must have this information, as the drip factor is one of the factors used in calculating the rate for a gravity infusion (see Appendix C). The only standard drip factor among manufacturers is for the "minidrip" set. These sets always have a drip factor of 60 drops (gtt)/mL (Fig. 4–8). Sets with larger drip factors are often called "macrodrip" sets (Fig. 4–8).

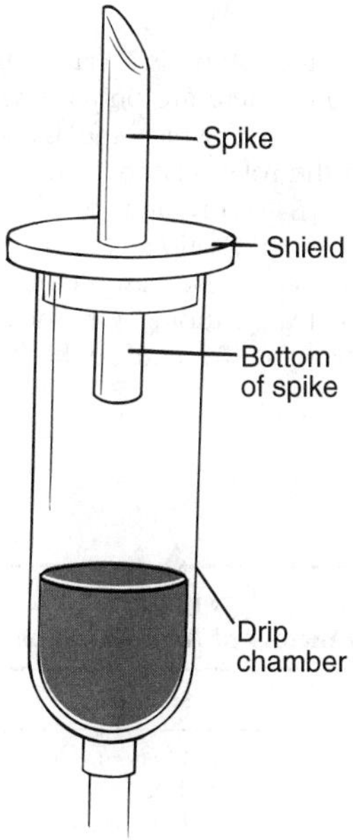


**FIGURE 4–7.** Components of an administration set tubing.

The nurse must consider the size of the drops when choosing an administration set. Minidrip sets are beneficial when regulating small volumes of fluids such as for a young child or elderly client. A physician's order for fluid to infuse at 40 mL/h is easier to regulate with a minidrip set than with a macrodrip set. When using a minidrip set the nurse counts 40 gtt/min to maintain this rate. To maintain a rate of 40 mL/h with a macrodrip set and a drip factor of 10 gtt/mL, the nurse must regulate the rate at approximately 7 gtt/min. This would be a very difficult task. Likewise, the nurse should use a macrodrip set when regulating a larger volume of fluid. In the case of a physician's order indicating an infusion to run at 125 mL/h with a macrodrip set of 10 gtt/mL tubing, the nurse regulates the fluid at about 21 gtt/min. To carry out the same order with a minidrip set, the nurse must regulate the tubing to deliver 125 gtt/min. This too is a very difficult job.

## TUBING

The next major piece of the administration set is the tubing. Administration set tubing runs from the bottom of the drip chamber to the connector device. Again, there is no standard among manufacturers in length of tubing, and the same manufacturer may make administration sets of multiple lengths. The diameters of the different tubings may differ from manufacturer to manufacturer as well.

## CLAMPS

Somewhere on the tubing is a clamping device that regulates the fluid flow. There are only a few different designs for clamps (Fig. 4–9), of which the most popular are the screw clamp and the roller clamp. The nurse may move either of these clamps to any area on the tubing when the clamps are in the open position.

**Screw Clamps.** The screw clamp consists of a hard plastic piece that encircles the tubing. On one side is a hard plastic screw with a flat end. To regulate the fluid flow the nurse

**TABLE 4–1**
**Drip Factors of Administration Sets**

| Manufacturer | Standard | Minidrip |
|---|---|---|
| Abbott | 15 gtt/mL | 60 gtt/mL |
| Cutter | 20 gtt/mL | 60 gtt/mL |
| McGaw | 15 gtt/mL | 60 gtt/mL |
| Travenol | 10 gtt/mL | 60 gtt/mL |

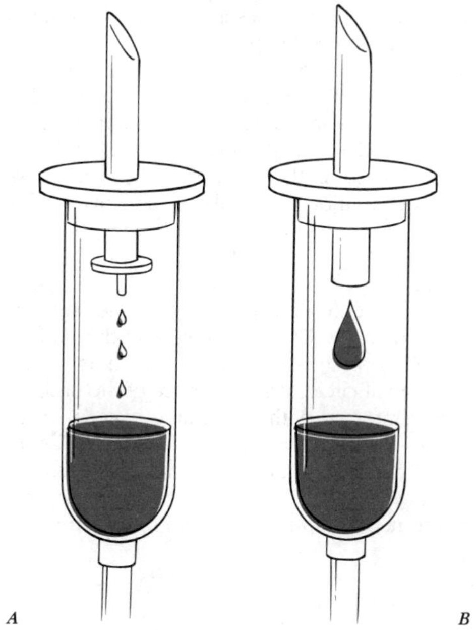


**FIGURE 4–8.** Administration set drip chambers. **A,** Minidrip chamber. **B,** Macrodrip chamber.

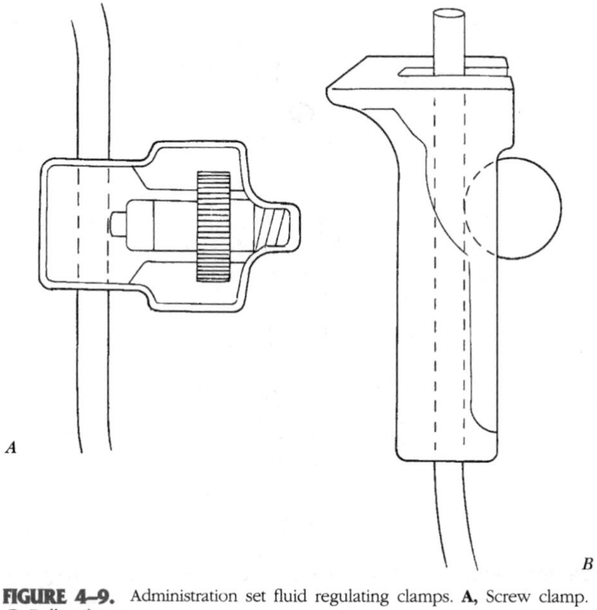


**FIGURE 4–9.** Administration set fluid regulating clamps. **A,** Screw clamp. **B,** Roller clamp.

turns the screw, which causes it to close off the tubing. The tubing may be closed completely or to the degree that accommodates the prescribed rate of delivery (see Fig. 4–9).

**Roller Clamps.** The roller clamp sits around the tubing. This device is a wheel that runs along an inclined plane. The wheel sits closer to the plane on the lower end than on the upper end. As the nurse rolls the wheel down, the tubing occludes, and this regulates the flow of fluid (see Fig. 4–9).

## FLASHBALL

Toward the end of the tubing, some administration sets have a piece of latex that connects the tubing to the connector. This piece is commonly known as the flashball. Frequently, small circles on the surface of the flashball highlight areas reinforced with self-sealing material (Fig. 4–10). If the nurse wishes to administer medications as an intravenous (IV) push, these areas permit a needle stick to gain access to the access device. After the injection the nurse removes the needle, and the material reseals to prevent any leaking.

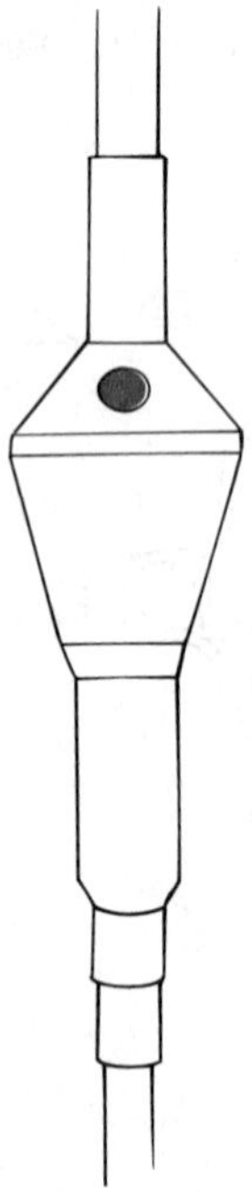

**FIGURE 4–10.** A flashball. Note the self-sealing target for IV push medications.

## CONNECTORS

At the end of the tubing is the connector. Although the designs of the connectors are varied, thankfully the dimensions are standard and attach to any female hub. Three types of connectors may be seen.

**Slip Tip.** The simplest connector is the slip tip. A slip tip is a male end that has a small circumference at the tip. The size gradually increases as it moves back toward the tubing or flashball. The nurse connects the slip tip to the access device or needle hub by pushing straight into the female end. To disconnect the tip the nurse rotates the connector about a quarter turn and pulls. Slip tip connectors may leak and are not recommended for long-term connections (Fig. 4–11).

**Luer Lock.** The next type of connector is the Luer lock connector. Like the slip tip, the Luer lock connector has a male end that inserts into the female end of the access device or needle hub. However, around the male end this device also has a threaded lip that the nurse screws into the hub. This generally prevents leaking but requires a little more time to secure, which may allow blood to leak out of the access device (Fig. 4–11).

**Slip Luer.** The last connector is the slip Luer. This device has a longer male slip than the plain Luer lock connector.

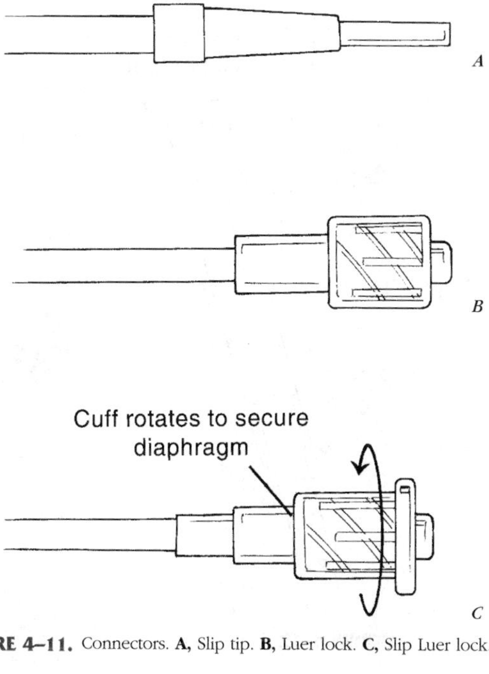


**FIGURE 4–11.** Connectors. **A,** Slip tip. **B,** Luer lock. **C,** Slip Luer lock.

The threaded Luer lip on this device turns freely, so the nurse can quickly make the connection with the slip tip and then secure the connection with the Luer lock (Fig. 4–11).

## Y-SITES

In addition to the flashball, administration sets sometimes have one or more Y-sites that the nurse may use to inject or drip medications and other fluids into this set. Sometimes called sidearms or injection ports, these sites may be located anywhere along the tubing. The Y-site is a hard, clear plastic tube. The lower end is an integral part of the set's tubing. The upper end is a rubber diaphragm. This diaphragm allows penetration with a needle and self-seals after removal (Fig. 4–12).

The nurse must clean both the Y-site and the flashball before inserting a needle through them. Appropriate cleansing agents include alcohol and povidone. The cleansing procedure is more than just a haphazard wipe; the nurse must apply some pressure while wiping to assure an adequate decontamination. In addition, the insertion sites do not accommodate an infinite number of penetrations and do not remain free from leaks. Some manufacturers rate their injec-

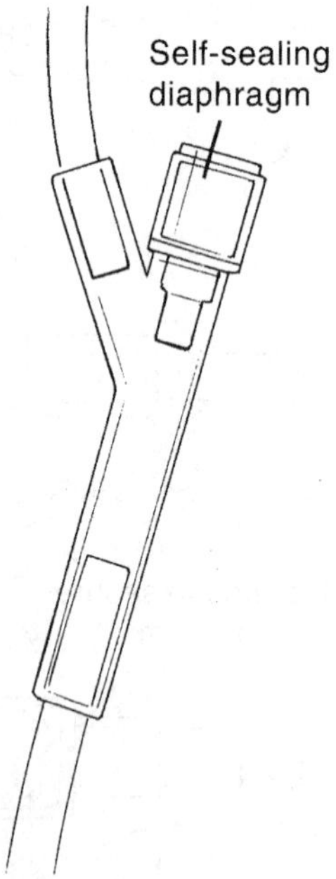


**FIGURE 4–12.** Administration set Y-site.

tion ports for a certain number of entries with a specific-size needle. It is advisable to use the smallest gauge needle that will accomplish the task.

## MISCELLANEOUS COMPONENTS

Some other additions to the administration set are on-off clamps, burettes, back-check valves, and passive flow regulators.

**On-Off Clamps.** There are two types of on-off clamps: slide and clip. These clamps are not appropriate for drip regulation because the level of control is poor. For this reason on-off clamps should only be used to open or close the administration set to flow.

***Slide Clamp.*** The slide clamp is a rectangular piece of plastic with a cutout in the shape of an elongated teardrop. The tubing passes through the cutout. As the tubing moves through the hole to the narrow portion, the lumen of the tubing is compressed until it is closed (Fig. 4–13).

***Clip Clamp.*** The clip clamp consists of a clip around the tubing. To close the clamp the nurse squeezes the sides of the clamp together. To open the clamp the nurse pushes up with his or her thumb under the tab (Fig. 4–13).

**Burettes.** A burette is a reservoir that is either incorporated into or added to the administration set. It sits below the drip chamber and above the regulation clamp. Burettes are frequently known by the name particular manufacturers give them such as Buretrol, Volutrol, or Soluset (Fig. 4–14). The reservoir holds between 100 and 150 mL of fluid. Written on the side of the reservoir are calibrations, usually in 1-mL increments, to assist the nurse with accurate measurement. Between the drip chamber and the burette is a clamp that controls the flow into the reservoir. At the top or bottom of the burette is a rubber cap that looks like the end of a "Y-site." Through this self-sealing cap the nurse can add any medications or additives ordered for the client. The burette is useful for mixing IV drugs for administration or for controlling the amount of fluid available for administration, a critical consideration in the care of the young child or the elderly.

To fill the burette the nurse closes the main clamp below the burette. Opening the clamp between the solution container and the burette allows fluid to flow into the burette. When the appropriate amount of fluid has infused into the burette, the nurse closes the clamp. At this point the infusion is regulated by the lower clamp. The nurse remembers that only the volume of fluid in the burette is available to infuse into the client. This is a valuable safety apparatus when the nurse is regulating fluids for an elderly client or young child because an inadvertent overinfusion of fluid in these clients can have very severe effects.

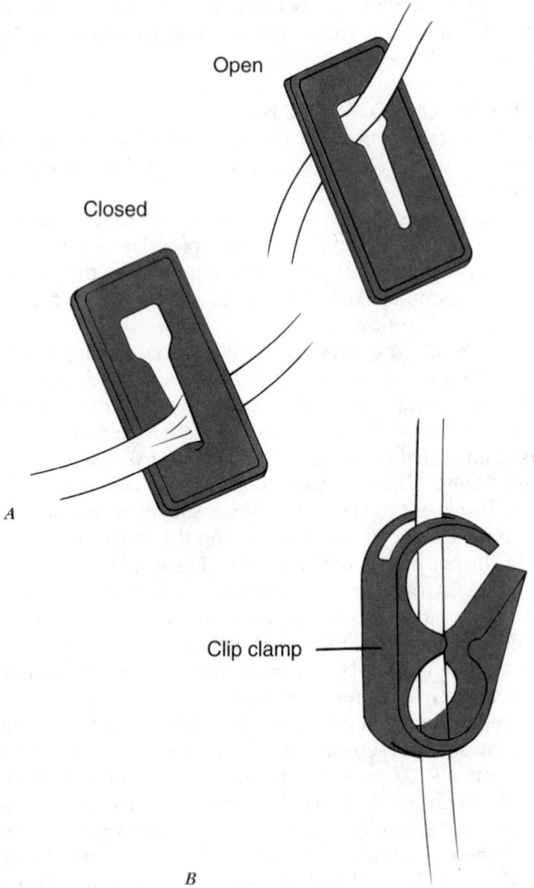


**FIGURE 4–13.** Administration set on-off clamps. **A,** Slide clamp. **B,** Clip clamp.

Burettes are beneficial not only in regulating the amount of fluid available for infusion but also when the nurse must mix medications for infusion. If the client is to receive an intermittent medication such as an antibiotic, the nurse fills the burette with the amount of fluid prescribed and then injects the appropriate amount of medication into the burette. After calculating the number of drops per minutes (gtt/min) at which the medication is to infuse, the nurse regulates the drip rate with the lower roller clamp.

**Back-Check Valves.** When present, a back-check valve is built into the administration set. This device functions as a one-way valve that allows fluid to travel away from the so-

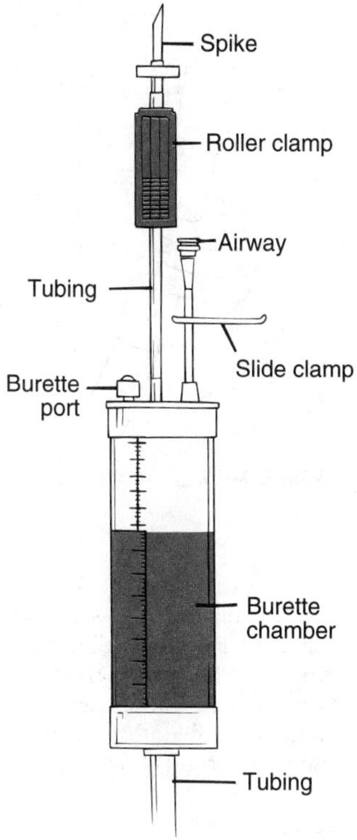


**FIGURE 4–14.** A burette or metered chamber.

lution container but prevents fluid from flowing upstream toward the container (Fig. 4–15). This is beneficial when the nurse is administering medications by IV push or piggyback through a Y-site. It assures that all of the medication being administered is given to the client at the time of the administration. Otherwise, the medication could be pushed upstream, enter the large volume parenteral (LVP) solution container, and be administered at the rate of the LVP.

**Passive Flow Control Devices.** When administering an LVP solution for hydration purposes or a medication whose rate is not critical, the nurse may employ a passive flow control device. These add-on devices look like an extension set with a dial (Fig. 4–16). The nurse uses this dial to set the administration to infuse at the appropriate rate in milliliters per hour. The nurse leaves any other clamps open, and the passive flow control device regulates the administration at the prescribed rate.

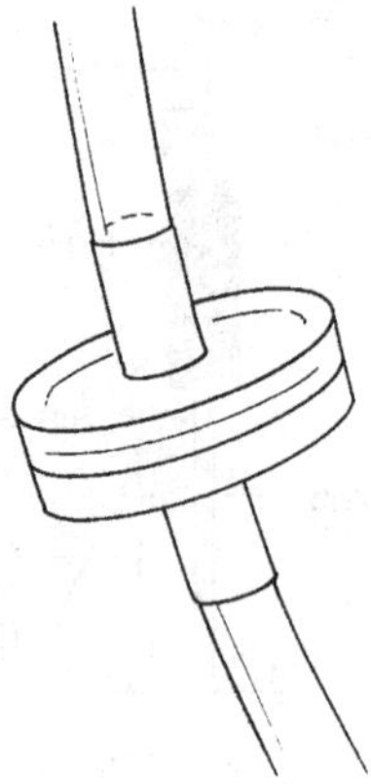

**FIGURE 4–15.** A back-check valve.

# FILTERS

Filters remove particulate matter suspended in the infusion solution while allowing the fluid to pass through to the client. The nurse may see filters of two types: membrane and depth. They may be "in-line" (an integral part of the administration set) or "add-on" (a filter that is separate and must be added to the administration set) (Fig. 4–17).

## Membrane Filters

A membrane filter has pores sized to prevent the passage of particles into the filter. These tiny pores capture any particles on the filter's surface. In some cases enough particles are trapped on the surface to prevent fluid flow. This is know as "loading." For this reason membrane filters are most effective as a "final filter" that is preceded by another filter.

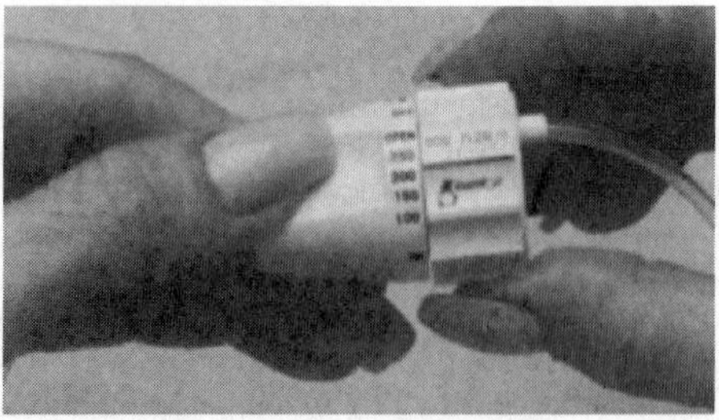

**FIGURE 4–16.** Passive flow regulator. (Courtesy of Medical Specialties Company, Inc.)

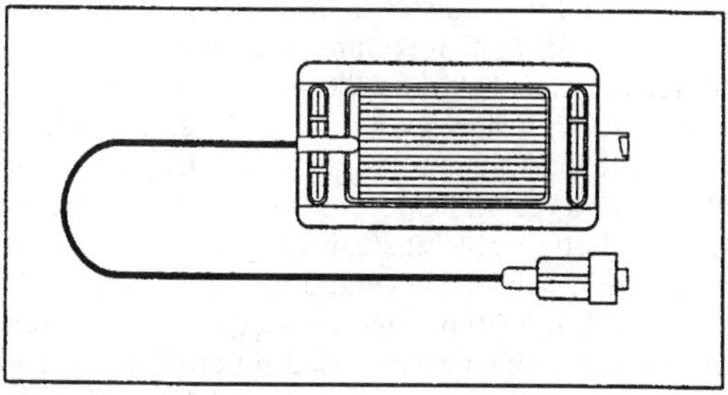

**FIGURE 4–17.** Membrane filters. (Courtesy of Pall Biomedical Products Corporation, East Hills, New York.)

## Depth Filters

A depth filter has a mazelike configuration. Any particles suspended in the fluid pass through the surface but become trapped in the multitude of passages as they travel through the device. An occasional particle may escape the maze and flow to the client. Because the filter surface does not become coated, depth filters are functional for longer periods than membrane filters.

This mechanical restraint is not the only way that depth filters work. Depth filters also have adsorption properties that cause the particles to adhere to the filter material itself without regard to size.

Membrane and depth filters are rated by the size of the smallest particle they hold back. A 0.22-μm filter retains any particles 0.22 μm and larger, as well as the organisms *Escherichia coli* and *Pseudomonas*.

Many filters on the market today also have air-eliminating properties. This provides protection against air embolism because the filter removes any air bubbles that may be above the filter in the administration set.

When selecting a filter, the nurse considers the structural configuration. Filters should be designed to provide maximal surface area for filtration inside the unit without adsorbing drug. Filters are rated as to the pressure they can withstand. This rating in pounds per square inch (lb/in$^2$ or psi) is an important consideration when using electronic infusion devices. If the pumping pressure is higher than the filter rating, the filter may crack, leaving the infusion system open to contamination.

Some controversy surrounds the use of filters. The Intravenous Nurses Society (INS) supports the use of filters for all infusions. The decision is based on the belief that by filtering infusion solutions the nurse can minimize client complications. INS believes 0.22-μm filters decrease the incidence of phlebitis by elimination of particulate matter, remove bacteria present in solutions, and eliminate any air bubbles from the administration set.

The Centers for Disease Control (CDC) disagree with the INS position. The CDC recommend against the routine use of IV filters as an infection control measure because contamination of the infusion solution itself is rare. The INS claim that filters prevent phlebitis is also controversial. Falchuk et al. (1985) found contradictory results in efficacy studies. Furthermore, although phlebitis can be painful, it is rarely life-threatening and can be prevented by other means. The National Coordinating Committee on Large Volume Parenterals determined that if filters were used routinely for every infusion the number of filters would exceed 100 million nationally. In view of this the use of IV filters becomes an issue of cost versus benefit.

The necessity of filters for the removal of particulate matter from commercially manufactured solutions is also questionable. Since the late 1970s, filtering of commercially prepared IV fluids is mandated during manufacturing. In practice admixed fluids may be filtered in the pharmacy during preparation particularly if the drug must be reconstituted or if it must be drawn from a glass ampule. However, if the pharmacy does not filter or if the nurse must reconstitute the drug or withdraw it from an ampule, filtering is recommended.

Another controversy surrounding filtering involves drug adsorption and, consequently, loss when filtered. Because of contradictory information in the literature, the National Coordinating Committee of Large Volume Parenterals in 1979 recommended against filtering when drugs are to be administered "in dosages or concentrations of less than 5 mcg. and/or when the total amount is less than 5 mg. over a 24 hour period."

## PIGGYBACKING

At times the client may require the infusion of intermittent medications while an LVP infuses. The medication container or minibag uses a shorter administration set, sometimes called a secondary set. The nurse attaches the secondary set to the LVP administration set with a needle into a Y-site. The actual medication administration relies on differential pressures created between the two containers when they are raised to different heights above the client. The medication container is hung higher than the LVP container (Fig. 4–18). As long as the nurse hangs the medication container so its lower level is above the highest level of the LVP container and the drip factors of the administration sets are either both macrodrip or minidrip, the laws of physics prevail and the medication container empties first. The LVP container begins dripping when the medication container is empty.

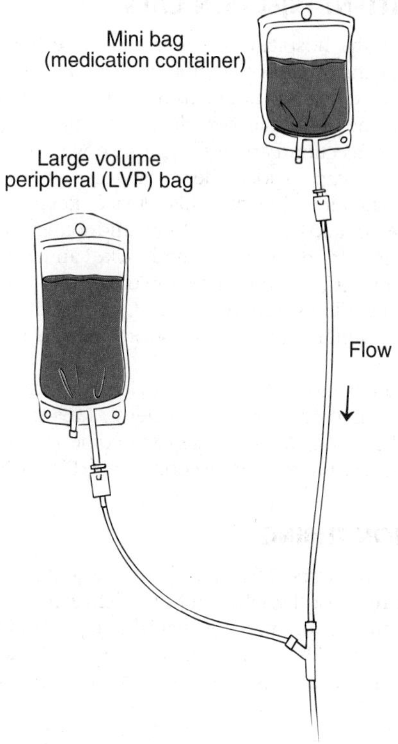


**FIGURE 4–18.** Piggybacking a minibag. (Adapted from Kee, J. L., & Marshall, S. M. [1992]. *Clinical calculations* [2nd ed., p. 132]. Philadelphia: W. B. Saunders.)

When piggybacking medications, the nurse must consider the compatibility of the medication with the LVP solution and the compatibility between piggybacked medications if the same secondary set is used for the administration of these medications.

Certain drugs are incompatible with some LVPs or their additives. Piggybacking these medications into incompatible solutions may cause the medication to precipitate (cause the formation of solid particles of the drug) or inactivate the drug. (See Appendixes F and G.) Phenytoin (Dilantin) piggybacked into any dextrose-containing solution precipitates. Amphotericin B (Fungizone) precipitates in any solution containing sodium chloride. Dopamine (Intropin, ♣Revimine) is inactivated in solutions with a high pH and must not be piggybacked into any solution with sodium bicarbonate.

## INTERMITTENT INJECTION CAPS

At times the hospitalized client and more frequently the client receiving infusions at home or in an ambulatory or long-term-care setting do not have continuous infusions. In these cases the infusion access device is "capped off" with an intermittent injection cap. Sometimes known as a "heparin" or "saline" or cap or lock (depending on what the agency uses to maintain patency), this device keeps the access device sterile and prevents blood and other body fluids from leaking from an open end. Like an administration set injection port, the intermittent injection cap is self-sealing after the needle is removed. Most of these devices are rated for a certain number of "sticks" before they require changing.

Fortunately, the ends of these devices are of universal size and fit the female end of any catheter or tubing designed for infusion therapy. Many of these caps come in Luer lock design to prevent them from disconnecting (Fig. 4–19).

## EXTENSION TUBING

At times the nurse may find that the equipment available is not just right for the infusion to be delivered. For these instances there are a number of available types and lengths of extension sets with a variety of devices on them. Some of these extension tubings have "Y-sites," whereas some may

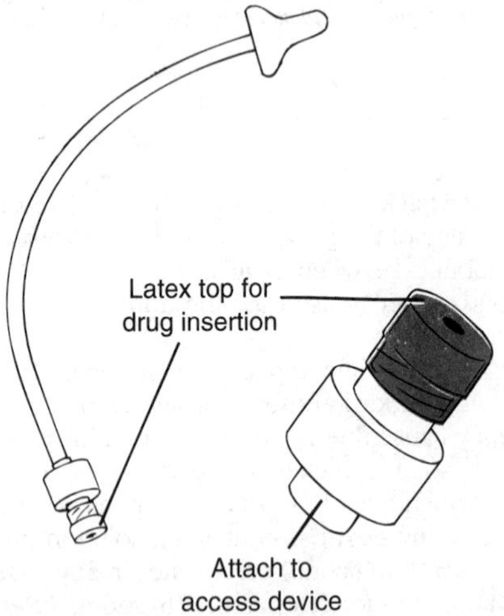


**FIGURE 4–19.** Intermittent injection cap. (From Kee, J. L., & Marshall, S. M. [1992]. *Clinical calculations* [2nd ed., p. 132]. Philadelphia: W. B. Saunders.)

only have filters. Others have a combination of both. Some are spiral like a telephone cord to provide extra length when necessary but prevent long lengths of tubing from draping on the ground (Fig. 4–20).

When choosing an extension set, the nurse must consider infection control issues. These and any other add-on devices increase the potential for infection due to the risk of separation. The INS suggests that these devices have a Luer lock design to secure them and that they be changed on the same schedule as the device to which it is attached or if its integrity is in question (INS, 1990).

The loop extension set with an intermittent injection port at the end is of particular use for home care clients, as most home care clients self-administer their intermittent medications. When used on a peripheral IV catheter, this device assists with shifting the pressure the client uses to pierce the intermittent injection cap to the extension set rather than the IV catheter site itself (Fig. 4–21). This type of extension set is also useful when administering intermittent medications to clients with fragile veins such as the elderly. Again, shifting the pressure the nurse uses to pierce the heparin or saline cap away from the catheter insertion site can prevent the nurse from dislodging the cannula during the procedure.

## NEEDLELESS OR NEEDLE-FREE SYSTEMS

In July 1992 the Occupational Safety and Health Administration's guidelines entitled "Occupational Exposure to Blood Borne Pathogens; Final Rule" was implemented. This document requires health care organizations to initiate engineering controls "that isolate or remove the blood borne pathogen hazard from the workplace" (see Appendix A). A number of new products are now available to decrease the nurse's exposure to contaminated needles. Some of these include devices that use recessed needles, whereas others include one-way valves or blunt plastic cannula. It is estimated that these systems can eliminate up to 80% of the traditional metal needles used in a hospital setting (Beason, 1993).

### Safsite System

The Burron Safsite Needlefree System is one of the systems that eliminates the use of needles for most infusion procedures. One of the advantages of this system is that it adapts to essentially any infusion system the health care institution currently uses. The heart of this system is a two-way valve that replaces the traditional intermittent injection cap (Fig. 4–22). One end of the valve is a male Luer lock that connects

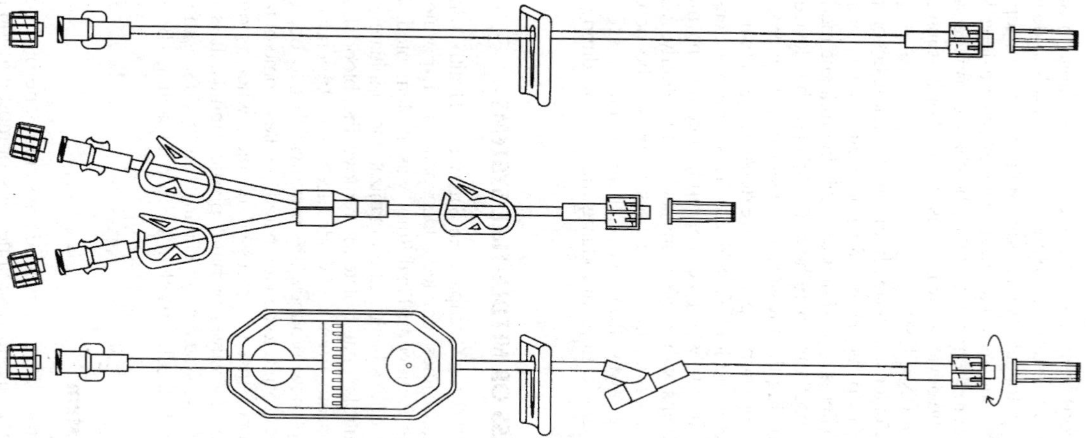

A

B

C

**FIGURE 4–20.** Extension sets. **A,** Extension set with slide clamp and Luer locks. **B,** Bifurcated extension set with pinch clamps and Luer locks. **C,** Extension set with filter, Luer locks, slide clamp, and injection Y-site. (Courtesy of Churchill Medical Systems, Inc., Horsham, Pennsylvania.)

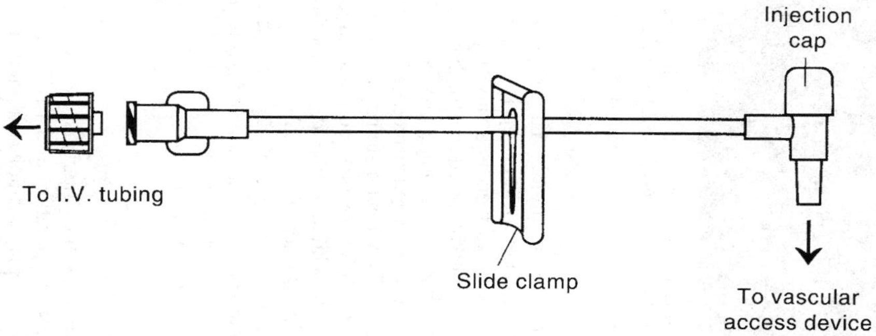

**FIGURE 4–21.** Loop extension set. (Courtesy of Churchill Medical Systems, Inc., Horsham, Pennsylvania.)

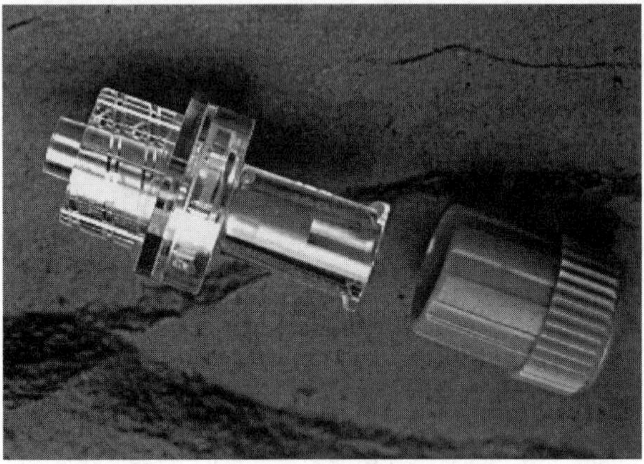

**FIGURE 4–22.** Burron Safsite Needlefree IV System valve and "deadhead." (Courtesy of B. Braun Medical, Inc., Bethlehem, Pennsylvania.)

to the female end of the cannula. The other is a female end that accepts slip tip, Luer lock, or slip Luer tip administration sets or extension sets, as well as a slip or Luer lock tip syringe. Like the intermittent injection cap, this valve is used to cap off infusion devices. The nurse may administer continuous, intermittent, bolus, or push medications and solutions through this valve. To maintain sterility of the system in between intermittent, bolus, or push administrations, the nurse caps the valve off with a sterile cap sometimes called a "deadhead" or "dead end" (Fig. 4–22).

The Safsite system has a multidose vial dispensing pin available. The nurse uses the dispensing pin to access multidose vials such as when drawing up heparin or 0.9% NSS flushes for heparin or saline locks.

## Interlink System

Another system is the InterLink IV Access System by Baxter Healthcare Corporation and Becton Dickinson Division. This system replaces traditional steel needles with a blunt, plastic cannula and preslit injection site. A family of InterLink products is available for intermittent and continuous therapy including syringe cannula, injection sites, catheter extension sets, vial access products, and primary and secondary IV sets (Fig. 4–23).

The vial access products include a universal vial adapter. This adapter has a spike that fits on a vial. The top of the adapter is the preslit injection site that accommodates the blunt plastic cannula.

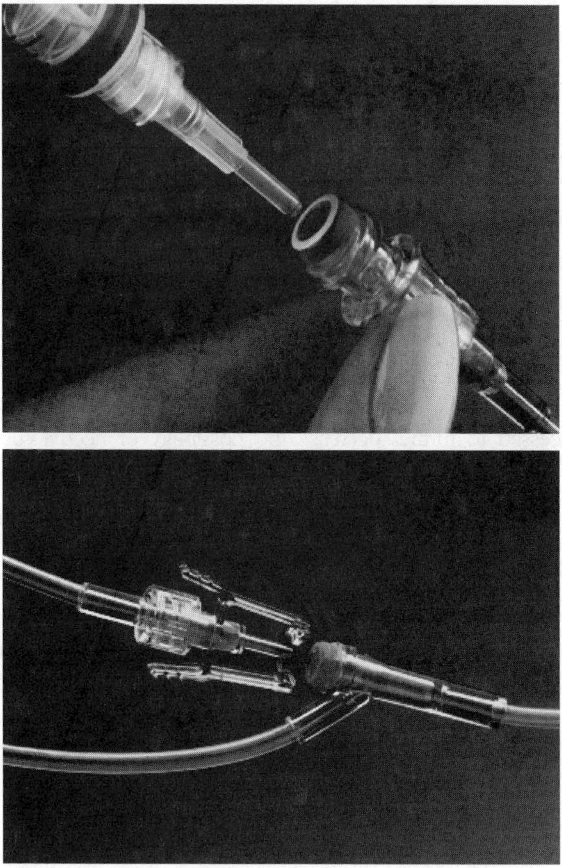

A

B

**FIGURE 4–23.** **A,** Syringe with InterLink blunt plastic cannula and preslit injection site. **B,** Secondary set with InterLink lever lock and preslit injection site for piggybacking.

## Clave System

The Clave is another needleless system. Developed by ICU Medical, this system uses the least number of pieces. The Clave consists of a cap, which at first appears to be a traditional intermittent injection cap. This cap actually incorporates a valve that slides the cap's diaphragm back into the cap when the male portion of a syringe or administration set depresses the diaphragm, allowing fluid to infuse. When the syringe or administration set is removed, the valve pushes the diaphragm back out so that it is flush with the cap. ICU Medical manufactures a multidose vial dispensing pin with the Clave port incorporated into the pin.

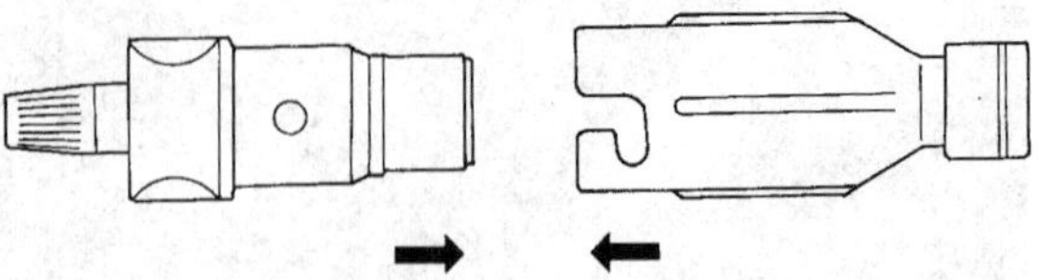


**FIGURE 4–24.** Ryan Medical Saf-T-Clik system.

## Saf-T-Clik System

The Saf-T-Clik System by Ryan Medical consists of a special prepierced injection cap and the Saf-T-Clik connector. The connector looks like a short needle with a blunt tip in the middle of a plastic tube. The blunt-tipped needle is recessed to further decrease the possibility of needle sticks (Fig. 4–24). A small opening on the side of the plastic tube connects to a small knob on the side of the injection cap. These two pieces connect with a "click," securely locking them together.

## SYSTEM EVALUATIONS

Nurses are frequently members of committees to evaluate new infusion systems. When evaluating new systems and equipment, the nurse should consider the following:

- Is the product a safe alternative for the client and nurse?
- Is the product reliable and durable?
- Does the product provide effective protection against accidental needle sticks?
- Can the product be disposed of easily and safely after use?
- Is the product packaged in such a way that it is easy to access while maintaining it sterile?
- Will a company representative be available to provide in-service support to all staff on each shift?
- In the case of new needleless systems, does the company have the capacity to provide your institution with enough equipment so that the new system or pieces of it will not be out of stock?
- If the system is to be used in the home, will the client and any other caregivers be able to use it without difficulty?

# CHAPTER 5
# Infusion Regulation Devices

*Marilyn Ferreri Booker*



The ability to regulate the rate and volume of infusions is critical to the safe and accurate administration of drugs and fluids to clients. Nurses have a choice of numerous devices designed to regulate infusions. Most are classified as either controllers or pumps and require either AC or battery as a power source (Table 5–1). Others fall into the new category of "elastomeric devices" and infuse via a pressure gradient rather than a power source.

Infusion regulation devices can save nursing time and prevent runaway infusions. Furthermore, infusion regulation devices reduce the incidence of infiltration and keep infusion access devices patent. The nurses and clients who use infusion pumps and controllers reap the benefits of some of the latest computer technology. Not every pump is appropriate for any situation. It is important for the nurse to consider the purpose of the infusion, the drug or solution, the client, the setting (hospital or home), and the type of access device the client has before deciding on a particular type of infusion regulation device.

## CONTROLLERS

A controller is a stationary (pole-mounted—attached to an intravenous [IV] pole) electronic device that can be classified as either nonvolumetric or volumetric. Nonvolumetric controllers rely completely on gravity for flow. A drop sensor attached to the drip chamber of the administration set regulates the flow (Fig. 5–1). Volumetric controllers also count drops and electronically convert the drops to mL/h. Because they

**TABLE 5–1**
**Comparison of Controllers and External Stationary Pumps**

| Criteria | Controller | Pump |
|---|---|---|
| Operation | Gravity or linear peristalsis | Piston syringe or peristalsis |
| Power source | AC with back-up battery | AC with back-up battery |
| Flow rates | Usually up to 400 mL/h | Can be up to 2000 mL/h |
| Access devices | Usually peripheral lines only | Any type of access device |
| Administration sets | May use straight line tubing | Usually dedicated tubing, although some newer models use straight line tubing |
| Pressure | Determined by fluid container head height | May be set by user or determined by pump manufacturer |
| Types of fluids or drugs | Low viscosity, no blood | Any viscosity. May be used for blood administration |
| Client population | Any but particularly elderly and neonates with fragile veins | All |

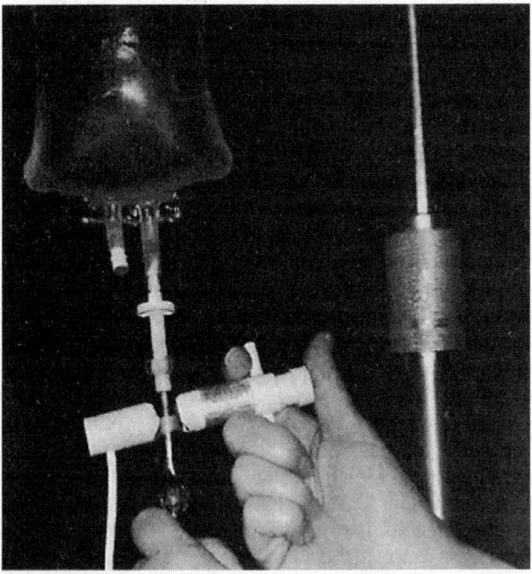

**FIGURE 5–1.** A drop sensor attached to the drip chamber of an administration set helps regulate flow. (From Bolander, V. B. [1994]. *Sorensen and Luckmann's basic nursing* [3rd ed., p. 1325]. Philadelphia: W. B. Saunders.)

count drops, which may and do vary in size, controllers are not as accurate as pumps. Volumetric controllers use linear peristalsis for flow. Linear peristalsis can be described as fingerlike projections intermittently walking across the administration set tubing. The nurse must thread the administration set tubing through guides that secure the tubing in the correct place (Fig. 5–2). Controllers that use linear peristalsis are not appropriate for administration of blood, as the intermittent squeezing of the administration set tubing can damage the blood cells.

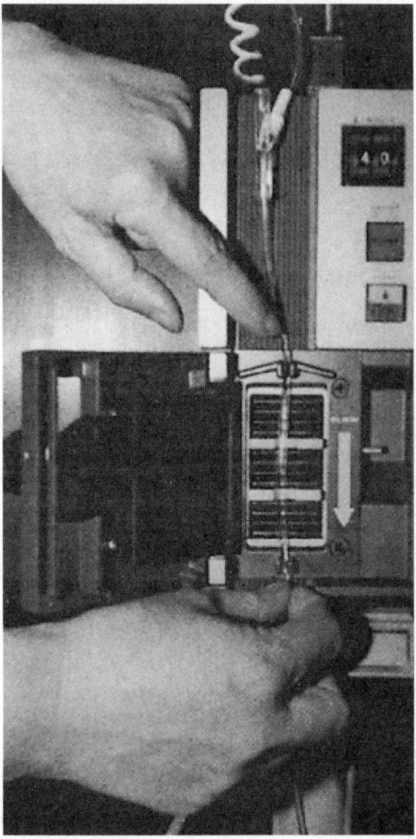

**FIGURE 5–2.** The nurse threads the administration set through guides, securing the tubing in place. (From Foster, R. L. et al [1989]. *Family-centered nursing care of children* [p. 920]. Philadelphia: W. B. Saunders.)

The maximum flow rate attainable with a controller is a product of the client's venous pressure and how high the infusion container is hung above the client's IV site. In general, the nurse can expect to administer up to 400 mL/h with a controller through a peripheral vein. A head height of at least 36 in (91.4 cm) is necessary to overcome peripheral venous pressure of 0 to 0.4 psi (pounds per square inch). Peripheral venous pressure of this level corresponds to between 0 and 20 mm Hg. Controllers may not be appropriate with some central venous catheters, depending on the client's central venous pressure and the solution being administered. Controllers are never appropriate to maintain flow on arterial lines, as arterial pressure is greater than gravity and blood backs up into the administration set. Any resistance to flow results in back pressure, causing an alarm to sound. For this reason, controllers are useful in the early detection of infiltrations. This is valuable when administering vesicant drugs such as doxorubicin (Adriamycin). Controllers are also useful when the client has small or fragile veins, as in the elderly client or neonate. Unfortunately, the sensitivity controllers have to any changes in pressure causes controllers to be responsible for many nuisance alarms. Clients may cause the alarm to sound by rolling over on their administration set tubings or changing positions.

## EXTERNAL PUMPS

Pumps may be either stationary (pole mounted), ambulatory (portable), or even implanted in the client. As their name indicates, these devices actually pump drugs or solutions under pressure. Stationary pumps may be nonvolumetric or volumetric. Nonvolumetric pumps count drops and because of this are inherently inaccurate due to the variation of drop size. There are three types of volumetric pumps available: syringe, cassette, and peristaltic.

### Syringe Pumps

Syringe pumps use a mechanism that closes the plunger at a selected mL/h rate. They find limited usage, usually only in neonatology, since infusing large volumes requires frequent syringe refilling (Fig. 5–3).

### Cassette Pumps

Cassette pumps use special sets that include a pumping chamber of exact volume. This volume is displaced by means of either a piston or a diaphragm at the selected mL/h rate. Cassette pumps require special techniques to prime the administration set (Fig. 5–4).

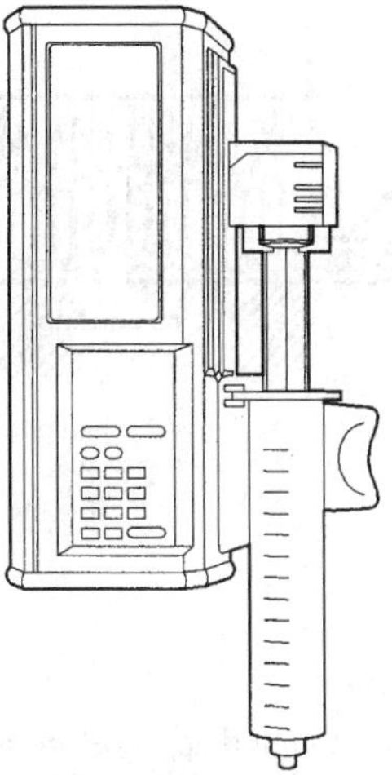

**FIGURE 5–3.** The Baxter syringe pump. (Courtesy of Baxter Healthcare Corporation, Niles, Illinois.)

## Peristaltic Pumps

Peristaltic pumps control rate by squeezing the tubing as described for linear peristaltic controllers. The administration sets of the newer peristaltic pumps are very elastic so that the tubing rebounds to its original shape after long periods of pumping. The administration sets of older pumps require that the nurse periodically readjust the tubing against the pumping mechanism to maintain the accuracy of the administration. Administration sets for peristaltic pumps usually prime the same way standard IV sets prime (Fig. 5–5).

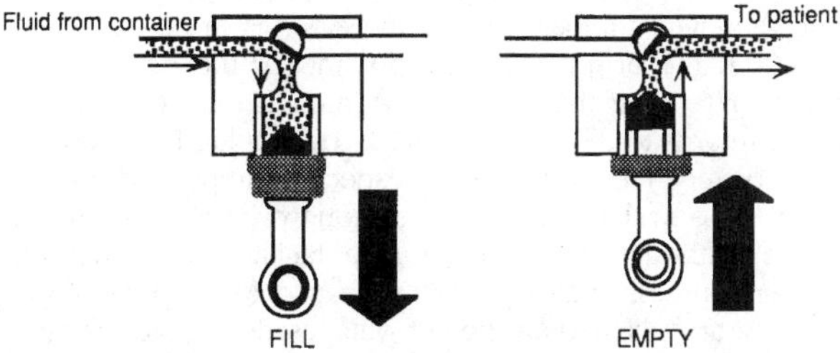


**FIGURE 5–4.** Schematic of a syringe cassette mechanism. (Courtesy of American Society of Health-System Pharmacists.)

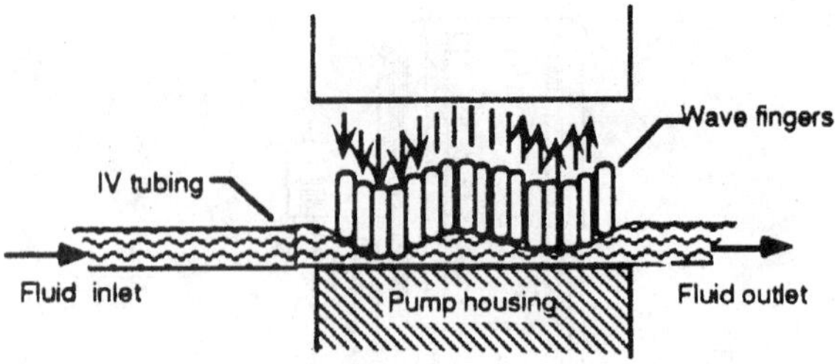


**FIGURE 5–5.** Schematic of linear peristaltic pumping mechanism. (Courtesy of American Society of Health-System Pharmacists.)

## Stationary Pumps

Stationary (pole-mounted) pumps are generally the most widely used infusion pumps (Fig. 5–6). These devices may be designed for general use or for more specific types of therapy such as patient-controlled analgesia (PCA). The following is a discussion of general features found on stationary volumetric pumps. Table 5–2 lists some of the more popular stationary pumps and their special features.

### PRESSURE

Most stationary pumps infuse at about 1.3 psi. Some pumps have variable occlusion pressure settings, which the nurse may program as either "high" or "low" or at a psi of between 4 and 25. A pump usually infuses at about 1.3 psi until it meets any resistance. The pump then attempts to overcome this resistance by increasing the pressure until it meets the previously set occlusion pressure limit. If the pump cannot overcome the resistance when it meets the preset occlusion pressure limit, it will alarm.

### POWER SOURCE

Stationary pumps use AC and have backup internal batteries. This allows the nurse to unplug the pump and maintain the client's infusion while the client is in other departments in the hospital. It is important for the nurse to remember to plug the pump back into the outlet when the client returns to the nursing unit, as battery life is not unlimited. Battery life evaluation is especially important for the client who will be using the stationary infusion pump at home. Although most health care facilities have backup power sources, homes generally do not. Many parts of the country are plagued by power outages during storms, and clients who are receiving home infusion therapy require adequate battery backup for their infusion pumps.

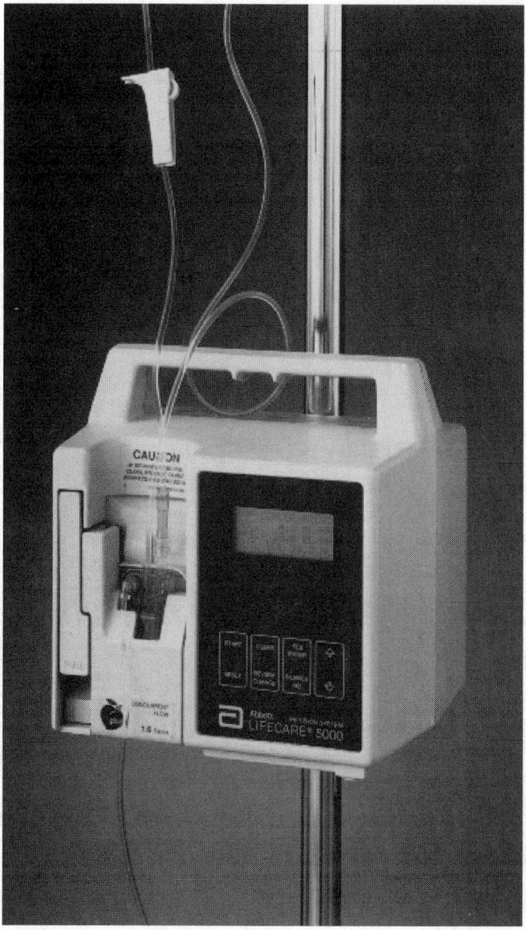


**FIGURE 5–6.** Stationary pole-mounted pump. (Courtesy of Abbott Laboratories, Abbott Park, Illinois.)

## TYPES OF INFUSION/RATE

A pump rather than a controller is required when the client is receiving viscous fluids such as total parenteral nutrition (TPN) or when very precise dosing is necessary, as in the case of dopamine or nitroglycerin. In areas, such as the emergency room, in which large volumes of fluids must be administered rapidly, a pump is invaluable. Some pumps can deliver up to 2000 mL/h. Pumps also allow low flate rate infusions. In general, controller or gravity systems do not infuse below 5 mL/h.

**TABLE 5–2**
**Popular External Stationary Volumetric Pumps and Their Features**

| Model and Manufacturer | Operating Principle | Operating Range | Features |
|---|---|---|---|
| IMED Gemini PC-1 | Linear peristaltic | Controller mode 0.1–500 mL/h<br>Pump mode 0.1–999 mL/h | Auto-taper, versa taper, dual rate piggybacking, tamperproof, data port for communication with remote monitoring system |
| IMED Gemini PC-2 | Linear peristaltic | Controller mode 0.1–500 mL/h<br>Pump mode 0.1–999 mL/h | Dual rate piggybacking, tamperproof, nurse call, data port for communication with remote monitoring system |
| IMED Gemini PC-4 | Linear peristaltic | Controller mode 0.1–500 mL/h<br>Pump mode 0.1–999 mL/h | Dual rate piggybacking, tamperproof, nurse call, programmable start time, four independent channels, data port for communication with remote monitoring system, |
| IMED Gemini PC-2TX | Linear peristaltic | 0.1–99.9 mL/h in 0.1 mL increments or 1–999 mL/h in 1 mL increments | Dual channel delivery, programmable start time, automatic drug dose calculation, data port for communication with remote monitoring system; can infuse directly from syringes for automated IV pushes |
| Baxer Flo-Guard 6201 | Linear peristaltic | 0.1–99.9 mL/h in 0.1 mL increments or 1–1999 mL/h in 1 mL increments | Uses standard Baxter administration set; automatic restart when occlusion is cleared, tamperproof, automatic piggybacking of secondary medications, alarm log of last 10 alarms, selectable options for customized control, data port for communication with remote monitoring system |
| Omni-Flow 4000 PLUS (Abbott) | Linear peristaltic | Macro 1.4–800 mL/h | Can infuse four different solutions, either simultaneously or at variable rates; has automatic line-purging, and computer interface |
| Sabratek | Linear peristaltic | Micro/macro: 0.1–999 mL/h | Uses any of a number of standard administration sets; variable rates, straight-line or step ramping, designed specifically for home care |

## ACCURACY

Any infusion regulator is accurate within certain specifications. These specifications are usually expressed as ± a certain percentage. An accuracy rating of ± 10% on a pump infusing fluids at a rate of 100 mL/h means the pump may actually be delivering the infusion anywhere between 90 and 110 mL/h. As long as the pump is delivering the fluids between these two values, the pump is performing within an acceptable accuracy rate based on the manufacturer's specifications. In general, the more precise the dosing, the smaller the acceptable margin of error. Higher margins mean larger variances in dosing. Most external pumps function at an accuracy rate of ± 2%.

## CONSISTENCY OF FLOW

Another consideration when evaluating an infusion pump is the consistency of flow. Even though two pumps may have identical accuracy ratings, they may not deliver flows of equal consistency. Different pumps split each milliliter into different numbers of parts. As an example, a pump that divides each milliliter into 600 parts, called a 600 parts per milliliter delivery, delivers a more consistent flow than a pump that divides each milliliter into only 200 parts. This can be very important when delivering vasopressers in critical care settings or in the care of very ill neonates.

## ALARMS

Many pumps have alarms that sound in the event of unauthorized tampering with the delivery parameters or if the door to the pump is opened. This is important for pumps used for confused clients or toddlers who cannot seem to get their fill of playing with buttons. Usually the pump must be placed in a "standby" or "stop" mode to reprogram the infusion parameters. Pumps have an alarm that sounds when the pump cannot overcome resistance. This is sometimes known as an occlusion alarm. Most stationary pumps have some type of electronic air in-line sensor that alarms when an air bubble of a predetermined size is in the administration set tubing. Many times pumps have an alarm that notifies the user of a electromechanical malfunction. When this alarm sounds, the pump must be sent to a biomedical technician for repair.

## PROGRAMMING

Programming infusion pumps entails setting infusion delivery parameters. The user usually completes this by using a keypad on the pump. For large-volume continuous peripheral infusions, those parameters are the minimum volume to be infused and the rate of the infusion in milliliters per hour or drops per minute. Some, more sophisticated stationary pumps can deliver multiple solutions at different rates or intermittent infusions, as in antibiotic delivery. Other pumps are designed for PCA and require the nurse to program continuous rates (also known as basal rates), bolus doses, and lock-out times. Administration of cycled parenteral nutrition requires programming a ramping schedule that includes a ramp up, a continuous rate, and a ramp down (Fig. 5–7). Most pumps keep track of the volume that was infused. This is helpful for the health care facility nurse who is keeping track of the client's intake and output. At the end of the shift the nurse can record what the pump reads for the volume infused. Many hospitals require that at the end of each shift the nurse clear out the volume infused. This helps to keep a correct record of the client's IV intake.

## ADMINISTRATION SET

Most stationary pumps require administration sets made for the particular pump (dedicated set) (Fig. 5–8). One of the newer models, the Sabratek, designed specifically for home care clients, is flexible in that the nurse may use either a Sabratek set or any of the major manufacturers' straight-line sets.

Some administration sets can be primed with the set loaded in the pump, whereas others use gravity to prime. Some require that the nurse hold the cassette upside down during the priming to eliminate all air from the set. It is very useful for the nurse to consult the administration set packaging when using a new set. The directions written on the package instruct the nurse in the proper priming and loading of the administration set. Completing these two procedures correctly is key to trouble-free pump usage. Before be-

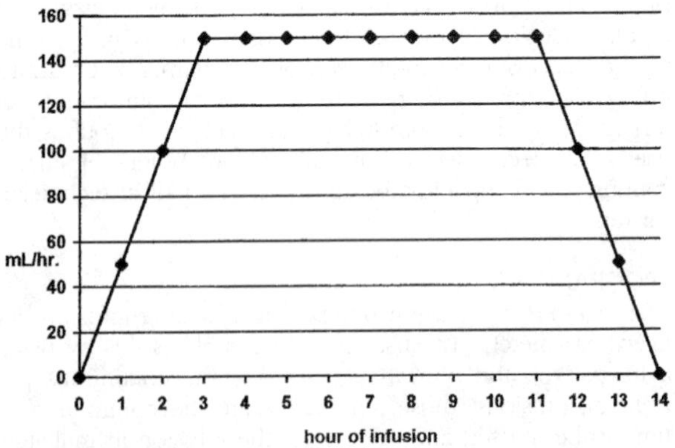


**FIGURE 5–7.** A typical programmed ramping schedule.

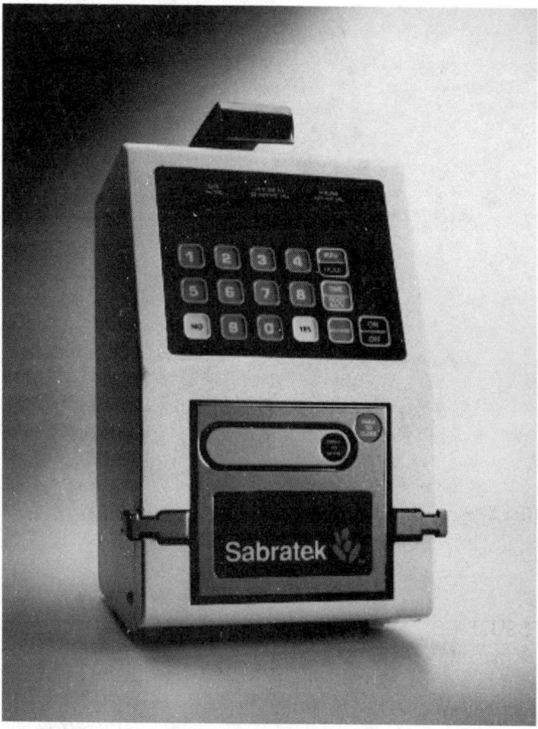


**FIGURE 5–8.** Some modern pumps, such as the Sabratek, are designed specifically for home care and use a straight-line administration set rather than a dedicated administration set. (Courtesy of Sabratek, Chicago, Illinois.)

ginning the infusion, the nurse should make sure that all clamps on the administration set are open. This avoids any faulty occlusion alarms.

The latest guidelines from the Centers for Disease Control indicate that administration sets should be changed every 72 hours unless the administration set is being used for parenteral nutrition administration. In this case, the administration set is changed every 24 hours. It is important that the nurse label the administration set with the date it was hung to avoid confusion among the rest of the staff.

## Ambulatory Pumps

Ambulatory pumps are generally used for home care clients. These pumps allow clients, who are able, to return to their normal activities while receiving infusion therapy (Fig. 5–9).

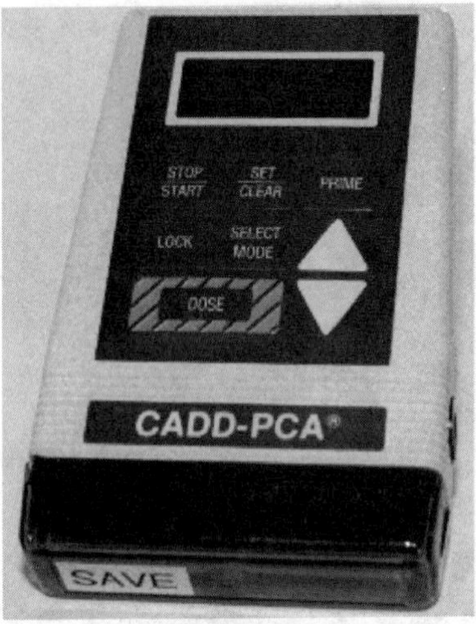


**FIGURE 5–9.** A continuous ambulatory drug delivery (CADD) pump. (Courtesy of Pharmacia, Minneapolis, Minnesota. Photograph courtesy of Monica Ridgely.)

## PRESSURE

Some ambulatory infusion pumps are variable pressure machines with a range between 8 and 20 psi. As with stationary pumps, when the pump continues to meet resistance at its highest occlusion pressure, it sounds an alarm to alert the user to a potential infiltration.

## POWER SOURCE

Ambulatory pumps operate on a variety of power sources. Most all can use one to two 9-V batteries. In addition, some use power packs that include rechargeable lead-acid or NICAD batteries. A few even have AC power adapters. The life of any battery in an ambulatory pump depends on how hard it must work to deliver the amount of fluid required. The larger the volume it must deliver each hour, the shorter the battery's life span. Some pump manufacturers list the approximate volume when fully charged or that new batteries can deliver at a certain rate such as, "Two 9-V batteries will deliver 4000 mL at 300 mL/h."

## TYPES OF INFUSION/RATE

In the early days of ambulatory pumps, each model was designed for a specific type of delivery mode. Many pumps continue to be used for specific delivery types. Recently though, ambulatory pumps are becoming as versatile as some of the stationary pumps in that they can administer intermittent infusions, PCA, and continuous infusions. Some can even automatically taper TPN infusions. The potential rates of any ambulatory infusion pump depend on the type of infusion for which the multidelivery mode pump is programmed or, in the case of the infusion-mode specific pump, the model type.

## ACCURACY

Not all ambulatory pumps claim an accuracy rate. Of those that do, most fall between ± 5% to 10%.

## PROGRAMMING

With most ambulatory pumps the nurse uses a keyboard for programming. In addition, one of the newer devices, the Verifuse system by Block Medical, uses computer software that prints out a bar code like the supermarket uses (Fig. 5–10). When it is time to program the pump, the user scans the bar code with the pump, and the optical reader in the pump sets the program. The user then checks the program using the pump's keypad. Another feature of this pump is the ability to monitor the pump's delivery via a computer modem over the client's telephone (Fig. 5–11).

## ADMINISTRATION SET

All ambulatory pumps use dedicated administration sets. Some ambulatory pumps such as the Pharmacia continuous ambulatory drug delivery (CADD) pumps use either a cassette reservoir (Fig. 5–12), which contains the medication, or a remote reservoir adapter (Fig. 5–13) for the administration of large-volume infusions such as hydration or TPN. Other

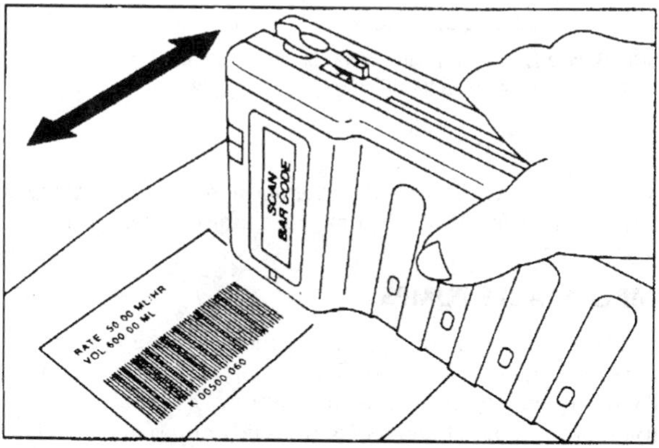


**FIGURE 5–10.** The Verifuse ambulatory pump uses bar code programming. (Courtesy of Block Medical, Carlsbad, California.)

2. Select **Status** from the Secondary menu; the computer will show:

```
Homebase/Verifuse Status
-------------------------------------------------
Exit=Esc, Print Status=Any other Key
Last Alarm - No Alarms Occurred
Low Volume Alarm At -- 245.0 ml
Volume Infused -------   1.7 ml
Volume To Be Infused - 250.0 ml
Current Rate --------- 10.0 ml/hr
Programmed Rate ------ 10.0 ml/hr
Elapsed Time --------- 000:10:23
Air In Line Detector - Off
Program Lock --------- Unlocked
Mode ----------------- Continuous

Connected with J. DEAN
Press 'C' to cancel call.
Calling Phone No    29
```

It will take a few seconds for the modem to begin to dial the phone number.

3. Once the computer system displays "Press <Esc> key to exit, or any key to print", your telephone can be picked up to talk with the patient. It will take a few seconds for the patient to come on the line.

   The patient can pick up the phone when the yellow and green phone lights on the Homebase have been flashing for a few seconds. It will take a few seconds for you to come on the line.

4. The infusion status report is not stored in memory; to print the infusion status report, press any key. The computer will show:

```
Start printing?
---------------
Yes
No
```

**FIGURE 5–11.** A typical status report of the client's infusion via telephonic transmission. (Courtesy of Block Medical, Carlsbad, California.)

pumps use a dedicated administration set, incorporating a cartridge that fits into the pump mechanism (Fig. 5–14).

## IMPLANTABLE PUMPS

Clients who require regional chemotherapy or continuous intraspinal narcotics are candidates for implantable pumps. There are two types of implantable devices currently available: the Infusaid (Intermedics Infusaid) pump and the SynchroMed infusion system (Medtronic). Both the Infusaid and the SynchroMed are implanted subcutaneously via laparo-

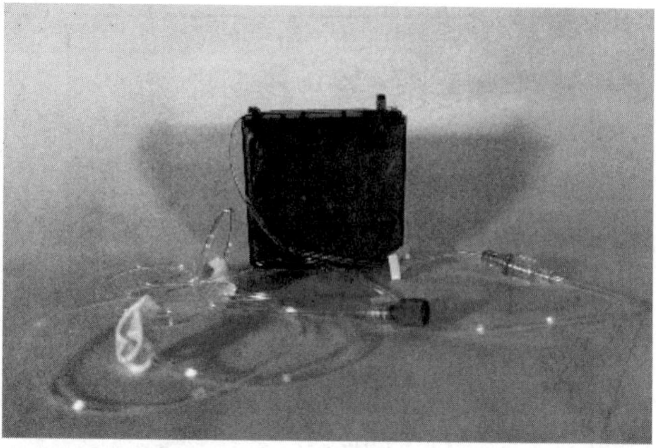

**FIGURE 5–12.** A cassette reservoir. (Courtesy of Pharmacia, Minneapolis, Minnesota. Photograph courtesy of Monica Ridgely.)

tomy in a pocket on the client's trunk (Fig. 5–15). Usual implant sites are the lower abdomen, the subclavicular area, or the subscapular area. Each pump has an attached catheter, which the surgeon threads to the target infusion site. If the client will be receiving antineoplastic drugs through the pump, the physician waits until the surgical site is healed before administering the drugs. For clients who will be receiving pain medication, pumps may be filled and treatment begun immediately.

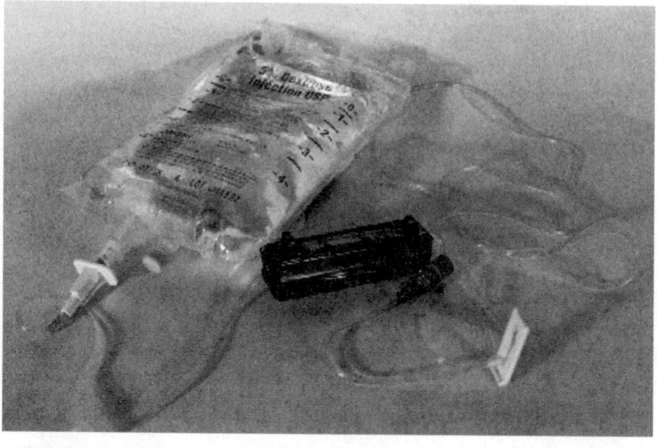

**FIGURE 5–13.** A remote reservoir. (Courtesy of Pharmacia, Minneapolis, Minnesota. Photograph courtesy of Monica Ridgely.)

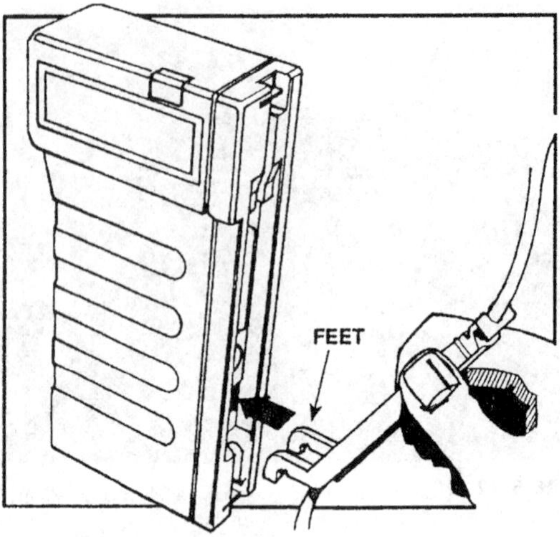


**FIGURE 5–14.** The Verifuse administration set cartridge. (Courtesy of Block Medical, Carlsbad, California.)

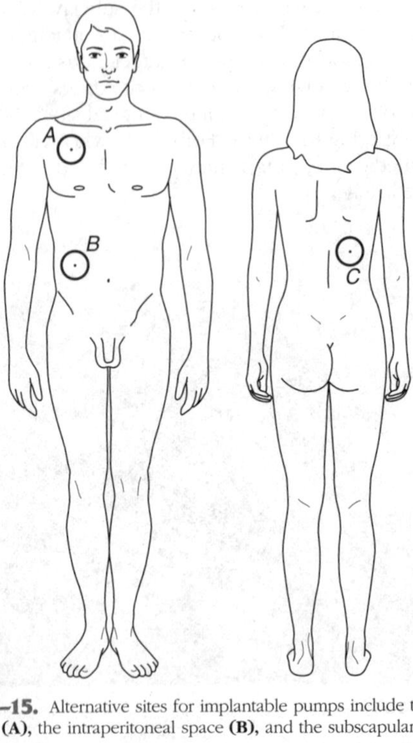


**FIGURE 5–15.** Alternative sites for implantable pumps include the subclavicular area **(A),** the intraperitoneal space **(B),** and the subscapular area **(C).**

## Infusaid

The Infusaid 400 pump measures 87 mm in diameter and 28 mm high. The Infusaid 400 has a 50-mL reservoir for medication. Other models have reservoir sizes between 22 mL and 50 mL and can deliver between 1 and 6 mL daily. After insertion, the physician gives the client an identification card that includes the model number and serial number of the client's pump. It is important for the client to keep this information in a convenient place so that his or her health care providers know what size medication reservoir the client's pump has.

The pump consists of two chambers (Fig. 5–16), one below the other, separated by a flexible metal bellows. The upper chamber is the medication chamber. The lower chamber contains the power source, which is Freon. When the medication chamber is filled, it exerts pressure on the Freon chamber, causing the Freon, which is in a gaseous state, to condense to a liquid state. As the Freon reaches body temperature, it returns to a gaseous state, causing it to expand. As it expands, the Freon chamber places pressure on the medication chamber, causing the drug to flow through an outlet filter and flow restrictor into the catheter for ultimate delivery to the client. The nurse or physician can administer boluses via a side port.

The rate of delivery is affected by altitude, the client's body temperature and blood pressure, and the concentration and viscosity of the medication. It is important that the nurse

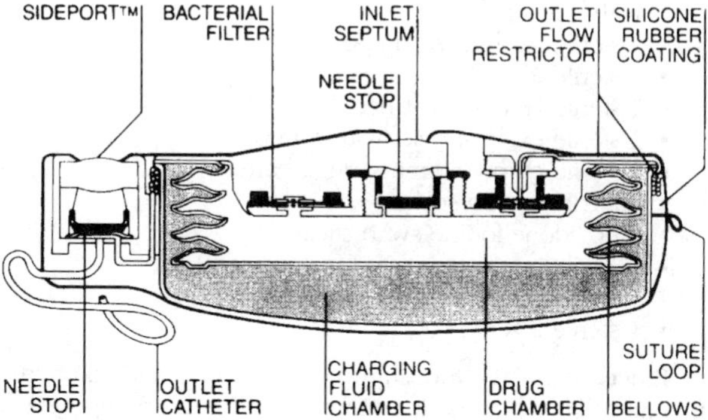


**FIGURE 5–16.** Cross section of the Infusaid implantable pump. (Courtesy of Shiley Infusaid, Norwood, Massachusetts.)

instruct the client carefully on discharge. The most important features of these instructions include the following:

1. Preventing any physical trauma to the pump insertion site
2. Abstaining from long hot baths, immersions in hot tubs, or sitting in saunas (Each of these activities may increase the client's body temperature and consequently increase the rate of medication infusion.)
3. Paying careful attention to any febrile episodes they experience
4. Discussing with the physician any proposed air travel, change in residence to an area with a significantly different altitude, or deep sea or scuba diving.
5. Reporting to the physician any side effects or complications related to either the drug or the pump
6. Keeping appointments with the physician or nurse for pump refilling

By knowing the pump model number and consequently the inherent pump infusion rate, the physician can plan for the appopriate rate of infusion by adjusting the concentration of the medication. If the client's medication rate must be changed, the concentration of the medication must be adjusted. The physician or nurse removes the "old" medication from the pump and refills the pump with medication in the "new" concentration.

## REFILLING THE PUMP

**Gathering the Supplies.** The following supplies are necessary to refill the Infusaid pump:

- 1 50 cc syringe of medication (depending on the size of the medication reservoir) in the appropriate concentration. (If the medication has been refrigerated, warm it to between room temperature and body temperature with a heating pad.)
- 1 sterile fenestrated drape
- 1 sterile towel
- 1 sterile Huber-point needle
- 1 sterile extension set with clamp
- 1 sterile empty 50-mL syringe barrel
- 3 alcohol swab sticks
- 3 povidone-iodine swab sticks
- 1 sterile pump template (as necessary)
- 1 pair sterile gloves
- 1 sterile 2 × 2

**Procedure.** The procedure consists of preparation, draining, and filling phases. It is important that the pump never be drained by aspirating, since the negative pressure would pull blood into the catheter, which may clot, possibly rendering the pump unusable.

*Preparation*

1. With the client lying flat, identify the outer edges of the pump by palpation.
2. Wash your hands and open the sterile towel, placing it on a clear surface.
3. Using sterile technique, place the opened sterile items on the sterile towel.
4. Apply the sterile gloves. Using the alcohol swabs, one at a time, cleanse the skin over the pump site in a circular motion working from the center out to the perimeter. Perform this same action with each alcohol swab.
5. Repeat this action with each of the three povidone-iodine swabs. Allow to dry.
6. Place the fenestrated drape over the pump site. Align the sterile template over the pump site as necessary.
7. Attach the Huber-point needle to one end of the extension set and the empty syringe barrel to the other.
8. Close the clamp and insert the needle into the pump's center septum perpendicular to the client's skin.

*Draining*

9. Open the clamp and allow the pump to completely drain (Fig. 5–17).
10. When the system stops draining, close the clamp and read the amount of fluid in the syringe barrel. Carefully remove the syringe barrel from the extension set. Record the volume returned, adding 1 mL to the volume to account for the amount of drug in the extension set.

*Filling*

11. Purge any air in the medication syringe and attach it to the extension set.
12. Open the clamp on the extension set and, using both hands, slowly inject 5 mL of drug solution into the pump. To assess proper needle placement, release the pressure and allow the fluid to back into the syringe. Continue to inject the drug into the pump in 5-mL increments until the entire volume has been injected.
13. While maintaining pressure on the syringe plunger, close the clamp on the extension tubing.
14. Remove the needle and apply pressure to the site with the sterile 2 × 2.

NOTE: If no fluid returns into the syringe barrel when the center septum is accessed, the possibility exists that the needle may be blocked, the pump is empty of all infusate, or the

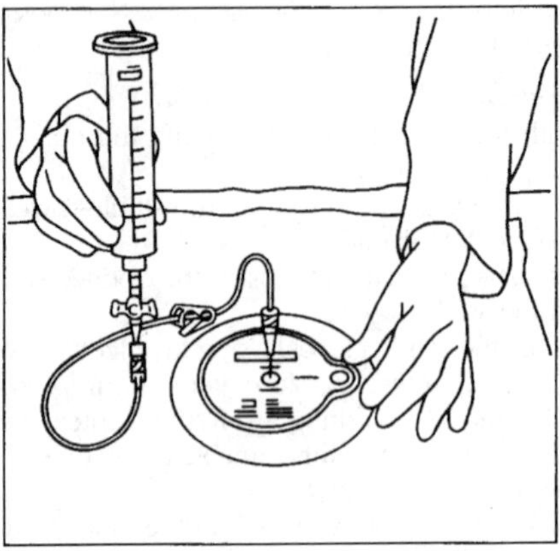

**FIGURE 5–17.** The nurse opens the clamp and allows remaining medication to empty into the syringe. (Courtesy of Pfizer Infusaid, Norwood, Massachusetts.)

septum may not have been penetrated. Disconnect the extension set and 50-cc syringe barrel, leaving the needle in place. Attach a 10-cc syringe filled with normal saline solution (NSS) to the extension set. Prime the extension set and reattach it to the needle. Slowly inject 5 mL of NSS into the pump. Release the pressure and observe for any fluid to return into the syringe. If no fluid returns, attempt to reinsert the needle into the pump. If repeated attempts fail, notify the physician of a possible pump failure.

## ADMINISTERING A BOLUS DOSE

**Gathering the Supplies.**

The following supplies are necessary to administer a bolus dose through the Infusaid pump:

- 1 medication syringe filled with the bolus medication at room temperature (limit the syringe to 3 to 5 mL)
- 1 sterile fenestrated drape
- 1 sterile towel
- 1 sterile Huber-point needle
- 1 sterile extension set with clamp
- 2 sterile 5-cc syringes filled with bacteriostatic water for flushing
- 3 alcohol swab sticks
- 3 povidone-iodine swab sticks
- 1 sterile pump template (as necessary)
- 1 pair sterile gloves
- 1 sterile 2 × 2

Procedure

*Preparation*

1. With the client lying flat, identify the outer edges of the pump by palpation.
2. Wash your hands and open the sterile towel, placing it on a clear surface.
3. Using sterile technique, place the opened sterile items on the sterile towel.
4. Apply the sterile gloves. Using the alcohol swabs, one at a time, cleanse the skin over the pump and the side port septum working in a circular motion from over the port to the periphery. Perform this same action with each alcohol swab.
5. Repeat this action with each of the three povidone-iodine swabs. Allow to dry.
6. Place the fenestrated drape over the pump site. Align the sterile template over the pump site as necessary.
7. Attach the Huber-point needle to one end of the extension set and a 5-cc bacteriostatic water-filled syringe to the other. Prime the extension set and close the clamp.
8. Insert the needle into the side port septum perpendicular to the client's skin.

*Injection*

9. Inject the rest of the bacteriostatic water to flush the catheter. Close the clamp and discard this 5-cc syringe.
10. Attach the medication syringe to the extension set. Open the clamp and slowly inject the medication at a rate not to exceed 10 mL/min. (Faster administration may damage the pump.) Close the clamp.
11. Remove the medication syringe from the extension set.
12. Attach the second bacteriostatic water syringe to the extension set. Open the clamp and flush the catheter. Close the clamp.
13. Remove the needle from the side port septum and apply pressure with the sterile 2 × 2.
14. Carefully record the procedure, including the drug, dose, and client's tolerance.

## SynchroMed Infusion System

The Medtronic SynchroMed infusion system consists of a pump, which measures about 70 mm in diameter and 28 mm in height (Fig. 5–18), a 20-mL reservoir, a catheter, a motor, a microprocessor, a radio receiver, and a lithium battery.

Sites of placement are the same as those appropriate for the Infusaid, and the client may receive chemotherapy or opioids via this pump as well. Depending on the rate and type of infusion, the pump battery lasts between 3 and 4 years before replacement is necessary. The pump has several warning tones that alert the client to the need to seek physician assistance. The soft high-pitched beeps occur several

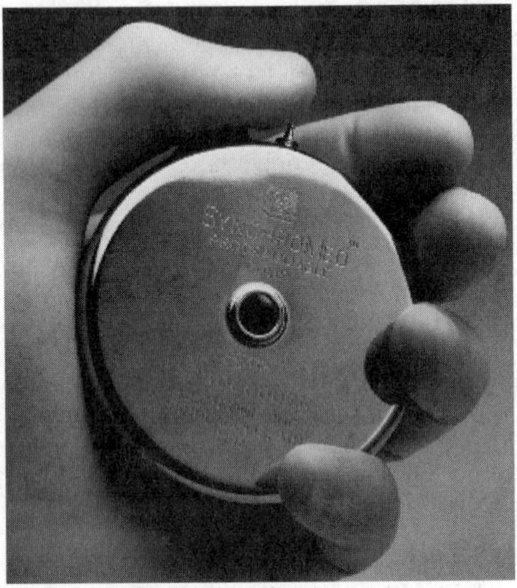

*A*

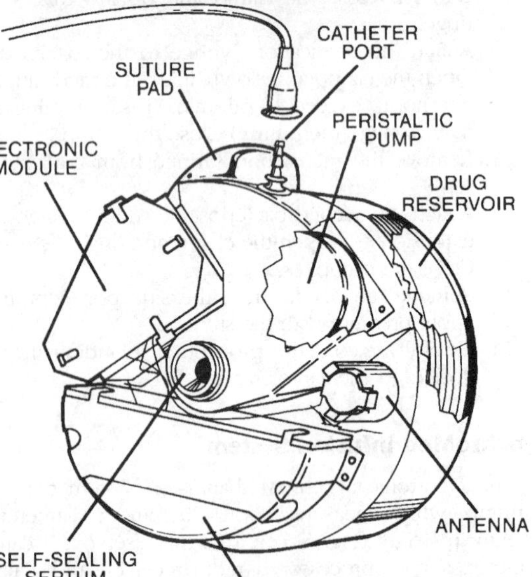


*B*

**FIGURE 5–18.** The SynchroMed infusion pump. (Courtesy of Medtronic, Minneapolic, Minnesota.)

times per minutes and indicate what is wrong. The warning tones may mean that the pump needs to be refilled, the battery should be checked, or the pump is not delivering the medication.

The SynchroMed pump requires an external component—the programmer (Fig. 5–19)—consisting of a computer, programming wand, and a printer. With the programmer, the clinician can noninvasively interrogate and program the SynchroMed pump in any increments from micrograms to millimoles. Infusion rates between 0.004 mL/h to 0.9 mL/h are possible. Possible infusion profiles include continuous hourly infusion, repeated bolus infusion with a specified delay, multistep dosing over programmed intervals, or single bolus infusions. The clinician can obtain a print out of all program information, which can be included in the client's medical record.

## ELASTOMERIC PUMPS

Mostly used in home care, elastomeric pumps are very useful for the administration of drugs prescribed for intermittent or very slow continuous administration (Fig. 5–20). The elastomeric system works by filling a ballonlike reservoir with the medication through a flow restrictor. The inherent rate and volume of the pump is a factor of the individual pump design. The Homepump Disposable Administration System is one of the more popular systems. These systems are manufactured with fill volumes between 50 mL and 375

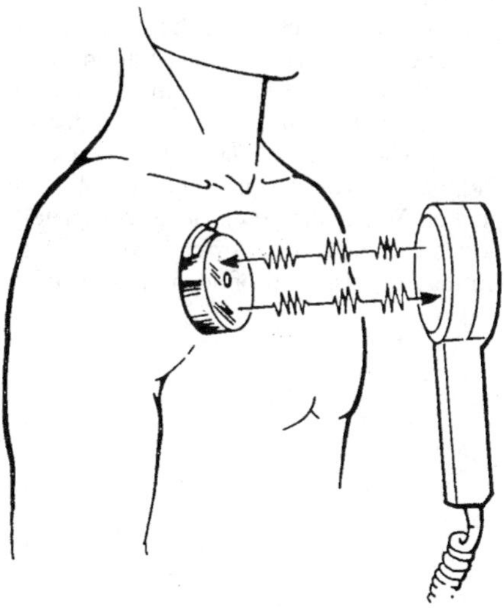

**FIGURE 5–19.** The programming head is used to program the client's infusion pump. (Courtesy of Medtronic, Minneapolis, Minnestoa.)

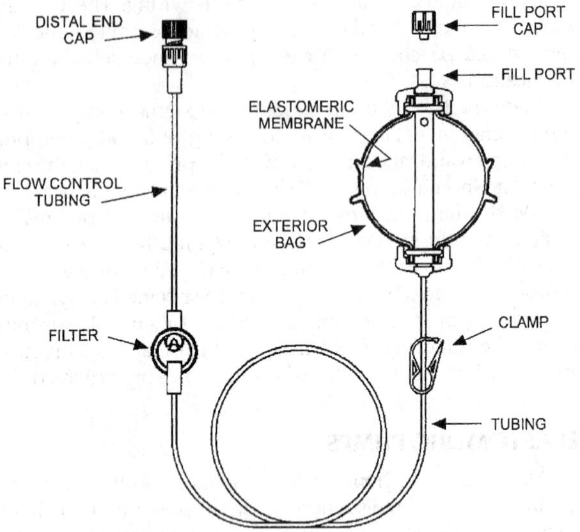


**FIGURE 5–20.** The Homepump Eclipse elastomeric pump. (Courtesy of Block Medical, Carlsbad, California.)

mL and rates between 2 and 200 mL/h. The accuracy of the system depend on the viscosity and temperature of the medicaiton. It is important that the solution be at room temperature for administration.

The system comes with an attached administration and a 0.22-$\mu$m in-line filter. The administration set tubing is clamped to maintain the pressure in the reservoir. When it is time to administer the drug, the clamp is opened and the tubing primed. The pump is attached to the client's infusion device, and the reservoir is small enough to be placed in the client's pocket. When the reservoir is completely deflated, the infusion is complete. The device is removed, and the entire system may be disposed of according to policy.

PART

# II

# TYPES OF INFUSION THERAPY

CHAPTER 6

# Peripheral Intravenous Therapy

*Marilyn Ferreri Booker*



## DESCRIPTION

The most common method of gaining access to the venous system is via the peripheral veins. Peripheral intravenous (IV) therapy involves the percutaneous insertion of a needle or flexible catheter into a peripheral vein. This differs from central venous therapy in that the tip of the catheter does not enter the superior vena cava.

Under most circumstances the peripheral veins provide the quickest and easiest approach to establishing a route for administering IV solutions and medications. These solutions or medications may be administered for therapeutic or diagnostic purposes. Replacement of fluid, electrolyte, and nutrient losses; administration of antiinfectives; blood and blood product transfusions; and medication administration can be infused via the peripheral vasculature. Diagnostic enhancing agents are also frequently administered via peripheral IV sites.

## SITE SELECTION

### Client Considerations

Assessment of the client's history and diagnosis, vein condition (including size and location), and type and duration of therapy are all important issues to consider. Client preference, whenever possible, also plays a role in determining the site for an IV.

#### HISTORY

The nurse considers a number of issues regarding the client when selecting an IV site. The nurse avoids using the side in which the client has had a mastectomy, or any type of axillary lymphatic dissection, because circulation in this arm is likely to be impaired. Cellulitis, lymphedema, or other compromising conditions also necessitate the use of the opposite limb. These conditions also impair circulation to and away from the area and leave the client at risk for local infection, which may easily become systemic. The arm of a dialysis client with an arteriovenous shunt or fistula should be avoided. Any insult to this area either mechanical or bacterial could render the shunt or fistula unusable.

#### CLIENT POSITIONING

The type of surgery scheduled may affect which arm should be used for the IV. Certain procedures require the client to be placed in a side-lying position. In these cases the nurse avoids using the arm that will be in the dependent position on the procedure table.

#### ACTIVITY

Consideration must be given to the client's activity level. A client who goes to physical therapy for instruction in the use of a walker will have difficulty performing the therapy with an IV in the hand. Both the physical therapy and the infusion will be more successful with an IV site above the wrist. Whenever possible, the nurse places the IV in the client's nondominant limb. This makes it easier for the client to maintain independence and participate in activities of daily living.

### Vein Considerations

The veins considered the most appropriate for peripheral IV therapy are the metacarpal, cephalic, basilic, and median veins, as well as their branches (Fig. 6–1).

Unless there are extenuating circumstances, such as trauma to the arms, the Centers for Disease Control (CDC) advise that only veins located in the upper extremities be

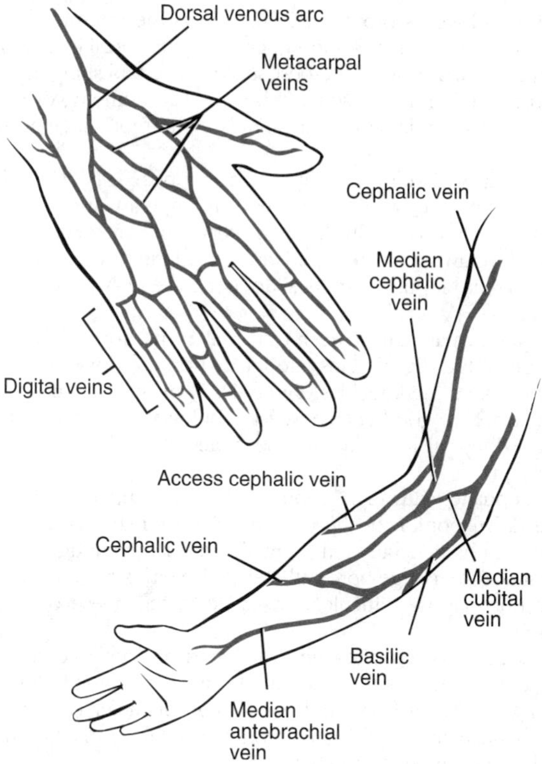


**FIGURE 6–1.** Peripheral veins appropriate for intravenous (IV) therapy in the older child and the adult.

used in adults. Use of veins in the lower extremities places the client at risk for thrombophlebitis and potential pulmonary embolism.

The nurse may be tempted to select the largest or the most superficial or visible veins for IV insertion. However, these may not be the most appropriate choice. The large veins, located in the antecubital space, although easy to encannulate, are best left for intermittent blood drawing. This is an area of flexion that could lead to the cannula's becoming dislodged, causing an infiltration, and the continual movement of the catheter in the vein can lead to a mechanical phlebitis. Immobilizing the joint for a lengthy infusion is uncomfortable for the client.

## CONDITION, SIZE, AND LOCATION

A systematic approach is best when determining a site for the client's IV. The nurse starts by assessing the most distal veins and works proximally. This allows the more proximal veins to be used for subsequent IV starts. Resilient, long, straight veins provide the best success in establishing access and providing the prescribed therapy. Hard, knotty, or sclerotic veins are difficult to encannulate and more likely to infiltrate.

When palpating a vein for a proposed IV site, the nurse must be sure that a vein and not an artery is selected. Arteries usually have thicker walls, are deeper, the blood return is more rapid and a brighter red, and the vessel has a pulse. Arteries do not have valves, whereas veins do.

**Metacarpal Veins.** The metacarpal veins, formed by the union of the digital veins, are located on the dorsum of the hand above the knuckles (Fig. 6–1). In most cases these are considered a good choice in establishing venous access because they dilate easily and the bones of the hand provide support.

**Cephalic Veins.** The cephalic vein runs up the arm on the radial portion of the dorsum of the forearm (Fig. 6–1). This vein is generally long, straight, and large enough to accommodate a large-bore catheter. This vein is readily palpable but may be difficult to visualize in the obese or hairy client.

**Accessory Cephalic Vein.** The accessory cephalic vein is the continuation of the metacarpal veins of the thumb. It runs along the radial bone and has a large diameter (Fig. 6–1). Clients usually find this a comfortable site for an IV because it does not impede mobility.

**Basilic Vein.** The basilic vein can be found on the dorsum of the forearm on the ulnar side (Fig. 6–1). This large vein travels toward the anterior of the arm just below the elbow. Because of its unobtrusive location, this vessel is often forgotten. To observe this vein the nurse asks the client to flex the elbow and bend the arm. The infusion nurse who is ready to declare that the client has no further peripheral access is likely to be pleasantly surprised at the size and condition of this vein.

**Median Antebrachial Vein.** The median antebrachial vein is located along the ulnar side of the forearm (Fig. 6–1). This vein may be smaller than other veins in the area. Clients may find this a painful site for an IV to be started, as there are numerous nerve endings in the area.

**Median Brachial and Median Cephalic Veins.** The median brachial and median cephalic veins are located in the antecubital fossa (Fig. 6–1). These large veins are not appropriate for infusions with short peripheral catheters, except as a last resort or in an emergent situation because the elbow must be immobilized, leading to discomfort for the client.

## Type and Duration of Therapy

### TYPE OF THERAPY

When selecting a site, the nurse must be aware of the type of infusion to be administered and the length of the therapy. Consideration is given to the rate at which the infusion is to be administered and the nature of the infusate (solution). For example, infusions such as packed cells require a large vein because of blood's high viscosity. Solutions or drugs with high osmolarity or very high or very low pH can be harsh and cause vein irritation. Because the larger veins have a higher volume of blood circulating through them, the solution becomes more dilute. This helps decrease the harmful effects of these agents on the vein. Rapid infusions of large volumes of fluid require the selection of a large vein. This is particularly important if the solution is administered under positive pressure such as with an infusion pump.

### DURATION OF THERAPY

The duration of therapy also influences the selection of an IV site. A one-time dose of IV push furosemide (Lasix, ✦Uritrol) can be given in any vein, but a continuous infusion of peripheral parenteral nutrition (PPN) requires a larger vessel to avoid complications.

# DEVICE SELECTION

## Considerations

The nurse considers the age and condition of the patient; the size, location, and condition of the available veins; and the type and duration of the infusion. The shortest, smallest gauge device that accommodates the vein, type of infusion, and duration of therapy is the nurse's best choice when selecting infusion catheters. Gauge refers to the internal and external diameter of the catheter. The larger the number, the smaller the catheter diameter.

As with most areas of health care, technology is moving so rapidly that new and updated brands of peripheral access devices are entering the market almost daily. Some are made of new materials marketed as increasingly more biocompatible or new coatings for catheters designed to provide easier insertion. Despite all the new materials, peripheral venous access devices fall into three categories: winged IV sets, or butterflies; over-the-needle catheters; and midline catheters.

## Winged IV Sets

Commonly known as a butterfly, winged IV sets come in two types: the winged metal needle and an over-the-needle flexible catheter (Figs. 6–2 and 6–3). Some practitioners consider these devices the easiest to insert. Both of these catheters have butterfly-type wings, which the practitioner grasps when inserting the device. When the insertion is completed, the wings lie flat against the skin and provide an excellent area for taping. Winged IV sets have small-bore flexible tubing between the wings and the end piece. This tubing comes in varying lengths up to 12 inches (30.5 cm). Some of these sets come with latex injection caps at the end, whereas others may have a female plastic adaptor or hub to attach an IV tubing, a syringe, or an injection cap. The wings and the plastic hub of the butterfly IV sets are color coded. This color coding indicates the size of the catheter gauge so that the nurse knows the size of the device without looking at the client record. Unfortunately, the industry is not consistent with this "coding" and a change in manufacturer probably means a different color coding system.

## WINGED METAL NEEDLE

The winged metal needle was the first device designed for infusion therapy. Made of a biologically inert metal such as stainless steel, the needle is sharp and coated with silicone for ease of insertion. The coating also decreases clot formation. Although metal catheters have a lower infection rate than catheters made of other materials, their lack of flexibility in the vein makes them prone to dislodge, causing infiltration. For this reason the Intravenous Nurses Society (INS)

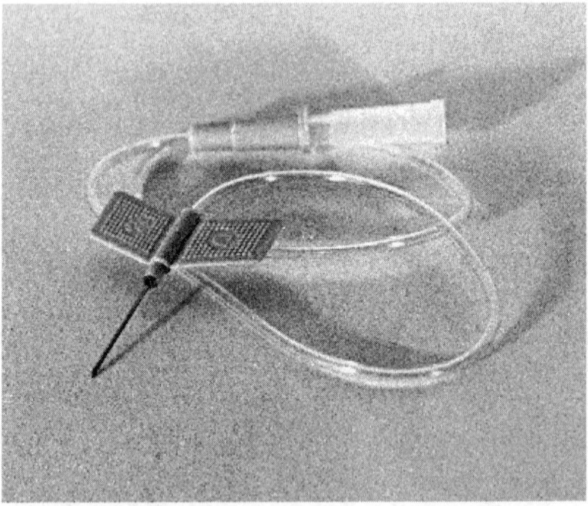

**FIGURE 6–2.** Winged metal butterfly needle. (Photograph courtesy of Monica Ridgely.)

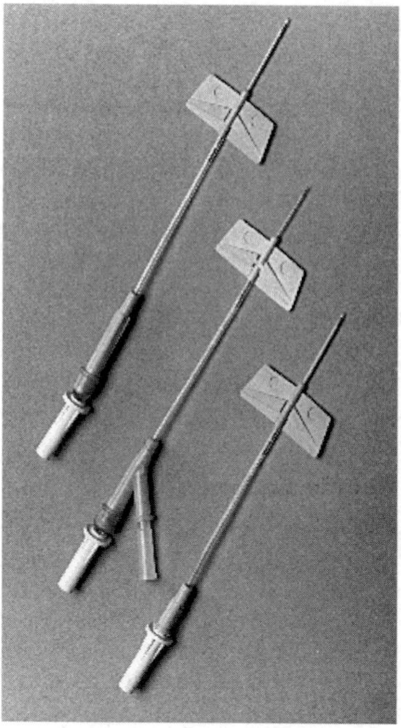

**FIGURE 6–3.** Over-the-needle flexible catheter butterfly. (Courtesy of Becton Dickinson Vascular Access, Sandy, Utah.)

suggests that use of these devices be limited to short-term or single-dose administrations such as a bolus of fluid or an IV push medication. These devices are about ¾ inch (2 cm) long and come in gauge sizes from 27G to 16G (Fig. 6–2).

## WINGED OVER-THE-NEEDLE CATHETER

The winged over-the-needle flexible catheter is a new variation of the metal butterfly. This catheter has a sharp needle that sits inside a flexible ¾- to 1-inch (2 to 2.5 cm) catheter made of a silicone-coated plastic. They are available in gauges ranging from 24G to 16G. The proximal end of the needle becomes a fine, very flexible metal stylet that runs the length of the attached tubing. At the hub is a hard plastic piece the nurse uses to pull the needle from the catheter after access has been established. The flexible plastic catheter remains in the vein. This catheter is radiopaque for radio-graphic visualization. These catheters may come with a latex injection cap attached or the nurse may add one if desired. Some of these catheters have a Y at the end. One arm of the Y has a latex injection cap used for intermittent piggyback infusions, whereas the other has a plastic adapter used for the client's continuous infusion. These catheters should be changed every 48 to 72 hours to avoid complications (Fig. 6–3).

### USES

Most solutions can be infused through winged IV sets as long as the gauge and the vein can accommodate the type and rate of the infusion. However, winged metal infusion sets should be limited to short-term infusions because of the potential for infiltration. Winged metal infusion sets are an excellent choice for drawing blood or administering one dose of an IV push medication. Because of cost considerations the winged metal set is the choice over the flexible over-the-needle winged set for these short procedures.

## Over-the-Needle Catheters

As with the winged infusion sets, there are many variations of the over-the-needle catheter. They differ in appearance and function. Over-the-needle catheters may be single or double lumen, have plastic or metal hubs, and be made of a number of different materials such as plastic or polyurethane. Some have small wings on either side of the hub with suture holes (Fig. 6–4).

A standard catheter is between ¾ and 3 inches (2 to 7.5 cm) long and ranges in gauge size from 14G to 26G. The longer, larger gauge sizes are generally used in the operating room or other critical care area where it may be necessary to administer large volumes of blood or other fluids very

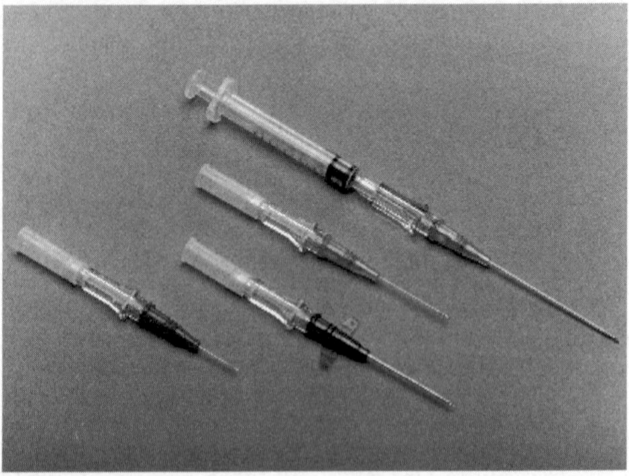

**FIGURE 6–4.** Over-the-needle catheter. (Courtesy of Becton Dickinson Vascular Access, Sandy, Utah.)

rapidly. The usual adult in the short-term care setting needs a catheter between 3/4 and 1 inch (2 to 2.5 cm) in length with a gauge size of about 22G or 20G. The nurse remembers that the shortest, smallest catheter that accommodates the vein and the infusion is best for the client.

The over-the-needle catheter consists of a needle inside the plastic catheter. The needle is removed after the venipuncture has been made and the plastic catheter remains inside the vessel. The female hub accommodates either IV tubing or an injection cap.

One of the newer over-the-needle catheters is made of an elastomeric polymer called Aquavene. This material expands when it becomes immersed in liquid. Within 1 hour after insertion the cannula of a 3/4-inch (2-cm) device, bathed in plasma, expands two gauge sizes and about 1/4 inch (0.5 cm) in length. Therefore, a 24G 3/4-inch (2-cm) catheter becomes a 22G 1-inch (2.5-cm) catheter. Because of the smaller size, clients report a less painful insertion, but the therapy benefits from the larger, longer cannula (Fig. 6–5).

## USES

Over-the-needle catheters can be used to infuse IV fluids, transfusions, and drugs. The nurse chooses the correct gauge and length to accommodate the client's age and the type and duration of therapy. Table 6–1 outlines the common gauge sizes of catheters and their uses and disadvantages.

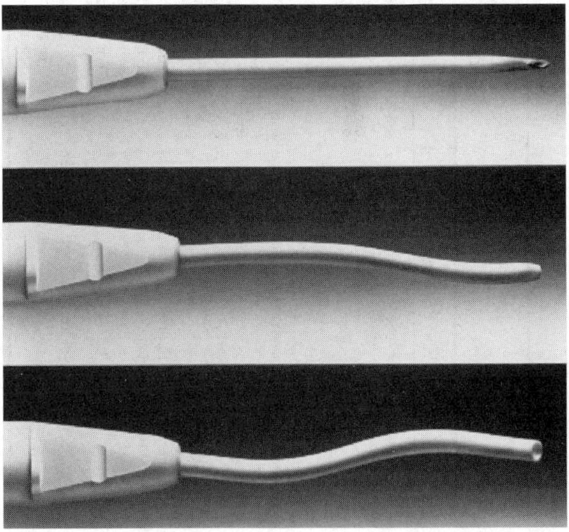

**FIGURE 6–5.** Streamline over-the-needle catheter. (Courtesy of Menlo Care, Menlo Park, California.)

**TABLE 6–1**
**Common Gauge Sizes of Catheters**

| Gauge | Client Considerations | Uses | Disadvantages |
|---|---|---|---|
| 16 | Adults | Major surgery and trauma<br>May give large volumes of fluid rapidly | Insertion painful<br>Large vein required |
| 18 | Adolescents and adults | Surgery<br>May give blood products and high-viscosity drugs | Insertion painful<br>Large vein required |
| 20 | Large children, adolescents, adults, and the elderly | Any setting<br>For the administration of fluids, blood, and drugs | Flow rate is slower than a larger gauge device |
| 22 | Toddlers, children, adolescents, adults, and the elderly | Any setting<br>For the administration of fluids, blood, and drugs | Flow rate is slower than a larger gauge device |
| 24 | Neonate, infants, children, adolescents, adults, and the elderly | Any setting<br>For small digital or metacarpal veins in adults<br>For scalp veins of infants<br>For the administration of fluids, blood, and drugs | Will not accommodate blood administration well<br>May be difficult to insert in adult with thick skin<br>Slow flow rates |
| 26 | Neonate, infants, children, and the frail elderly | Any setting<br>For scalp veins of infant and neonates<br>For the administration of fluids, blood, and drugs | Very slow flow rates |

## Midline Catheters

In recent years a new term, *midline catheters,* has been coined to describe a catheter that is longer than the traditional peripheral line but shorter than a central line. Midline catheters are usually placed in one of the large veins of the upper arm: the basilic or cephalic. There are two different types of midline catheters: an over-the-needle winged set and a through-the-needle catheter.

### OVER-THE-NEEDLE WINGED SET

The over-the-needle winged set is made of Aquavene, an elastomeric polymer (Fig. 6–6). This device is a 6-inch (15-cm) catheter, which, when hydrated, expands two gauge sizes and up to 1 inch (2.5 cm) in length. The catheter is encased in a plastic sheath to maintain sterility during insertion. After the vein is encannulated with the needle, the needle is withdrawn through the catheter into a plastic casing that is removed and discarded after the insertion is completed. The catheter is advanced by pulling up on a tab proximal to the butterfly wings. This unique system allows for a completely bloodless procedure (Fig. 6–7).

### THROUGH-THE-NEEDLE CATHETERS

Through-the-needle catheters may either have a breakaway needle or a plastic peel-away sheath to encase the nee-

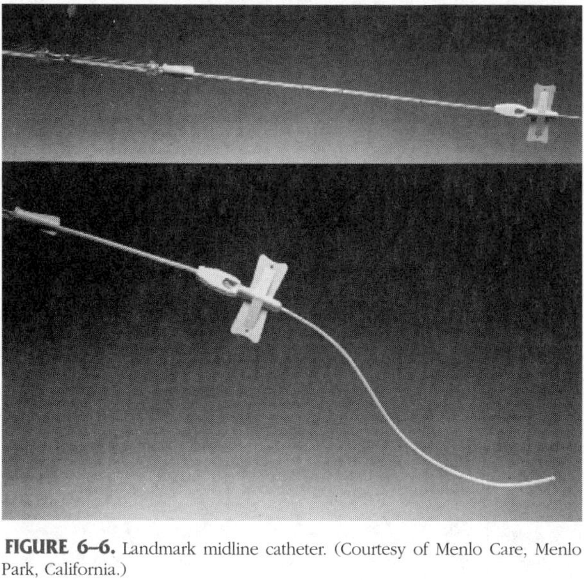

**FIGURE 6–6.** Landmark midline catheter. (Courtesy of Menlo Care, Menlo Park, California.)

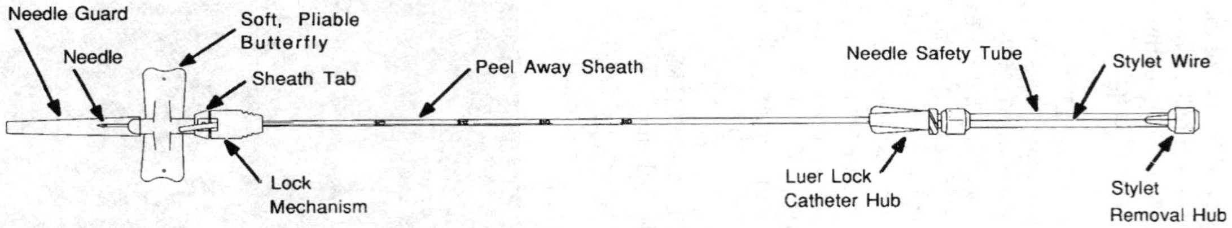


**FIGURE 6–7.** The nurse gently pulls up on the sheath tab proximal to the wings. (Courtesy of Menlo Care, Menlo Park, California.)

1 **INSERTION**

Squeeze butterfly wings upright.
(Pebble side against fingers)
Perform venipuncture.
Check for flashback.
Advance to butterfly hub.

2 **REMOVAL OF STYLET**

Release butterfly wings and hold flat.
Release tourniquet.
While holding needle safety tube, withdraw stylet fully until needle tip is enclosed in safety tube.

3 **ADVANCEMENT**

Hold butterfly wings flat.

Pull sheath tab slowly forward to advance catheter to desired initial length.

4 **REMOVAL OF SHEATH**

Continue to hold butterfly wings.

Lock catheter in place by firmly pulling back on remaining extension tubing.
Cut sheath.

5 **COMPLETION**

Remove needle safety tube and attach IV tubing or heparin lock to luer lock.
Secure and dress site per institution policy.
Immobilize arm for 30 minutes.

**FIGURE 6–7.** *Continued*

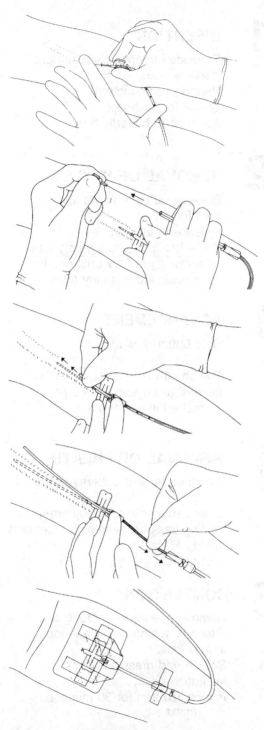

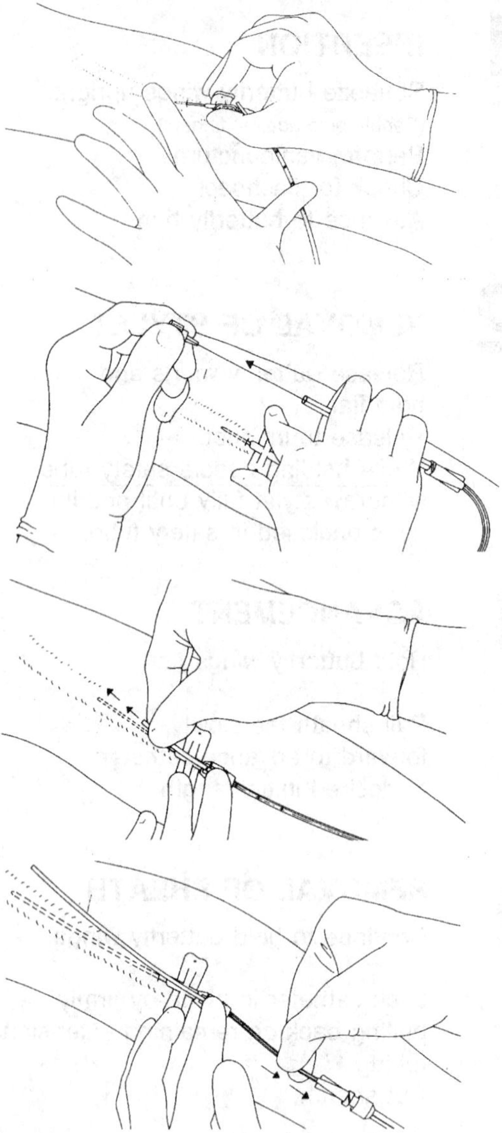

**FIGURE 6–7.** *Continued*

dle after the catheter is advanced through it. The INS believes there is a risk of puncturing and shearing the catheter during insertion, and therefore these catheters are not recommended for routine peripheral venous access. However, they, like the over-the-needle midline catheter, have a place in long-term peripheral IV therapy (Fig. 6–8).

Through-the-needle catheters come in varying lengths from 8 to 22 inches (20.5 to 56 cm). They are usually inserted into the cephalic or basilic veins. After measuring the client's arm the nurse chooses a catheter of the appropriate length. The catheter has measurements along its length to indicate how much of the catheter has been inserted. The entire catheter is not always threaded into the vein if the catheter is longer than desired. A portion of the distal end may be left outside and affixed to the skin. The INS recommends this method rather than altering the tip by cutting it.

One of the problems of a through-the-needle catheter is that the needle used to access the vein is usually much larger than the catheter itself. After the catheter is threaded and the needle removed or broken away, there is frequently leaking around the site because the hole made by the needle is larger than the catheter can accommodate. This may provide a source for bacteria to enter the client's system.

## USES

Dwell times of up to 6 weeks and longer have been documented with midline catheters. For this reason they are appropriate for longer term therapy such as seen in the treatment of endocarditis with IV antibiotics. This catheter is appropriate for IV fluids, drugs, and transfusions. Because of their length, these catheters are not likely to become dislodged. They are particularly ideal for infusing caustic drugs because of the large vessels in which they are placed.

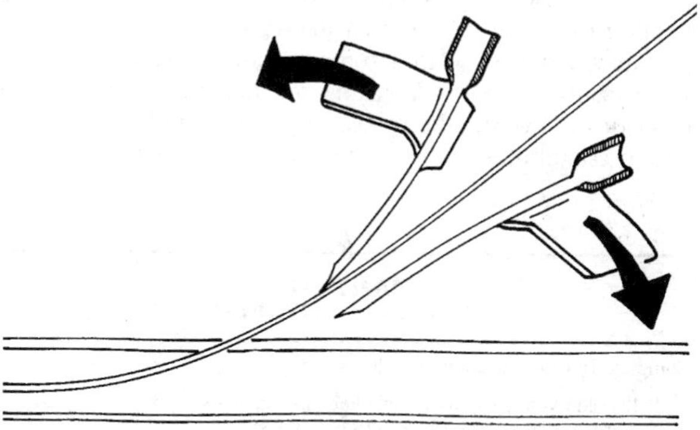

**FIGURE 6–8.** Peel-away sheath introducer of a through-the-needle catheter. (Courtesy of Gesco International, San Antonio, Texas.)

## INSERTION TECHNIQUE

There is a series of steps associated with the insertion of an IV access device. The nurse prepares the client, gathers and prepares the appropriate supplies, performs the IV insertion, and documents the procedure in the client's medical record.

### Client Preparation

After checking the client's chart for allergies and the IV orders, the nurse prepares the client for the IV insertion (Table 6–2). Taking time to prepare the client is important to the success of the IV insertion. Some clients have not had experience with IV therapy and may be anxious or fearful. Anxiety can cause vasoconstriction, making the venipuncture more difficult for the nurse and more painful for the client. A client who knows what to expect during the procedure can assist the nurse by relaxing and cooperating.

The nurse greets the client by name and makes introductions. The nurse's confident, professional, but friendly demeanor is an important factor in making the client feel comfortable. The nurse explains the procedure in simple, easy-to-understand terms. The purpose for IV insertion and how the IV impacts on the client's movement and ability to participate in his or her care is part of the discussion. Providing time for the client to ask questions helps allay any fears. The nurse listens carefully as the client expresses any concerns.

The nurse prepares the environment for the IV insertion. It is important to provide privacy for the client during the procedure. The nurse requests that visitors step into the hall and draws the curtain around the client's bed. It is usually more convenient for the client to wear a hospital gown if a continuous IV is ordered for the hospitalized client. Any jewelry in the area of proposed IV site is removed. The nurse places the client in a comfortable position and adjusts the lighting to illuminate the area intended for the IV. It is important for the nurse to assume a comfortable position too when starting the IV. Adjusting the bed height or using a chair or the over-the-bed table to provide the best work situation contributes to the success of the IV insertion.

**TABLE 6–2**
**Anatomy of an IV Order**

Complete IV orders include the following:

1. Solution to be infused including any additives
2. Total volume or total dose to be infused
3. Rate of infusion in mL/h or mg/h

## Gathering Supplies

### CONTINUOUS INFUSION

- Keeping in mind the criteria discussed earlier in this chapter, select the appropriate infusion device.
- If the physician has ordered a continuous IV solution, arrange to obtain the bag or bottle of the IV fluid, and administration set, and an IV pole.
- Obtain a filter and a pump or controller, depending on agency policy.
- Some agencies provide IV start kits that include all the supplies the nurse needs to prepare the IV site and dress it after the insertion is completed. The IV device is not included, but a tourniquet and nonsterile gloves generally are. If the agency does not supply these kits, gather a pair of nonsterile gloves, a tourniquet, skin cleansing material, tape, sterile 2 × 2s, and a transparent dressing
- Cleanse the site. The INS states that tincture of iodine, 1% to 2% iodophor, 70% isopropyl alcohol, or chlorhexidine are appropriate skin cleansing materials. These should be in single-use size, and any remaining solution is discarded after the procedure.

### INTERMITTENT INFUSION

- If the physician's order indicates an intermittent infusion device (sometimes called a heparin or saline lock) is to be placed, the IV fluid, IV pole, and administration set are not necessary.
- An intermittent injection cap, 2- or 3-cc syringes with 22G 1-inch (2.5-cm) needles, a vial of normal saline, and a vial of whatever concentration of heparin stated in agency policy are needed.

## Preparing Supplies

### CONTINUOUS INFUSION

1. As with any IV procedure, wash your hands with soap and water. Some agencies use special antibacterial soaps for this purpose.
2. Open the administration set package, remove the administration set, and close the roller clamp. If agency policy states that a filter must be used and the administration set does not have one, add the filter now.
3. Examine the solution container, observing for any cracks, leaks, or particulate matter. Note the expiration date. If there are any questions about the integrity of the container or solution, discard it and obtain another.

4. Remove the administration set spike cover and spike the IV solution container.
5. Hang the IV container on the IV pole. If your agency uses time strips preprinted by the IV solution manufacturer, place the time strip next to the volume graduations along the length of the solution container and mark the infusion times according to the directions listed on the time strip. If preprinted time strips are not available, a piece of tape the length of the solution container will suffice. Place the tape next to the volume graduations along the length of the solution container. With a pen make a mark on the tape at the top of the solution container fluid level. Using the volume graduations on the solution container as a guide, make the next mark on the tape at the level that the fluid will be after 1 hour of infusion. (For example, if the physician's orders state that the 1 L of solution should infuse at 100 mL/h, the first tape mark will correspond to the 1000 mL graduation on the solution container. The next tape mark will correspond to the 900 mL graduation on the solution container.) Continue marking the tape at the corresponding solution container volume graduations until the last infusion level is marked. Next, mark the time that the container will be hung next to the first tape mark. Place the time corresponding to 1 hour later at the next fluid level mark. Continue marking the times in this manner until each fluid level is marked with a corresponding time that is 1 hour later than the previous volume level time. A time strip marked with corresponding infusion times allows the nurse to quickly determine if the infusion is running at the correct rate. Even infusions on controllers or pumps should be time stripped (Fig. 6–9).
6. If using a pump that allows priming the administration set while on the pump, follow the manufacturer's instructions. If using a controller or gravity, slowly open the roller clamp and prime the tubing. If the tubing has an in-line filter or one has been added, hold the filter upside down to remove all air.
7. Continue priming the tubing until all air is removed. Close the roller clamp.
8. If a pump or controller is used, perform the setup procedure now.

## INTERMITTENT INFUSION

1. As with any IV procedure, wash your hands with soap and water. Some agencies use special antibacterial soaps for this purpose.
2. Draw up 3 mL of saline into one of the 3-cc syringes and carefully recap the needle.

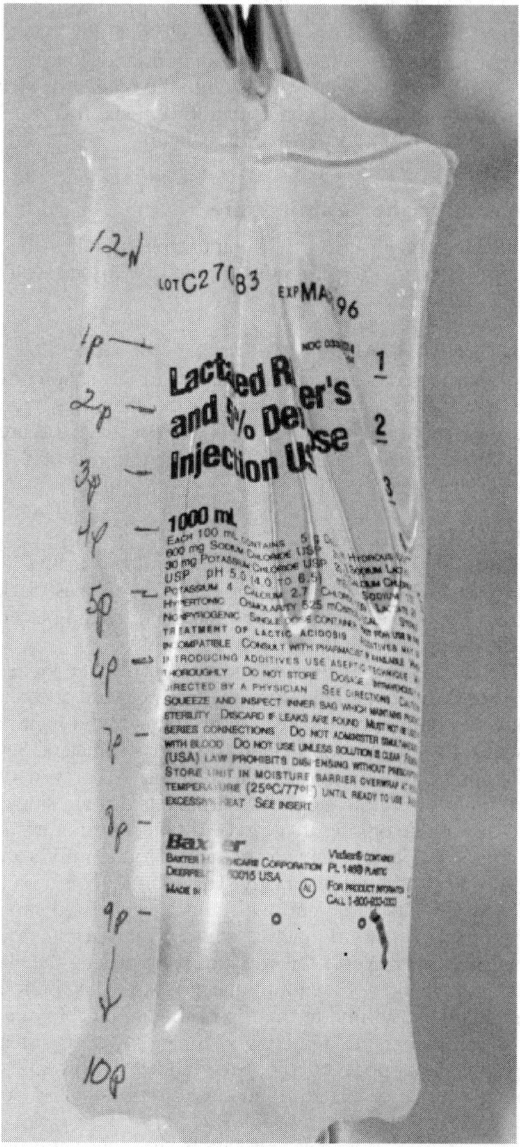


**FIGURE 6–9.** All large-volume parenteral (LVP) containers should be time stripped, even if they are running on an infusion control device. (Photograph courtesy of Monica Ridgely.)

3. Open the injection cap package and place it near the work site. Take care not to contaminate the male end of the injection cap if it is not equipped with a cap.
4. If the agency uses heparin as the final flush to maintain patency, draw up the amount and concentration stated in the agency policy into the other 3-cc syringe. The amount and concentration of heparin is usually 1 to 3 mL of 10 to 100 U/mL heparin.

## Performing the Venipuncture

Performing a successful venipuncture requires that the nurse selects an area, distends the vein, and inserts a cannula inside the vein.

### SELECTING THE AREA

Using the criteria established earlier in this chapter, select the area for the catheter insertion. If the client has hair over the area, clip the hair with scissors. Do not shave this area as any nicks or razor burn exposes the client to potential infection in this area.

### DISTENDING THE VEIN

Trapping blood in the vein engorges it and makes it easier to see and feel. This also provides for the "flashback" of blood in the IV device chamber that confirms the placement of the device during the insertion process.

To distend the vein, place a tourniquet about 6 inches (15 cm) above the intended puncture site. The tourniquet should be wide enough to prevent it from rolling into a tight band. Usually a width of about 1 inch (2.5 cm) is sufficient. Several different types of tourniquets are available. To prevent cross-contamination the INS prefers tourniquets that are single use and disposable or ones that can be disinfected after each use.

One type of disposable tourniquet is found in IV start kits or can be purchased separately. This tourniquet is a piece of latex about 1 inch (2.5 cm) wide and 15 inches (38 cm) long (Fig. 6–10). This tourniquet is "stretchy" and accommodates most limb sizes. Apply this tourniquet by placing the client's limb in the center of the tourniquet and stretching both ends, bringing them around to the top of the limb. Cross one end over the other as though tying a string. However, instead of bringing the upper end completely under the lower, leave a "tail." Removal of this tourniquet is accomplished by pulling up on the "tail."

A blood pressure cuff can also be used as a tourniquet. Although this equipment is not disposable, it can be disinfected. Apply the cuff as you would to obtain a blood pressure reading but about 6 inches (15 cm) above the intended IV site. Inflate the cuff to a pressure between the client's sys-

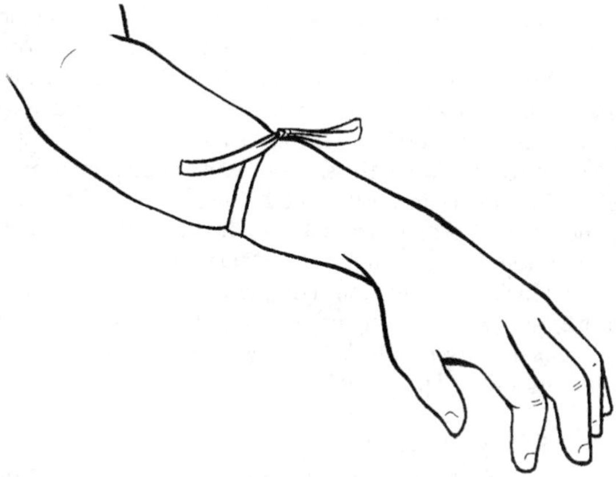

**FIGURE 6–10.** The nurse applies the tourniquet to the client's arm above the intended puncture site.

tolic and diastolic pressure. Using a blood pressure cuff as a tourniquet is ideal for clients with large arms, as the cuff will not roll. Remove the cuff by pulling up on the top flap as you normally would, but do not wait for the pressure to be released.

After applying the tourniquet, palpate the pulse distal to the tourniquet placement to ensure that arterial flow has not been interrupted. Facilitate distending the vein by asking the client to clench and unclench his or her fist a few times. A properly distended vein feels full, round, and "bouncy."

If these actions do not distend the vein satisfactorily, remove the tourniquet and request that the client place his or her arm in the dependent position for a few minutes. Replace the tourniquet on the limb before moving the arm to the original position.

Clients who are suffering from peripheral vasoconstriction such as those who are cold, hypotensive, or in shock may require further steps to obtain vein distention. In these cases, applying a warm compress to the area or rubbing the limb gently toward the tourniquet may encourage venous filling.

## PREPARING THE SKIN

Prepare the skin over the vein with the cleansing agent used in your agency by cleaning in a circular motion from the intended penetration site out about 2 inches (5 cm). Allow the cleansing agent to air dry. This provides an antibacterial barrier around the penetration site (Fig. 6–11).

## ADMINISTERING A LOCAL ANESTHETIC

Although the INS does not recommend administering a local anesthetic, some physicians order a local anesthetic for their clients during the IV device insertion. The usual choice of local anesthetic is 0.1 mL of 1% lidocaine without epinephrine. Be certain that the client is not allergic to lidocaine. Draw up the drug, using a tuberculin syringe for precise measurement. Cleanse the skin and insert the tip of the 27G needle at about a 30-degree angle just to the side of the intended puncture site. If the vein is deep, insert the needle directly over the intended puncture site. Remember that this is an intradermal and not an IV injection. Inject enough of the drug into the tissue to create a small wheal. The client may complain of a stinging feeling. Remove the needle. Gently rub the wheal with an alcohol swab to facilitate absorption. When you insert the IV device, the client should feel pressure but not pain.

## ANCHORING THE VEIN

Place the thumb on your nondominant hand approximately 1½ to 2 inches (4 to 5 cm) below the intended insertion site and pull the skin taut against the direction of the insertion. This stabilizes the vein between the skin and the tissue below and keeps it from rolling.

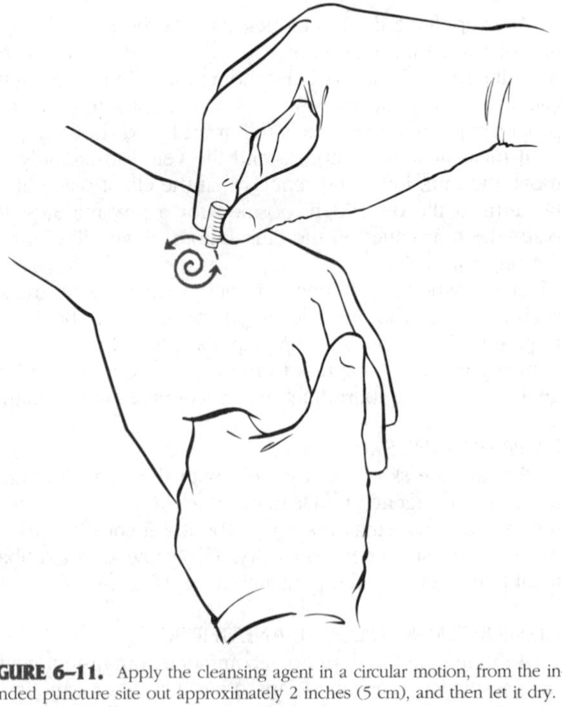

**FIGURE 6–11.** Apply the cleansing agent in a circular motion, from the intended puncture site out approximately 2 inches (5 cm), and then let it dry.

## HOLDING THE CATHETER

No matter what type, all catheters are held with the bevel up. This allows the sharpest side of the needle to puncture the skin first, making the penetration less traumatic. When using a winged IV set, grasp the wings between the thumb and first two fingers of your dominant hand and squeeze the wings together (Fig. 6–12). Over-the-needle catheters are held by the plastic end of the stylet, not the hub of the catheter (Fig. 6–13).

## INSERTING THE CATHETER

There are two methods for inserting a catheter into a vein: direct and indirect.

**Direct Method.** Hold the catheter in your dominant hand as discussed. Stabilize the vein as described. Pierce the skin over the vein at about a 30-degree angle and observe for a flashback of blood. This indicates a successful venipuncture. Immediately lower the angle of the needle to avoid puncturing the back wall of the vein. The direct method is also used for encannulating deep veins, but the insertion angle may need to be increased.

**Indirect Method.** After stabilizing the vein with your nondominant hand, hold the catheter in your dominant hand as described. Enter the skin just next to the vein at a 30-degree angle. Drop the catheter parallel to the skin and angle the catheter toward the vein, entering it from the side. This method is preferred when there is concern about injuring the back wall of small fragile veins.

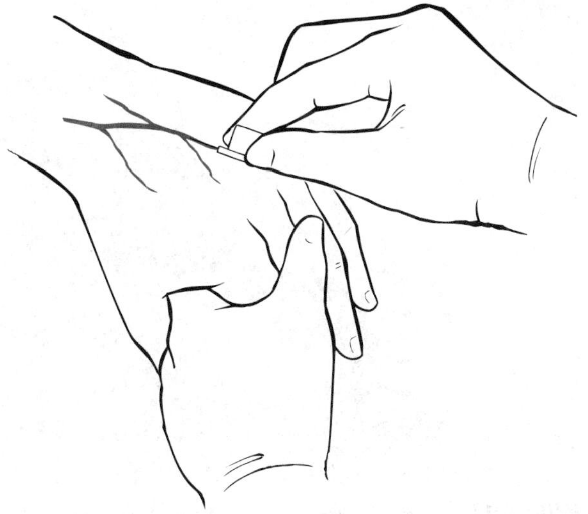

**FIGURE 6–12.** Squeeze the wings together between the thumb and forefinger.

## ADVANCING THE NEEDLE

After establishing that the needle is in the vessel, advance the catheter further into the client's vein. The technique used to do this depends on the type of device used and the vein condition.

**Winged IV Sets.** For easily visualized veins, carefully advance the catheter to the wings. Remove the tourniquet and attach the IV tubing or intermittent injection cap.

If the veins appear fragile, the catheter may be "floated" into the vein. Remove the tourniquet and attach the IV fluids or the saline syringe. Infuse the fluids or inject the saline. This expands the vessel and allows for gently advancing the catheter further into the vein. Observe the site carefully for any signs of infiltration.

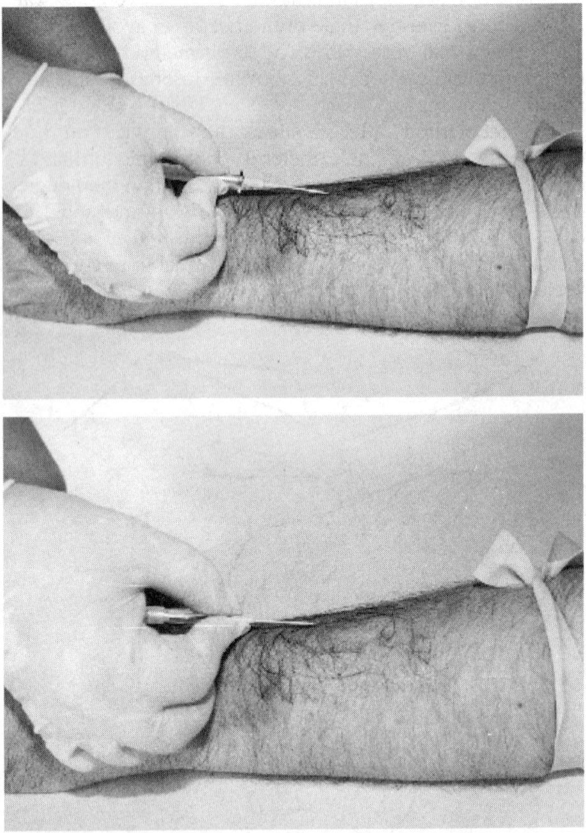

*A*

*B*

**FIGURE 6–13.** For greater control, hold the catheter by the plastic end of the stylet **(A),** not by the hub of the catheter **(B).** (Photograph courtesy of Monica Ridgely.)

If the winged IV set is the over-the-needle type, carefully remove the stylet by securing the wings with one hand, grasping the plastic end of the stylet with the other, and gently pulling it toward you until the needle is completely removed from the set.

**Over-the-Needle Catheter.** To advance the over-the-needle catheter, some nurses use the nondominant hand to push the catheter into the vein while stabilizing the stylet with the dominant hand. This avoids advancing the needle any further into the vein, possibly causing damage to the intima of the vessel (Fig. 6–14). Other nurses continue to hold the skin taut with the nondominant hand. Using the thumb and second finger to stabilize the stylet, place the forefinger against

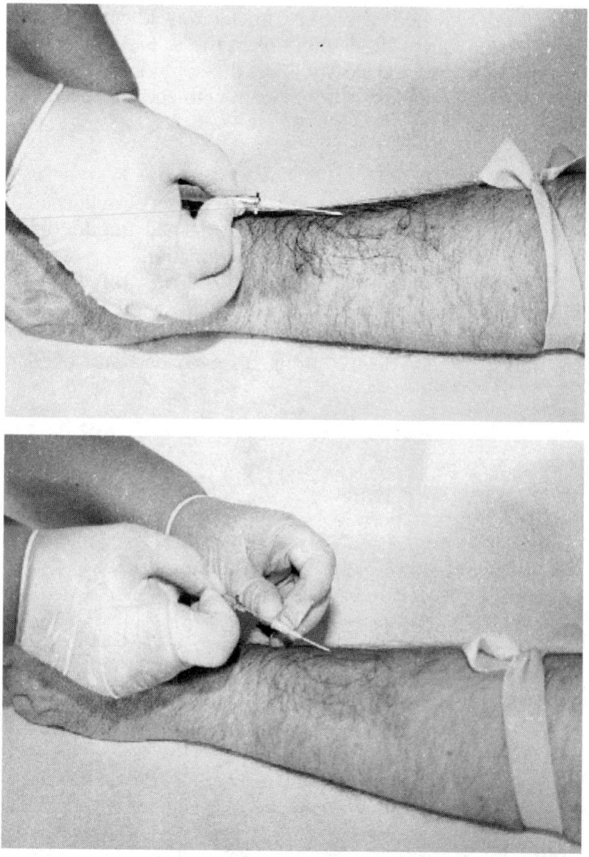

A

B

**FIGURE 6–14.** **A,** Holding the stylet with the dominant hand, piece the skin and enter the vein. **B,** With the nondominant hand, advance the catheter over the stylet. (Photograph courtesy of Monica Ridgely.)

the catheter hub and push the catheter into the vein over the needle. Place the thumb of your nondominant hand above the catheter site to decrease any bleeding. Remove the rest of the stylet. Remove the tourniquet and attach the IV tubing or the intermittent injection cap.

If the veins are fragile, "floating" the catheter into the vein as described with the winged IV sets is possible. Be certain to remove the tourniquet before infusing or injecting any solution. Failure to do so may cause the vein to rupture.

## COMPLETING THE INSERTION

If the client is to receive a continuous infusion, adjust the infusion rate with the roller clamp or the electronic control device.

If the client is to receive an intermittent infusion and the line was not flushed when the catheter was advanced, clean the injection cap with alcohol, insert the saline syringe into the injection cap, and slowly inject the solution. In agencies that use heparin, flush the catheter with the prepared heparin syringe.

## DRESSING THE IV SITE

Some institution policies include the use of antibacterial ointment at the IV insertion site. Apply a small amount of the ointment at the catheter insertion site junction.

**Securing a Catheter With a Hub.** To secure an IV catheter with a hub, tear a piece of ½-inch (1.3 cm) wide, 3-inch (7.5 cm) long tape. Carefully place the tape sticky side up under the hub of the IV device. Bring up each end and overlap

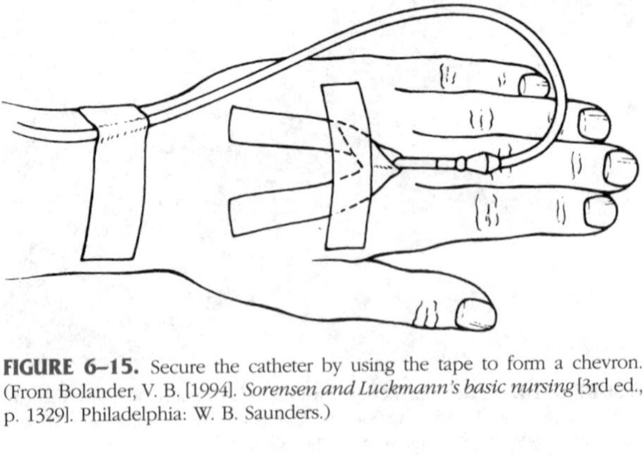

**FIGURE 6–15.** Secure the catheter by using the tape to form a chevron. (From Bolander, V. B. [1994]. *Sorensen and Luckmann's basic nursing* [3rd ed., p. 1329]. Philadelphia: W. B. Saunders.)

them in a chevron fashion (Fig. 6–15). Avoid applying the tape directly over the skin-cannula junction site. Place another piece of ½-inch (1.3 cm) wide, 2-inch (5-cm) long tape across the hub. Some agency policies state that gauze dressings are used to cover the IV site. Others provide for transparent semipermeable membrane (TSM) dressings (Fig. 6–16). In either case apply the dressing, maintaining aseptic technique. Secure the gauze dressing with tape along all edges in a picture frame fashion. The TSM dressing is self-securing. With another piece of tape, label the site with the date, time, catheter gauge and length, and your initials.

**Securing the Winged Catheter.** The procedure for securing a winged IV catheter is very similar to that for securing a catheter with a hub. Instead of bringing the tape up in a chevron, the wings are used to secure the catheter in a U-shaped formation (Fig. 6–17). The balance of the procedure is as described above.

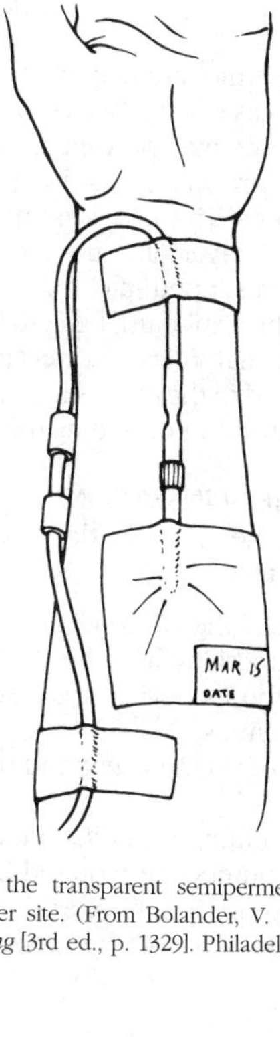


**FIGURE 6–16.** Apply the transparent semipermeable membrane (TSM) dressing over the catheter site. (From Bolander, V. B. [1994]. *Sorensen and Luckmann's basic nursing* [3rd ed., p. 1329]. Philadelphia: W. B. Saunders.)

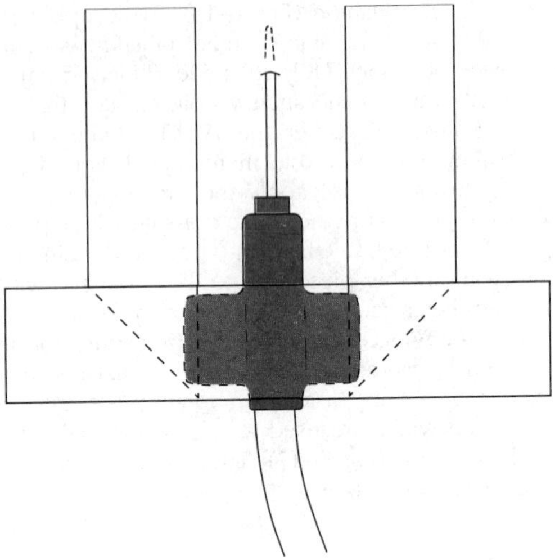

**FIGURE 6–17.** Winged catheters are secured by taping the catheter in a U shape.

## ARMBOARDS

In some cases an armboard may be necessary. The use of an armboard in the case of an IV site close to a joint or for a client who is confused may prevent an infiltration of the IV.

Choose an armboard that is just long enough to prevent flexion at the joint. Most armboards are made of a thick cardboard covered with a layer of foam and encased in plastic. The armboard is then slipped into a sleeve of soft paper

When applying the armboard, be certain that the limb will be able to assume an anatomically correct position. Apply tape to secure the armboard to the client's arm, taking care to avoid covering the insertion site or occluding the vein above the site.

## DOCUMENTING THE IV INSERTION

After completing the insertion, document the following in the client's medical record:

- Date and time of the procedure
- Type, gauge, and length of the IV device
- Site in which the IV device was inserted
- Number of attempts
- Instruction given to the client and indication of client's understanding
- The IV solution hung including additives, amount, rate, and container number (if required by the agency)
- The type of pump or controller
- The name and title of the person performing the procedure

If an intermittent catheter is inserted, naturally there is no IV solution or pump or controller information to document; however, the nurse documents the type and amount of flush used to maintain patency.

## PERIPHERAL IV THERAPY MAINTENANCE

Now that the peripheral IV therapy is initiated, the nurse attends to maintaining the therapy. Maintenance includes monitoring and documentation. Maintenance may include dressing changes, adding IV solution containers, changing the administration set, and rotating IV sites. IV maintenance may also include converting the continuous infusion to an intermittent infusion device, maintaining this device, and discontinuing the infusion device.

### Monitoring and Documentation

The frequency with which the nurse monitors the IV therapy is usually outlined in the agency's policies. In any case the nurse considers the therapy, the client's condition, and the practice setting. Unstable clients are usually placed in critical care areas to receive constant monitoring of their responses to therapy. In addition, the critical care nurse assesses the cannula site and flow rate every 15 minutes to assure proper functioning. No matter what the therapy, client condition, or type of medical facility setting, the nurse should evaluate the client at least once each hour.

The nurse documents any pertinent data derived from the assessment. These data include but are not limited to the condition of the IV site, the infusion rate, and clinical data about the client—vital signs, appearance, and response to therapy. In the home setting, clients and their caregivers are instructed in monitoring the IV site for redness, swelling, and patency.

### Dressing Changes

The nurse changes the dressing using sterile technique. The frequency of the dressing changes depends on the integrity of the present dressing and the type.

#### GAUZE DRESSING

Using sterile technique, the nurse changes a gauze dressing every 48 to 72 hours in conjunction with the IV administration set change. The nurse also applies a new gauze dressing any time the integrity of the present dressing is compromised.

To change the gauze dressing, the nurse gathers sterile 2 × 2's, bacteriostatic ointment (if indicated in agency policy), the appropriate skin cleansing material, tape, and nonsterile and sterile gloves.

1. Wash your hands and open the 2 × 2's, using the tear-down packing to maintain sterility.
2. Put on the nonsterile gloves.
3. Carefully loosen the tape at the perimeter of the gauze dressing.
4. Remove the dressing and discard it.
5. Observe the site for redness, swelling, and tenderness. If none of these are present, proceed. If any of these symptoms are observed, remove the IV cannula and establish another site.
6. Remove the nonsterile gloves and put on the sterile gloves.
7. Using the skin cleansing material, carefully clean around the insertion site, working in a circular motion from the insertion site out while holding the IV tubing or injection cap in your nondominant hand to avoid accidentally pulling the catheter out. Allow to air dry.
8. If agency policy dictates, apply a small amount of antibacterial ointment.
9. Cover the IV site with the sterile 2 × 2 and tape along the perimeter.
10. Document the procedure in the client's record, including the appearance of the site and the type of dressing.

## TRANSPARENT SEMIPERMEABLE MEMBRANE DRESSING

It is undetermined how frequently the water-resistant, air-permeable TSM dressings require changing. The INS suggests that the nurse replace TSM dressings in conjunction with the IV administration set change every 48 to 72 hours (INS, 1990).

To change the TSM dressing the nurse gathers the following: nonsterile gloves, skin cleansing material, sterile gloves, and a new TSM dressing.

1. Wash your hands and put on the nonsterile gloves.
2. Holding the IV tubing or injection cap with your nondominant hand, gently remove the old TSM dressing.
3. Although the site has been visible through this dressing, assess the site for redness, swelling, or tenderness. If any of these are present, remove this catheter and reestablish the IV site in another area. If none of these symptoms are present, proceed.
4. Remove the nonsterile gloves and put on the sterile gloves.
5. Carefully clean around the IV insertion site with the cleansing material while holding the IV tubing or in-

jection cap to avoid accidentally removing the catheter. Allow to air dry.
6. If agency policy dictates, apply a small amount of antibacterial ointment to the insertion site.
7. Place the new TSM dressing over the site.
8. Document the procedure in the client's medical record, including the appearance of the site and the type of dressing.

## Adding IV Solution Containers

To avoid bacterial growth, no IV solution should hang for longer than 24 hours. Check the physician's order and secure the next IV container ordered. Check this container for cracks, leaks, or particulate matter. Note the expiration date. Place a time strip along the length of the solution container.

Slow the present IV rate and open the new IV solution container. Take the old solution container from the IV pole and, holding the container upside down, remove the administration set spike and avoid contamination. Keep the spike above the client's heart. Spike the new solution container according to the manufacturer's instructions. Hang the new container on the IV pole and reset the rate. Document the procedure in the client's medical record. Include the type and amount of the solution, any additives, and the administration rate. Some agencies use IV flow sheets for this purpose. Follow the agency's policy.

## Changing the Administration Set

The CDC indicate that the nurse change the IV administration set every 48 to 72 hours unless the infusion is parenteral nutrition. Change parenteral nutrition administration sets every 24 hours. Change the administration set any time it becomes contaminated or if there is question about its integrity. INS suggests that administration set changes be coordinated with the hanging of a new IV solution container or an IV site rotation. This maintains the IV setup as a "closed system" and decreases the opportunity for contamination.

Some facilities use flow sheets for routine nursing care. Document the procedure as outlined in the agency's policy.

### ADMINISTRATION SET WITH SOLUTION CONTAINER CHANGE

To change the administration set with the IV solution container, gather the following: a new administration set, the next solution container ordered, gloves, a sterile 2 × 2, tape or label, and a pair of hemostats.

1. Wash your hands.
2. Spike the new solution container with the new administration set and prime it. If the administration set must be primed on the pump, take the old set off the pump and slow the rate with the roller clamp. Place the new set on the pump and perform the priming procedure now.
3. Put on your gloves and place the 2 × 2 under the junction of the catheter hub and the administration set. This provides a sterile field for the procedure and absorbs any fluid or blood drops when the administration set is detached.
4. With your nondominant hand, place the hemostats around the hub of the catheter. Be careful not to tighten the hemostats to the point of cracking the hub.
5. With your dominant hand, close the roller clamp on the old administration set and quickly detach it from the catheter hub by twisting it in a counterclockwise direction. Make sure that the catheter hub is stable.
6. Continue to hold the hemostats on the catheter hub. Drop the old administration set and take the end of the new administration set, remove the cap, and insert it into the catheter hub. Be certain that this connection is secure.
7. Adjust the rate and label the tubing with the date, time, and your initials. Document the procedure in the client's medical record.

## ADMINISTRATION SET CHANGE WITH SITE ROTATION

Changing the administration set and the IV site requires that the nurse gather a new administration set and the equipment to establish a new IV site.

1. Wash your hands.
2. Slow the rate of the present IV. If using a pump, remove the administration set from the pump and use the roller clamp to adjust the rate. Open the new administration set.
3. Holding the IV solution container upside down and above the client's heart, carefully remove the old spike from the container.
4. Take the cap from the spike of the new IV set and cover the exposed spike from the old IV set with it. Spike the IV container with the new administration set.
5. Discontinue the present IV catheter (see procedure below) and discard this equipment.
6. Prime the tubing and label it with the date, time, and your initials. Follow the procedure for starting an IV. Remember to document the procedure in the client's medical record.

## Rotating the IV Site

To prevent IV-related complications, peripheral IV sites are rotated every 48 to 72 hours. In cases in which venous access is limited this may not be feasible. In these situations the nurse notifies the physician that the client's access does not permit routine IV site changes. This allows the physician to make some decisions regarding the client's therapy. These may include changing the route of medication or fluid administration or making preparations for the placement of a central venous access device. If the physician wishes to continue using the present site, the physician should indicate this in the form of an order. In any case the nurse monitors the site carefully for any signs of IV-related complications described later in this chapter. If complications are detected, the nurse removes the IV device and notifies the physician if necessary. It is important that all documentation about the IV site observations and discussions with the physician about the IV infusion be accurate, complete, and timely.

## Converting the Continuous IV to an Intermittent Device

An intermittent device, usually called a heparin or saline lock, maintains venous access without continuously infusing IV fluids. The nurse may administer IV medications or draw blood using an intermittent device. In cases when fluid overload is a concern, an intermittent infusion device provides rapid access to the client's vascular system without giving unnecessary fluids. Home infusion therapy is usually administered via an intermittent infusion device.

To convert a continuous IV infusion to an intermittent device, gather an injection cap, one or two 3-cc syringes with 1-inch (2.5-cm) 22G needles, gloves, a sterile 2 × 2, a vial of normal saline for injection, a vial of heparinized saline in the concentration outlined in policy, alcohol preps, and hemostats. Some agencies maintain intermittent de-vice patency using saline flush only, others with heparin. Consult agency policy. (For a further discussion see Research Box 6–1.)

1. Wash your hands and put on the gloves.
2. Stop the IV infusion.
3. Draw up the amount of saline and heparin dictated by agency policy.
4. Using the saline syringe, prime the injection cap.
5. Place the sterile 2 × 2 under the catheter hub.
6. Secure the catheter hub with the hemostats, taking care not to crack the hub.
7. Holding the hub stationary, carefully disconnect the administration set from the catheter by twisting the set counterclockwise.

**RESEARCH BOX 6–1**

*Goode, C. J., et al. (1993) Improving practice through research: The case of heparin vs. saline for peripheral intermittent infusion devices.* MEDSURG Nursing, *2(1), 23–27.*

There is controversy surrounding the flushing of intermittent infusion devices. This controversy involves whether the device should be maintained using a saline or heparin flush and how frequently the device should be flushed. Furthermore, if heparin is appropriate, how much and in what concentration?

Nurses at the University of Iowa Hospitals and Clinics used meta-analysis to determine that for clients at least 28 days old, saline is just as effective as heparin for maintaining patency, decreasing phlebitis, and increasing the duration of placement in peripheral lines. The nurses also determined that decreasing the frequency of flush to every 12 hours had no effect on the longevity of the peripheral line.

**Nursing Implications**

Nurses at the University of Iowa Hospital and Clinics and at other agencies have revised their intermittent peripheral catheter flushing policies as a result of nursing research studies such as this one. These findings highlight the value of nursing research in identifying cost and time saving measures that do not sacrifice the quality of client care. In addition, these findings suggest opportunities for further nursing research such as the following: Will daily flushing of peripheral lines provide the same results of patency and duration as twice-a-day flushing? Is heparin necessary to maintain patency of central lines? Do central lines require daily flushes?

8. Remove the set and quickly attach the injection cap to the catheter hub.
9. Clean the injection cap with alcohol and flush the catheter with the rest of the saline solution, observing the site for any infiltration.
10. If agency policy dictates, flush the device with heparin.
11. Document the procedure.

## Intermittent Device Maintenance

To maintain the intermittent device the nurse flushes the catheter routinely or after each use. Agency policies differ in how this aspect of the client's care is handled. Some facilities flush with a heparinized saline solution once a day, others require an every 8-hour flush. In all cases the nurse flushes the catheter after each use for medication administration. This prevents thrombus formation at the end of the catheter.

## Discontinuing the Infusion Device

At the end of therapy or when rotating the IV site, the nurse removes the infusion device. To discontinue the infusion device the nurse gathers gloves, a sterile 2 × 2, and a Band-Aid.

1. Wash your hands and put on the gloves.
2. Stop the infusion if one is running.

3. Carefully remove the dressing and any tape on the IV device.
4. With your nondominant hand, place the 2 × 2 over the insertion site. A dry sterile gauze is recommended, as the anticoagulant properties of alcohol cause the site to bleed.
5. With your dominant hand, pull the infusion device toward you flush with the skin.
6. As you remove the device, apply pressure on the insertion site with the 2 × 2.
7. Examine the device, making certain that the entire length of the catheter has been removed.
8. Continue to apply pressure to the site for about 2 minutes or until the bleeding stops. This prevents a hematoma or bleeding from the site.
9. After the bleeding stops, apply a Band-Aid.
10. Document the procedure.

## COMPLICATIONS

Vigilant nursing care is the key to decreasing the incidence of complications associated with peripheral IV therapy. The nurse maintains strict aseptic technique in all handling of the equipment and the catheter site. The nurse inspects all equipment and infusion containers for any sign of cracks or leaks. Frequent monitoring and clear, concise documentation assist the health care team in delivering safe and effective therapy.

Another determinant in achieving positive outcomes in peripheral IV therapy is client education. A well-educated client can alert the nurse to any signs of difficulty in the early stages of the untoward event, before the situation becomes serious. The nurse instructs the client that the infusion therapy should not cause pain or physical discomfort. The client is aware that at the first sign of any change, he or she notifies the nurse.

Unfortunately, even with conscientious nursing care and well-informed clients, peripheral IV therapy can be associated with complications. These untoward events may be local or systemic in nature. The local complications include infiltration, extravasation, phlebitis, hematoma, local infection, catheter embolism, and venous irritation. Systemic infection, air embolism, circulatory overload, speed shock, and allergic reaction are the more serious, systemic complications of peripheral IV therapy.

### Local Complications

#### INFILTRATION

**Definition.** Infiltration is defined as the infusion or seepage of IV solution or medication into the extravascular tissue.

The seriousness of this occurrence is determined by the type of fluid or medication, the concentration, and the volume of the infiltrated infusate. The severity can range from a small amount of edema caused by the seepage of an isotonic solution to a large area of tissue necrosis from the infiltration of a concentrated antibiotic.

**Cause.** Infiltration occurs when the venous access device either partially or completely dislodges from the vein or perforates it.

**Signs and Symptoms.** One of the first signs the nurse may observe is a sluggish IV rate. Another sign is the increasing edema at the site. Inspection of the same area of the opposite limb confirms that fluid is leaking into the adjacent tissue. Some nurses believe that when applying negative pressure with a syringe or when lowering the infusion container below the heart, if a blood return is obtained, there is no danger of infiltration. However, if the catheter bevel has only partially perforated the vein, some of the infusion may be entering the vein while the rest is infusing into the tissue. Although a blood return is present, the line is infiltrated. To verify an infiltration the nurse applies a tourniquet above the IV site to restrict venous flow. If the fluid continues to infuse, the client has an infiltration, and the nurse removes the IV catheter immediately.

The client with an infiltration may complain of burning, tenderness, or pain at the site. The client may state that the skin feels tight over the infiltration. The nurse notes that the area of the infiltration is cooler than the adjacent skin and may be blanched.

**Treatment.** If the infiltration is recent, an ice pack to the area may prevent any further infiltration. If the infiltration is larger in size, warm, moist heat assists the reabsorption of the fluid.

**Documentation.** The nurse documents the infiltration by describing the appearance of the site and the fluid or medication involved. All nursing actions are also recorded on the client's record. Most agency policies require that the nurse completes an incident report and notifies the physician.

**Prevention.** The nurse prevents infiltrations by well stabilizing the IV catheter, using the smallest catheter that accommodates the vein and the infusion, avoiding IV placement over areas of flexion, and frequently monitoring the site.

## EXTRAVASATION

**Definition.** Extravasation is the accidental administration of a vesicant solution or medication into the surrounding tissue. A vesicant is an agent capable of causing or forming a blister or tissue destruction, such as dopamine (Intropin).

**Cause.** The causes of extravasation are the same as those for infiltration; the IV catheter either completely or partially dislodges from the vein or perforates it.

**Signs and Symptoms.** Vesicant drugs are extremely damaging to the surrounding tissue. The nurse may note the same signs and symptoms seen in infiltration. The client may complain of stinging, burning, or pain at the catheter site. Redness may occur around the needle. Swelling may be present immediately or appear up to hours later.

**Treatment.** The Oncology Nursing Society (ONS) states that the treatment of extravasation appears to be related to the concentration of the drug, the amount of the drug extravasated, and the individual tissue responses. Some of these agents have well-documented antidotes that are given IV, subcutaneously, or topically. In each case the nurse immediately stops the infusion. The nurse leaves the catheter in place and attempts to aspirate any drug from the site with a syringe. The physician is notified immediately.

**Documentation.** The nurse documents the extravasation, including the type and suspected amount of drug and the evaluation of the site. The documentation in the record includes any nursing actions taken and the client's response. The nurse follows agency policy regarding the completion of an incident report.

**Prevention.** To prevent extravasation the nurse monitors the IV site frequently. The nurse avoids inserting IV devices into veins over areas of flexion and determines that the IV catheter is well secured. Using the smallest catheter that accommodates the vein and the infusion assists the nurse in preventing extravasation. When administering a vesicant drug IV push, the nurse gives the drug through the side arm of a running IV device. Although this does not preclude extravasation, the drug will be more dilute if extravasation occurs, limiting the severity of damage.

## PHLEBITIS

**Definition.** Phlebitis is actually an inflammation of the vein. Phlebitis may run along the length of a vein.

**Cause.** Some of the causes of phlebitis include the insertion technique, the condition of the patient, vein condition, type and pH of medication and solutions or compatibility, filtration, and gauge, size, length, and material of the catheter.

**Signs and Symptoms.** Early in phlebitis the client may complain of pain around the catheter. If the nurse does not intervene by changing the site, the injury progresses and the client with phlebitis may complain of pain at the tip of the catheter and along the vein. The nurse may note that the vein appears red and inflamed along the length. The client may spike a temperature. In the later stages of phlebitis the client's vein becomes hard and cordlike. Phlebitis can predispose the client to a local infection, which may become systemic.

**Treatment.** The nurse removes the catheter at the first sign of phlebitis. Warm compresses may decrease the client's discomfort.

**Documentation.** The nurse documents the incidence of phlebitis. The following phlebitis scale provides the nurse with a consistent method of measuring the severity of the phlebitis.

1+ Pain at the site, erythema, or edema; no streak; no palpable cord
2+ Pain at the site, erythema, or edema; streak formation; no palpable cord
3+ Pain at the site, erythema, or edema; streak formation; palpable cord

If the phlebitis is severe and the client has a temperature, notify the physician. Many agencies require that the nurse complete an incident report as well.

**Prevention.** To prevent phlebitis the nurse changes the site of the IV catheter every 48 to 72 hours. The nurse avoids the veins in the lower extremities because they are susceptible to trauma and subject to venous stasis. They are therefore more likely to develop phlebitis. When infusing irritating solutions or solutions with high osmolality, the nurse uses veins that are large enough to provide adequate blood flow around the catheter. A well-anchored catheter prevents movement in the vein, causing irritation, damage to the intima, and clot formation. The nurse adheres to strict aseptic technique when inserting the catheter.

## HEMATOMA

**Definition.** Hematoma is the leaking of blood into the surrounding tissue.

**Cause.** A hematoma can occur during the IV insertion if the catheter pierces the back of the vein. Clients who are receiving anticoagulant therapy or who have faulty coagulation ability are susceptible to hematoma development during the IV insertion process.

**Signs and Symptoms.** The nurse observes a discolored area of bruising around the IV site. The client may complain of pain at the site. The area may or may not be swollen.

**Treatment.** At the first sign of discoloration around the insertion site, the nurse removes the IV device and applies pressure. If the size of the area is stable, warm soaks assist the hematoma to resolve.

**Documentation.** The nurse measures the size of the hematoma and documents it in the client's record along with any interventions.

**Prevention.** To prevent hematoma the nurse carefully advances the catheter at an angle parallel to the client's skin. Again, selection of the smallest lumen catheter that accommodates the vein and the infusion avoids hematoma formation.

## LOCAL INFECTION

**Definition.** A local infection is contamination, usually bacterial, at the IV site.

**Cause.** A local infection is usually the result of a break in aseptic technique either during the IV insertion or in the handling of the sterile equipment.

**Signs and Symptoms.** An infected IV site appears red, swollen, and warm. The client may complain of tenderness at the site. The nurse may observe a purulent or malodorous exudate. Left untreated, the client can develop a septic phlebitis and subsequent septicemia.

**Treatment.** After removing the catheter, the nurse allows the site to bleed for a few seconds to observe for any purulence from the vein. A 2 × 2 is used to express any discharge. The nurse sends the catheter tip for culture. The site is cleansed with an antibacterial solution and covered with a dry sterile dressing. In the case of septic phlebitis, surgical intervention to strip the vein may be necessary.

**Documentation.** The nurse documents the appearance of the site and any exudate noted. If the infection is severe, the nurse notifies the physician, who makes arrangements for any further treatment. An incident report is completed per agency policy.

**Prevention.** Strict aseptic technique whenever the nurse cares for the IV site is the key to prevention. Attention to monitoring and maintenance of the site and IV equipment prevents the occurrence of infection. The nurse carefully inspects all IV solutions and medications before hanging them and changes infusion containers every 24 hours.

## CATHETER EMBOLISM

**Definition.** Catheter embolism occurs when a shaving or piece of the IV catheter breaks off and floats freely in the vessel.

**Cause.** Catheter embolism can occur if the needle of an over-the-needle catheter is reinserted into the catheter or if the catheter of a through-the-needle catheter is inadvertently pulled back through the catheter. When the nurse administers an IV push drug or flushes an intermittent infusion device, the needle may clip the inside of the catheter and cause a fragment of the catheter to break off.

**Signs and Symptoms.** Clients who have a catheter embolism experience a decrease in blood pressure and complain of pain along the vein. The client's pulse is weak, rapid, and thready and the nurse may note cyanosis of the nail beds and circumorally. The client may lapse into unconsciousness.

**Treatment.** The nurse discontinues the catheter and applies a tourniquet high on the limb of the catheter site. The nurse inspects the catheter for any rough edges and notifies the physician. A radio-graph is taken to determine the presence of any catheter pieces. Surgical intervention to remove the pieces is necessary.

**Documentation.** The nurse documents the incident in the client's medical record and on the agency's incident report. The documentation includes the client's condition, the nursing actions, and the appearance of the catheter removed.

**Prevention.** Catheter embolism is preventable. When inserting an over-the-needle catheter, the nurse never reinserts the needle into the catheter. The nurse avoids pulling a through-the-needle catheter back through the needle during the insertion or maintenance. When administering a drug or flushing an intermittent infusion device, the nurse uses the shortest needle that will puncture the injection port. A 1-inch (2.5-cm) needle is generally sufficient.

### VENOUS IRRITATION

**Definition.** Venous irritation is inflammation along the vein that is usually rate or infusion related. Without intervention, venous irritation may become phlebitis.

**Cause.** The infusion of hyperosmolar, high- or low-pH solutions or irritating drugs in a high concentration leads to venous irritation.

**Signs and Symptoms.** Venous irritation may cause the client to complain of achiness or tightness along the vein. The nurse notes that the vein may be darkened or reddened along its length.

**Treatment.** Decreasing the rate of the infusion may assist with the pain. The nurse discusses the problem with the pharmacy and requests that the drug concentration be decreased. The addition of a buffer to high-pH solutions may be possible.

**Documentation.** The nurse documents the client's symptoms and nursing interventions.

**Prevention.** The nurse starts the IV infusion in a large vessel if the administration of irritating drugs or solutions is anticipated.

## Systemic Complications

### SYSTEMIC INFECTION/SEPSIS

**Definition.** A systemic infection occurs when pathogenic organisms enter the client's circulation.

**Cause.** Systemic infection may result from poor aseptic technique or contaminated infusions or if the catheter site is not changed routinely.

**Signs and Symptoms.** Early symptoms of sepsis include fever, chills, headache, and general malaise. If left unattended, the client may experience severe infection, which may lead to vascular collapse and death.

**Treatment.** At the first suspicion of sepsis, the nurse changes the entire infusion system, from solution to the IV device. The nurse notifies the physician, obtains cultures as ordered, and administers the medications the physician orders. If the infusate is suspected as the cause, the nurse sends a specimen of the solution to the laboratory. The nurse monitors the client for any signs of worsening condition and reports findings to the physician.

**Documentation.** The nurse documents the client's symptoms and all interventions. Continuous monitoring and documentation of the client's condition is critical to the client's outcome.

**Prevention.** Meticulous aseptic technique is necessary to avoid sepsis. The nurse carefully inspects all IV solutions and their containers before hanging them. If the integrity of the dressing or any IV equipment is questionable, it is changed or discarded. The nurse changes the client's IV site every 48 to 72 hours.

### AIR EMBOLISM

**Definition.** The entry of air into the client's circulatory system is an air embolism. Air embolism is unusual in clients with peripheral IV infusions.

**Cause.** Empty IV solution containers, air in the tubing, and loose IV connections can cause air embolism.

**Signs and Symptoms.** The client experiencing air embolism complains of chest or shoulder pain, back pain, and dyspnea. The nurse notes a sudden drop in blood pressure, cyanosis, and a weak, thready pulse. The client may lose consciousness.

**Treatment.** At the first signs of air embolism the nurse positions the client on his or her left side in the Trendelenburg position. The nurse monitors the client closely, taking frequent vital signs, and notifies the physician. The nurse maintains the IV site and obtains oxygen should the physician order it.

**Documentation.** The nurse documents all observations and interventions in the client's medical record and on the agency's incident report.

**Prevention.** The use of Luer lock connections for all IV devices and equipment assists in preventing air embolism. The nurse carefully monitors the IV infusion to avoid air in the administration set. When adding a new IV container to the administration, the nurse assures that there is fluid in the drip chamber. Using an electronic control device that sets off an alarm when the infusion is completed or when air is detected in an administration set assists the nurse in preventing the entrance of air to client's circulatory system.

### CIRCULATORY OVERLOAD

**Definition.** The disruption of fluid homeostasis with excess fluid in the circulatory system is called circulatory overload.

**Cause.** The infusion of fluids at a rate greater than the client's system can accommodate results in circulatory overload.

**Signs and Symptoms.** The client with circulatory overload may complain of shortness of breath and cough. The nurse notes that the client's blood pressure is elevated, there may be puffiness around the eyes, and edema in dependent areas. The client may have engorged neck veins and moist lung sounds. The nurse may find that the client's intake is far greater than the output. (Also see Chapter 13, Fluids and Electrolytes.)

**Treatment.** The nurse slows the IV rate and notifies the physician. Placing the client in a sitting position may assist with his or her breathing. The nurse monitors the client's vital signs and administers oxygen as ordered. The physician may order a diuretic, which the nurse administers as ordered.

**Documentation.** The nurse documents the client's symptoms and any intervention. If the client receives a diuretic, the nurse carefully maintains intake and output records.

**Prevention.** Intake and output should be monitored in clients receiving continuous IV infusions. As soon as the nurse notices an imbalance between the intake and output, the physician is notified so that the fluid therapy may be adjusted.

## SPEED SHOCK

**Definition.** Speed shock is a systemic reaction that occurs when a substance, unfamiliar to the body, is rapidly infused into the circulatory system.

**Cause.** Speed shock may occur with the rapid administration of drugs or bolus infusions. The rapid infusion causes the level of the drug in the system to reach toxic proportions quickly.

**Signs and Symptoms.** The client may complain of lightheadedness or dizziness and tightness in his or her chest. The nurse may note that the client has a flushed face and irregular pulse. Without medical intervention the client may lose consciousness and go into shock and cardiac arrest.

**Treatment.** The nurse discontinues the drug infusion immediately and hangs D5W to keep the vein open. The nurse monitors the client carefully and notifies the physician for further treatment orders.

**Documentation.** The nurse documents the client's symptoms, including vital signs, level of consciousness, and response to treatment.

**Prevention.** Before administering an IV push medication the nurse is aware of the appropriate rate for the administration. Speed shock from the administration of medication drips is prevented by the use of electronic infusion devices. If an electronic infusion device is not available, the nurse uses a pediatric (minidrip) infusion set to closely monitor the IV rate.

### ALLERGIC REACTION

**Definition.** A local or general response to an allergen is termed allergic reaction.

**Cause.** In IV therapy an allergic reaction may be in response to the tape, cleansing agent, drug, solution, or IV device.

**Signs and Symptoms.** The client having a local reaction may exhibit a wheal, redness, or itching at the IV site. In the case of a general reaction the client may complain of itching, runny nose, and tearing. The nurse may note bronchospasm, wheezing, and a truncal rash. Without treatment, the client may experience anaphylaxis, a severe reaction that may include agitation, convulsions, shock, and death.

**Treatment.** For local reactions the treatment is the removal of the irritant. The nurse removes the dressing and any tape and redresses the site with hypoallergenic supplies. If the drug or solution is suspected as the allergen, the drug is discontinued. The client is treated symptomatically with antihistamines. For an anaphylactic reaction the nurse stops the infusion immediately, maintains a patent airway, and notifies the physician. The nurse maintains the IV line with a solution of D5W to keep the vein open. Oxygen is administered as indicated. The physician may order antihistamine, steroid, or antiinflammatory drugs. The physician may order 0.2 to 0.5 mL of 1:1000 epinephrine subcutaneously stat and every 3 to 4 minutes as necessary.

**Documentation.** The nurse documents the client's symptoms, vital signs, treatment, and response in the client's medical record. The drug or solution is added to the client's allergy record on the nursing unit and in the pharmacy. An incident report is completed per agency policy.

**Prevention.** The nurse listens carefully to the client when completing the admission history and physical examination. Any and all allergies are documented in the record and the front of the chart and sent to the pharmacy for their records. The nurse checks the client's allergy record before administering any drug. The nurse considers the possibility of any cross-allergies among medications in the same or similar classes.

## LIFE SPAN CONSIDERATIONS

### Infants and Children

IV therapy in infants and children presents the nurse with unique challenges. These challenges include considerations for the type of therapy, the child's stage of growth and development, and locating veins in the smaller child.

## TYPE OF THERAPY

Infants and children are prescribed IV therapy to replace fluids and electrolytes, to administer antibiotics and other drugs, and to administer nutrients. Although these therapies are the same as those generally given to adults, the administration can be more complex because a child who appeared stable just hours previous may deteriorate rapidly and present with a life-threatening condition.

## GROWTH AND DEVELOPMENT

The nurse's ability to identify the child's stage of growth and development and provide the appropriate preparation or diversion determines the success of the procedure.

After explaining the procedure to the child's parents, the nurse asks the parents if they would like to stay. The nurse allows the parents to decide. Some may feel that their presence during the procedure may comfort their child. Others may worry that their child may sense their anxiety and become more frightened. Whatever their decision, the nurse respects it.

The nurse never asks the parents to participate by restraining the child in any way. Their presence is for the child's comfort. The nurse requests another staff member to hold the child during the procedure. Never tell the child that his or her parents' presence is predicated on the child's behavior. The child must feel free to express any feelings he or she has about the procedure.

Although the child's hospital room is not home, it should be a place where the child can go to feel safe and comfortable. For this reason, unpleasant or painful procedures are best completed in a treatment or procedure room.

Table 6–3 outlines the developmental stage and accompanying tasks for children. More tips for the nurse are included.

## SITE SELECTION

As with adults or older children, the nurse selects the most distal site on the limb. This preserves more proximal sites for use later in the therapy if necessary. Again, resilient, long, and straight veins are the best choice for a successful IV start. Avoiding the areas over a joint is even more important with young children than with the adult, as the young child is more active and is less likely to keep from flexing the joint during the therapy. The site that requires the least restraint during the therapy is the best. Appropriate IV sites in infants and children include the metacarpal and cephalic veins in the upper extremities; the dorsalis pedis and great saphenous veins in the lower extremities; and the temporal, posterior auricular, and metopic veins in the head.

**TABLE 6–3**
**Developmental Stages and Accompanying Tasks for Children**

| Age | Developmental Stage/Task | Behavior During Procedure | Actions | Tips |
|---|---|---|---|---|
| Infant (0-1 y) | Oral-sensory<br>Develop trust | Crying, gasping, may vomit | Staff to hold<br>Offer pacifier | Do not feed for 1 h before procedure |
| Toddler (1-3 y) | Muscular-anal<br>Autonomy | Withdraw, kick, cry, hit, and scream | Staff to hold<br>Give simple explanations prior to procedure | Allow expression of anger by providing stuffed animals to hit or throw |
| Preschool (3-5 y) | Initiative | May direct aggression at the nurse | Explain procedures just before undertaking | Allow child to "start IV" on toy<br>Provide diversion in form of magic |
| School age (6-11 y) | Industry | May behave "bravely" during procedure | Explain procedures to be done early in day if possible<br>Ask family assistance to reinforce teaching | Allow opportunity for questions<br>Teach relaxation techniques |
| Adolescence (12-18 y) | Puberty | Similar to adult behavior | Explain procedure giving as many opportunities for decision making as realistic | Teach relaxation techniques<br>Provide privacy during procedure |

**Upper Extremity Veins.** The primary upper extremity veins are the metacarpal and the cephalic veins (Fig. 6–18).

***Metacarpal Veins.*** As in adults, the metacarpal veins on the back of the hand provide a good choice for a child's IV site. These veins dilate well and are supported by the bones of the hand.

***Cephalic Veins.*** Running from just above the thumb around to the inner aspect of the forearm and up to the antecubital fossa, the cephalic vein provides the nurse with another option for an IV site. These veins are large and well secured by connective tissue.

**Lower Extremity Veins.** The lower extremity veins include the dorsal pedis and the great saphenous veins (Fig. 6–19).

***Dorsalis Pedis Veins.*** Although not suggested for use in the older child and adult, the dorsalis pedis veins are a potential IV site in the younger child or infant. Located on the anterior of the foot, these veins are formed by the union of the digital veins of the toes. Like the metacarpal veins of the hands, they dilate easily and are well supported by bony structure. Use of these veins impedes the child's ability to walk. For this reason

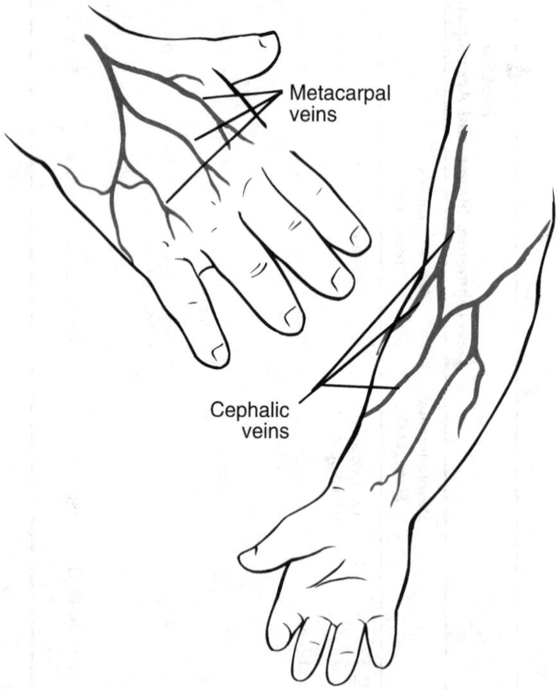


**FIGURE 6–18.** Suitable upper extremity veins in the child.

the nurse tries to reserve their use for children who are not walking, generally those under the age of 9 months. As with any IV site, the nurse pays special attention to immobilizing the site in the proper anatomic position.

*Great Saphenous Vein.* Another lower extremity vein is the great saphenous vein. This large vessel is the longest vein in the body. It is located just above the inner malleolus and proceeds up the inner leg to the femoral vein. This vein is generally used for emergency access in children, but its use may be necessary if other IV sites are inaccessible.

**Scalp Veins.** The scalp veins appropriate for use in IV therapy include the temporal, the posterior auricular, and the metopic veins (Fig. 6–20). Some health care facilities routinely use scalp veins for infants under the age of 9 months. These veins are superficial and therefore easier to see than those in the upper and lower extremities, which are imbedded in fatty tissue in this age group. As with veins in the extremities, the nurse inserts the catheter, directing it toward the heart.

*Temporal Veins.* The temporal veins are located on either side of the head in front of the ears. They are large and relatively easy to encannulate. The nurse uses caution to avoid puncturing the temporal artery.

*Posterior Auricular Veins.* Located behind the ears, the posterior auricular veins are another choice for IV therapy in the infant. Although these veins are not as large as the temporal veins, they do not pose the risk of arterial puncture that the temporal veins do.

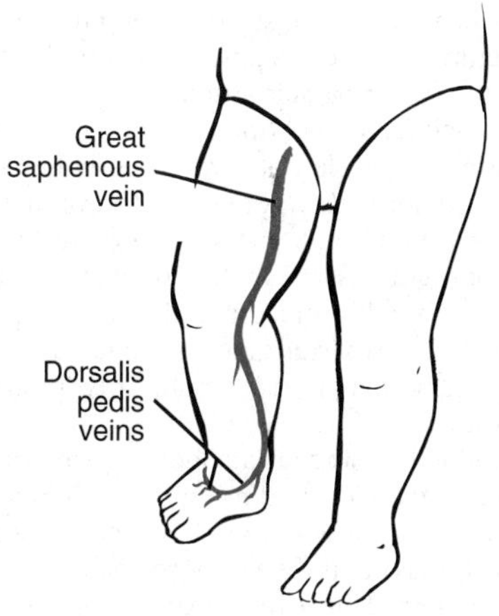


**FIGURE 6–19.** Suitable lower extremity veins in the child.

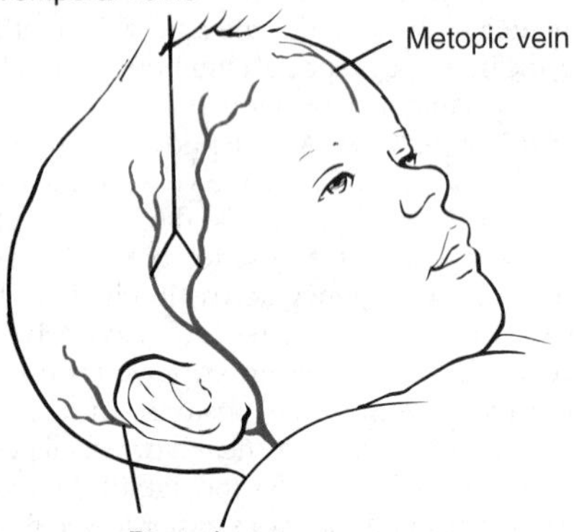


**FIGURE 6–20.** Scalp veins can be used in infants less than 9 months old.

*Metopic Vein.* The metopic vein runs down the middle of the forehead. The vein is easily visible and poses minimal risk to the infant. Parents may prefer the nurse to use this vein. Because of its location away from the hairline, the infant does not require a haircut.

## SPECIAL TECHNIQUES FOR INFANTS AND CHILDREN

**Scalp Veins.** Instead of a tourniquet, the nurse uses a rubber band to distend the scalp veins of the infant. A tab of tape applied to the rubber band allows the nurse to remove it with one hand after the IV cannula is inserted.

Have a staff member place his or her hands on either side of the infant's head to keep it steady during the insertion. Another staff member should keep the child's body still. To protect the IV catheter after it is inserted, some nurses tape over the site a disposable cup with the bottom cut out. This keeps the IV insertion site visible but away from little hands.

**Neonate.** The nurse may not need a tourniquet to start an IV infusion for a neonate if the veins are easily visible. Increasing venous congestion in the neonate's fragile veins may cause them to roll or bleed into the skin on penetration.

**Dark Skin.** To assist visualizing the veins of children with dark skin, the nurse may find it helpful to wipe the selected area with povidone-iodine (Betadine).

**Chubby Child.** Pressing an alcohol preparation pad with the thumb over the anticipated route of the vein in a chubby baby or toddler may allow the nurse to see the vein as it refills with blood, making the vein more visible.

**Newborn or Very Thin Child.** Darkening the room and placing a flashlight or using a special transluminator under the hand or limb of the newborn or very thin child may assist the nurse in finding a suitable vein. Care must be taken to avoid burning the infant. The tender, thin skin of the newborn cannot withstand the same temperatures adult skin can. This technique also assists in identifying veins in the child whose hands have been darkened with hematomas from previous IV attempts. The vein should appear darker than the bruise.

**Inserting the Catheter.** When inserting the IV device in a small vein, some nurses approach the vein with the catheter bevel side down. This keeps the catheter from piercing the lower wall of the vein, which would cause infiltration.

**Equipment.** To avoid fluid overload the nurse uses an electronic infusion device or burette for all continuous infusions for the infant and child.

## Elderly

The elderly are another special group for whom the nurse provides peripheral IV therapy. Elderly clients receiving IV therapy have special needs. The normal aging process presents changes in the skin and vessels that require the nurse's attention.

### SKIN AND VESSEL CHANGES IN THE ELDERLY

As people age, they lose subcutaneous fat. The dermis thins, and the density and amount of collagen lessen. Elastin fibers just below the dermis become more abundant but less effectively organized. The fine elastin fibers in the dermis disappear. This accounts for the decreased elasticity of the skin.

For these reasons the elderly person's skin may be described as loose, thin, and transparent. The veins appear tortuous and large because of inadequate venous pressure. The veins are likely to roll, as there is little connective tissue to hold them. The veins themselves become more fragile. These changes may require the nurse to alter the insertion technique.

### SPECIAL TECHNIQUES FOR THE ELDERLY

If the client's veins appear large and tortuous, using a tourniquet may increase venous congestion and cause blood to leak around the puncture site into the surrounding tissue. Instead of using a tourniquet, the nurse holds the client's arm in a dependent position. This may fill the veins sufficiently for the IV start.

To stabilize large, tortuous veins for the IV insertion it may help to place the tourniquet below the proposed IV site. After cleansing the skin, the nurse places the tourniquet below the site just tightly enough to keep the skin from moving. Lifting the tourniquet with one hand, the nurse pulls the

**TABLE 6–4**
**Special Nursing Considerations for Elderly Clients Receiving IV Therapy**

- Do not use hand veins for starting an IV line, as these veins are too small and limit the elderly client's mobility and ability to perform activities of daily living (ADL's).
- Use the smallest gauge IV catheter possible, preferably 21G or smaller. (May use a 24G catheter to deliver up to 100 mL/h).
- Do not use a rubber tourniquet or Penrose drain; a blood pressure cuff is easier on the client's skin.
- Take the time to find the most suitable vein.
- Use strict aseptic technique; the elderly client typically is immunocompromised.
- Do not slap the arm to help visualize the vein.
- Use a decreased angle for insertion of the catheter (5 to 15 degrees).
- Set the flow rate of IV medications, especially antibiotics, to no more than 100 mL/h; for clients with congestive heart failure or renal failure, set the rate at 50 mL/h.
- Use a protective skin preparation before applying a transparent dressing over the IV insertion site; dry gauze pads may be best for clients with tissue-thin skin. (Newer products such as Primapore are better for the client's skin.)
- Cover the IV dressing with flexible netting or if netting is unavailable, use minimal tape or an elastic bandage to secure the dressing and protect the site; keep the needle insertion site visible at all times.
- Do not use soft wrist restraints on the arm with the IV catheter in place.
- Do not use the client's foot for starting an IV line because lower extremity circulation may be impaired.

skin down with the other and traps it with the tourniquet, without snapping the tourniquet against the skin. Quickly the nurse inserts the catheter and releases the tourniquet.

Because the elderly client's skin may be fragile, the nurse takes special care with the IV site dressing. Tape directly on the elderly client's skin can tear the skin on removal, placing the client at risk for infection. TSM dressings are generally less damaging to this sometimes paper-thin skin. Other special considerations for the elderly client receiving IV therapy can be found in Table 6–4.

CHAPTER 7

# Central Venous Therapy

*Marilyn Ferreri Booker*



## DESCRIPTION

Central venous therapy involves the placement of a flexible catheter into one of the client's large veins. The tip of the catheter is situated in the superior vena cava or the right atrium of the heart. The placement may be accomplished by direct insertion (percutaneous stick) into either the chest or arm veins or by surgical insertion in the case of tunneled catheters or implanted ports.

Drugs, fluids, nutrients, enhancing agents, blood, and blood products may be infused through a central IV line. At times a central venous catheter (CVC) is inserted because the client's peripheral venous access is inadequate for the duration or type of IV therapy required. In some clients a CVC allows the nurse to measure and monitor central venous pressure (CVP) (Fig. 7–1). In other cases a CVC is inserted to ensure venous access when at-home IV therapy is prescribed.

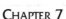

1. Position the water manometer so that the zero mark or the air-fluid interface is at the same height as the phlebostatic axis.

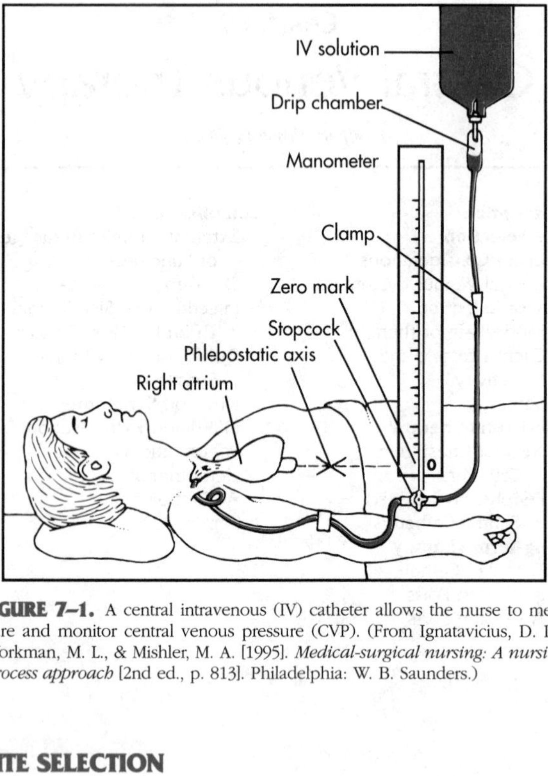


**FIGURE 7–1.** A central intravenous (IV) catheter allows the nurse to measure and monitor central venous pressure (CVP). (From Ignatavicius, D. D., Workman, M. L., & Mishler, M. A. [1995]. *Medical-surgical nursing: A nursing process approach* [2nd ed., p. 813]. Philadelphia: W. B. Saunders.)

## SITE SELECTION

### Client Considerations

Some clients who have had central lines previously or who have sustained thrombosis of one or more of the central veins may have a limited selection of veins for catheter insertion.

Physicians are usually hesitant to place a central catheter by direct insertion into the chest veins of clients who suffer from chronic obstructive pulmonary disease because the direct insertion of a catheter into the chest veins can be complicated by pneumothorax. This misadventure, serious in any client, can be particularly dangerous in clients who have compromised pulmonary function.

Physicians may have a difficult time inserting catheters into the chest veins of clients who are obese or who have other anatomic changes such as superior vena cava syndrome, obstruction of the subclavian veins, tumor blockage,

2. Turn the stopcock as shown to fill manometer with IV fluid.
3. Turn the stopcock as shown to record the CVP. With each respiration, the fluid level in the manometer should fluctuate. When the level has stabilized, read the highest level of the fluid column.
4. Return the stopcock to the position shown to resume the flow of IV fluid to the client.

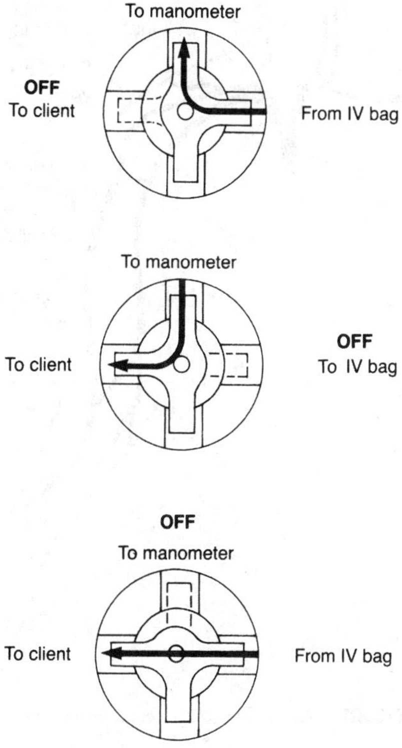


**FIGURE 7–1.** Continued

bilateral radical neck dissection, or trauma to the upper torso. Each of these conditions makes identifying landmarks and advancing catheters difficult. In such cases the physician can place the catheter through the saphenous vein and advance it into the inferior vena cava.

## Central Venous System

The following veins comprise the anatomic structure known as the central venous system. Figure 7–2 shows the

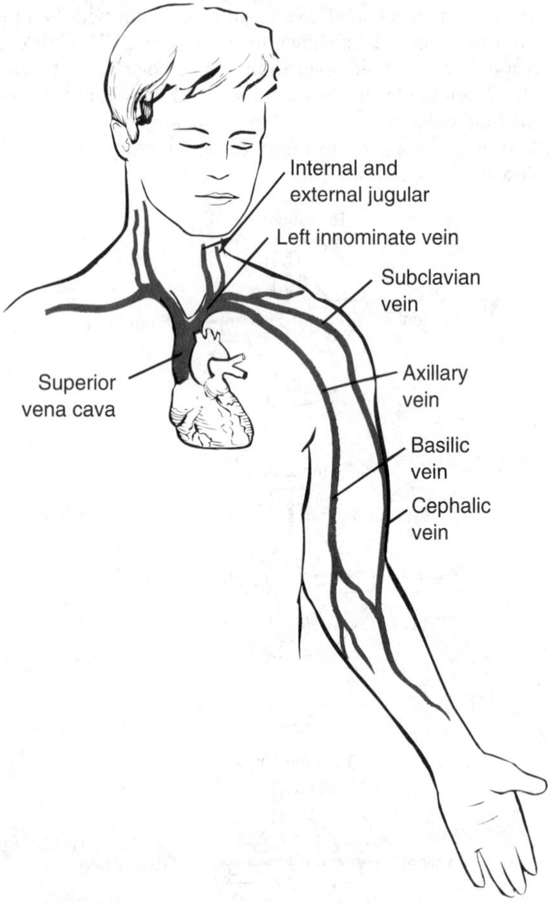


**FIGURE 7–2.** Anatomy of the central venous system.

location of each of these vessels. Although all these veins are not the target for the catheter tip, the physician advances the catheter through them on its way to the superior vena cava or right atrium.

## CEPHALIC VEIN

The cephalic vein ascends along the outer edge of the biceps muscle to the upper aspect of the arm. It then passes between the pectoralis major and deltoid muscles. It terminates in the axillary vein with a descending curve just below the clavicle.

## BASILIC VEIN

The basilic vein is larger than the cephalic vein. It passes up the arm in a straight path along the inner side of the biceps muscle. The basilic vein terminates in the axillary vein.

## AXILLARY VEIN

The axillary vein is an extension of the basilic vein. As it ascends, it increases in size. The axillary vein ends just beneath the clavicle at the outer edge of the first rib. Here it becomes the subclavian vein.

## EXTERNAL JUGULAR VEIN

On the side of the neck the external jugular vein is easily recognized. This vein connects to the subclavian vein along the center of the clavicle.

## INTERNAL JUGULAR VEIN

The internal jugular vein initially descends behind and then to the outer side of the internal and common carotid arteries. The internal jugular vein joins the subclavian vein at the base of the neck. At this point the left subclavian vein receives the thoracic duct, whereas the right subclavian vein receives the right lymphatic duct.

## SUBCLAVIAN VEIN

The subclavian vein is a continuation of the axillary vein. The subclavian vein extends from the outer edge of the first rib to the inner end of the clavicle. Here it unites with the internal jugular vein to form the innominate vein.

## RIGHT INNOMINATE VEIN

The right innominate vein (approximately 1 inch [2.5 cm] in length) passes vertically down and joins the left innominate vein just below the cartilage of the first rib.

## LEFT INNOMINATE VEIN

The left innominate vein is about 2.5 inches (6 cm) long and larger than the right innominate vein. It runs left to right in a downward angle across the anterior of the upper chest. It joins the right innominate vein to form the superior vena cava.

## SUPERIOR VENA CAVA

The upper portion of the largest vein in the body, the superior vena cava receives all the blood from the upper half of the body on its way to the heart. It is short, about 2.5 to 3 inches (6 to 8.5 cm) long and initiates below the first rib near the sternum on the right. From there the superior vena cava descends vertically and slightly to the right. It empties into the right atrium of the heart.

## DEVICE SELECTION

Although most types of central line placement are not within the realm of nursing practice, nurses perform vital roles in the preparation and instruction of the client and maintenance of the catheters. In addition to the client's medical history and condition of the central veins, the type of therapy and its duration and the client's lifestyle, activity, and setting in which the therapy is to be administered are all important considerations for the physician, nurse, and client when deciding on the correct type of catheter for a particular client.

### Mode/Rate of Administration

The client's type of therapy may impact the number of lumens the catheter should have. Most CVCs come with one, two, three, or four lumens. Multiple-lumen catheters allow for the infusion of more than one concurrent administration. Frequently, one lumen of the catheter is designated for the infusion of nutritional support fluids (total parenteral nutrition [TPN]), whereas the other lumen(s) is (are) used to infuse other fluids, blood products, or medications. Because blood sampling for venous specimens is possible through most CVCs, one lumen may be designated for obtaining blood.

The use of multiple-lumen catheters for nutritional support is a controversial subject. Multiple studies have shown a higher incidence of catheter-related sepsis in clients receiving TPN with multiple-lumen catheters than with clients receiving TPN with single-lumen catheters (Clark-Christoff, 1992; Hilton, 1988). Despite this research, in practice, nurses find that multiple-lumen catheters are used for TPN and other infusions, as well as for blood drawing. Frequently, the insertion of a single-lumen CVC solely for TPN may not be practical for other reasons. The client with cancer may have no other veins available for peripheral access. Clients who are critically ill may require so many infusions that no other choice exists than to use a multiple-lumen catheter for the nutritional support and the other critically needed infusions. In these cases the physician has usually determined that the risks associated with the multiple-lumen catheter are less than the benefits to the client's care. Nurses who care for these clients must be aware of this potential complication; whenever possible, the lumen used for TPN should be left exclusively for that purpose.

Another issue with multiple-lumen catheters is the administration of incompatible drugs and solutions simultaneously through separate catheter lumens. Although this practice has not been documented to be harmful, neither has it been documented to be safe and effective. See Research Box 7–1.

**RESEARCH BOX 7–1**

*Collins, J. L., Lutz, R. J. (1991). In vitro study of simultaneous infusion of incompatible drugs in multilumen catheters.* Heart and Lung, *20(3), 271–277.*

Researchers at the National Institutes of Health (NIH) designed an in vitro (laboratory) study using a double-lumen catheter with adjacent holes and a triple-lumen catheter with offset and staggered holes. Phenytoin (Dilantin) and TPN were chosen for the study because of their rapid and observable precipitation when mixed.

Each run of the TPN and phenytoin (Dilantin) through a double-lumen catheter resulted in clouds of precipitate near the tip of the catheter, and a solid clump of crystals formed on the tip itself. When either drug alone was infused through one lumen, no precipitate formed.

Infusions through the triple-lumen catheter with these same agents netted no immediate precipitate, although a thin white film formed near the mouths of the proximal and middle side holes when phenytoin was infused through them. The film was most pronounced on the middle hole when TPN was infused simultaneously through the proximal hole.

**Nursing Implications**

The results of this study have implications for the nursing care of clients with multiple-lumen catheters. Incompatible drugs should not be administered simultaneously with double-lumen catheters. When administering incompatible drugs simultaneously through triple- or quadruple-lumen catheters, the nurse should use the lumens with the most distal holes as designated near the catheter lumen hub.

The duration of the therapy affects the type of catheter chosen for a particular client. Clients whose therapy will last a relatively short time (6 weeks or less) can usually receive this therapy through a direct insertion catheter placed in the chest, neck, or arm veins. Clients receiving many weeks or cycles of chemotherapy or TPN probably require a long-term tunneled catheter or surgically placed port.

## CLIENT LIFESTYLE AND ACTIVITY

The client who will receive infusions for a long period of time or who has an active lifestyle may not want an external catheter. These clients frequently prefer surgically implanted ports. These catheters are completely internal, and there is only evidence of the catheter when it is accessed for an infusion. This feature keeps the client from being constantly reminded of his or her illness by a catheter exiting from the chest.

As a safety measure, clients who are confused and who require long-term infusions may benefit from an implanted port over a catheter that exits from the chest. When the catheter is not accessed for an infusion, there is nothing for the confused client (who may forget that the catheter is there) to pull on. Therefore this prevents the confused client from inadvertently injuring himself or herself by pulling out the catheter.

## Setting

When determining which type of catheter to place for the home care client, the physician, nurse, and client should also consider the capabilities and limitations of the client both socially and financially. Long-term external catheters require more care and maintenance than surgically implanted ports. The external catheters require more frequent flushing and dressing changes than implanted ports and therefore are more expensive in terms of time and money. These are considerations for any group of clients but particularly for the elderly who may have to depend on the home health nurse to provide maintenance care for the CVC.

Clients who are in long-term care facilities can benefit from central lines because they are easier to use and require less staff time for maintenance while ensuring venous access. Table 7–1 outlines generic care requirements for each type of central vascular access device. Individual agency policies may differ, and the nurse is advised to follow those protocols.

## SHORT-TERM THERAPY

Clients requiring CVCs for less than 6 to 8 weeks generally have catheters placed directly through the skin and into the vein. The insertion site for this type of catheter may be into one of the neck veins (the internal or external jugular),

**TABLE 7–1**
**Central Venous Catheter Generic Maintenance Schedule**

| Catheter | Flush | Frequency | Dressing Change |
|---|---|---|---|
| Hickman, Broviac | 2.5 mL 10 U/mL heparinized saline | Each day | 3 times per week for 6 weeks; then once each week |
| Groshong tip | 5 mL 0.9% NSS | Each week | 3 times per week for 6 weeks; then once each week |
| Direct insertion | 2.5 mL 10 U/mL heparinized saline | Each day | 3 times per week |
| Port | In use: 2.5 mL 10 U/mL heparinized saline | Each day | Each week with needle changes |
| | Not in use: 5 mL 100 U/mL heparinized saline | Each month | None |
| PICC | 3 mL 100 U/mL heparinized saline | Each day | 3 times per week |

PICC = peripherally inserted central catheter.

a chest vein (the subclavian), or an arm vein (the basilic or cephalic).

## Neck or Chest Vein Catheters

A number of different catheters made of a variety of materials are available for insertion into the neck or chest veins. Some are made of different types of polyurethane, whereas others are made of Silastic. The catheters range in length from 6 inches (15 cm) to 12 inches (30 cm) and in size from 4F to 7F. During the insertion process the physician measures the appropriate length of the catheter based on anatomic landmarks. Because of the anatomy, longer catheters are usually required for left-sided insertions. In the average client a 6-inch (15-cm) catheter reaches the superior vena cava when placed in the right or left subclavian or the right internal jugular vein. A left-sided approach through the jugular vein usually requires an 8-inch (20-cm) catheter.

Most single-lumen catheters have a hole at the distal end of the catheter. Most multiple-lumen catheters have holes at the end of the catheter as well as one, two, or three holes (depending on the number of lumens) on the sides of the catheter in staggered positions approximately 1 inch (2.5 cm) apart. Except for the holes on the side, this part of the catheter appears the same on single- and multiple- lumen catheters. In the multiple-lumen catheter the body of the catheter (the part inserted into the client) is actually a sheath that surrounds all the lumens, making it appear to be a single-lumen catheter, but each lumen is truly separate with no communication between the lumens. At the point where the catheter enters the skin the catheter usually has a tab for sutures. From this tab the catheter may have one or more "tails," one for each lumen. At the end of each "tail" is a female hub that accepts a slip, Luer lock, or slip Luer connection. Just proximal to the female hub, mutliple-lumen catheters have the name of the lumen listed on them. The distal lumen exits through the hole at the end of the catheter. The median lumen exits at the hole on the side of the catheter that is most distal, and the proximal lumen exits through the side hole most proximal. The hubs of the catheter are usually color coded, but the color coding is not standard across manufacturers, and the nurse must check for the lumen labels.

### CLIENT EDUCATION

Client education can easily be accomplished at the client's bedside. The staff nurse may be asked to assist or the agency may have a team whose responsibilities include the insertion of central lines. In either case a well-prepared client can assist with making the insertion a success.

The nurse describes the procedure to the client, allaying any fear of pain and explaining that the client should only feel a pressure in the insertion area. Many agencies require signed consent forms for clients in whom a central line is to be placed. The nurse follows the agency's policy regarding this. Instructions to the client include alerting the physician or nurse should the client develop any respiratory difficulty.

## GATHERING SUPPLIES

Catheters are available individually or in insertion kits. The outside packaging lists supplies included in the kit and the size and length of the catheter.

If a kit is not available, to insert the catheter the physician generally requires the supplies listed below. Unless this is an emergency placement, the physician should use full aseptic technique, including hand washing, sterile gloves, mask, hat, and gown. The nurse discusses with the physician which approach he or she will use and, using either the criteria outlined above or the physician's request, obtains the following:

- Catheter of the appropriate size and length
- Suitable antiseptic material to wash and prepare the skin
- Two 18-gauge 1- to 1½-inch (3.75-cm) needles
- 25-gauge ⅝-inch (1.6-cm) needle
- Local anesthetic such as 1% lidocaine (Xylocaine)
- Three sterile drapes or barriers (two nonfenestrated and one fenestrated)
- Solution to flush each catheter lumen (usually 0.9% normal saline solution [NSS])
- Alcohol preps
- Three or four sterile 4 × 4's
- Scalpel
- Requested suture material
- Two or three (each) 5- and 10-cc syringes.

If the client is to receive IV fluids when the catheter is placed, the nurse has the solution with the IV tubing primed and ready for infusion. Any medication administration is delayed until the catheter placement is verified by radiography, unless this is an emergency placement. If the catheter is not to be used immediately, the nurse supplies the physician with an intermittent injection cap for each catheter lumen if they are not provided with the catheter or kit. The appropriate flushing solution is also needed to maintain patency.

## CLIENT PREPARATION

If the physician elects a subclavian approach, the nurse adjusts the client's bed or the procedure table to a Trendelenburg position. The client's head is turned away from the proposed insertion site at about a 45-degree angle. A rolled sheet is placed between the client's shoulders along the upper thoracic vertebral column. The client drops his or her shoulders posteriorly. The client's arms should be at his or her sides; the client is instructed to reach for his or her toes.

If the physician plans an internal jugular approach, the nurse places the client in the Trendelenburg position with his or her head extended and turned 45 degrees away from the proposed insertion site.

## ASSISTING WITH THE PROCEDURE

The nurse's role in the insertion procedure is threefold: (1) provide support and comfort, (2) assess the client, and (3) assist the physician. Frequently, the client's face and head are covered with the sterile drape or barrier during the procedure. This can be frightening to the client. It is helpful for the nurse to explain what the physician is doing at each part of the procedure, as this may help the client to relax.

The physician may ask the nurse to open packages of syringes and 4 × 4's or other supplies and drop the contents onto the sterile field. This keeps the item sterile so there is no contamination when the physician uses it with his or her sterile-gloved hands. The nurse holds the vials of lidocaine (Xylocaine) or 0.9% NSS upside down so that the physician can insert the needle and draw up the medication or solution. The field must not be contaminated during the procedure. The nurse never hands anything directly to the physician. The nurse opens each item using the tear-down packaging and drops it onto the sterile field.

## SUBCLAVIAN VEIN APPROACH

There are many ways an individual physician may choose to insert a central line. This outline describes one method the nurse may see for the subclavian approach.

1. The physician prepares the catheter by priming each lumen with 0.9% NSS in a syringe. This helps to avoid air embolism during the insertion procedure.
2. The physician usually inserts the catheter about $\frac{3}{8}$ inch (1 cm) below the curve at the midpoint of the clavicle.
3. As the anesthetic is administered, the physician uses the $\frac{5}{8}$-inch needle to raise a skin wheal. The physician punctures the anesthetized skin with one hand while pressing gently into the suprasternal notch with the other hand. The physician advances the needle in a horizontal direction underneath the clavicle, aiming for the site marked by his or her index finger.
4. Many physicians prefer to locate the subclavian vein initially with a small-diameter needle attached to a syringe. The needle is then withdrawn, and an 18-gauge needle on a syringe is inserted and passed along the same path.

When venous access is verified by the ability to easily aspirate blood, the syringe is removed, and a guide wire is inserted through the needle. Guide wires may have depth markings to measure the wire's advancement. It is especially important for the nurse to carefully monitor the client's pulse during guide wire and catheter placement. Arrhythmias or cardiac puncture are most likely to occur during these parts of the procedure.

5. At this point the physician removes the needle, leaving the guide wire in place. The physician makes a small incision in the skin at the insertion site with the scalpel. A dilator slides over the guide wire to enlarge the passage. The dilator is then removed. While firmly holding the guide wire, the physician threads the catheter over it and advances the catheter to a graduation on the catheter previously determined to be the desired length.
6. The physician flushes each catheter lumen to maintain patency, using the amount and solution outlined in agency policy, and sutures the catheter to the client's skin through the suture holes on the tab. Antibiotic ointment is applied to the insertion site, and the area is covered with a sterile dressing.
7. Unless it is an emergency, the physician may request that the nurse infuse nonmedicated IV fluids at a rate just rapidly enough to keep the vein open (KVO) until catheter placement is verified by radiography. In an emergency the client is stabilized, and the radiography is performed when the client no longer requires lifesaving procedures.
8. The nurse documents the procedure, including the number of attempts at insertion, the sites, the size and gauge of catheter inserted, and the client's tolerance of the procedure.

If the attempt to encannulate the subclavian vein is not successful, the physician obtains a chest x-ray examination before attempting insertion into the opposite subclavian vein. This x-ray examination is necessary to rule out any clinically undetected pneumothorax or hemothorax.

## INTERNAL JUGULAR VEIN APPROACH

Use of the internal jugular approach is associated with less risk of pneumothorax than is the subclavian route. Because of the anatomy, a right-sided approach is preferred.

1. The physician prepares the catheter by priming each lumen with 0.9% NSS in a syringe. This helps to avoid air embolism during the insertion procedure.
2. As with the subclavian approach, the physician may use a small locator needle. After withdrawing this nee-

dle, an 18-gauge needle on syringe is inserted near the medial border of the clavicular head of the sternocleidomastoid muscle.

3. The physician palpates and displaces the common carotid artery to the side while advancing the needle under the muscle toward the thoracic inlet at a 30-degree downward angle. The needle enters the vein just above the thoracic inlet.
4. At this point the physician passes the guide wire through the needle lumen to the appropriate length.
5. The 18-gauge needle is removed, and the dilator is threaded over the wire.
6. After removing the dilator, the physician advances the catheter over the guide wire into position.
7. The physician flushes each catheter lumen to maintain patency per agency policy and sutures the catheter to the client's skin through the suture holes on the tab. Antibiotic ointment is applied to the insertion site, and the area is covered with a sterile dressing.
8. Unless it is an emergency, the physician may request that the nurse infuse nonmedicated IV fluids at a rate just rapidly enough to KVO until catheter placement is verified by radiography. In an emergency the client is stabilized, and the radiography is performed when the client no longer requires lifesaving procedures.
9. The nurse documents the procedure, including the number of attempts at insertion, the sites, the size and gauge of catheter inserted, and the client's tolerance of the procedure.

### EXCHANGING THE CATHETER

If the client's therapy exceeds the initially intended time frame or if it is determined that a catheter with a different number of lumens is needed, the catheter may be changed. The physician can accomplish this by inserting a guide wire into the catheter and removing the catheter. A fresh catheter is then inserted over the guide wire, and the guide wire is removed. As with the initial insertion, this procedure is completed under strict aseptic technique.

## Peripherally Inserted Central Catheters

The peripherally inserted central catheter (PICC) is a relatively new device that provides reliable central venous access. Also known as long arm or long line catheters, the PICC can be inserted at the bedside. The procedure can be performed by a physician or in some states by a registered nurse certified to perform it. The potential complications associated with these devices are fewer and less severe than those found with chest and neck central line placement.

These catheters are available from a number of manufacturers in sizes ranging from 23- to 16-gauge and 7¾ to 23½ inches (20 to 60 cm) in length. PICC lines are made of polyvinyl chloride, silicone, polyethylene, and polyurethane. They can be inserted using guide wires, stylets, or introducers. The catheters can be purchased in kits or as a single item.

PICCs are usually single lumen and have a hole at the distal end of the catheter. The Catheter Technology Corporation, however, manufactures a Groshong PICC, which has a slit-valve opening (Fig. 7–3).

## CLIENT EDUCATION

The catheter insertion can be performed at the bedside. As with any procedure, the nurse explains to the client what to expect to see and feel during the insertion process. The nurse encourages the client to ask questions, and the nurse answers using terms understandable to the lay person. If the agency requires a signed consent form, the nurse obtains it.

## GATHERING SUPPLIES

The supplies required for the insertion include the following:

- PICC
- Introducer needle
- Dressing material
- Suitable antiseptic material to wash and prepare the skin

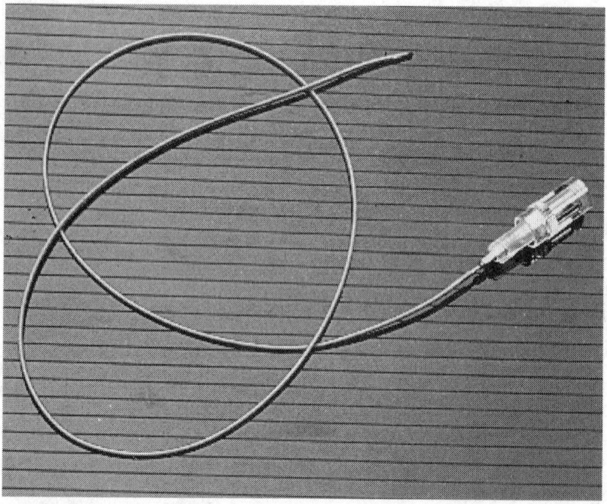

**FIGURE 7–3.** A Groshong peripherally inserted central catheter (PICC). (Courtesy of Bard Access Systems, Salt Lake City, Utah.)

- A sterile 2 × 2 package
- Two sterile 4 × 4 packages
- Two pair of sterile gloves
- A fenestrated drape
- Two nonfenestrated drapes
- Tape measure
- 4-inch (10-cm) extension tubing
- Injection cap
- Stainless steel half-covered forceps (smooth)
- Two 10-cc syringes with 21-gauge needles
- Alcohol preps
- Steri-strips
- Tape
- 10-mL vial of 0.9% NSS
- 5-mL vial of heparin 100 U/mL (or concentration specified in agency policy)
- Tourniquet
- Mask, goggles, and gown

## CLIENT PREPARATION

The nurse positions the client on the client's back. The client's arm intended for the catheter insertion is abducted to a 90-degree angle. The client positions his or her head toward the insertion site.

## PROCEDURE

There are some differences in the insertion procedures for each manufacturer's PICC. They are minor, but the nurse is advised to read the package insert of the individual catheter to assure safety.

Following is a generic procedure.

1. Wash your hands well with the antimicrobial scrub your agency uses.
2. Apply a tourniquet approximately 4 inches (10 cm) above the antecubital fossa. Assess venous access. If the client's basilic, cephalic, and median cubital veins are sclerosed, they may not be used for the insertion. Assess the other arm. If all veins are acceptable, the basilic vein is preferred, as it is generally straighter than the other veins and its lumen widens as it becomes the axillary vein. After making your choice, release the tourniquet.
3. Using the tape measure, determine the insertion length. Measure from the antecubital site up the arm to the shoulder and across to the midclavicular area. Continue to the sternal notch and down to the third intercostal space. This measurement determines the length of the catheter for superior vena cava placement.
4. Use one nonfenestrated drape as a sterile field on which to open and drop the supplies.
5. Don sterile mask and gloves. Place the second nonfenestrated sterile drape under the client's arm.

6. Prepare the insertion site from midupper arm to mid-lower arm with the alcohol prep sticks, followed by the povidone-iodine prep sticks. Use each stick once, cleaning in a circular motion from the insertion site out. Allow the povidone-iodine to air dry.
7. Place the fenestrated drape over the cleansed arm with the hole positioned over the intended insertion site.
8. Prime the extension set with 0.9% NSS and attach the intermittent injection cap if necessary.
9. Reapply the tourniquet around the upper arm, taking care not to contaminate the fenestrated drape.
10. Remove your gloves and put on a new pair of sterile gloves.
11. Using the introducer needle provided with the catheter, perform the venipuncture.
12. Thread the catheter through the needle about 2 to 3 inches (5 to 7.5 cm), taking care not to withdraw or pull back on the catheter through the needle (Table 7–2).
13. Using a sterile 4 × 4, release the tourniquet.
14. Continue to advance the catheter until you reach the predetermined length.
15. Place your thumb about 2 inches (5 cm) above the insertion site and apply pressure to secure the catheter as the introducer needle is removed.
16. Slowly withdraw the introducer needle until it is outside of the client's skin. Press the wings of the needle together until they snap. Peel the needle from around the catheter.
17. Using the Steri-strips, secure the catheter, making a chevron with the strip. Apply a Steri-strip across the

**TABLE 7–2**
**PICC Line Precautions**

While threading the catheter through the introducer needle, the nurse must not withdraw or pull the catheter back through the needle. This could cause the needle to shear the side of the catheter. Any small pieces of the catheter that may break off could lead to a catheter embolism.

Applying pressure near the end of the introducer needle could cause the needle to cut or shear the catheter.

Because these catheters have such small lumens, infusion pump settings should be kept below 15 psi. Higher pressure can cause the catheter to rupture. Using a small tuberculin-type syringe may cause pressure levels that could rupture the catheter. Larger syringes such as 10-mL syringes produce less pressure than tuberculin-type syringes and may be used safely.

From Masoorli, S., & Angeles, T. (1990, January). PICC lines: The latest home care challenge. *RN*, pp. 44–51. Copyright © 1990 Medical Economies, Montvale, N.J. Reprinted by permission.

ends of the chevron, keeping the insertion site visible. Apply a small amount of antimicrobial ointment at the insertion site and cover the site and Steri-strips with a small transparent semipermeable membrane (TSM) dressing.

18. Attach the NSS-primed extension set to the end of the catheter and flush with 3 to 5 mL of heparinized saline in the concentration used by the agency.
19. Coil any remaining catheter tubing and place a large transparent dressing over the catheter and extension tubing connection.
20. Send the client for an x-ray for physician verification of catheter position.
21. Document the procedure in the client's medical record.

## LONG-TERM THERAPY

Clients who require infusions for more than 6 weeks should have a long-term catheter placed. Several types of catheters are used for longer term therapies. These catheters can be tunneled or implanted such as the port.

### Tunneled Catheters

Currently, three types of tunneled catheters are available for surgical placement in the client with the need for longer term venous access. They are the Broviac, Hickman, and Groshong catheters. The original tunneled right atrial catheter (Broviac) was developed by Dr. Belding Scribner and associates in the late 1960s. This was a single-lumen catheter designed primarily for use in the administration of TPN. In 1975 Dr. Robert O. Hickman modified the Broviac catheter by making it larger bore. Between 1978 and 1984 the Hickman-Broviac catheter was developed, and the mid-1980s saw the development of triple-lumen catheters. As the 1990s unfold, quadruple-lumen catheters are becoming more available.

Each of these catheters is similar in design and insertion technique. All are made of polymeric silicone (Silastic) material and are available in single, double, triple, and quadruple lumen. The catheters are usually 42 to 90 cm in length before the physician trims them during insertion. Each has a Dacron cuff that sits about 12 inches (30 cm) from the external end of the catheter (Fig. 7–4). This cuff sits under the skin where fibrous tissue develops around it. The tissue development secures the catheter in place and produces a physical barrier to the migration of organisms up the tunnel and into the circulatory system.

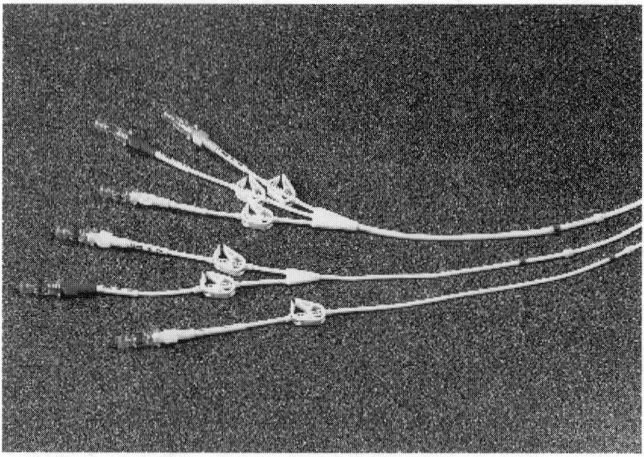

**FIGURE 7–4.** Hickman peripherally inserted central catheters (PICCs). (Courtesy of Bard Access Systems, Salt Lake City, Utah.)

## VITACUFF ANTIMICROBIAL CUFF

Some physicians are now attaching a second cuff to the catheter to provide protection against CVC-related infections. This second cuff, called a VitaCuff Antimicrobial Cuff (Davol), can be attached to any CVC during insertion and is attached just under the skin at the insertion site of direct insertion catheters or at the exit site of tunneled catheters. The VitaCuff is a device comprising two concentric layers of material (Fig. 7–5). The outer layer encourages tissue in- growth into the outer porous matrix of the cuff for creation of a bacterial barrier at the skin interface. This matrix is impregnated with silver ions, which provide an antimicrobial effect at the insertion site. This cuff is initially in a compressed state for ease of insertion. After placement, the matrix absorbs the normal body fluids and expands to approximately twice the original size. The antimicrobial activity lasts for about 4 to 6 weeks.

## HICKMAN AND BROVIAC CATHETERS

The external portions of the Hickman and Broviac catheters have a reinforced area on each lumen. When the catheter is not being used for infusions or during intermittent injection cap changes, the lumens are clamped at the reinforced area to avoid air embolism. Only clamps provided with the catheter or clamps without teeth may be used to clamp the catheter lumens. The use of a traditional Kelly clamp or other clamp with teeth cuts through the catheter similar to a pair of scissors cutting paper. This places the client at risk for air embolism, infection, and exsanguination.

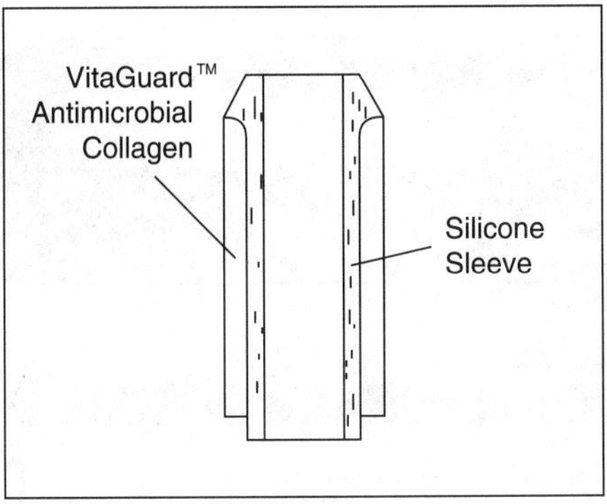


**FIGURE 7–5.** The VitaCuff antimicrobial cuff. (Courtesy of Bard Access Systems, Salt Lake City, Utah.)

## GROSHONG CATHETER

The distal tip of the Groshong catheter is not open as in the Hickman and Broviac catheters. The Groshong catheter's tip is closed and rounded. On the side of the catheter body is a slit-valve (Fig. 7–6). This valve can assume three positions: a neutral or closed position, an aspiration or negative pressure position, and an infusion or positive pressure position. Because the valve on this catheter is naturally closed, the Groshong catheter is not supplied with clamps, and manufacturer's instructions state that if the catheter is clamped, the valve can be rendered ineffective. The Groshong catheter requires only a weekly flush with 5 mL of 0.9% NSS when not in use because the valve keeps blood from backing up into the catheter.

## CLIENT EDUCATION

The nurse describes the procedure to the client and encourages questions. Explanations of the procedure including what the client will feel and hear during the insertion are given in terms the lay person can understand. Generally, an operating room or a minor surgical room is used for the insertion procedure. Tunneled catheters can be placed on an outpatient basis and the client discharged to home or a long-term-care facility a few hours after the insertion.

## INSERTION TECHNIQUE

Catheter insertion was originally performed via cephalic, external, or internal jugular vein cutdown. Since the 1980s the catheter is inserted percutaneously using a "peel-away" catheter introducer with placement into the right atrium or superior vena cava at the atrial caval junction through the cephalic vein. It is then tunneled subcutaneously and exits

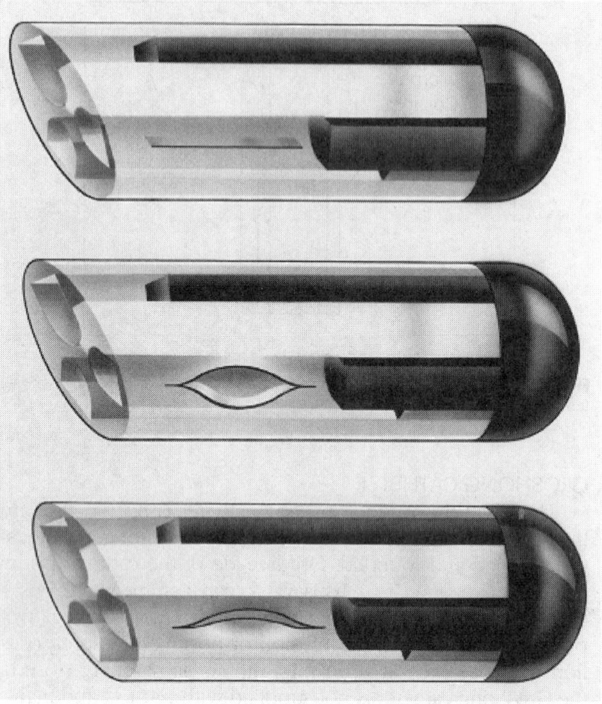

**FIGURE 7–6.** Distal tip of the Groshong catheter, with slit valve at the side of the catheter body. (Courtesy of Bard Access Systems, Salt Lake City, Utah.)

on the chest at about the third intercostal space. Catheter placement is verified by x-ray before the catheter is used.

## Implanted Ports

Ports are implanted subcutaneously to provide access to the venous system. Ports have several advantages over external venous access devices. There is less risk of infection and less interference with the client's normal daily activities. There is minimal threat to body image since the client with an implanted port has no external reminder of his or her illness.

Clients who experience needle phobia may find the need for accessing the port through the skin with a needle to be a significant disadvantage.

Implantation of a port into a client with a known infection or a client with inadequate body tissue to support the device is contraindicated. Placement of the portal body under skin that has been irradiated or under a mastectomy site is not recommended.

Implanted ports consist of a portal body, a central septum, a reservoir, and a catheter (Fig. 7–7). The portal body can be made from stainless steel, titanium, polysulione, or in a combination. The height of the portal body ranges from 9.8 to 17 mm with the base diameter ranging from 16.5 to 40 mm. Port weights range from 2.1 to 28.8 g. Internal volumes or reservoirs inside the portal body range from 0.2 to 1.47 mL. On the base are two to eight suture hole sites.

Most venous ports are inserted with the portal body implanted subcutaneously in a pocket at the clavicular area (Fig. 7–8). Some newer types of venous ports have the portal body implanted subcutaneously at the antecubital fossa. The catheters from these ports are threaded up the basilic or cephalic veins much like the PICC line.

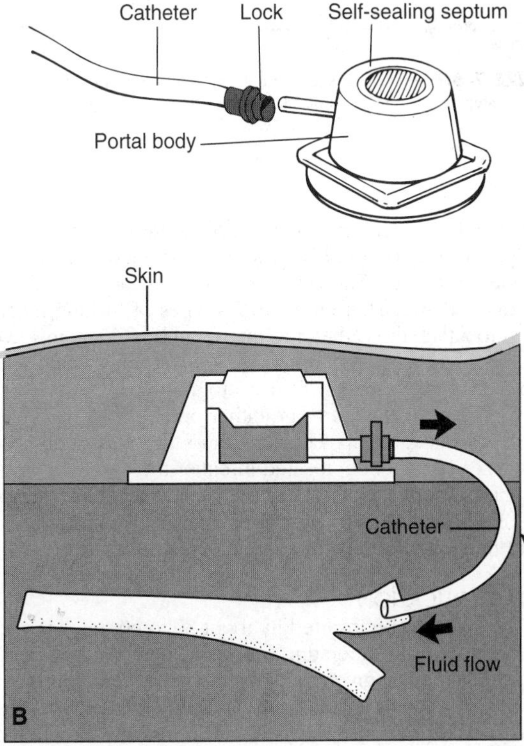


**FIGURE 7–7.** Implantable access device. (From Bolander, V. B. [1994]. *Sorensen and Luckmann's basic nursing* [3rd ed., p. 1326]. Philadelphia: W. B. Saunders.)

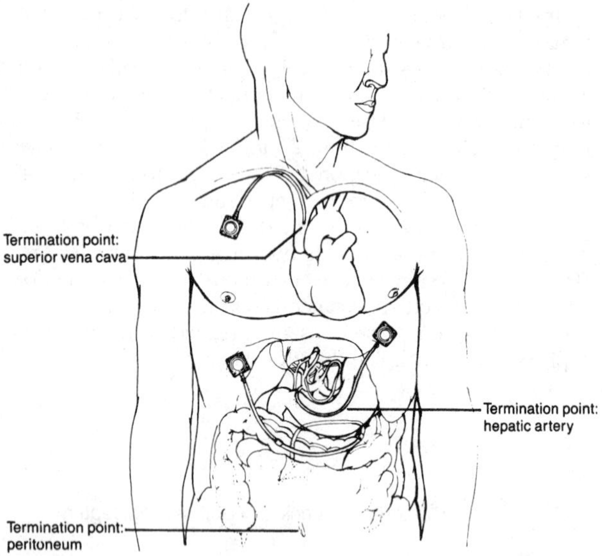


**FIGURE 7–8.** Termination sites for implanted infusion ports. (Courtesy of SIMS Deltec, Inc., St. Paul, Minnesota.)

Several manufacturers make double-lumen ports. These devices have two portal bodies, each attached to a separate catheter (Fig. 7–9). The catheters can be made from silicone or polyurethane. There are various types of locking mechanisms to attach the catheter to the portal body. The inside diameters of venous ports range from 1 to 1.6 mm with the external diameters ranging from 1.6 to 4.6 mm.

The distal tips of ports are either open ended or utilize a Groshong slit-valve tip. The septum of the port is composed of self-sealing silicone, located in either the center or on the side of the portal body. These self-sealing septa are rated by the number of needle punctures they can withstand. The usual range is from 1000 to 2000 needle punctures.

## CLIENT EDUCATION

The port can be inserted in about 30 to 60 minutes while the client is in the operating room and under local anesthesia. Clients may be given medication to relax them during the procedure. When the procedure is complete, the client has a small incision over the clavicular area closed with either staples or sutures. The client's port requires a dressing only when it is accessed for infusion. At other times no dressing is needed.

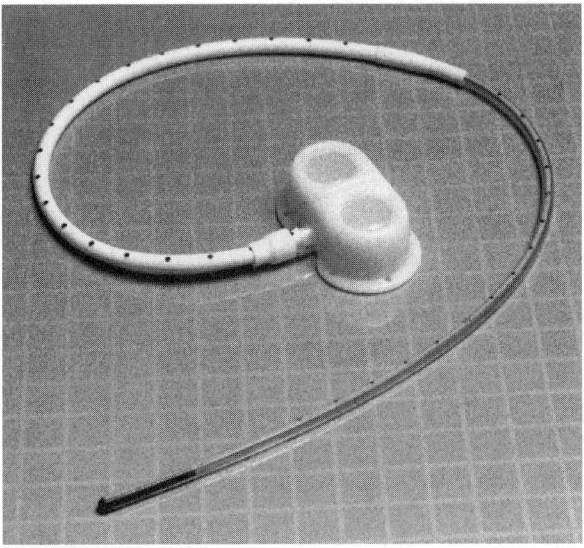

**FIGURE 7–9.** Double-lumen port. (Courtesy of Bard Access Systems, Salt Lake City, Utah.)

## INSERTION TECHNIQUE

Physicians currently use two techniques to insert ports: cut-down method or the percutaneous method, using a guide wire and a tear-away introducer. The CVC is introduced through a venotomy into the subclavian, cephalic, or exterior jugular vein, and under fluoroscopy the catheter tip is placed in the superior vena cava above the junction of the right atrium. The proximal end is subcutaneously connected to the portal body implanted in the infraclavicular fossa above the pectoralis major fascia.

Antecubital ports are placed using the same procedure as described above except that the physician uses the basilic, cephalic, or axillary vein to access the superior vena cava.

The PAS Port (Deltec) (Fig. 7–10) is a unique antecubital port that can be implanted using a sensor wire–catheter tracking system, while the client is at the physician's office or in bed in the hospital. This precludes the necessity of fluoroscopy. The device comes preassembled with a sensor wire that is introduced into the vein and advanced into the superior vena cava. The physician uses the locator wand's visual and audible signals and external anatomic landmarks (the third rib and sternum) for guidance in determining the location of the catheter tip. After the catheter is placed, the portal body is subcutaneously implanted below the antecubital fossa.

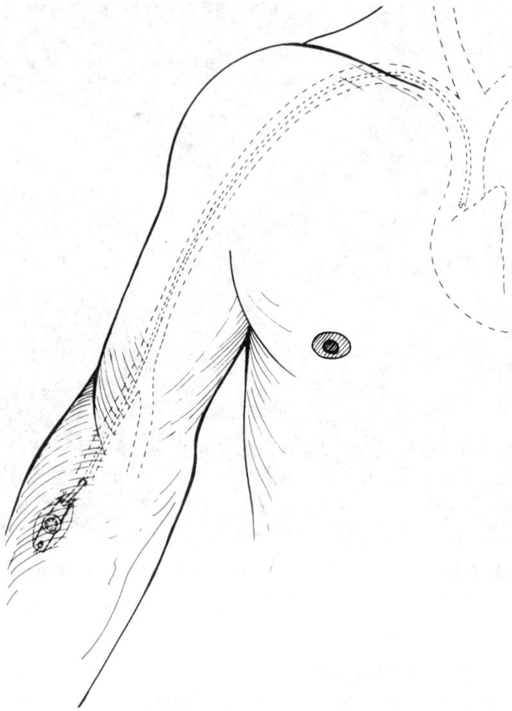

**FIGURE 7–10.** Anatomic location of PAS Port. (Courtesy of SIMS Deltec, Inc., St. Paul, Minnesota.)

## Accessing Ports

### CLIENT PREPARATION

Explain the procedure to the client in terms the lay person understands. Describe what the client will feel such as the wetness and coldness of the cleansing material and a needle stick. Position the client on his or her back with the port area and about 6 inches (15 cm) surrounding the port exposed.

### EQUIPMENT

Only Huber-point needles are appropriate for use in accessing a port (Fig. 7–11). The angle of the bevel of these needles prevents coring of the portal septum. Huber-point needles are available in various lengths and sizes. Some have a 90-degree bend along the needle shaft that allows them to sit flush with the skin while the port is accessed during an infusion. Many of these needles come with an extension set

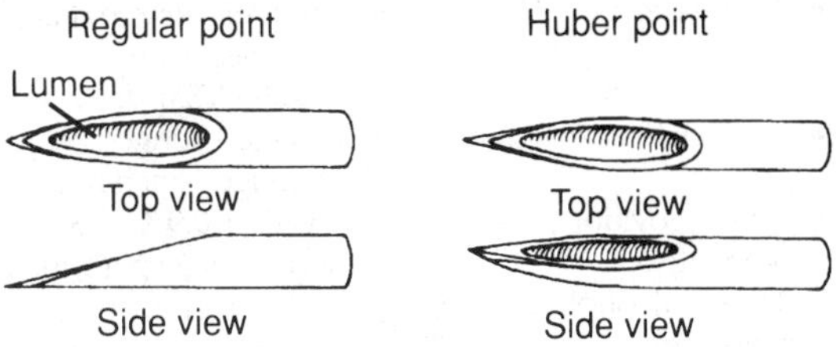


**FIGURE 7–11.** Needle points. Only Huber-point needles are appropriate for accessing a port. (From DeWit, S. C. *Rambo's nursing skills for clinical practice* [4th ed., p. 924]. Philadelphia: W. B. Saunders.)

that easily accepts an intermittent injection cap or IV tubing and butterfly wings on either side of the needle. The nurse may see other Huber-point needles that are straight. These are appropriate for the monthly maintenance flush required to maintain patency of the venous port.

A recent innovation in Huber-point needles is the foam-covered base that eliminates the need for a gauze under the needle holder (Fig. 7–12).

## GATHERING SUPPLIES

To access a port for infusion the nurse needs the following supplies:

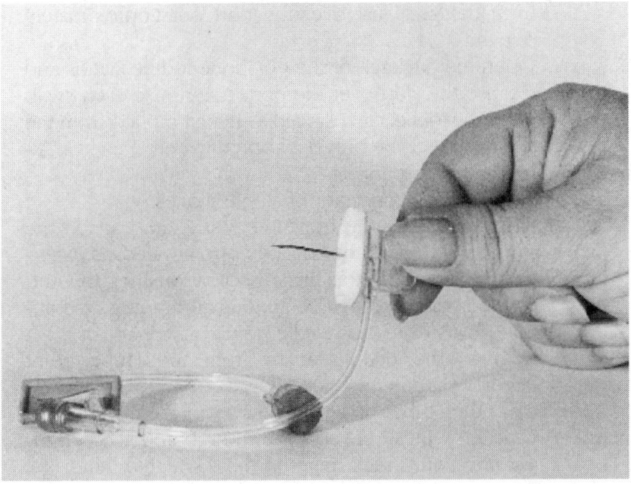

**FIGURE 7–12.** Huber-point needle with foam-covered base, which eliminates the need for a gauze under the needle holder. (Photograph courtesy Monica Ridgely.)

- A 90-degree Huber-point needle of appropriate length
- Two pairs of sterile gloves
- Three povidone-iodine prep sticks
- Three alcohol-acetone prep sticks
- A nonfenestrated drape or sterile barrier
- A 2 × 3 TSM dressing
- A 10-cc syringe with a 22-gauge 1-inch needle
- A vial of 0.9% NSS
- Sterile 2 × 2 split gauze

## PROCEDURE

1. Wash your hands with the antiseptic agent provided by the agency.
2. Open the sterile barrier.
3. Tear down the packages of the Huber-point needle, TSM dressing, and syringe and drop each supply onto the sterile barrier.
4. Open a pair of sterile gloves and put them on.
5. Maintaining your dominant hand sterile, hold the vial of 0.9% NSS in your nondominant hand. With the syringe in your dominant hand draw up approximately 5 mL of sterile 0.9% NSS. Place the filled syringe back on the sterile barrier.
6. Remove and discard the gloves.
7. Locate the portal body by palpating the area.
8. Open the package of the alcohol-acetone prep sticks and cleanse the skin over the port. Use each swab stick once, cleansing in a circular motion from the area just over the port out approximately 3 inches.
9. Open the package of the povidone-iodine swabs and cleanse the skin over the port. Again, use each swab stick only once, cleansing in a circular motion from the area just over the port out approximately 3 inches. Allow the area to air dry.
10. Put on the second pair of sterile gloves.
11. Remove the needle from the syringe and attach the syringe to the end of the Huber-point needle's extension set. Prime the extension set by pushing the end of the syringe plunger until a small amount of solution drops from the needle point.
12. Remove the needle guard from the Huber-point needle.
13. Hold the Huber-point needle in your dominant hand with the wings between your thumb and second finger and your index finger at the 90-degree bend.
14. With your nondominant hand, isolate the port between your second and third fingers to stabilize the portal body.

15. Insert the needle into the center of the port septum in one straight motion, pushing down until you feel the back of the portal body. Do not rock the needle back and forth. As the needle enters the port, you will feel a resistance as the needle pierces the septum, then no resistance as the needle passes through the reservoir, and then a stop as the needle hits the back of the portal body.
16. Release the needle and aspirate with the syringe until you get blood back in the extension set.
17. When the insertion is verified by the ability to aspirate blood, flush the needle with the 0.9% NSS in the syringe. Flushing should be easy and require little pressure on the syringe plunger.
18. Apply the TSM dressing over the accessed port. If the wings of the Huber-point needle do not sit flush with the skin, place a sterile gauze under the wings to stabilize them and then apply the dressing.
19. Close the clamp on the extension set, remove the syringe, and attach the primed IV administration set to the end of the extension set. Adjust the rate on the infusion.

## COMPLICATIONS

All vascular access devices have a risk of complication. The key to prevention of most of these complications is expert nursing care. The nurse follows strict aseptic technique in the handling of the catheter and all infusion supplies and equipment. Careful assessment and adherence to all care protocols and agency policies and procedures assist the nurse in providing the care the client with a central vascular access device requires.

Client/caregiver education helps prevent complications. Many clients require maintenance care of their catheters in a site other than a health care setting. Frequently this requires that the client or a significant other take responsibility for the care of the catheter. Therefore, it is imperative that the nurse educate the client or caregiver in all aspects of catheter care.

Some of the potential complications associated with central vascular access devices are due to improper insertion, some to mechanical failure, and still others are due to infection.

### External Catheter Breakage or Puncture

**Definition.** The catheter may have damage at any point along the external body. This damage can be in the form of tiny pin holes or a complete breaking of the catheter.

**Cause.** Damage may be caused by using large-bore or long needles through an intermittent injection cap or using scissors near the catheter. Catheter damage may be the result of clamping the catheter with clamps that have teeth (Kelly clamp) or flushing the catheter against a closed clamp.

**Signs and Symptoms.** The catheter may have pin holes in the catheter body near the hub, or there may be a "blow-out" hole between the clamp and injection cap. The catheter may actually be in two pieces. The nurse or client may notice leaking during or after flushing.

**Treatment.** The nurse clamps the catheter between the client and the damaged area(s). Using the appropriate repair kit, the physician or trained nurse repairs the catheter. If the repair is unsuccessful, the catheter is removed.

**Documentation.** The nurse documents the catheter damage and any treatment in the client's record.

**Prevention.** To avoid catheter damage only needles less than 1 inch (2.5 cm) in length and less than 21 gauge should be used for flushing. All sharp objects and scissors are kept away from the catheter. All caregivers should remember that when flushing, if any resistance is met, the caregiver STOPS flushing and assures that the catheter clamp is open. The caregiver tapes the extra catheter length to the client's chest or arm in a manner that avoids the possibility of damage to the catheter.

## Occlusion

**Definition.** Catheter obstruction that may prevent infusion or withdrawal through the catheter is called occlusion.

**Cause.** The occlusion of the catheter may be due to a thrombus development; lipid deposits; precipitation of drugs, minerals, or electrolytes; or a malposition of the catheter.

**Signs and Symptoms.** Fluid may or may not infuse. It is likely that the catheter will not draw. The client may complain of discomfort in the shoulder, neck, or arm at the insertion site. Nurse may observe edema in the client's neck or shoulder and an increase in collateral circulation over chest area.

**Treatment.** The client should turn side to side, raise arms over the head, and cough and deep breath. These actions may move an extraluminal clot from the lumen outlet hole. The nurse may attempt a gentle push-pull technique with a 0.9% NSS syringe attached directly to the catheter hub. A venogram may be necessary to determine the size and location of the occlusion. If the occlusion is secondary to a blood clot, the physician may order thrombolytic administration; if the occlusion is from drug precipitate, the physician may order hydrochloric acid or ethanol solution (see Table 7–3). If these measures are unsuccessful, the catheter must be removed.

**Documentation.** The nurse documents all information obtained from the client assessment, techniques used, and results of any trouble-shooting efforts.

**Prevention.** The caregiver follows appropriate flushing protocol. Some physicians may order low-dose oral anticoagulant therapy for clients with CVCs. The nurse flushes with ample 0.9% NSS especially between incompatible drugs. The caregiver tapes any extra length of catheter to the client's chest or arm in a manner that avoids tugging on the catheter.

**TABLE 7–3**
**Evaluation of Silastic Catheter Patency**

When the nurse is unable to infuse or withdraw through a Silastic catheter, a catheter occlusion may be the cause. In certain situations, catheter patency has been restored using thrombolytic agents, ethyl alcohol, hydrochloric acid, or sodium bicarbonate. Before attempting to restore patency pharmacologically, the following steps should be taken to ensure that the catheter is not merely kinked or malpositioned.

1. Verify placement of the tip by x-ray.
2. Review the procedures, medications, and solutions for which the catheter was used.
3. Check for mechanical obstruction such as kinking or occlusive sutures.
4. Observe the client for swelling of the head, face, neck, and arms and distended collateral circulation over the chest.
5. Manually flush the catheter by attaching a 10-mL syringe directly to the catheter and attempting to flush with 5 mL 0.9% NSS. If unsuccessful, attempt to aspirate.
6. If the catheter can be irrigated but not aspirated, reposition the client side to side or sitting to lying. Try a smaller syringe (5 or 3 mL). Have the client assist with changing the intrathoracic pressure by raising the arms and waving side to side, coughing or deep breathing with slow exhale, or performing the Valsalva maneuver.
7. If these manipulations are successful and blood can be aspirated, flush the catheter vigorously with 10 to 20 mL of 0.9% NSS and resume the IV fluid administration or cap the catheter and heparinize according to agency policy.

If the catheter can be flushed but not aspirated, it is likely that the catheter may have developed a fibrin flap or sheath at the catheter tip. Left untreated, the flap or sheath may calcify and make both aspiration and infusion impossible. Treatment with thrombolytics such as streptokinase or urokinase usually restores patency by lysing the thrombus.

If the catheter can not be irrigated or aspirated, attempt to determine the cause by reviewing what drugs and solutions have been infused through the catheter. TPN prepared as a total nutrient admixture (TNA or three-in-one solution) has been known to cause the development of a waxy lipid material on the end of the catheter that causes infusion as well as aspiration difficulties. In these cases, patency can be reestablished by using a lipid solvent solution of 70% ethyl alcohol. A volume equal to the catheter volume is instilled and allowed to dwell for 1 to 2 hours.

The inability to infuse or aspirate may also be caused by the infusion of poorly soluble or incompatible medications into the CVC. This may result in the formation of a precipitate that occludes the catheter. Frequently, solubility can be improved by altering the pH. If a precipitate of medications or minerals is suspected, it must first be determined if increasing or decreasing the pH improves solubility.

*Continued*

**TABLE 7–3**
**Evaluation of Silastic Catheter Patency Continued**

If the medications are acidic or solubility can be improved by decreasing the pH, 0.1N HCl acid can be administered. This formula has been successfully used to clear occlusions of etoposide crystals and calcium phosphate precipitate and an occlusion due to the sequential administration of amikacin, piperacillin, vancomycin, and heparin.

If the occlusion is suspected of being the result of the administration of basic medications, increasing the pH may improve solubility. In these cases the use of sodium bicarbonate ($NaHCO_3$) has been reported to clear an occlusion caused by clavulanic acid–ticarcillin (Ticar), oxacillin (Bactocill), and heparin and even a phenytoin (Dilantin) occlusion.

Knowing whether to increase or decrease the pH to restore patency is frequently difficult. In a clinical situation, if changing the pH one way does not restore patency, it is reasonable to try changing the pH in the other direction before resorting to removing the catheter.

To administer the pharmacologic agent use the following procedure:

1. Obtain the pharmacologic agent from the pharmacy.
2. Cleanse the catheter hub and cap junction with povidone-iodine solution and allow to dry.
3. Draw up the appropriate amount of agent (catheter volume specific) into a 1-mL syringe.
4. Clamp the catheter and remove the cap.
5. Attach the syringe to the catheter hub.
6. Unclamp the catheter and slowly inject the pharmacologic agent into the catheter. If the catheter does not inject easily, instill the agent with a gentle repeated push-pull action.
7. Clamp the catheter, remove the syringe, and apply a sterile cap.
8. Allow urokinase to dwell from 30 to 60 minutes; ethyl alcohol, hydrochloric acid, or sodium bicarbonate for 60 minutes.
9. At the end of the appropriate dwell time, cleanse the cap or catheter junction with povidone-iodine solution and allow to dry.
10. Remove the cap and attach a 10-mL syringe to the catheter. Attempt to aspirate the agent and blood.
11. If able to aspirate easily, remove between 3 and 6 mL of blood. Clamp the catheter.
12. Discard the aspirated blood and vigorously flush the catheter with 0.9% NSS. Reclamp the catheter.
13. Resume the IV administration as ordered or heparinize and cap the catheter according agency policy.

If this procedure is unsuccessful, it may be repeated. If the second attempt is still unsuccessful, allow the pharmacologic agent to dwell overnight. In multiple-lumen catheters each lumen probably must be treated.

From Holcombe, V. J., Forloines-Lynn, S., & Garmhausen, L. W. (1992). Restoring patency of long-term central venous access devices. *Journal of Intravenous Nursing, 15*(1), 36–41.

## Infection: Exit Site, Tunnel, Thrombus, Port Pocket

**Definition.** Infection is the invasion and multiplication of microorganisms in a body tissue, causing local cellular injury.

**Cause.** Infection is caused by a breach of aseptic technique or lack of dressing integrity.

**Signs and Symptoms.** The caregiver observes redness, drainage, edema, or tenderness at the exit site. Temperature may be above 38°C. Laboratory data may indicate increased white blood cell count (WBC), increased polymorphonuclear leukocytes (polys) and mononuclear phagocytes (monos). The nurse may be asked to draw blood cultures from the catheter and from a peripheral site. This assists the physician in determining if the infection is truly from the catheter or if the infection is from another site.

**Treatment.** The physician may order antibiotic therapy. If a thrombus is present, the physician may prescribe a thrombolytic agent. The catheter may be removed and another catheter inserted (see Research Box 7–2).

**Documentation.** The nurse records all observations, client's vital signs, and any treatments.

**Prevention.** The nurse maintains strict adherence to aseptic technique in all dealings with the catheter. The nurse highlights this aspect when instructing the client/caregiver in the care of the client's catheter.

## Dislodgment (Twiddler's Syndrome)

**Definition.** A catheter that has moved out of the superior vena cava or right atrium is said to have dislodged.

**Cause.** Catheters may become dislodged because of insecure taping, pulling on the catheter length, or trauma.

**Signs and Symptoms.** The external catheter length may be longer or shorter than the original length. There may be edema or drainage at the exit site. On palpation, the nurse

### RESEARCH BOX 7–2

*Mukau, L., Talamini, M. D., Sitzman, J. V., et al. (1992). Long-term central venous access vs. other home therapies: Complications in patients with acquired immunodeficiency syndrome.* Journal of Parenteral and Enteral Nutrition, *16(5), 455–459.*

Staff at Johns Hopkins Hospital, Baltimore, Maryland, followed 127 home care clients with 140 silicone CVCs. Fifty-six of the clients had acquired immunodeficiency syndrome (AIDS); 44 of the clients without AIDS were receiving home parenteral nutrition; and 27 non-AIDS clients received home antibiotic therapy. Catheter-related sepsis was higher among the AIDS population ($P < .01$) and in the clients receiving parenteral nutrition ($P < .05$) compared with those receiving antibiotics. Prior catheter infections and AIDS were the most significant predictors of catheter infection ($P < .01$).

Fourteen of the infected catheters were salvaged by antibiotic therapy (37.8%) after the initial episode of infection. Of these catheters six (42.9%) had recurrent multiple infections.

**Nursing Implications**

When caring for clients who require long-term CVCs, the nurse should ascertain if the client's catheter has a history of infection. This may help in predicting the client's likelihood of developing catheter-related sepsis. If the catheter becomes infected, treatment with antibiotics and catheter removal should be considered for any client who requires the catheter for longer than 30 to 60 days.

may feel coiling under the skin at the tunnel. The client's neck veins may be distended.

**Treatment.** The catheter may require removal and reinsertion.

**Documentation.** The nurse documents the external catheter length daily to assist with identifying catheter dislodgment.

**Prevention.** The external lengths of all catheters are looped and securely taped to the client's chest or arm to protect the catheter from pulls and other trauma. The caregiver avoids unnecessary hand manipulation of the portal bodies.

## Pinch-off Syndrome

**Definition.** Pinch-off syndrome is a partial catheter obstruction sometimes found with tunneled catheters placed in the subclavian vein.

**Cause.** Pinch-off syndrome occurs as the catheter enters the space between the clavicle and the first rib because of the pincher action of the clavicle and the first rib.

**Signs and Symptoms.** The caregiver may report postural resistance to flushing or infusing solutions. A chest x-ray shows a narrowing of the catheter ("pinch-off sign") as it passes over the first rib and beneath the clavicle. If undetected, the narrowing may lead to catheter fracture and infraclavicular discomfort and swelling at the time of medication injection.

**Treatment.** At the first sign of positional resistance to flushing, the nurse notifies the physician. After verification by x-ray, the physician removes the catheter. Reinsertion of the catheter at a more peripheral position is then appropriate.

**Documentation.** The nurse documents the ease of flushing and infusing of medications in the client's record.

**Prevention.** Physicians inserting tunneled catheters should enter the axillary vein at the midclavicular location.

## Infiltration/Extravasation

**Definition.** Infiltration is the inadvertent infusion or seepage of medications or fluids into the extravascular tissue. The seriousness is determined by the type of fluid or medication, concentration, and volume of the infiltrated infusate. Extravasation is the infiltration of vesicant solution or medication.

**Cause.** Infiltration is caused by a fracture of the catheter in the tunnel or the malposition of the catheter tip out of the vein. If a port is used, the Huber-point needle may have backed out of the portal body.

**Signs and Symptoms.** The tissue develops erythema or edema and has a spongy feeling. The catheter has no blood return, and IV solution does not free flow. The client may complain of pain with infusion.

**Treatment.** Discontinue infusion immediately. Notify physician and apply a warm compress if nonvesicant. If vesicant, notify physician and use manufacturer's recommended antidote. Obtain x-rays if physician requests them.

**Documentation.** The nurse records all signs and symptoms identified, approximation of amount of infiltrate/extravasation, and assessment of appearance of tissue. Notation of all treatments and client tolerance is made.

**Prevention.** The nurse always flushes the catheter with 0.9% NSS before administering medications. Assess for ease of flushing and blood return.

## Pneumothorax

**Definition.** Pneumothorax is the presence of air in the pleural cavity, resulting in the collapse of the lung on the affected side.

**Cause.** Pneumothorax occurs in approximately 5% of clients who have catheters inserted by direct subclavian approach. It also occurs when the physician punctures the pleura with a needle of the catheter during insertion of the catheter.

**Signs and Symptoms.** The client usually complains of pain on inspiration and expiration; dyspnea, apprehension, and diminished breath sounds over the affected side are often present. If untreated, pneumothorax may lead to hypoxia and shock. In some cases the client may be asymptomatic, and the pneumothorax is diagnosed during the postinsertion chest x-ray.

**Treatment.** The physician inserts a chest tube to reexpand the lung. Reexpansion may occur in a few hours or a few days.

**Documentation.** The nurse records all client signs and symptoms, as well as treatment and client tolerance. Careful records of chest tube drainage are maintained.

**Prevention.** The lung apex rises higher in the left neck than it does in the right. Therefore, the use of a right-sided subclavian approach is preferred over the left-sided approach, as this is less likely to cause a pneumothorax. Cachectic patients, those with minimal soft tissue between the clavicle and the apex of the lung, are more likely to develop pneumothorax. The arm or neck approach is preferred in these clients.

## Hemothorax

**Definition.** Hemothorax is the presence of blood in the pleural cavity.

**Cause.** Generally, hemothorax is caused by puncture of the subclavian vein or artery during catheter insertion.

**Signs and Symptoms.** Signs and symptoms are similar to those of pneumothorax, but initial symptoms are more likely to be dyspnea and tachycardia instead of pain.

**Treatment.** Same as pneumothorax.

**Documentation.** Same as pneumothorax.

**Prevention.** The use of the small needle and guide wire prevents the puncture or laceration of the back wall of the subclavian vein or artery and the parietal pleura.

## Air Embolus

**Definition.** The inadvertent entrance of air into the vascular system is called air embolus.

**Cause.** Air may enter the vasculature through an unprimed catheter during placement, through the end of an unclamped catheter, or during the removal of the catheter.

**Signs and Symptoms.** The nurse can auscultate a loud churning sound over the precordium. The client may complain of chest pain and anxiety. The nurse may find the client has tachycardia, hypotension, and hypoxia.

**Treatment.** The nurse places the client on his or her left side in a Trendelenburg position (Durant position). This relieves pulmonary vascular obstruction. The physician orders 100% oxygen.

**Documentation.** The nurse documents the signs and symptoms, treatment, and client's response to these interventions.

**Prevention.** Air embolus is avoidable. Nursing interventions such as maintaining a closed catheter system, placing the client in a Trendelenburg position for catheter placement and removal, and having the client perform the Valsalva maneuver when the system is open are all actions that assist in preventing air embolism.

## Sepsis

**Definition.** The invasion and multiplication of microorganisms in the blood stream is called sepsis.

**Cause.** Sepsis is caused by the breach of aseptic technique in dealing with the catheter or the seeding of the catheter with microorganisms from another site of infection.

**Signs and Symptoms.** The client may complain of fever, chills, headache, and general malaise. The nurse may note hypotension and tachycardia and in some cases vomiting. If untreated, the client may lapse into coma and circulatory collapse, which can lead to death (Table 7–4).

**Treatment.** Supportive therapy includes fluids and maintenance of cardiac output. The physician orders blood cul-

**TABLE 7–4**
**Identifying Catheter-Related Sepsis**

At times, despite excellent nursing care of the client's CVC, the client may develop signs and symptoms of sepsis. Frequently, the CVC is the first origin considered for the septic event, and in many cases the catheter is removed. In some cases the CVC may be the cause of the client's morbidity; however, this is not always the case. Removal of the catheter without positive identification of the site of the infection is expensive in terms of cost and further morbidity for the client. Mosca et al., (1987) described the following procedure to determine the presence of true catheter-related sepsis. It is a quantitative blood-culturing method.

1. Paint the connection between the administration set and the client's catheter with povidone-iodine solution and allow it to dry.
2. Disconnect the administration set and attach a sterile 10-mL syringe to the catheter. Withdraw 10 mL of blood and discard this sample.
3. Attach a new 10-mL syringe to the catheter and withdraw another 10 mL of blood specimen.
4. Cleanse the surface of the rubber stopper of an Isolator tube (Isolator, DuPont Company, Wilmington, Delaware) with alcohol and allow it to dry.
5. Inject the blood sample into the Isolator tube and send it to the laboratory for incubation and analysis.
6. Perform this procedure on blood from each lumen of the catheter and on blood from a peripheral venipuncture.

After 16 to 18 hours of incubation the laboratory determines the number of microbial colonies growing on each plate. If microbial colony counts from the catheter are greater than or equal to five times more than that of the peripheral blood, a central catheter-related sepsis is the diagnosis. Of course, treatment with antimicrobials is begun as soon as the specimens are obtained.

From Mosca, R., Curtas, S., Forbes, B., et al. (1987). The benefits of isolators cultures in the management of suspected catheter sepsis. *Surgery, 102,* 718–723.

tures from the catheter and from a peripheral site to determine if the catheter is truly the source of the infection. The nurse administers antibiotics and possibly steroids per the physician's order. In most cases, at the earliest possible opportunity, the physician removes the catheter and either replaces it with another catheter or administers the therapies through a peripheral IV catheter.

**Documentation**. Careful recordation of all observations, treatments, and client response to interventions is necessary.

**Prevention**. Maintenance of strict aseptic technique in the handling of the catheter and all supplies is essential. Clients who are immunocompromised, very young, or elderly are at risk for catheter-related sepsis.

# CHAPTER 8
# Subcutaneous Therapy

*Donna D. Ignatavicius*



## DESCRIPTION

Subcutaneous infusion therapy has been used as an alternative to intravenous therapy for many years. In the past fluids for rehydration were administered subcutaneously when intravenous access was not available. This method was referred to as hypodermoclysis. In recent years subcutaneous infusions have been used primarily for drug administration, especially opioids for pain management and insulin for control of diabetes mellitus.

Continuous subcutaneous infusion (CSQI or CSCI) is gaining increased popularity, particularly for clients in alternative care settings such as nursing homes and the client's home. In some countries, such as Canada, CSQI has largely taken over from continuous intravenous infusion for pain management because it enables clients to be managed on an outpatient basis (Moulin et al., 1992).

## CLIENT CONSIDERATIONS

Candidates for CSQI include clients who fit one of the following criteria:

- Are unable to take oral medications; e.g., have dysphagia, gastrointestinal obstruction, or malabsorption
- Have intractable nausea and vomiting
- Require parenteral medication but have poor venous access
- Require subcutaneous injections for greater than 48 hours
- Have a need for prolonged use of parenteral medication
- Need a continuous level of medication to control pain

- Cannot cope with the expense of intravenous therapy
- Are confused or depressed

CSQI is used most often for delivering opioid analgesics for clients with cancer. Between 60% and 90% of clients with advanced disease require an opioid analgesic to control their pain (Foley, 1985). In studies comparing the analgesic effect and side effects of subcutaneous and intravenous hydromorphone (Dilaudid), there was no significant difference (Moulin et al., 1991, 1992).

## PREPARATION FOR CSQI OF OPIOID ANALGESICS

The first step in preparing for CSQI of opioid analgesics is dose calculation. The pharmacist usually calculates the drug dose, but in some agencies the physician or nurse may determine the appropriate dose.

First, the client's previous 24-hour opioid requirement is determined. Next, this number is divided by the conversion factor for the subcutaneous route and then divided by 24 for the hourly infusion rate needed for CSQI in milligrams per hour (Table 8–1). An equianalgesic chart is used for accurate conversion to the subcutaneous route. The concentration of the drug is usually equal to or less than 1 mL/h; higher volumes may cause site irritation (McLaughlin-Hagan, 1990).

The next step in preparing for CSQI is to obtain the appropriate equipment. The equipment, especially the analgesia pump, may be different than that used in the hospital. The nurse involves the family or other caregivers in each step of teaching the client about the equipment and care for the CSQI. Most clients and families find that this drug administration technique is easier to learn than others.

## INSERTION TECHNIQUE

### Gathering Supplies

For a subcutaneous infusion, the nurse needs a 25- to 27-gauge (G) butterfly (winged) needle with infusion set (see Chapter 6 for a complete description) or a Sub-Q-Set subcutaneous infusion set (Baxter). The Sub-Q-Set has a 27G nee-

**TABLE 8–1**
**Example of Opioid Conversion for Subcutaneous Infusion**

| |
|---|
| MS Contin 45 mg b.i.d. = 90 mg/d (oral dose) |
| Conversion ratio of oral: subcutaneous = 3:1 |
| Total 24-hour subcutaneous requirement = 90 mg/3 = 30 mg per dose |
| Hourly subcutaneous infusion = 30 mg/24 h = 1.25 mg/h |

dle that is about ½ inch (1 cm) long. It is attached to a disk that lays flat against the skin after insertion (Fig. 8–1).

Alcohol sponges, waterproof tape, transparent semipermeable membrane (TSM) dressing (e.g., Tegaderm), and a portable (ambulatory) infusion pump filled with the prescribed amount of analgesic are also obtained. Most analgesia pumps have a feature that allows the programming of extra (bolus) doses. If this feature is not available, a three-way stopcock or T-connector may be used to administer extra doses.

One of several types of portable infusion pumps may be selected, depending on the client's needs, convenience, availability, and cost. The selected pump should deliver accurate doses and be easy for the client or caregiver to use. For safety, the pump should have a lock-out interval and an alarm system. It should also enable the client to administer a loading dose and extra doses if needed (see Chapter 5 for complete discussion of pumps).

One of the smallest, most convenient pumps is the Travenol infusor, a plastic, disposable cylinder that may be clipped to the client's clothes. This elastomeric balloon pump is about 6 by 1 inch (16 by 2.5 cm) and weighs about 3 oz (90 g) when filled with the drug. It can deliver a total volume of 48 mL in 24 hours at a fixed rate of 2 mL/h. Hydromorphone (Dilaudid) and morphine sulfate are commonly used opioid analgesics. The major disadvantage of the Travenol infusor is that it can only be used for a 24-hour period.

Other pumps, such as the programmable Pharmacia CADD-PCA or the Cormed pump, tend to be more complicated and weigh more than the Travenol pump. These

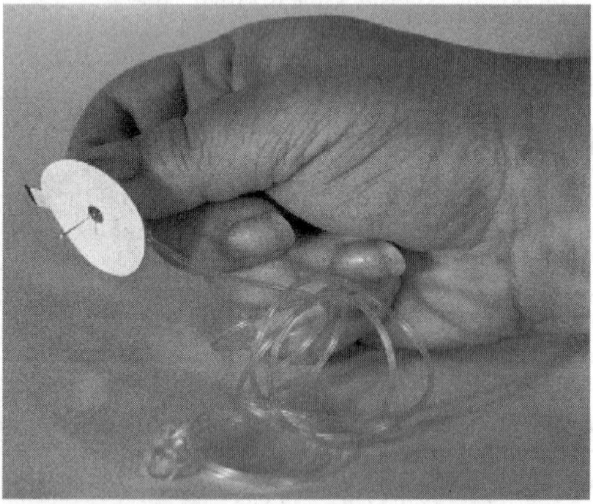

**FIGURE 8–1.** The Baxter Sub-Q-Set infusion set has a 27-gauge, ½-inch needle attached to a disk that lays flat against the skin. (Photograph courtesy of Monica Ridgely.)

pumps are carried in a holster around the client's waist or in a pocket. The Cormed pump is simpler and less expensive than the Pharmacia pump but may need a nurse or other health care professional for troubleshooting if problems occur. From a cost perspective, studies have shown that the programmable pumps, such as the Pharmacia CADD-PCA, are more cost-effective than disposable pumps, such as the Travenol infusor (Moulin et al., 1992).

## Performing the Subcutaneous Puncture

When performing the subcutaneous puncture, the nurse can use any area of the body that has sufficient subcutaneous tissue. Sites for needle insertion include the abdomen, thigh, upper arm, and supraclavicular area (upper chest). These areas allow the client to see the insertion site and cause minimal discomfort. For ambulatory clients the upper chest is a preferred site because it allows for unrestricted client mobility (Fig. 8–2).

Before insertion, the nurse primes the needle with the drug to be infused. The selected site is properly cleansed with alcohol, and the butterfly needle is inserted into the subcutaneous tissue at a 35- to 45-degree angle. The Sub-Q-Set needle is inserted at a 90-degree angle because it is shorter than the butterfly needle. The nurse anchors the needle with waterproof tape and covers the insertion site with a TSM dressing. (The procedure for applying a TSM dressing is described in Chapter 6.)

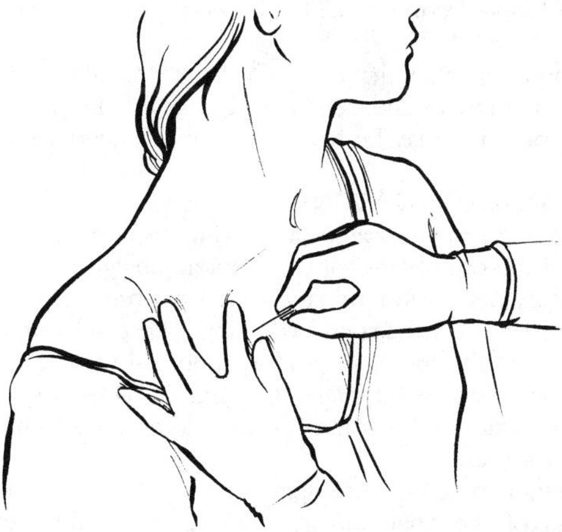

**FIGURE 8–2.** Insertion of a 23-gauge butterfly needle into the tissue of the upper chest. (From McLaughlin-Hagan, M. [1990]. Continuous subcutaneous infusion of narcotics. *Journal of Intravenous Nursing, 13,* 119–121.)

# SUBCUTANEOUS THERAPY MAINTENANCE

## Monitoring and Documentation

CSQI therapy may be started in the hospital in preparation for discharge to home or nursing home. After initiation of CSQI, the nurse monitors vital signs according to health care agency policy. Pain assessment is an essential part of client monitoring. The client is asked to rate his or her pain on a 0 to 5 scale, with 0 representing no pain and 5 representing the worst possible pain. If the client experiences pain with CSQI, the dosing may need to be changed or another drug may need to be used. Dose titration may require rapid dose escalation, but this increase is usually well tolerated by the client experiencing cancer pain. The client's pain level and vital signs are documented in the medical record.

The nurse also monitors for and documents the presence of complications that can result from CSQI. These complications include insertion site irritation and systemic complications related to drug therapy.

## Complications of CSQI

### INSERTION SITE IRRITATION

As with any needle insertion into the skin, the subcutaneous needle can cause local skin irritation, manifested by erythema, heat, or swelling. This complication is prevented by rotating the insertion sites at least every 7 days. For clients experiencing neutropenia from cancer therapy, more frequent rotation is needed, usually every 2 to 3 days.

If signs of inflammation are present, the nurse or other caregiver removes the needle and changes the site. Ice or heat application may be helpful for the inflamed site.

### SYSTEMIC COMPLICATIONS

Systemic problems associated with CSQI are usually the result of the drug being infused. Opioid analgesia can cause respiratory depression, urinary retention, pruritus, confusion, drowsiness, and nausea and vomiting. These side effects are not common. Serious respiratory depression is extremely rare in opioid-tolerant clients (Moulin et al., 1992). Nausea and vomiting can be controlled by adding an antiemetic to the infusion dose.

Another potential problem with CSQI is the ineffectiveness of the analgesic in relieving pain. Although not common, this complication may necessitate a change to central venous or intraspinal administration of the opioid analgesic.

**TABLE 8–2**
**Client/Family Education for Continuous Subcutaneous Infusion**

- Check the needle insertion site several times a day for redness, swelling, and warmth.
- Rotate the site every 2 to 7 days, depending on the client's health status.
- Inspect the equipment frequently; make sure the infusion rate is correct.
- Keep a record of extra bolus doses.
- For opioid analgesic administration, monitor the client's pain level.
- For insulin administration, monitor the client's blood glucose.
- Observe the client for side and toxic effects of drug therapy such as sedation in the client receiving an analgesic.
- Contact the health care provider if questions or problems occur.

## SUBCUTANEOUS INSULIN ADMINISTRATION

The procedure for continuous subcutaneous insulin therapy is very similar to that described for continuous opioid analgesia. Sites for needle placement typically include the thigh, upper hip, abdomen, and lower back.

The insulin pump must be able to deliver basal regular insulin doses every few minutes and bolus doses for mealtimes and during illness or at other times when blood glucose increases. Most pumps hold a syringe that delivers doses of 0.1 U or more by a mechanical driver that is computer programmed. Several types of pumps are available. One popular insulin pump, the MiniMed, is about the size of a deck of cards and looks like a beeper. It has four buttons that are used to program the pump: the *M* button is for the *m*eal bolus; the *B* button sets the *b*asal rate; the *A* button *a*ctivates the pump to carry out the set program; and the *T* button is used to set the *t*ime of day for insulin administration.

The client's blood glucose must be monitored carefully to prevent episodes of hyperglycemia or hypoglycemia. As with CSQI for opioid administration, the client's insertion site may become inflamed. Site rotation usually prevents this complication.

## CLIENT/FAMILY EDUCATION

The nurse teaches the client and family/caregiver about CSQI, especially if the client will be using CSQI at home (Table 8–2). The nurse ensures that they thoroughly understand the purpose of the therapy and how the equipment works. The client or caregiver is taught how to inspect and rotate the sites. Demonstration of how to insert the needle and use the pump is essential before the client is discharged to home. The nurse shows the client how to change the pump battery and how to stop and start the infusion. The nurse teaches the client and caregiver who to contact if questions or problems arise. A complete discussion of the care of the pump is found in Chapter 5.

CHAPTER 9

# Central Nervous System Therapy

*Marilyn Ferreri Booker*



Central nervous system infusion therapy involves the administration of drugs into the epidural space or intrathecally. In epidural therapy the physician or nurse administers the drug into the epidural space outside of the dura mater. The drug then diffuses into the cerebrospinal fluid (CSF). Intrathecal therapy differs from epidural therapy in that in intrathecal therapy the practitioner administers the drug directly into the CSF. This is an important distinction for the nurse to be aware of because differences exist among state boards of nursing in relation to intrathecal drugs. Some boards of nursing believe that intrathecal drug administration is a physician function, whereas others agree that a nurse, well-educated in the technique, can administer this therapy.

## EPIDURAL THERAPY

### Description

Epidural therapy involves the administration of medications into the epidural space of the spinal column. Located between the wall of the vertebral canal and the dura mater, the epidural space consists of fat, connective tissue, and blood vessels that protect the spinal cord (Fig. 9–1). Opioids administered epidurally slowly diffuse across the dura mater to the dorsal horn of the spinal cord. There they lock onto opiate receptors and block pain impulses from ascending to

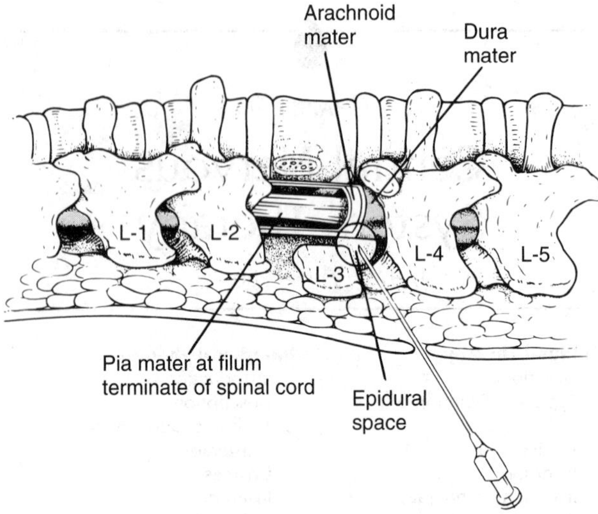


**FIGURE 9–1.** Epidural therapy involves the administration of medications into the epidural space of the spinal column. (From Ignatavicius, D. D., Workman, M. L., & Mishler, M. A. [1995]. *Medical-surgical nursing: A nursing process approach* [2nd ed., p. 398]. Philadelphia: W. B. Saunders.)

the brain. The client receives pain relief from the level of the injection downward. Table 9–1 outlines some opioids commonly administered epidurally and common dosages for postoperative pain relief, their lipid solubility, onset of action, and duration of action. In contrast, local anesthetics administered epidurally work on the sensory nerve roots in the epidural space to block pain impulses. The client perceives no pain in the areas served by these nerves.

**TABLE 9–1**
**Epidural Opioids**

| Drug | Dose | Lipid Solubility (Octanol/ Water) | Onset (Minutes) | Duration (Hours) |
|---|---|---|---|---|
| Morphine | 2–7 mg | 1.4 | 30–60 | 6–24 |
| Hydromorphone | 0.6–1 mg | 20 | 10–15 | 6–12 |
| Meperidine | 50–100 mg | 39 | 12–18 | 6–10 |
| Fentanyl | 50–100 mcg | 813 | 4–6 | 2–3 |
| Sufentanil | 10–50 mcg | 1800 | 5–10 | 3–6 |

From Ginsberg B. et al. (1993, May). Managing postoperative pain with epidural analgesia. *Pharmacy Times,* pp. 92–101.

## Type and Duration of Therapy

The most common uses of epidural therapy are for the relief of acute postoperative pain, chronic pain, and the pain associated with labor and delivery. The purpose of the therapy plays an important role in determining whether a local anesthetic or an opioid drug will prove more efficacious. Table 9–2 compares the efficacy of opioid and local anesthetics administered epidurally.

## Devices

The nurse may see four different types of epidural catheters, each with different indications for use.

### PERCUTANEOUS CATHETER

The indications for a temporary percutaneous catheter include temporary pain relief such as postoperatively or during labor and delivery, for clients with end-stage cancer, or for determining if the client with chronic pain will respond to epidural therapy. Because not all chronic pain responds to epidural analgesia or anesthesia, it is prudent to determine the individual client's response before inserting a more permanent catheter. The physician usually places a temporary catheter as a trial to determine the client's response. Once the efficacy of epidural therapy is confirmed, the physician places one of the more permanent epidural catheters.

**Description.** The epidural catheter consists of a flexible nylon catheter that is threaded through a spinal needle after the tip of the spinal needle is placed into the epidural space. The external end of the catheter has a standard female Luer lock hub, which accepts an intermittent injection cap (Fig. 9–2). The physician usually tapes the length of the catheter securely to the client's back and loops the length of the catheter over the client's shoulder for easy access.

**TABLE 9–2**
**Comparison of Efficacy of Epidural Opiates and Epidural Local Anesthetics**

| Type of Pain | Opiates | Anesthetics |
|---|---|---|
| Surgical pain | Partial relief | Complete relief |
| Labor pain | Partial relief | Complete relief |
| Postoperative pain | Good relief | Complete relief |
| Cancer pain | Good relief | Variable relief |

Data from Waldman, S.D. (1990). Practical Considerations in the Use of Spinal Opioids in the Management of Cancer Pain. Lecture.

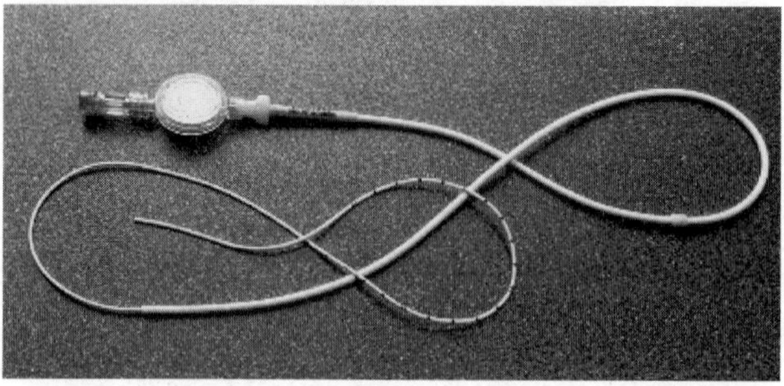

**FIGURE 9–2.** Epidural catheter. (Courtesy of Bard Access Systems, Salt Lake City, Utah.)

## SUBCUTANEOUS TUNNELED CATHETER

More permanent than the percutaneous catheter, the subcutaneous tunneled epidural catheter is made of Silastic material and is indicated for clients in whom epidural therapy has proved to be effective and who have a life expectancy of weeks to months.

**Description**. The subcutaneous tunneled catheter is longer than a temporary epidural catheter. As the name describes, the catheter is usualy tunneled subcutaneously from the point where it exits the spine to an area on the

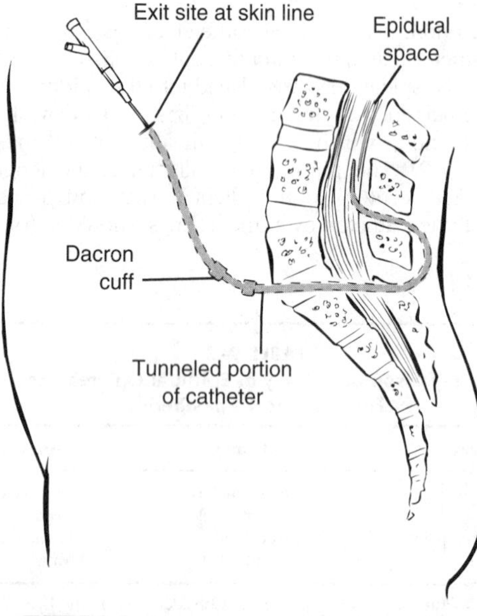


**FIGURE 9–3.** Subcutaneous tunneled epidural catheter.

client's trunk, usually just above the waist on the client's side (Fig. 9–3). The tunneled area has a Dacron cuff similar to that found on subcutaneously tunneled central venous catheters. This cuff prevents the migration of microorganisms along the catheter into the epidural space.

## TOTALLY IMPLANTABLE RESERVOIR OR PORT

An epidural port is more expensive than the subcutaneous tunneled catheter. The physician usually places an epidural port in clients who respond to epidural therapy and have a life expectancy of months to years. Another indication for the implanted port is the client who is confused and repeatedly pulls out his or her subcutaneous tunneled catheter.

**Description.** The implanted epidural port or reservoir appears identical to a venous or arterial port. The epidural port has a catheter and a portal body that the surgeon places over a bony prominence such as the spine itself or one of the lower anterior ribs (Fig. 9–4). To gain access to an epidural port the nurse uses the same procedure outlined in Chapter 7.

## TOTALLY IMPLANTABLE INFUSION PUMP

A totally implantable infusion pump, the most expensive method of administering epidural therapy, is indicated for clients who have a life expectancy of months to years.

**Description.** The implantable infusion device consists of a catheter whose tip sits in the epidural space at the appropriate level. The catheter is tunneled subcutaneously and attached to the pump, which is usually implanted in a pocket in the abdominal region or chest wall (Fig. 9–5).

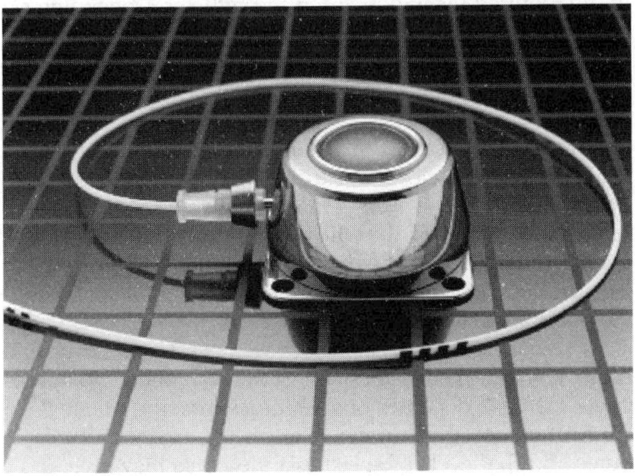

**FIGURE 9–4.** PORT-A-CATH Implantable Epidural Access System, a totally implantable port. (Courtesy of SIMS Deltec, Inc., St. Paul, Minnesota.)

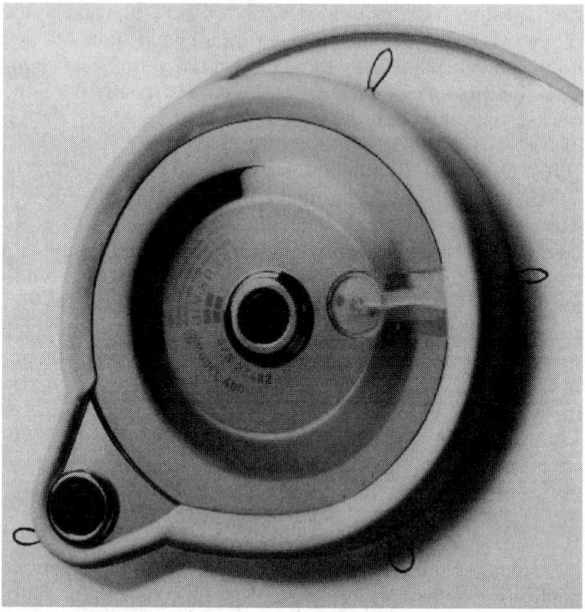

**FIGURE 9–5.** Totally implantable infusion pump. (Courtesy of Shiley Infusaid, Norwood, Massachusetts.)

## Insertion

Epidural catheters are placed by physicians. Usually neurosurgeons or anesthesiologists, physicians specially trained in the required technique, insert the catheter. Depending on the type of catheter and its purpose, the procedure may take place in the operating room or at the bedside.

### SITE

The goal for catheter insertion is the placement of the tip of the catheter as close to the spinal level requiring analgesia as appropriate. This is generally between T-11 and S-3. Lumbar placement is the safest and most popular site. The needle enters below L-1, which is where the spinal cord ends in most people. This eliminates the possibility of spinal cord trauma during placement.

For anesthesia, the height of the block (how far up the spinal column the anesthesia must travel to affect the appropriate nerves) depends on the procedure the client is to have. Table 9–3 lists common areas of surgery and procedures and the levels of anesthesia the nurse may see.

The physician can alter the extent of the block (the affected area) by manipulating the position of the needle or

**TABLE 9–3**
**Levels of Anesthesia Used in Common Operations and Procedures**

| Height of Block | Operations/Procedures |
|---|---|
| T-4 | Upper abdominal surgery |
| T-6 | Cesarean section |
| T-8 | Lower abdominal surgery |
| T-10 | Labor pains and bladder or inguinal hernia surgery |
| T-12 | Lower limb surgery |

From Hoerster, W., Kreuscher, H., Niesel, H.C., Zenz, M. (1990). *Regional Anesthesia*. St Louis: Mosby–Year Book.

the volume of the drug. The degree of block (the amount of analgesia or anesthesia) is a product of the concentration of the local anesthetic. For the surgical anesthesia the physician uses a 0.5% to 0.75% solution. For the treatment of somatic (body) pain a 0.25% to 0.5% solution is necessary for relief.

## Insertion Technique

There are two possible approaches the nurse may see used when the physician is attempting to place a temporary epidural catheter: the midline approach or the paramedian approach.

### MIDLINE APPROACH

In the midline approach the client is placed on his or her side. The physician locates L-4, which is at the same level as the top of the iliac crest. From there the physician can identify the space between L-2 and L-3 or L-3 and L-4. The nurse may assist the physician by helping the client roll into a fetal position. This position widens the space between the spinous processes and allows for easier needle placement (Fig. 9–6).

After cleaning the skin with a surgical scrub to the intended area, the physician administers a local anesthetic intradermally between the two spinous processes. The nurse may warn the client that he or she may experience a burning sensation from the local anesthetic.

The physician inserts the spinal needle with the obturator into the spine, holding the needle at a right angle to the skin, and then advances the needle into the intraspinal ligament. The physician removes the obturator and attaches a syringe to the needle. Some physicians prefer a syringe with air in it, whereas others use a syringe with preservative-free 0.9% normal saline solution (NSS). The physician uses the "loss of resistance" technique to advance the needle through the liga-

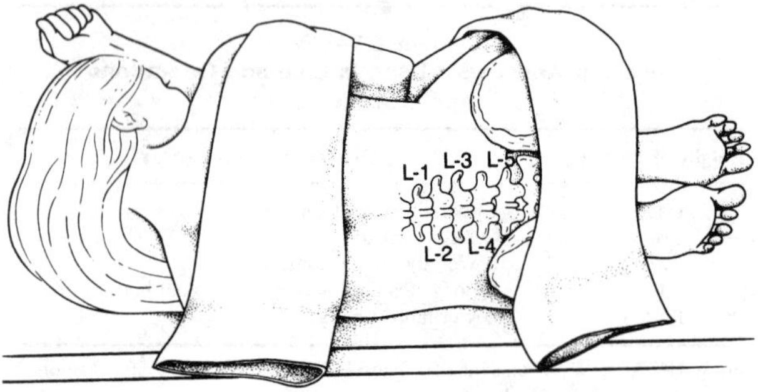


**FIGURE 9–6.** Positioning for midline approach for temporary epidural catheter insertion. (From Ignatavicius, D. D., Workman, M. L., & Mishler, M. A. [1995]. *Medical-surgical nursing: A nursing process approach* [2nd ed., p. 398]. Philadelphia: W. B. Saunders.)

mentum flavum, a tough layer of ligament, and into the epidural space.

## PARAMEDIAN APPROACH

The procedure for the paramedian approach is similar to that of the midline approach except that in the paramedian approach the physician inserts the needle approximately 1.5 to 2 cm lateral to the midline at the level of the spinous process below the chosen intervertebral space. The physician aims medially and upward. The first firm structure the physician should encounter using this approach is the ligamentum flavum. Just as with the midline approach the physician removes the obturator from the needle and attaches a syringe filled with either air or preservative-free 0.9% NSS. Again, the "loss of resistance" technique is used to advance the needle through the ligamentum flavum into the epidural space.

## CHECKING PLACEMENT

Before inserting the catheter the physician checks the needle placement to assure that the needle is truly in the epidural space. The physician accomplishes this by removing the syringe from the end of the spinal needle and observing any fluid that drips. Correct epidural placement is indicated by no or little fluid dripping from the end of the needle. If a steady stream of clear fluid flows, the physician has placed the tip of the needle into the subarachnoid space. This action changes the type of therapy from epidural to intrathecal. Unless the physician wishes to administer spinal (intrathecal) anesthesia, the needle must be removed and another site attempted. If blood flows from the needle, the needle is in an epidural vein. In this case also the needle must be removed and an insertion in another site attempted.

### INSERTING THE CATHETER

After assuring correct placement the physician threads the catheter through the needle and into the epidural space. If the catheter is for surgical or obstetric anesthesia or any other type of temporary procedure, the catheter is inserted 2 to 3 cm. For epidural analgesia the catheter is inserted 4 to 5 cm. The needle is then withdrawn by removing it over the catheter. Before injecting any medication the physician again observes for CSF or blood from the catheter. This can be accomplished by withdrawing with a syringe or by holding the end of the catheter below the level of the insertion site.

### SECURING THE CATHETER

The length of the external portion of the catheter is securely taped to the client's back and looped up over the shoulder. An intermittent injection cap is attached. It is important that the catheter be labeled EPIDURAL. Some clients with epidural catheters may also have central venous catheters. As both catheters are similar in appearance, one can easily be mistaken for the other. Inadvertent administration of drugs or solutions intended for intravenous (IV) administration into the epidural catheter could result in the client's death.

## Administering Medications

The physician administers the first dose of anesthesia or test dose. Usually, 3 to 5 mL of the appropriate concentration of local anesthetic or analgesia is administered while the physician observes the client carefully for at least 5 minutes.

Epidural drugs and the diluents used in their preparation must be preservative free. The epidural space can accommodate no more than 15 mL/min (Hansberry et al., 1990).

The rate at which a drug diffuses into the CSF depends on the lipid solubility of the drug. Drugs with higher lipid solubilities such as fentanyl (Sublimaze) diffuse faster and have a shorter duration of effect than drugs with lower lipid solubilities such as morphine.

Another factor determining the analgesic duration of spinally administered opioids is the total dosage. There is a direct relationship between the number of milligrams administered and the duration of effect. The only dose-limiting factor in epidural drug administration is the side effects the client exhibits. Table 9–4 is a comparison of some of the side effects clients may experience with either epidural opiates or epidural local anesthetics.

**TABLE 9–4**
**Comparison of Side Effects of Epidural Opiates and Local Anesthetics**

| | Epidural Opiates | Epidural Local Anesthetics |
|---|---|---|
| Cardiovascular | No postural hypotension<br>Minor changes in heart rate | Postural hypotension<br>Decrease in heart rate |
| Respiratory | If respiratory side effects occur, may be early at 1–2 h because of systemic absorption or late at 6–24 h after dose because of migration to brain | Usually unimpaired |
| Central nervous system | Sedation may be marked<br>Convulsions absent | Sedation absent to mild<br>Convulsions possible because of rapid vascular absorption<br>Sensory losses<br>Motor weakness |
| | Urinary retention<br>Pruritus<br>Nausea and vomiting | Urinary retention<br>Pruritus rarely occurs<br>Nausea and vomiting rarely occurs |

Data from Waldman, S.D. (1990). Practical considerations in the use of spinal opioids in the management of cancer pain. Lecture.

## LOCAL ANESTHETICS

Local anesthetics block pain signals primarily in the dorsal root ganglion, before they enter the spinal cord. They have a more generalized effect, affecting motor and sensory pathways in addition to pain. Soft touch, temperature, and position sense are blocked by local anesthetics, as are motor fiber and neural mechanisms that maintain vascular tone (sympathetic nervous system). These effects are dose dependent.

## NARCOTICS

Narcotics specifically block pain pathways inside the spinal cord by occupying opiate receptors in the dorsal horn. Opiate receptors have been identified in many sites in the central nervous system, the brain (cortex), brain stem (thalamus), and the substantia gelantinosa of the dorsal horns in the spinal cord. These receptors are specific for both endogenous and exogenous opiates. Exogenous opiates such as morphine mimic the action of endogenous opiates and inhibit pain pathways to the brain, thus altering the perception and emotional response to pain. Narcotics do not cause sympathetic and motor blockade.

There is some absorption of narcotic from the epidural space into the general circulation. However, levels of narcotic in the CSF average approximately 100 times those in the plasma. The long-term pain relief achieved is attributed to the drug in the spinal cord, not to the drug in the blood. The analgesia is prolonged because the narcotics must diffuse out of the CSF into the blood stream for excretion by the liver and kidneys.

## Administration Technique

Always check a temporary catheter's placement before administering any medications. Carefully disconnect the intermittent injection cap from the catheter and attach a sterile syringe. Gently aspirate the fluid from the catheter. If the catheter is in the proper place, no fluid or blood will be aspirated from the catheter.

### CONTINUOUS INFUSION

1. Gather the following supplies: Pump and IV pole (if stationary pump is used) Tubing with an in-line 0.22-mm filter or a separate 0.22-mm filter
   Labels that read EPIDURAL
   Tape
2. Attach the filter to the tubing if necessary.
3. Check the infusion bag to ensure that it contains the correct drug and solution and that each is appropriate for epidural infusion. Remember, both must be preservative free. Connect the tubing to the infusion bag or cassette and load the pump according to the manufacturer's instructions.
4. Prime the tubing and filter with the solution.
5. Attach the tubing to the catheter.
6. Label the front of the pump and the infusion bag or cassette with a label reading EPIDURAL to keep all other caregivers from confusing the epidural line with an IV line.
7. Tape over all injection ports on the tubing to safeguard against accidental injection into the epidural catheter.
8. Set or program the pump to deliver the prescribed dosage of drug.
9. Begin the infusion.
10. Monitor the client carefully for any complications.

## Complications

See Table 9–4 for a list of side effects the nurse may observe when administering epidural opiates and local anesthetics.

## INFECTION

**Definition.** Infection is the invasion and multiplication of microorganisms into body tissues or fluids.

**Cause.** Infection is caused by the disruption of the "closed" medication administration system (no openings between the medication and the client) or the lack of strict aseptic technique during handling of the catheter or medications.

**Signs and Symptoms.** Observe the client for inflammation, swelling, tenderness, local warmth, or drainage from the catheter insertion site. Instruct the client to report any headache, stiff neck, or temperature of greater than 101°F (38.3°C) to the nurse or physician.

**Treatment.** The physician may order antibiotics to be administered epidurally or intravenously. The catheter may be removed.

**Documentation.** The nurse records all observations and client statements about his or her condition.

**Prevention.** The nurse and physician exercise strict aseptic technique during the insertion of the catheter and when handling the tubings, connections, and medications. Epidural catheter dressings are changed every 72 hours. Epidural tubings and filters on continuous infusions are changed every 48 hours. Once opened, infusion solutions expire in 24 hours. If lines are accidentally disconnected, the nurse does not reconnect them. The entire infusion system must be changed. If the tip of the catheter becomes disconnected and contaminated, the nurse caps it and notifies the physician who inserted the catheter.

## MISPLACEMENT OR MIGRATION

**Definition.** The catheter can become misplaced at the time of placement or can move or become kinked after placement.

**Cause.** Failure to tape the catheter securely to the client's back causes misplacement.

**Signs and Symptoms.** When checking placement the nurse aspirates either clear free-flowing solution (CSF), indicating a migration into the subarachnoid space, or blood, indicating a catheter migration into a blood vessel. Clients who inadvertently receive local anesthetics directly into the subarachnoid space may experience high or total spinal block and convulsions or cardiovascular depression. Clients who receive local anesthetics intravenously may experience toxic reactions with convulsions.

**Treatment.** The physician usually removes the catheter. If the aspirated fluid is CSF, the physician may adjust medication dosages to accommodate intrathecal administration.

**Documentation.** The nurse observes and documents any changes in catheter length or aspirated fluid.

**Prevention.** The nurse carefully and securely tapes the catheter to the client's back.

## INTRATHECAL THERAPY

### Introduction

In the early 1960s, clients with central nervous system neoplasms required intermittent lumbar punctures (LPs) for chemotherapy administration. Dr. A. K. Ommaya (1963) described a device that provides a method of sterilely gaining access to the ventricular CSF using a subcutaneously implanted reservoir. This device, the Ommaya reservoir, has spared numerous clients the need for multiple LPs.

### Description

Intrathecal therapy through an Ommaya reservoir involves the administration of medications directly into the CSF. Unlike epidural therapy, intrathecal therapy is not dependent on diffusion to move the drug into the CSF.

### Type and Duration of Therapy

The Ommaya reservoir provides physicians with direct intrathecal access for the administration of chemotherapeutic drugs in the treatment of CSF malignancies or the prevention of metastasis to the CSF. Clients with infections in the CSF may receive antibiotics through the Ommaya reservoir. Analgesics administered via the Ommaya reservoir are very effective in the treatment of severe, chronic cancer-related pain in some patients resistant to other pain relief modalities. The reservoir may be used for measuring CSF pressure, draining excess CSF, or sampling CSF for laboratory studies.

Unless there are complications, the Ommaya reservoir should function for months and in some cases years. Up to 200 punctures are possible without leakage.

### Devices

The Ommaya reservoir consists of two pieces: a mushroom-shaped self-sealing dome made of silicone and a catheter that attaches to the dome. The end of the catheter is placed in one of the lateral ventricles. The reservoir is attached and placed beneath a flap in the client's scalp (Fig. 9–7). Some convertible models of the reservoir have a side outlet tube that can be used as a shunt to remove excess CSF in the client with increased intracranial pressure.

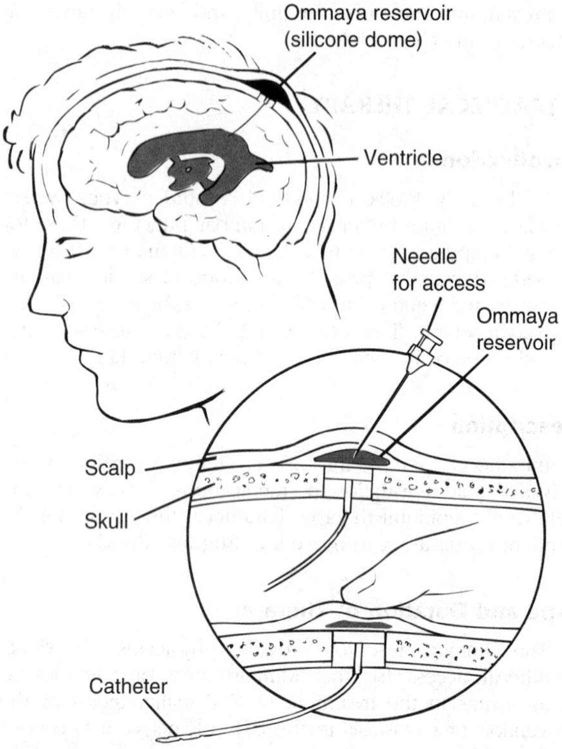


**FIGURE 9–7.** The Ommaya reservoir is a self-sealing dome attached to a surgically implanted catheter. The dome is pressed to release medication into the lateral ventricle.

## Insertion

The insertion of the Ommaya reservoir is a surgical procedure that can be completed using local or general anesthesia, depending on the client's condition and the client's and surgeon's preference. After shaving the hair from the placement area, the surgeon makes a burr hole in the client's skull. The surgeon guides the catheter through a "silent" area of the nondominant frontal lobe and into the lateral ventricle. (The nondominant frontal lobe is chosen to minimize the potential for neurologic deficit.) Intraoperative radiography confirms correct placement. The reservoir is inserted over the burr hole and attached to the catheter. The surgeon sutures the scalp flap over the reservoir, which makes a soft bulge on the client's scalp of about 1½ inches (3.5 cm) (Fig. 9–7).

## Postoperative Site Care

The client returns from the operating room with a pressure dressing over the insertion site. After 24 hours this dressing is replaced with a 4 × 4 to protect the area until the sutures are removed. The nurse reminds the client to avoid any trauma to the area. Approximately 1 week after reservoir placement the client may shampoo his or her hair as long as this area is washed gently. The client may allow hair to grow back over the area except for a spot about the size of a quarter that must be kept shaved for the injections. Forty-eight hours after placement the reservoir may be used for injection or drainage.

## Administering Medications

### CHEMOTHERAPY

Some drugs such as methotrexate and cytarabine (ARA-C, Cytosar-U) are effective against CSF neoplasms. Because they do not cross the blood-brain barrier when administered intravenously, for effective treatment these drugs must be given intrathecally. Unfortunately, these medications cause both central nervous system and systemic side effects when administered in this manner. Clients may complain of headache, fever, nausea, and vomiting. Some clients may exhibit changes in mental status such as confusion or disorientation. These neurologic effects are usually transient and subside after 30 to 60 minutes.

### ANALGESICS

Intrathecal morphine sulfate via an Ommaya reservoir alleviates intractable cancer pain. Doses may be as small as 0.25 to 1 mg injected into the CSF. Only preservative-free morphine (such as Duramorph PF or Infumorph) diluted in preservative-free 0.9% NSS should be used for intrathecal injection. Clients report relief of pain within 2 to 30 minutes with a duration of relief from 12 to 52 hours. Usually the morphine is injected every 24 hours, but in severe cases the nurse may observe dosing as frequently as every 4 to 6 hours. After the client is stabilized on a dosage of intrathecal morphine, the client may be discharged to the care of home health nurses. In some cases very motivated family members may be trained to administer the drug to the client.

## Administration Technique

1. Gather the following supplies:
   Sterile gloves
   Sterile drape
   Sterile 2 3 2 gauze sponges
   23- or 25-gauge butterfly needle or 22-gauge LP needle

Sterile tubes for specimens
Alcohol swab sticks
5-mL syringes
Safety razor
Povidone-iodine swab sticks

2. Before administering any chemotherapeutic agent, check for the following parameters: blood urea nitrogen (BUN) greater than 20; white blood cell count (WBC) less than 2.5; platelets less than 100,000 or on a downward trend. Observe the client for any mouth ulcers. If any of these conditions exist, do not administer the medication and notify the physician of your findings.
3. Assess the client's vital signs and neurologic status including orientation, level of consciousness, pupils, and presence of headache.
4. Dilute the drugs with nonbacteriostatic sterile water, preservative-free 0.9% NSS, or Elliot B's solution. The pH and chemical composition of these solutions are compatible with CSF. As with epidural medications, avoid the use of solutions with preservatives, as they may irritate the meninges. Draw the diluted drugs into a syringe.
5. Place the sterile barrier under the client's head. If the client's reservoir is attached to a shunt for drainage, close the valve to the off position.
6. Shave the area over the reservoir.
7. Don the sterile gloves.
8. Clean the site with the povidone-iodine swab stick in a circular motion from the center outward. Allow the povidone-iodine to dry.
9. Attach the butterfly or LP needle to the empty 5-mL syringe.
10. Holding the needle and syringe in your dominant hand as you would a dart, puncture the reservoir, inserting the needle at an oblique angle. Slowly withdraw an amount of fluid equal to the volume of the drug to be infused.
11. Carefully disconnect the syringe and maintain its sterility. Add the medication syringe to the needle.
12. Slowly instill the medication into the reservoir.
13. Remove the needle and place the sterile 2 × 2's over the puncture site, applying gentle pressure.
14. Gently "pump" the reservoir three times by gently pushing down and releasing while maintaining your finger over the area. You should be able to feel the CSF fill the reservoir. This assures adequate circulation of the medication through the CSF.
15. After any leaking has stopped, clean the puncture site with alcohol swabs.

16. Instill the CSF in the 5-mL syringe into the specimen tubes and send for any tests the physician has ordered. Physicians usually request a culture and sensitivity of the CSF with each treatment.
17. Instruct the client to lie flat in bed for 30 minutes after the procedure.
18. Observe the client for any immediate side effects. These may include nausea, vomiting, headache, dizziness, or adverse drug reactions. Monitor vital signs and neurologic status carefully. If the client exhibits any side effects and they do not subside within 15 minutes, notify the physician.
19. If the client's reservoir was attached to a shunt for drainage, you may reopen the shunt after 4 hours.
20. Observe the client for any complications.

## Complications

### INFECTION

**Definition.** Infection is the inadvertent injection of microorganisms into the CSF.

**Cause.** Intrathecal administration of drugs by repeated injection places the client at risk for infection of the reservoir and the entire central nervous system.

**Signs and Symptoms.** Observe the client for inflammation, swelling, tenderness, local warmth, or drainage from the injection sites. Instruct the client to report any headache, stiff neck, or temperature of greater than 101°F (38.3°C) to the nurse or physician. If the nurse observes that the aspirated CSF appears cloudy, specimens should be sent for culture and sensitivity evaluations.

**Treatment.** Intrathecal antibiotics usually eliminate infection in the reservoir and the central nervous system. In extreme cases the Ommaya reservoir may be removed.

**Documentation.** The nurse records all observations and client statements about his or her condition.

**Prevention.** The nurse maintains strict aseptic technique during the injection of medications and instructs the client in the importance of protecting the reservoir site from trauma and keeping it clean.

### MISPLACEMENT OR MIGRATION

**Definition.** The catheter can become misplaced at the time of placement or can move or become kinked after placement.

**Cause.** The cause of misplacement is unknown.

**Signs and Symptoms.** When "pumping" the reservoir the nurse observes no or very slow filling. (Do not "pump" the reservoir if the client's neurologic status is unstable. In some cases the client may exhibit new neurologic symptoms.)

**Treatment.** The physician requests a computed tomography (CT) scan to determine catheter location. If the scan shows that the catheter is displaced, the catheter is either repositioned or removed.

**Documentation.** The nurse observes and documents the client's neurologic status frequently.

**Prevention.** None.

# CHAPTER 10
# Arterial Therapy

*Marilyn Ferreri Booker*



## DESCRIPTION

Establishing arterial access involves the insertion of a needle or catheter into an artery. The nurse may see arterial access used for three very different purposes: (1) blood sampling for arterial blood gases (ABGs), (2) hemodynamic monitoring, and (3) intraarterial chemotherapy (IAC). For a discussion of hemodynamic monitoring, the nurse is referred to a text on critical care nursing.

The purpose of the procedure determines the member of the health care team who performs the insertion. More and more nurses are performing arterial punctures to obtain blood for laboratory studies and to establish an arterial line ("art line" or "A-line") for hemodynamic monitoring. In some settings respiratory therapists or pulmonary function technicians may draw ABGs to determine the concentration of oxygen and carbon dioxide in the client's blood. Depending on the artery used, hemodynamic monitoring lines may require a physician to perform the placement. If the arterial access is for IAC, a physician establishes the line.

## BLOOD SAMPLING

### Site Selection

For arterial blood-sampling the small radial and ulnar arteries lie close to the surface of the skin and are easier to encannulate than the larger, deeper brachial arteries (Fig. 10–1). The radial artery is the preferred site for extracting an ABG specimen because of its accessibility. However, the nurse may use the ulnar or the brachial arteries as well. Other potential sites include the femoral, dorsalis pedis, and tibial ar-

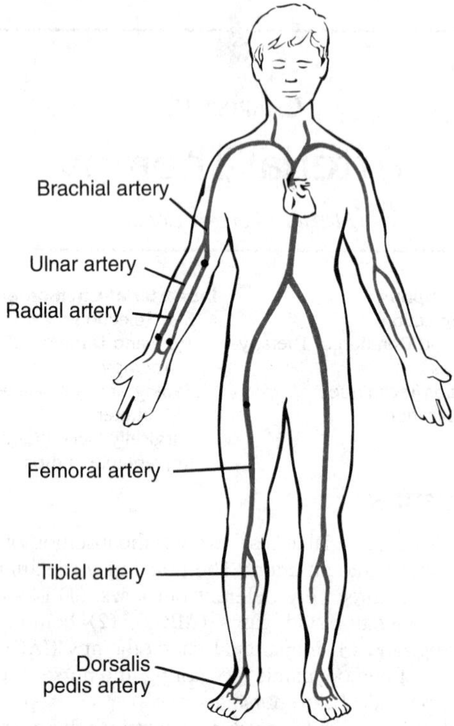


**FIGURE 10–1.** Common sites for arterial blood sampling.

teries. In the neonate the umbilical artery is a potential site (Milliam, 1988). Table 10–1 outlines some of the advantages and disadvantages of each site.

When preparing to perform an arterial puncture for blood sampling, the nurse carefully assesses the client's circulation in the extremity to be used. Arterial sites in extremities that are blanched, cold, swollen, or discolored or that have had multiple previous punctures are not appropriate selections. The nurse avoids areas in which the client complains of numbness or tingling. The nurse can use Allen's test to assess the circulation of the radial, ulnar, or brachial arteries (Table 10–2).

## Type and Duration of Therapy

In addition to blood sampling for ABGs, blood samples for other studies can also be obtained via the arterial route if they are needed. This saves the client the discomfort of an additional needle stick into a vein and saves the nurse time

**TABLE 10–1**
**Advantages and Disadvantages of Arterial Blood Sampling Sites**

| Artery | Advantages | Disadvantages |
|---|---|---|
| Brachial | Largest artery in the lower arm; close to surface in thin or elderly patients; extension of the arm stretches the artery; easy to puncture with direct, perpendicular approach; pulsation sometimes visible; easy access provides good visibility after puncture | Can be deep in muscular or obese arms; may be difficult to stabilize if surrounding tissues are loose; traumatic puncture more likely to damage nerves and ligaments than puncture in a wrist site; may be difficult to find if previously bruised, edematous, or hardened from repeated punctures |
| Radial | Close to the surface, easily palpable; area of papability wider on thin people; can check site easily; easy to stabilize when patient is uncooperative | Pulsation difficult to palpate if client has short, obese arms or deeply situated vessels; site may be bruised or artery hardened from previous punctures |
| Ulnar | Fairly close to surface; accessible; convenient; good alternative when radial artery has several previous punctures | Palpation difficult if artery is small or deep; difficult to keep wrist extended if patient is uncooperative or has spastic flexion |
| Femoral | Relatively large artery, easy to palpate and puncture; allows a more direct, perpendicular approach of the needle; easy to locate when patient is supine; arterial spasm during needle insertion rare | Site (groin) at risk of contamination; potentially embarrassing for client; if client is obese, an assistant must retract pendulous abdomen or skin folds to expose puncture site; hematoma may go undetected when site is covered with bedclothes; possible to puncture femoral vein accidentally because of its proximity to femoral artery |
| Dorsalis pedis, tibial | Can be used as a last resort | Rarely used for blood sampling; small; hard to locate; risk of compromising lower extremity circulation |

**TABLE 10–2**
**Allen's Test**

1. With the client sitting or lying in the supine position, face the client so the inner aspect of his or her hand is easily visible.
2. Palpate the radial and ulnar arteries of the client's wrist and compress them with the thumb or fingers to occlude the blood flow.
3. While continuing to compress the arteries, ask the client to open and close his or her fist forcibly. The client's hand should lose color or look blanched.
4. Ask the client to relax his or her hand so the fingertips are visible. The fingers should not be hyperextended.
5. Release the radial artery and watch for reactive hyperemia (capillary blush) of the inner hand. The blush starts at the base of the thumb and spreads across the palmar arch toward the base of the fifth finger.

The result is considered normal if the capillary blush is completed within 5 to 6 seconds. This confirms that circulation to the hand is adequate. If any portion of the hand does not fill within 5 to 6 seconds, the continuity of the palmar arch is considered incomplete, and the radial artery is not an appropriate choice for arterial puncture.

Repeat this test, compressing the radial and ulnar arteries. When the ulnar artery is released, the reactive hyperemia should spread across the palmar arch, starting at the fifth finger and extending to the base of the thumb.

The client whose circulation of both the radial and ulnar arteries is compromised should not have a catheter placed in the brachial artery.

as well. Blood for the other studies should be labeled "arterial blood," since pH and some electrolytes differ in arterial samples. Arterial punctures for blood sampling are usually episodic, so the nurse withdraws the needle after the specimen has been collected.

## Devices

A number of different types of arterial blood sampling kits are available on the market. Most of these have heparinized syringes, and others have an air venting system that allows the blood to displace air as the syringe fills to a preset level. These kits also have some type of cap or rubber stopper to attach to the end of the syringe after the specimen is drawn. If heparinized syringes are not available, the nurse heparinizes the specimen syringe by drawing up about 0.5 to 1 mL of any heparin concentration into a tuberculin or 3-mL syringe.

A short, 23- or 25-gauge 1-inch (2.5-cm) butterfly needle with 8 to 12 inches (20 to 28 cm) of tubing attached is a good choice for most arterial punctures. The butterfly needle is lightweight enough to sit in the artery without moving, and tubing allows the nurse to place the syringe on the bed next to the client so that the nurse's hands are free to change syringes if other blood specimens are being collected during the procedure. This extra tubing prevents trauma to the artery during the manipulation.

If the client is obese, a 1-inch (2.5-cm) needle may not reach the artery. In this case the nurse may need to use a 1½-inch (3.8 cm) 21-gauge needle instead. Changing syringes for the collection of other specimens is very difficult with this setup. In this case the nurse may wish to attach an extension set to the needle hub and add the syringe to the end of the extension set. This allows the nurse to change syringes without traumatizing the artery.

## Insertion Technique

### CLIENT PREPARATION

As with any procedure, the nurse explains the procedure to the client. Enlisting the client's assistance in remaining still during the procedure ensures less trauma to the artery and increases the likelihood of a successful arterial puncture.

If the ABG is being drawn to measure the effects of a change in oxygen therapy or to monitor the client after oxygen has been discontinued, the nurse waits 20 to 30 minutes after the change in therapy or discontinuation of oxygen to draw the specimen. This allows time for the body to assimilate the change in therapy.

### ADMINISTERING A LOCAL ANESTHETIC

Because arterial punctures can be very painful, some agencies use a local anesthetic for those clients who are not allergic. An injection of 0.1 to 0.2 mL of 1% lidocaine (Xylocaine) injected directly over the artery with a 27-gauge ⅝-inch (1.6 cm) needle usually anesthetizes the area sufficiently. The nurse inserts the full length of the needle at a 30-degree angle and withdraws the needle slowly while injecting the anesthetic. Massaging the area with an alcohol prep assists with absorption of the medication. The lidocaine (Xylocaine) also acts to relax the walls of the artery and decreases the likelihood of arterial spasm, which is common in small arteries such as the radial and ulnar.

### PUNCTURING THE ARTERY

1. After washing your hands and putting on gloves, palpate the selected artery with the middle and forefingers of your nondominant hand to locate the area of the strongest pulsation. Care should be taken not to obliterate the pulse.
2. Position the client's extremity over a rolled towel to hyperextend the area. This stretches the artery and brings it closer to the skin surface.
3. Prepare the skin over the artery with the cleansing agent used in your agency by cleaning in a circular motion from the intended penetration site out about 2 inches (5

cm). Allow the cleansing agent to air dry. This provides an antibacterial barrier around the penetration site.

4. Grasp the butterfly wings between the thumb and forefinger of your dominant hand; the bevel should be up as though performing a venipuncture. If using a $1\frac{1}{2}$-inch (3.8-cm) needle with an extension set attached, the needle is held at the hub with the bevel up.
5. While palpating the artery with the nondominant hand about $\frac{1}{2}$ inch (1 cm) above the intended penetration site, insert the needle with a quick smooth motion into the area of pulsation. Bright red blood entering the tubing confirms successful needle placement. (A poorly oxygenated client's blood appears dark red.)
6. If you have not penetrated the artery, pull the needle back without removing it and attempt to puncture the artery again. If this attempt is unsuccessful, remove the needle and try another site.
7. While keeping the needle steady in the artery, hold the syringe up to allow it to fill. If the syringe is not vented, pull up on the plunger to 1 mL; 0.5 to 1 mL of blood is all that is required for ABG analysis (0.3 mL for infants).
8. If other specimens are to be drawn, carefully release the needle and change syringes.

## REMOVING THE NEEDLE

1. After all the specimens are collected, place a sterile 2 × 2 (5 × 5 cm) gauze over the penetration site and apply firm pressure.
2. Remove the needle in one swift movement. Hold the gauze firmly in place for at least 2 minutes. If the client is receiving anticoagulants (heparin or warfarin), you may need to apply pressure for a few minutes longer.
3. Apply a pressure dressing and leave it in place for 6 hours.
4. If bleeding persists, apply an ice pack.

## PREPARING THE SPECIMEN

1. Cap the ABG specimen with the cap provided in the kit and agitate the specimen to heparinize it.
2. Holding the syringe in the upright position, tap the sides of the syringe to allow any air in the specimen to rise to the top. If there are any bubbles, uncap the syringe and, holding a gauze to the tip of the syringe, gently push on the syringe plunger to expel any air into the gauze.
3. Recap the syringe, label the specimen, and place the specimen in a plastic bag with ice or in a paper cup with ice. The ice slows metabolic changes in the specimen. ABG specimens must be analyzed within 15 minutes of collection.

#### DOCUMENTATION

The nurse documents the procedure, including the oxygen conditions under which the specimen was drawn and the client's tolerance of the procedure. If any other specimens were obtained during the arterial puncture, that notation is included in the client's medical record.

### Complications

#### HEMATOMA

Hematomas are usually secondary to trauma to the arterial wall during the needle insertion, but they can be due to inadequate pressure over the puncture site. Using the smallest gauge needle available lessens the risk of this complication.

#### SCLEROSIS

Repeated punctures in the same arterial site may cause scarring of the arterial wall and narrowing of the arterial lumen. Whenever possible, using different arteries or at least different sites along an artery decreases the potential for the client to develop this complication.

#### INFECTION

As with any invasive procedure, infection is always a risk. To avoid infection the nurse must use strict aseptic technique during the procedure and apply only sterile dressings to the penetration site.

## INTRAARTERIAL CHEMOTHERAPY

### Site Selection

Site selection for IAC differs from that of blood sampling in that the artery encannulated is specific to the diseased organ or structure. The nurse is most likely to see IAC used to treat a localized inoperable tumor in the liver, head, neck, or bones. Liver tumors are usually treated through the hepatic artery or branches of the celiac artery. The nurse may see the external carotid artery used in the treatment of head and neck tumors and the internal carotid artery used for the treatment of brain tumors.

The physician places the catheter in a main artery that feeds the target organ or structure, and antineoplastic agents are infused. Administering chemotherapy in this manner allows a high concentration of drug to be delivered to the tumor site before it is diluted in the circulatory system or metabolized in the liver or kidneys. Furthermore, a high drug concentration can be achieved at the tumor site with lower systemic drug levels and consequently fewer systemic side effects. Enough drug is available systemically, however, to treat undetected micrometastases.

Clients receiving IAC may receive treatments on an intermittent or continuous basis. Some clients receiving intermittent chemotherapy are admitted to the hospital for 5 days every month for their IAC. Some of the agents administered arterially include floxuridine (FUDR), fluorouracil (5-FU), and mitomycin (mitomycin-C, MTC, Mutamycin).

Whether the client is receiving intermittent or continuous treatment, the infusion must be run on an electronic infusion pump, since the use of a controller or gravity flow will not overcome arterial pressure and blood will back up the tubing.

## Type and Duration of Therapy

IAC can be administered through catheters placed radiographically or surgically. Generally, the length of the therapy regimen and number of treatments determine which type of catheter will be used.

## Radiographically Placed Catheter

### DESCRIPTION

Clients who are having intermittent IAC for a limited time usually have catheters placed by the radiologist in the x-ray department. Placement of the arterial catheter in this manner requires no general anesthesia, and the client experiences only minor discomfort for a short period. These catheters are generally made of a vinyl polymer or Teflon. The client may be hospitalized for about 5 days for catheter placement and administration of chemotherapy. After each chemotherapy cycle the catheter is removed, and the client is discharged until the next cycle is due.

### CLIENT PREPARATION

As with any procedure the physician or nurse explains the procedure to the client. The client may have laboratory and x-ray studies before the procedure. Some centers only allow the client to have clear liquids before the scheduled procedure. While the catheter is in place, the client will not be able to shower or sit in a tub, so the client should shower or bathe before the catheter insertion. The client is taken to the x-ray department on a stretcher. The procedure generally takes between 1½ to 2 hours. During the procedure the client must lie flat and still on the procedure table. The physician may order a medication to assist the client to relax during the insertion.

## ANESTHESIA

Clients usually receive a local anesthetic before the catheter is placed.

## PLACING THE CATHETER

The radiologist places a needle into the artery and threads the catheter over the needle. The client's arterial anatomy is visible during the procedure by angiography. The client may have several vessels supplying the tumor site or the target vessel can not be infused without infusing other adjacent vessels. When this occurs, the radiologist may elect to occlude these other vessels by injecting Gelfoam or metal coils through the catheter. Embolizing the arteries in this way may cause the tumor to necrose or shrink without the chemotherapy. The body absorbs Gelfoam within a few days, reestablishing circulation. Metal coils, however, provide permanent vascular occlusion.

Until the body establishes collateral circulation, the client may complain of general malaise and pain in the area occluded. It is important for the nurse to know if embolizing agents were used so that the nurse appropriately recognizes the cause for these symptoms.

## CHECKING PLACEMENT

After the catheter is placed, the radiologist usually checks the placement of the catheter by injecting contrast dye through the catheter and taking x-rays. The patient may complain of a burning sensation or a warm feeling as the dye moves through the catheter.

## DRESSING THE SITE

When the radiologist is certain the catheter is correctly placed, a sterile transparent dressing is applied to the insertion site. At times, the physician may place adhesive tape to the adjacent limb and then suture the catheter to the adhesive tape to keep the catheter in place. The area is then covered with a transparent dressing.

## DOCUMENTATION

The nurse documents the integrity of the dressing and the length of the catheter external to the insertion site. Continuous monitoring and documentation of these parameters can alert the physician to possible catheter displacement. The nurse also checks and documents the presence and quality of the pulse distal to the catheter insertion site to assess the circulation to the client's arm or leg.

## COMPLICATIONS

**Catheter Displacement.** Displacement of the catheter is the most common problem associated with temporary arterial catheters for chemotherapy. If the client's activity orders include bathroom privileges, the nurse accompanies the client to the bathroom, making sure there is no pull on the catheter.

If the catheter becomes displaced, the client may experience signs and symptoms that include dyspepsia, excessive nausea and vomiting or diarrhea, gastric pain from peptic ulcers, or upper abdominal pain from pancreatitis. The physician may order the chemotherapy infusion temporarily discontinued while a heparinized saline solution is infused and antacids or cimetidine (Tagamet) are administered.

**Subintimal Tear.** If the patient complains of pain near the target organ during infusion, it may be a sign of subintimal tear (separation of the intima and media of the arterial wall). This can happen from manipulation during placement and can cause a postponement of the chemotherapy for up to 8 weeks until the tear heals. Sometimes the chemotherapeutic agent itself can cause irregularities of the arterial wall.

**Arterial Occlusion.** Arterial occlusion is usually avoided by including heparin in the chemotherapy infusion or by administering 650 mg of aspirin twice daily. Even with this precautionary treatment the nurse may observe transient or permanent loss or decrease in the client's pulse distal to the insertion site. The nurse must report this finding immediately. If the diagnosis of arterial embolus or thrombus is made, the radiologist either removes the catheter or attempts to irrigate it. Clients generally tolerate the injection of clotted materials into the liver, but if the catheter is placed into an artery supplying an organ other than the liver, it should not be irrigated. In these cases a fibrolytic enzyme preparation, urokinase (50,000 U/mL), usually in an amount equal to the catheter volume is instilled into the catheter. Each agency has its own protocol for the use of urokinase (Abboki-nase, Abbokinase Open-Cath) to open clotted catheters. The procedure usually involves waiting a period of time after the instillation and then aspirating the dissolved clot. Clients usually do not exhibit any side effects other than an occasional transient fever from urokinase administration in these doses.

## Surgically Placed Catheter

### DESCRIPTION

Some clients receiving continuous chemotherapy or long-term intermittent chemotherapy require long-term catheters placed surgically. These catheters are usually made of Silastic, a material that resists becoming brittle with age. Early in the history of this type of therapy the catheter was placed into the gastroduodenal or inferior epigastric artery, then brought through a separate stab wound on the abdominal wall.

Since the development of the subcutaneously placed port, the more common surgically placed arterial catheters are implantable ports, similar to the venous ports discussed in Chapter 7 (see Fig. 7–8). With these catheters the entire access system is internal, so the possibility of trauma to the catheter is minimized.

Clients with surgically placed catheters may receive their chemotherapy via a portable infusion pump at home or are admitted to the hospital each time the next cycle of chemotherapy is due.

Other clients have implantable infusion pumps placed into the subcutaneous tissue in the abdomen. An internal arterial catheter connects to the pump. Medication is injected into the pump reservoir by placing a needle through the abdomen and into a port on the pump. Medication infuses into the artery at a preprogrammed rate (see Fig. 5–18). The client can resume a normal lifestyle while receiving therapy.

The clients who will receive outpatient IAC should be willing to receive chemotherapy in an environment without readily available medical assistance, have a willing and able caregiver, and be responsible enough to manage the administration.

## CLIENT PREPARATION

Clients preparing for a surgical placement of an arterial catheter require preoperative preparation similar to any other surgery. The client probably is given nothing by mouth (NPO) after midnight the night before the scheduled surgery. If an external catheter is inserted, the client will not be able to get the surgical site wet for up to 5 days. The catheter exit site must remain covered with a sterile dressing for up to 6 weeks to avoid infection. This dressing is changed three times each week.

The surgeon uses radiography during the procedure to visualize the arterial vasculature. If the tumor site or target vessel is supplied by a number of other arteries, these may be occluded using Gelfoam or metal coils as in the radiographically placed catheter.

## ANESTHESIA

Because surgical placement of an arterial catheter is more involved than radiographical placement and requires at least one incision, clients may receive general anesthesia or intravenous sedation with local anesthesia.

## PLACING THE CATHETER

After preparing the site the surgeon makes an incision through the skin to cut down to the artery. Arterial ports are most commonly placed in the hepatic artery. The gastroduodenal artery is encannulated with the catheter, and the tip is advanced to the junction of the gastroduodenal and common hepatic arteries. The port is subcutaneously implanted over the lower rib cage.

Unlike venous ports this device is not recommended for blood drawing because of the high pressure within the artery and the increased chance for clotting. As in the case with venous ports, the nurse accesses these devices only with Huber-point needles to avoid coring the port diaphragm.

## CHECKING PLACEMENT

Because the surgeon can see the vessels as he or she works on them, there is no need to check the catheter placement with radiography and contrast media (dye).

## DRESSING THE SITE

After the surgery the client is discharged from the operating room with a dry sterile dressing over the suture or staple line. The surgeon will provide orders for dressing care.

When the port is accessed and in use, a sterile dressing is required to maintain sterility of the accessed site and to assist with keeping the port needle in place.

## DOCUMENTATION

The nurse documents the client's condition on return from the operating room, making special note of the client's

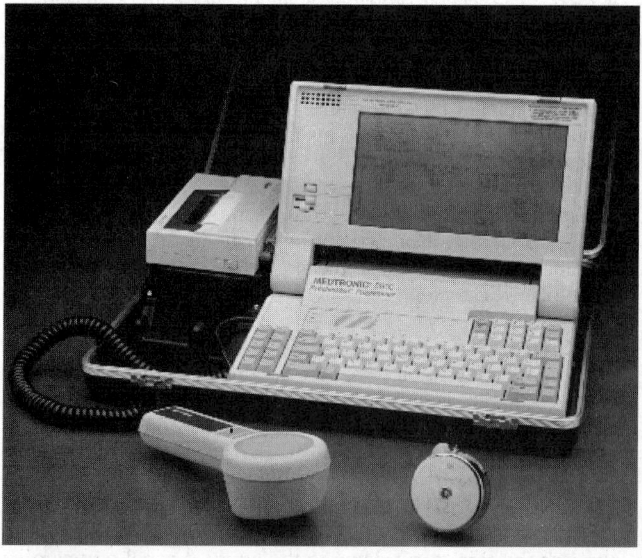


**FIGURE 10–2.** The SynchroMed Infusion System pump can be programmed via radio signals to dispense medication through a catheter at a specific body site. (Courtesy of Medtronic, Inc., Minneapolis, Minnesota.)

bilateral dorsalis pedis arterial pulses. The client may return from the operating room with a heparin infusion running. The nurse maintains the infusion and documents the amount and concentration of the drug running.

### COMPLICATIONS

**Occlusion.** If a clot should obstruct the catheter, the physician will probably order the use of urokinase.

## Implantable Pumps

Another alternative for arterial therapy is the implantable infusion pump. These pumps' descriptions and procedures for use are discussed in Chapter 5. The pumps are surgically implanted in a pocket of subcutaneous tissue in the lower abdomen or the chest. A surgically placed silicone catheter is attached to the pump and tunneled to the target infusion site. One of the pumps, the Infusaid, delivers the chemotherapeutic agent at a preset rate based on the pump's model number. Another pump, the SynchroMed Infusion System, is telemetrically programmed by the health care team to deliver the medication at the prescribed rate (Fig. 10–2).

CHAPTER 11

# Intraperitoneal Therapy

*Marilyn Ferreri Booker*



## DESCRIPTION

Intraperitoneal (IP) therapy is the administration of therapeutic agents (cytotoxic drugs and biologic response modifiers [BRMs]) into the peritoneal cavity. This method of drug administration is receiving renewed attention in cancer research, as pharmacokinetic evaluations and clinical trials verify the advantages of this approach for tumors confined to the peritoneal cavity.

The peritoneal cavity generally acts as a tumor refuge separated from the blood stream by a cellular enclosure similar to that of the blood-brain barrier. The barrier protects the tumor by not allowing systemic chemotherapy to penetrate the peritoneum adequately. IP therapy allows for the administration of a high concentration of antineoplastic agents directly to tumor sites in the peritoneal cavity. This enhances the drug's penetration and cell kill while restricting systemic effects. The drug stays in the peritoneum and allows a continued attack on the tumor with a clearing 10 times slower than if administered intravenously or intraarterially (Swenson, 1986). IP therapy provides for greater antitumor effect with fewer toxic side effects such as myelosuppression, nephrotoxicity, and neurotoxicity. Peak drug levels that could not be tolerated systemically can be achieved intraperitoneally.

## CONSIDERATIONS

### Disease Site

IP therapy is effective in treating cancers limited to the peritoneal cavity. Carcinomas of the ovaries and fallopian tubes generally meet this criterion. These cancers are usually confined to the peritoneal cavity when they are diagnosed and are limited to this region even as the disease progresses to the end stage. Clients with these cancers seldom experience morbidity or mortality from distant metastases. IP therapy has also been given for other cancers confined to the IP cavity such as colon/rectal, endometrial, gastric, bladder, breast mesothelioma, sarcoma, germ cell, and cancers of unknown origin (Laffer et al., 1988; Markman et al., 1985).

### Type of Therapy

Chemotherapeutic agents and BRMs are two types of drugs given in IP therapy.

#### CHEMOTHERAPEUTIC AGENTS

Chemotherapeutic agents cause tumor destruction by directly affecting the tumor cells. Chemotherapeutic drugs are used in IP therapy as single agents or in combination with other agents. Table 11–1 lists some of the drugs studied to date.

#### BIOLOGIC RESPONSE MODIFIERS

Sometimes called biotherapy, the use of BRMs is a fairly recent development in the treatment of cancer. BRMs are agents or approaches that modify the body's biologic response to tumor cells with therapeutic benefit. Some research has shown that some BRMs possess direct cytotoxic properties (Borden, 1984), but most act by enhancing the body's immune response. This action may be by activating

**TABLE 11–1**
**Chemotherapeutic Drugs**

| Generic | Trade Names/Synonyms |
|---|---|
| Cisplatin | Platinol, Platinol-AQ, CIS, CDDP |
| Doxorubicin | Adriamycin PFS, Adriamycin RDF, Rubex, ADR |
| Methotrexate | Folex, Folex PFS, Abitrexate, methotrexate LPF, Mexate, Mexate-AQ, MTX |
| Cytarabine | Cytosar-U, cytosine arabinoside, ARA-C |
| Vidarabine | Vira-A, ara-A, Adenine arabinoside |
| Etoposide | VePesid, VP-16-213 |
| Melphalan | Alkeran, L-PAM, phenylalanine mustard |
| Mitomycin | Mutamycin, mitomycin-C, MTC |
| Fluorouracil | Adrucil, 5-fluorouracil, 5-FU |

natural killer (NK) cells, lymphokine-activated killer (LAK) cells, and cytotoxic T cells. These effector cells perform the actual tumor destruction. The BRMs administered intraperitoneally include bacille Calmette-Guérin (BCG), *Corynebacterium parvum,* monoclonal antibodies, interferons, interleukin-2 (IL-2), LAK cells, and tumor necrosis factor (TNF) (Markman, 1987; Lotze et al., 1986; Bookman, 1989). Most often, these have been given as single agents; however, recently there has been research using these drugs in combination or concomitantly with chemotherapeutic agents.

## DEVICES

There are three types of IP access devices most commonly seen: temporary indwelling catheters, semipermanent indwelling external catheters, and implantable IP ports. As with any medical device, there are advantages and disadvantages associated with each type.

### Temporary Indwelling Catheters

#### DESCRIPTION

Temporary indwelling catheters include the temporary peritoneal dialysis catheter, paracentesis catheters, and a 16- or 18-gauge over-the-needle intravenous (IV) catheter.

#### ADVANTAGES

Many temporary indwelling catheters may be inserted and removed at the bedside. The temporary catheters are relatively inexpensive. Because these catheters are only inserted for a short period of time, they are less likely to develop fibrous sheaths or infections. Also because these catheters are removed before the client leaves the medical facility, he or she will not require home care.

#### DISADVANTAGES

Temporary indwelling catheters are associated with an increased risk of visceral perforation. This catheter is not recommended for cyclic therapy because of the necessity for placing the catheter with each treatment. Clients with these catheters require extra precautions when moving, as displacement of the catheter is likely.

### Semipermanent Indwelling External Catheters

#### DESCRIPTION

Three types of indwelling external catheters include the Tenckhoff catheter, the Gore-tex catheter, and the column-disk catheter (Fig. 11–1). The Tenckhoff catheter is a soft,

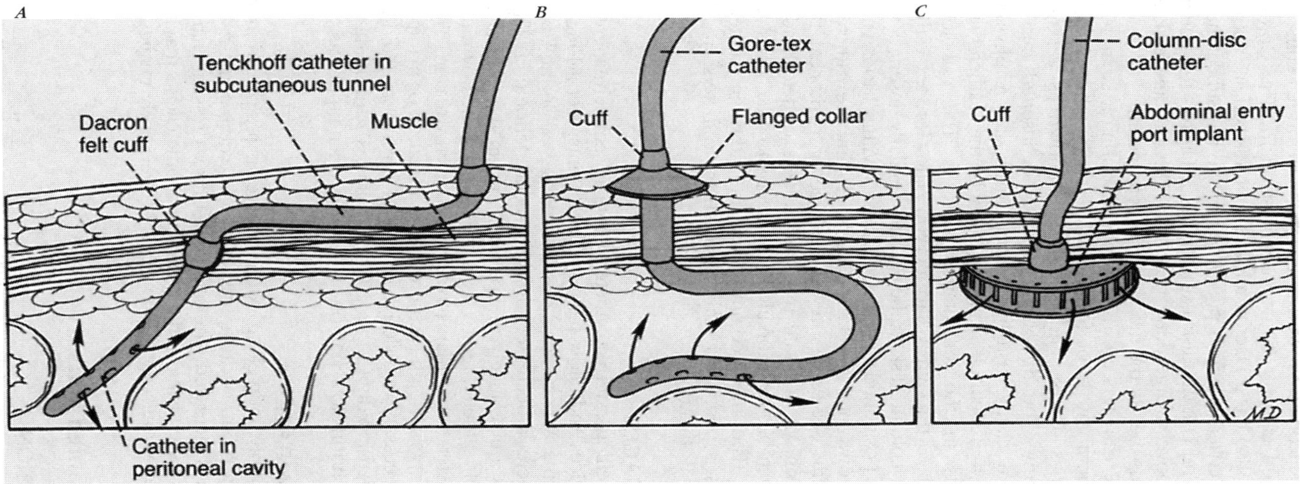


**FIGURE 11–1.** Three types of indwelling external catheters. **A,** Tenckhoff catheter. **B,** Gore-tex catheter. **C,** Column-disk catheter. (From Black, J. M. & Matassarin-Jacobs, E. [1993]. *Luckmann and Sorensen's medical surgical nursing: A psychophysiologic approach* [4th ed., p. 1511]. Philadelphia: W. B. Saunders.)

flexible silicone tube with one or two Dacron felt cuffs. The two-cuffed catheter is the current standard. The Gore-tex catheter also has a Dacron felt cuff, but this cuff sits above a flanged collar, which is positioned in the the subcutaneous tissue. The column-disk catheter has a Dacron felt cuff located above a large entry port disk. The cuff and disk are placed just below the fascia in the peritoneum.

These catheters are usually placed during a laparotomy. The laparotomy is performed to determine the extent of the client's disease and is therefore known as a staging laparotomy. The tip of the catheter is inserted into the peritoneal cavity, usually at the tumor site. A physician placing a Tenckhoff catheter tunnels the catheter with the cuffs in the subcutaneous tissue. The catheter is externalized through a stab incision. The Gore-tex catheter and the column-disk catheters are similarly inserted with the cuffs positioned as described above. Within 1 to 2 weeks, tissue grows into the Dacron cuffs, affixing the catheter in place. This serves to prevent leakage of peritoneal fluid, medication, or dialysate from around the catheter and inhibits microbial invasion along the tract into the client's peritoneum. The most common use of indwelling external catheters is peritoneal dialysis, but these catheters are also used for IP therapy.

#### ADVANTAGES

Indwelling external catheters serve as semipermanent access devices and allow for cyclic treatments over a long period of time. When such catheters are inserted during laparotomy, there is decreased risk of visceral perforation. These catheters are relatively inexpensive, and in the case of the Tenckhoff catheter, removal can be accomplished by pulling the catheter rather than through a surgical excision. These catheters permit high-pressure forced irrigation or manipulation if necessary to dislodge or loosen fibrin clots. Fluid can be instilled rapidly (2 L in 10 to 15 minutes), and in the absence of fibrin clots, peritoneal fluid can drain rapidly as well.

#### DISADVANTAGES

Preferably, indwelling external catheters are placed in the operating room. Because the catheter is external, the risk of infection is increased. The catheter requires dressing changes to the exit site, using sterile technique. Some clients may find this catheter unacceptable in terms of their body images.

### IP Implanted Ports

#### DESCRIPTION

Like other models of implanted ports, the totally implanted subcutaneous IP port has two major components: a portal body and the Silastic catheter. The portal body has a self-sealing silicone rubber septum that allows access to the chamber by the insertion of a noncoring needle through the skin and into the chamber (see Fig. 7–8). The physician inserts the catheter through a small incision near the umbilicus into the peritoneum, with the catheter tip placed into the right or left gutter prerectally. A distal Dacron cuff is tethered to the rectus abdominis muscle fascia. The rest of the catheter is tunneled subcutaneously to the portal body, which is placed subcutaneously in a pocket beneath the skin and sutured to the fascia of the muscles overlying an anatomic area that provides support and stability, usually the lower rib cage below the breast.

#### ADVANTAGES

Like the indwelling external catheters the IP port is a semipermanent device that provides access for cyclic therapy over a long period of time. The port must be surgically placed, thereby decreasing the potential for visceral perforation. Because there is no external catheter, the incidence of infection is lower than with external devices, and no home catheter maintenance is required. The absence of an external catheter also positively influences client acceptance of the device.

#### DISADVANTAGES

The IP port requires surgical placement and surgical removal. The device itself is more expensive than either the temporary catheter or the indwelling external catheters. The catheter does not tolerate forced irrigation or manipulation to dislodge or loosen clots. The manufacturer recommends that pressure not exceed 40 psi (pounds per square inch). Clients with needle phobias dislike the required needle stick each time the port is accessed.

## ADMINISTRATION OF THERAPY

Many different protocols are presently prescribed for administration of therapeutic agents intraperitoneally. Some clients may receive therapy for 24 hours a week for 16 weeks; others receive a 24-hour infusion for 7 days, every other week, for eight cycles; and still others may receive therapy every 4 weeks for six cycles.

No matter what the frequency and number of cycles the client is to receive, each treatment usually consists of three phases: the instillation phase, the dwell phase, and the drain phase (Fig. 11–2).

### Instillation Phase

The instillation phase is the shortest of the three phases. During instillation the therapeutic agent is infused through

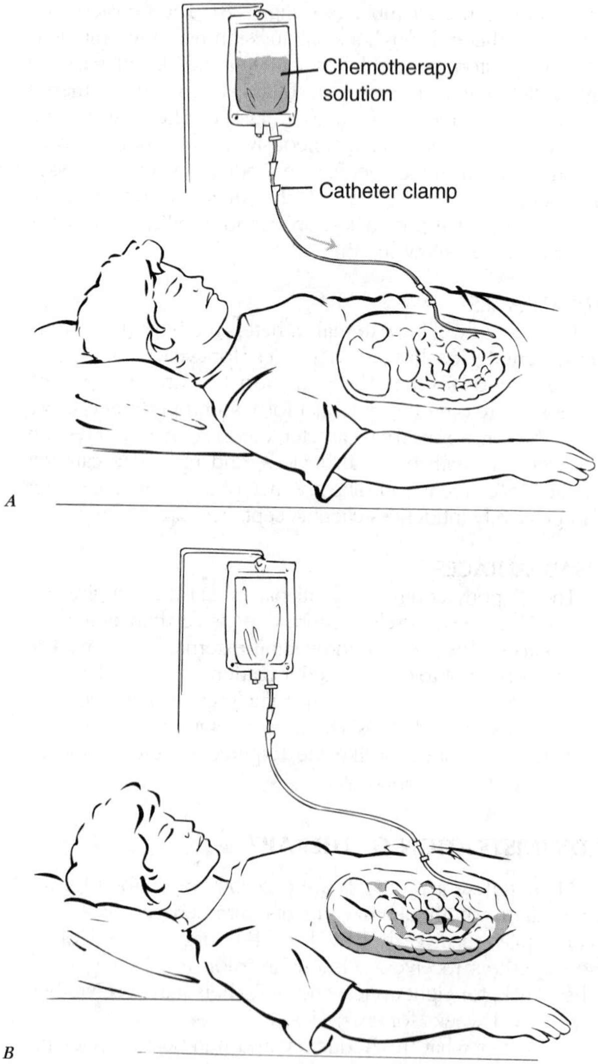


**FIGURE 11–2.** Chemotherapy administration. **A,** Installation phase. The therapeutic agent is infused into the peritoneal cavity. **B,** Dwell phase. The catheter clamps are closed, and the therapeutic agent is held in the peritoneal cavity.

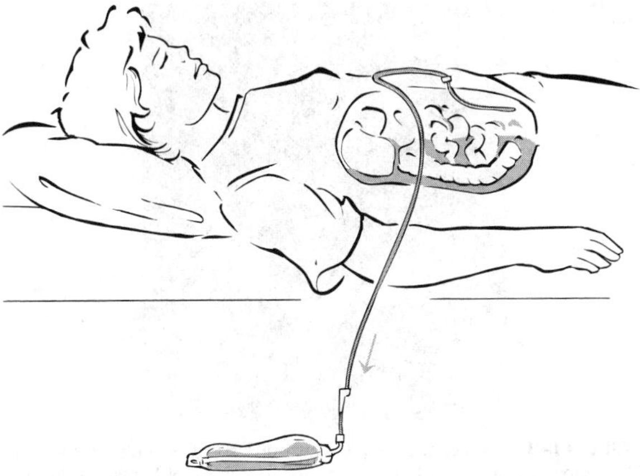


**FIGURE 11–2.** C, Drain phase. The solution container is hung below the level of the client, and the clamps are opened, allowing the medication to drain into the container.

the catheter into the peritoneal cavity. The drug is usually mixed in 1 to 2 L of an isotonic solution. The solution infuses via gravity usually over 15 to 20 minutes.

### Dwell Phase

The longest of the three phases is the dwell phase. During this phase the therapeutic agent rests in the peritoneal cavity. The nurse assists the client in changing position to allow the solution to come in contact with all the peritoneal surfaces. This contact allows for maximal therapeutic effect. The dwell time may last from 2 to 6 hours, depending on the protocol.

### Drain Phase

During the drain phase the solution is allowed to drain by gravity or a mild suction apparatus into a sterile container. This process is usually completed within 2 hours.

Some protocols allow the fluid to remain in the peritoneal cavity. About 80% of peritoneal fluid is absorbed by portal circulation. The drug is partially detoxified by the liver before entering systemic circulation. This reduces the systemic toxicities usually associated with the individual drugs. This process of reabsorption generally takes 24 hours.

## ADMINISTRATION EQUIPMENT

In protocols that require draining the therapeutic solution after the dwell phase, a closed administration set is used.

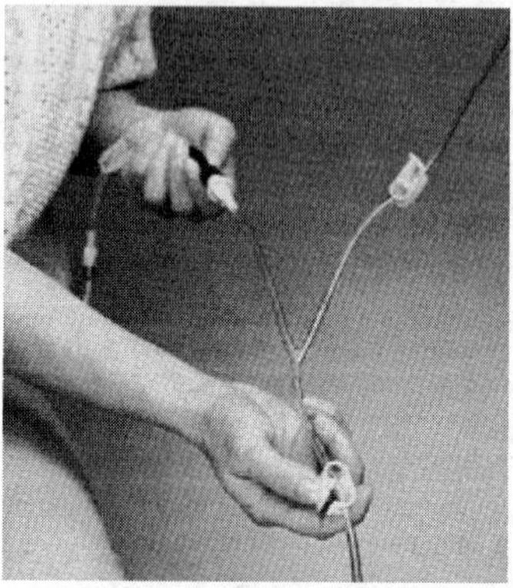

**FIGURE 11–3.** The continuous peritoneal dialysis set includes a Y-system with clamps that direct the flow of the fluid. (Courtesy of Baxter Healthcare Corporation, Deerfield, Illinois.)

Similar to a disposable continuous ambulatory peritoneal dialysis (CAPD) set, a closed administration set incorporates a Y-system with clamps that direct the flow of the fluid (Fig. 11–3). The afferent arm has a spike like a regular infusion administration set. The therapeutic agent is administered through this arm into the client's peritoneum. The efferent arm is attached to a sterile drainage bag. Between these two arms is the tubing that connects to the client's peritoneal catheter. During the instillation phase the roller clamps on the tubing from the drug and the tubing to the client are opened while the clamp on the tubing to the drainage bag is closed. This directs the fluid to the client. During the dwell phase, all roller clamps are closed to keep the therapeutic agent in the peritoneum. If there is a drain phase, the roller clamp on the tubing from the drug is closed while the clamps on the tubing from the client and the tubing to the drainage bag are open. This directs the fluid flow from the client to the drainage bag.

## PREPARING THE CLIENT

### Peritoneal Perfusion Scan

In some oncology centers, clients have a peritoneal perfusion scan before the first treatment and at intervals during the therapy series. This initial scan documents the uniformity or nonuniformity of the peritoneal cavity. Follow-up scans evaluate any changes in fluid distribution after several IP treatments by identifying loculations (small cavities) or adhesions and any measurable disease at that point in therapy.

To prepare the client for the scan the nurse infuses 2 L of body temperature normal saline solution (NSS) containing radiopaque dye into the peritoneal cavity via the client's peritoneal access device. The client then has a computed tomography (CT) scan. The fluid is drained from the client's peritoneal cavity as described in the procedure below.

## ADMINISTERING IP THERAPY

### Instructing the Client

The nurse describes the procedure to the client before administering the therapy. The description includes the drugs to be given and their dosages, as well as potential side effects and their management. After the treatment the client's abdominal girth is likely to be larger than before the treatment. For this reason the nurse instructs the client to wear garments that fit loosely around the waist.

### Administering the Drug

1. Warm the drug infusion to room or body temperature as described in agency policy.
2. Don gloves and access the peritoneal port as described in Chapter 7. If the client has a Tenckhoff catheter, cleanse the catheter as described in agency policy.
3. Flush the catheter with 10 mL of 0.9% NSS. (Some agencies prefer preservative-free saline.)
4. Prime the administration set with the drug solution.
5. Attach the administration set to the client's peritoneal access device.
6. Open the clamps on the tubing that runs between the infusion container and the client. Make sure the clamp between the drainage bag and the client is closed.
7. Infuse the drug solution into the client's peritoneum over 15 to 20 minutes. Slow the rate if the client complains of discomfort. Administer analgesics as ordered if necessary. If the flow is sluggish, assist the client in rolling from side to side to improve flow. Irrigating the catheter with 0.9% NSS may improve flow. If you are sure the catheter is patent, administer the drug via an IV infusion pump to assist with the instillation.
8. Close all clamps and allow the drug solution to dwell for the prescribed time, usually 2 to 6 hours.
9. During the dwell time, assist the client in changing position every 15 to 20 minutes to assure that the entire peritoneal surface is bathed in the solution.

10. Observe the client for shortness of breath. Position the client in a high Fowler position to alleviate any respiratory distress. If it is severe, the physician may prescribe oxygen therapy.
11. At the end of the dwell time if the protocol includes draining the therapeutic solution, open the clamps between the client and the drainage bag.
12. Turn the client side to side to promote drainage.
13. If the drainage is inadequate, instruct the client to perform the Valsalva maneuver and apply moderate pressure to the client's abdomen with your hand.
14. After 2 hours, flush the catheter with 10 mL of 0.9% NSS. If the catheter is a port, follow this with 10 mL of 100 U/mL heparinized saline solution.

## COMPLICATIONS

### Leakage Around Site

**Definition.** Ascitic fluid or drug solution leaks around catheter.

**Cause.** Leakage may be due to incomplete healing of tunneled tract or failure of scar tissue to grow into the Dacron cuffs, especially in the presence of abdominal pressure due to ascites.

**Signs and Symptoms.** Exit site dressing is wet.

**Management.** Assessment of the exit site area is performed at least every 8 hours. Before administering any treatment the nurse withdraws or drains ascitic fluid. This decreases abdominal pressure.

**Documentation.** The nurse documents the appearance of the area and the dressing every 8 hours.

**Prevention.** Allowing the tissue at the Dacron cuffs on the Tenckhoff catheter to heal for about 2 weeks before using the catheter for IP therapy usually eliminates the potential for leakage.

### Exit Site Infection

**Definition.** Exit site infection is indicated by redness, tenderness, and warmth of the tissue around the catheter site with or without exudate. It is more frequently seen with Tenckhoff catheters than with ports.

**Cause.** Exit site infection is caused by contamination of the exit site area, usually with skin flora.

**Signs and Symptoms.** See Definition.

**Management.** The nurse assesses and documents the client's symptoms and obtains a culture of the areas around the catheter exit site. The client requires frequent skin care and dressing changes, using sterile technique. The physician may prescribe an antimicrobial ointment with the dressing changes.

**Documentation.** Careful recording of all signs and symptoms, treatments, and the client's response is appropriate.

**Prevention.** While the client is in the hospital, the exit site is maintained with a sterile dressing. During the first 2 weeks after insertion the client requires daily dressing changes with povidone-iodine solution and a dry sterile dressing. If after 2 weeks there is no sign of infection, the client may wash the area daily with soap and water in the shower and cover the site with a dry sterile dressing. Taping the catheter to the client's abdomen prevents accidental pulling, which can lead to irritation and subsequent infection.

## Microbial Peritonitis

**Definition.** Inflammation of the peritoneal membranes from the invasion and proliferation of microbes is called microbial peritonitis.

**Cause.** Microbial peritonitis is caused by contamination of the peritoneal access device or the administration system.

**Signs and Symptoms.** The client may have a fever greater than 100°F or may complain of abdominal pain or tenderness. The nurse may or may not note abdominal rigidity and rebound tenderness. The peritoneal fluid is usually cloudy (although this may be a desired symptom, indicating the presence of lymphokine-activated killer (LAK) or natural killer (NK) cells in the client receiving BRMs). There is usually an elevated white blood cell count (WBC) in the peritoneal fluid, or the client's blood count may indicate an increase in the WBC.

**Management.** Monitor the client's vital signs every 4 hours. When obtaining and handling peritoneal fluid specimens for culture and sensitivity, the nurse maintains sterile technique to avoid contaminating the specimen. The physician usually prescribes antimicrobials intravenously or intraperitoneally.

**Documentation.** The nurse carefully documents all observations and actions, including the appearance of the peritoneal fluid and the client's symptoms.

**Prevention.** In all dealings with the client's catheter the nurse maintains strict sterile technique, including washing hands with an antimicrobial soap before handling the system, scrubbing all connections with povidone-iodine solution before separating them, and wearing sterile gloves when opening any connections in the system. When possible, the nurse minimizes accessing the system to reduce the chance of contamination. The nurse changes solution containers and bags every 24 hours; but for long therapies the tubing is changed every 7 days (Zook-Enck, 1990).

## Chemical Peritonitis

**Definition.** Inflammation of the peritoneal lining caused by the antineoplastic agent is called chemical peritonitis.

**Cause.** Chemical peritonitis is caused by contact irritation of the antineoplastic agent.

**Signs and Symptoms.** The client may exhibit all the signs and symptoms of a microbial peritonitis with the exception of bacterial growth. The onset is generally after the instillation of the drug and may persist for a period of time after completion of the therapy. If it is severe, chemical peritonitis may require a delay in further treatment or a discontinuation of treatment. In addition, severe chemical peritonitis can lead to microbial peritonitis and sepsis.

**Management.** Assessment of the client, including vital signs every 4 hours and a pain assessment, is important. The physician usually prescribes analgesics to treat the pain.

**Documentation.** Documentation of all assessments assists in determining the severity of the peritonitis.

**Prevention.** Warming the IP solution assists with decreasing the client's pain. If the client experienced chemical peritonitis with a previous treatment, the physician may alter the drug dosing with subsequent treatments.

## Occlusion

**Definition.** Occlusion is the inability to administer fluid into the peritoneum or withdraw fluid from the peritoneum (one-way valve effect).

**Cause.** Occlusion is caused by formation of fibrous sheaths or fibrin clots or plugs inside the catheter or around the tip; compartmentalization of fluid due to adhesions; or twisting, kinking, or displacement of the catheter.

**Signs and Symptoms.** Fluid does not infuse or drain from the peritoneum.

**Management.** At the first sign of sluggish instillation or drainage the nurse notifies the physician. The nurse checks the tubing for kinks, making certain that all appropriate clamps are open. Keeping the drainage bag below the client's abdomen aids in draining fluid from the peritoneum. Having the client change position may encourage instillation or drainage. If an indwelling external catheter is used, forceful irrigation and aspiration (a "push-pull" irrigation technique) with 10 mL of 0.9% NSS may help. This manipulation is inappropriate through a peritoneal port, as any pressure exceeding 40 psi may cause the catheter to shear from the port. The physician may attempt to remove the occlusion by inserting a sterile stylet into the catheter. In some cases, particularly if the client has a peritoneal port, the physician may prescribe a drip of 25,000 IU of urokinase in 250 mL 0.9%

NSS to infuse over 4 hours in an attempt to lyse the clots or sheath.

**Documentation.** In the client's medical record the nurse documents any procedures (both successful and unsuccessful) used to clear the occlusion.

**Prevention.** Irrigating the catheter with 30 to 50 mL 0.9% NSS before and after administering therapy or withdrawing any fluid assists with keeping the catheter patent. Maintaining the drainage bag below the catheter site aids in drainage.

CHAPTER 12

# Intraosseous Infusion

*Marilyn Ferreri Booker*



A previously used and reemerging method of gaining access to the vascular system is via the intraosseous approach. This method provides rapid access to the vascular system in critically injured clients. Clients who are critically ill or injured frequently develop circulatory collapse, making the health care team's ability to gain direct access to the venous system difficult or impossible.

Intraosseous access involves the insertion of a rigid needle with an inner stylet into the client's bone marrow cavity. This procedure is generally seen in trauma units, emergency departments, or at an accident site. Prehospital providers, such as emergency medical technicians (EMTs) and paramedics, or physicians usually perform the procedure. But in some areas of the country, infusion nurses who have completed advanced training such as the Pediatric Advanced Life Support (PALS), Advanced Cardiac Life Support (ACLS), and the Advanced Trauma Life Support (ATLS) courses may initiate this therapy (Manley, 1988).

## SITE SELECTION

### Client Considerations

#### AGE

Because the objective of therapy is to gain access to the rich vascular network located in the long bones, intraosseous infusions are generally best used in the child under the age of 6 years (Wheeler, 1988). The red spongy bone marrow found in this age group is replaced by yellow bone marrow as people age, rendering the long bones inadequate as a route to the vascular system in the adult. By the time the client reaches the age of 18 years, red bone marrow and consequently hematopoietic activity are found only in the vertebrae, ribs, skull, pelvis, and the most proximal portions of the extremities (Manley, 1988).

In the past 10 years, however, there has been expansion in the use of intraosseous infusion, and the technique is occasionally used in adults as well as children. As the technique is more widely researched, the nurse may see intraosseous infusions in adults more frequently.

## HISTORY

Children with a history of bone disorders such as osteopenia (decrease in the mass per volume of bone) or osteogenesis imperfecta (inherited condition causing brittle bones) are not candidates for intraosseous infusions. Inserting a needle through the bone of a client with these types of bone disorders results in trauma to the bone and possible permanent disabilities.

## PRESENT CONDITION

Intraosseous infusion is generally used for very ill children or those who have sustained some trauma such as from a car accident or fire. Therefore, consideration is given to any bone fractures or burns in the area of proposed needle insertion. Neither these areas nor the area beneath infected tissue (cellulitis) is an appropriate site for needle insertion. The infusion of fluid or drugs through a needle inserted into a fractured bone causes an infiltration of the infusate. Passing a needle through infected tissue can seed bacteria in the bone, resulting in osteomyelitis.

## SITE CONSIDERATIONS

Virtually any bone is a potential insertion site in the young child. However, the distal tibia, the proximal tibia, and the distal femur are areas of choice. These locations allow easy accessibility. In view of the fact that this access is used for children who are in a life-threatening condition or who have undergone cardiac arrest, these sites can be initiated without interruption of lifesaving techniques such as airway management or cardiac compressions.

Of these locations the one most often recommended is the anterior medial aspect of the tibia. This area is flat and easily accessible. The cortex of the bone and the tissue over this area are thin. This location also lacks other strutures such as large muscle groups, blood vessels, or nerves (Manley, 1988).

## Type and Duration of Therapy

The infusion site also may be used to aspirate blood from the medullary cavity and to monitor changes in arterial pH and $Paco_2$. Access to this information without having to draw blood from an elusive artery during cardiac arrest is very beneficial during resuscitative efforts. Once the client is stabilized and the veins are accessible, the nurse or physician initiates a traditional central venous or peripheral intravenous (IV) line to administer the child's therapy.

Fluids that have been successfully administered intraosseously include 5% and 10% dextrose in water (D5W and D10W); blood products, including packed red blood cells, plasma, and whole blood; Ringer's lactate; and saline solutions. The list of drugs includes antibiotics, anticonvulsants, atropine, catecholamines, mannitol, dextrose and sodium bicarbonate, digoxin, dopamine, dobutamine, lidocaine (Xylocaine), and succinylcholine (Manley, 1988; Drigger et al., 1991). Absorption rates of drugs and fluids administered intraosseously are similar to those achieved with peripheral or central venous administration (Neufeld et al., 1986; Drigger et al., 1991).

# DEVICES

Although theoretically any needle may be used to access the medullary space, certain considerations make some needles superior to others.

Standard hypodermic and butterfly needles are readily available in emergency departments and on emergency rescue vehicles. However, these needles may become clogged with bone deposits during the insertion. Also, these needles tend to have thin walls that cause them to wobble or bend during the procedure. Although spinal needles have a removable stylet, their thin walls cause them to bend. Bone marrow needles generally work well. They have a removable stylet and thicker walls, but the shaft is usually longer than necessary and may become dislodged after the insertion.

Features of needles well-suited for intraosseous infusion include a removable stylet that screws into the cannula to keep the needle from retracting during insertion, a short shaft to eliminate accidental dislodgment after placement, an adjustable guard to stabilize the needle at skin level, and graduations along the needle to guide the practitioner during the insertion. Two commercially available needles fit this description: the Jamshidi Disposable Modified Illinois Sternal/Iliac Bone Marrow Aspiration Needle (Baxter, Valencia, California) and the disposable intraosseous infusion needle by Cook Critical Care (Bloomington, Indiana) (Wheeler, 1988).

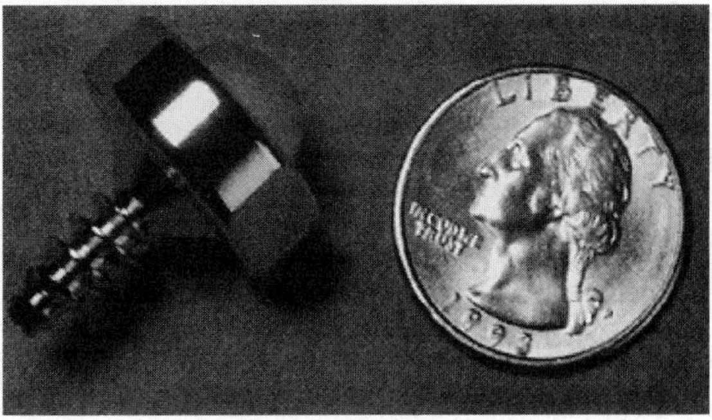

**FIGURE 12–1.** Osteoport. (Courtesy of LifeQuest Medical, Inc., San Antonio, Texas.)

An 18-gauge needle is best for infants up to the age of 8 months, whereas older children require a 15- to 16-gauge needle (Wheeler, 1988).

Osteoport is a new and improved intraosseous needle from LifeQuest Medical, Inc. (Fig. 12–1). The Osteoport is similar to a subcutaneous venous access device in that it is implanted under the skin and the practitioner accesses the device's septum with a needle through the skin. Because it must be surgically implanted, the placement of the Osteoport has no value as a field procedure, but it is appropriate for placement in hospitalized clients who require alternate vascular access. The Osteoport consists of a 1-inch titanium or stainless steel needle with a self-sealing septum. Along the sides of the shaft are threads that allow for precise placement in the marrow and keep the device from moving. The Osteoport can be placed while the client is under general or local anesthesia. The Osteoport is indicated for clients whose vascular access is exhausted and who require no more than 30 days of infusion therapy.

## INSERTION TECHNIQUE

The role of the nurse in intraosseous therapy varies with the health care setting. In some areas the nurse may insert the cannula and maintain the site. In other areas the nurse may be limited to assisting the physician or other health care practitioner during the insertion. In all cases the nurse should be prepared to maintain the site, identify complications, and administer drugs or fluids.

### Client Preparation

Once the decision to insert an intraosseous needle is made, the procedure itself takes from 30 to 60 seconds.

## Performing the Insertion

As with any invasive procedure, the practitioner inserts the intraosseous needle under strict aseptic technique.

### PREPARING THE SKIN

The nurse prepares the area over the intended insertion site by cleansing the area with the institution's approved cleansing agent. The nurse cleans the area with a circular motion from the intended penetration site out about 2 inches (5 cm) and allows the area to air dry before inserting the needle. This provides an antibacterial barrier around the insertion site.

### ADMINISTERING A LOCAL ANESTHETIC

In the case of a client who is unconscious or who has had cardiac arrest, a local anesthetic is not needed. For a conscious client a local anesthetic is injected into the skin and periosteum before needle insertion.

### INSERTING THE NEEDLE

The nurse assists the practitioner inserting the needle by stabilizing the extremity. The practitioner inserting the needle holds the needle between the first and second fingers of his or her dominant hand with the thumb against the top of the device (Fig. 12–2). With the bevel of the needle away from the joint, the practitioner penetrates the skin and directs the needle at a 10- to 15-degree angle away from the epiphyseal plate. Firm, downward pressure with a rotary or "screwing" motion is applied until there is less resistance or a "pop" felt. The needle does not need to be advanced any further. To do

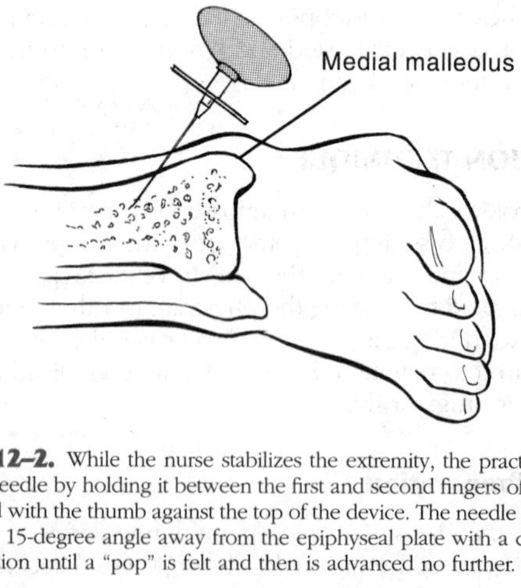


**FIGURE 12–2.** While the nurse stabilizes the extremity, the practitioner inserts the needle by holding it between the first and second fingers of the dominant hand with the thumb against the top of the device. The needle is directed at a 10- to 15-degree angle away from the epiphyseal plate with a downward rotary motion until a "pop" is felt and then is advanced no further.

so may cause the needle to puncture the other side of the bone.

#### CHECKING NEEDLE PLACEMENT

To check placement the stylet is removed and a syringe attached to the cannula hub. Aspiration of bone marrow, similar in appearance to blood, confirms placement. In some cases it may be difficult to aspirate bone marrow. If this occurs and the needle is firmly in place, the nurse flushes the cannula with 2 to 3 mL of sterile 0.9% normal saline solution (NSS) while palpating the extremity for infiltration. There may be slight resistance felt such as that of inflating the balloon on a Foley catheter. More resistance than this could mean that the bevel of the needle has not penetrated the bone's cortex or may be lodged against the opposite cortex. The practitioner may attempt to adjust the cannula position. In the event of extravasation the needle should be removed and this bone not used for further infusions.

After the nurse determines that the cannula placement is correct, the access may be used for the administration of fluids or medications.

#### DRESSING THE SITE

Because this cannula is not intended for long-term therapy, it is doubtful that the site will require dressing changes. After insertion, the needle should require very little in the way of securing it to the skin because it is firmly anchored into the cortex of the bone. A dry sterile dressing with 4 × 4's or a transparent semipermeable membrane (TSM) dressing maintains the area sterile. The nurse changes this dressing if it becomes soiled or wet.

#### DOCUMENTATION

After the procedure, the nurse documents the following:

- Date and time of the procedure
- Type, gauge, and length of the intraosseous cannula
- Site in which it was inserted
- The infusion solution hung, including additives, amount, rate, and any medications administered
- The type of pump or controller (if applicable)
- The name and title of the person performing the procedure (if applicable)
- The nurse's name and title

### Administration

#### FLUIDS

Administration of fluids by gravity may be slow at first probably because of the clogging of the cannula with bone marrow contents or densely packed cells in the marrow cavity. The flow rate can be increased by flushing with 5 to 10 mL of sterile 0.9% NSS to clear the cannula, but flow rates are not as rapid as through an IV line (Spivey, 1987). Flow rates of 10 mL/min with gravity and 41 mL/min with 300 mm Hg pressure bag have been demonstrated with a 13-gauge needle in the medial malleolus of calves (Shoor et al., 1972). If no other alternatives exist, volume resuscitation may be accomplished by starting another intraosseous infusion site in the opposite limb.

#### DRUGS

Drugs may be administered by intraosseous push or infusion. When administered by push, the initial peak level is usually not as high as that with an IV push, but within minutes these levels correspond favorably (Spivey, 1987). The nurse may enhance the achievement of earlier drug peak levels by flushing the cannula with 10 mL of 0.9% NSS after administering the drug. This additional volume may cause the drug to enter the peripheral circulation more rapidly. Furthermore, serum levels of drugs administered by the intraosseous route tend to be elevated longer than when administered intravenously. However, this fact should not alter drug dosages (Spivey, 1987).

## MAINTENANCE

Because intraosseous infusion therapy is usually initiated on clients who require resuscitative efforts, there is generally no actual maintenance schedule. These clients are surrounded by the health care team until they are stable or it is determined that emergency efforts are no longer appropriate.

When hanging intraosseous infusion solutions and administering intermittent medications, the nurse follows the same procedure as for IV therapy (see Chapter 6).

### Monitoring and Documentation

The nurse monitors the site for any signs or symptoms of complications at the insertion site and documents any pertinent data derived from this assessment. These data include but are not limited to the condition of the site, the drugs or fluids used (including the infusion rate), and clinical data about the client (vital signs, appearance, and response to therapy).

### Discontinuing the Device

As soon as venous access can be established, the intraosseous cannula should be removed. After removing the dressing the nurse loosens the cannula from the bone by carefully rotating it. When this is accomplished, the nurse removes the cannula by pulling it straight out in one motion. The nurse applies pressure to the site for several minutes with a dry sterile gauze.

The nurse places a dry sterile dressing over the site. Daily observation and sterile dressing changes are the only other nursing care required.

## COMPLICATIONS

As with any invasive procedure, complications can occur. Fortunately, complications with this therapy are uncommon, most are associated with technique, and the risk of complications decreases as the practitioner gains more experience.

### Improper Needle Placement

Improper needle placement is the most common complication associated with technique. The nurse may observe infiltration of fluids or medications if there is either insufficient penetration into the marrow or accidental penetration into the other side of the bone.

### Needle Obstruction

If there is any delay in flushing the cannula or initiating the infusion after insertion, the cannula may become clotted with bone marrow. Repeating the aspiration with increased force or rotating the needle may clear the clots from the cannula. If these actions are not successful, it may be necessary to remove the cannula and initiate the therapy in another site (Wheeler, 1988).

### Osteomyelitis

Osteomyelitis is a complication of great concern. However, in more than 4000 cases of intraosseous therapy, only 0.6% of clients developed infections in the bone. In most of these cases, either the intraosseous cannula was left in for over 24 hours or the client had bacteremia before the insertion (Spivey, 1987). Osteomyelitis could have been avoided in those clients with prolonged cannula insertion by removing the cannula as soon as other vascular access could be established.

### Embolization

As with any orthopedic procedure the potential exists for a fat embolus or bony fragments to enter the peripheral circulation (Manley, 1988). The nurse observes the client for any respiratory distress, tachycardia, hypertension, tachypnea, fever, or petechiae. Laboratory data indicate an increased sedimentation rate and decreased red blood cell and platelet count.

## Damage to the Bone

In general, there is no permanent damage to the bone marrow or the bone itself with an intraosseous needle. After removal of the intraosseous cannula a round defect can be seen on x-ray, but by 6 weeks this is barely visible (Manley, 1988).

## Compartment Syndrome

There is some indication that in rare instances intraosseous infusions may cause compartment syndrome. Compartment syndrome is a condition in which increased tissue pressure in a confined anatomic space causes decreased blood flow. There is a report (Vidal et al., 1993) of a 1-month-old infant admitted to a community hospital for fever and irritability. The infant received fluids through a bone marrow needle inserted into the lower right leg. Fluids were infused over a 2-day period. Fluid collection was noticed in the infant's right foot after removal of the needle. The right foot was also cool to the touch. The infant's leg became progressively more swollen and discolored over a 3-day period. The infant was diagnosed with compartment syndrome, and the leg was amputated after no improvement in circulation occurred.

PART

# III

# Parenteral Fluids and Transfusion Therapy

# CHAPTER 13
# Fluids and Electrolytes

*Donna D. Ignatavicius*



Infusion therapy is often administered to maintain fluid and electrolyte balance in the body or to correct fluid and electrolyte imbalances. The nurse must fully recognize the significance of these imbalances when caring for clients receiving infusion therapy.

## FLUID AND ELECTROLYTE BALANCE

Body fluids and electrolytes are found throughout the body for cellular function. The total amount of fluids, primarily water, in an average adult male is 40 L, or 57% of the total body weight (Guyton, 1991). Fluids can be divided into intracellular and extracellular fluid compartments.

### Fluid Compartments

*Intracellular fluid* is contained within the cells of the body and accounts for approximately two thirds of all body fluid. The fluid of each cell contains its own mixture of different substances, but the concentration of the substances is similar from one cell to another.

*Extracellular fluid* can be further divided into three compartments: interstitial fluid, intravascular fluid, and transcellular fluid.

#### INTERSTITIAL FLUID

Interstitial fluid (ISF) is the fluid (including lymph fluid) around or between cells. Fluid and electrolytes move freely between this compartment and the intravascular space.

### INTRAVASCULAR FLUID

Intravascular fluid (IVF) is the fluid within the blood vessels, or plasma. The average blood volume for an adult is 5 L, of which 3 L is plasma. The remaining 2 L consists of red blood cells (erythrocytes), white blood cells (leukocytes), and platelets (thrombocytes).

### TRANSCELLULAR FLUID

Transcellular fluid (TCF) is found in many places within the body because it is secreted by epithelial cells. Examples of TCF include cerebrospinal fluid, intraocular fluid, digestive fluids, and synovial fluid.

## Fluid Gain and Loss

Water is necessary for life. Although people can live for several weeks without food, they can survive only a few days without water. Water is vital to the body for temperature regulation, blood volume maintenance, nutrient and electrolyte transport, and cellular metabolism. Body fluids, hormones, and electrolytes work together to maintain fluid balance.

Although body water is gained and lost every day, the net amount of body fluid remains fairly constant. Water is available for the body through food ingestion, oxidation, and water consumption as a liquid or as part of beverages. Water is lost from the body through the urine, skin, lungs, and feces. In an adult, about 2 L of water is gained and lost each day.

Many hormones and body systems help control fluid balance when the body experiences a health problem. For example, if a person has a fever, the kidneys conserve water and sodium in the body by decreasing urinary output. Conversely, if fluid intake is excessive, the kidneys eliminate additional water and sodium to maintain fluid balance. Sometimes these systems are unable to compensate for changes in fluid volume.

Although there are many ways to assess a person for fluid imbalance, body weight is one of the best indicators. A weight gain or loss without a change in diet or activity usually indicates water retention or loss. A weight gain of 2.2 lb (1 kg) is approximately equivalent to a gain of 1 L of water. A loss of 2.2 lb (1 kg) represents a loss of 1 L of water.

## Solutes in the Body

Solutes are substances that are dissolved in solution, called a *solvent*. The primary solvent in the body is water. The solutes are electrolytes and nonelectrolytes.

### ELECTROLYTES

Electrolytes are substances that carry an electric charge and can conduct an electric current when they are dissolved in solution. *Cations,* such as potassium, carry a positive charge. *Anions,* such as chloride, carry a negative charge. The primary intracellular cation is potassium ($K^+$), and the primary intracellular anion is phosphate. The major extracellular cation is sodium ($Na^+$), and the major anion is chloride ($Cl^-$).

As shown in Table 13–1, electrolytes are measured in milliequivalents per liter (mEq/L). The normal range for each of several important electrolytes is specified. In addition, the primary function of each electrolyte is listed.

## NONELECTROLYTES

Nonelectrolytes do not carry an electric charge or have the ability to conduct electricity. Examples of these substances include glucose, creatinine, and albumin. Some nonelectrolytes such as creatinine and urea are toxic wastes found in low concentrations in the blood and high concentrations in the urine. Other nonelectrolytes such as glucose and albumin are needed by cells to function and are often replaced by infusion therapy when their levels become too low.

**TABLE 13–1**
**Major Body Fluid Electrolyte Concentrations and Functions**

| Electrolyte | Serum Concentration (mEq/L) | Major Functions |
|---|---|---|
| Sodium ($Na^+$) | 136–145 | Maintenance of plasma osmolarity<br>Generation and transmission of action potentials<br>Maintenance of acid-base balance<br>Maintenance of electroneutrality |
| Potassium ($K^+$) | 3.5–5.0 | Regulation of intracellular osmolarity<br>Maintenance of membrane electrical excitability<br>Maintenance of plasma acid-base balance |
| Calcium ($Ca^{2+}$) | 4.5–5.5<br>8.0–10.5 mg/dL | Cofactor in blood-clotting cascade<br>Excitable membrane stabilizer<br>Provision of strength and density to teeth and bones<br>Essential element in contractile processes in cardiac, skeletal, and smooth muscle |
| Chloride ($Cl^-$) | 96–106 | Maintenance of plasma acid-base balance<br>Maintenance of plasma electroneutrality<br>Formation of hydrochloric acid |

From Ignatavicius, D. D., Workman, M. L., & Mishler, M. A. (1995). *Medical-surgical nursing: A nursing process approach* (2nd ed., p. 255). Philadelphia: W. B. Saunders.

## Transport of Fluids and Electrolytes

All solutes and water molecules are in constant motion. These substances can cross cell membranes by one of four mechanisms: diffusion, active transport, filtration, and osmosis.

### DIFFUSION

Diffusion is the random movement of substances through a solution or gas. Substances typically move from an area of high concentration to an area of lower concentration across a cell membrane. Simple diffusion occurs if the substance (such as water, oxygen, and urea) is small enough to readily cross a cell membrane. Facilitated diffusion occurs if the substance is too large to cross the membrane alone, i.e., it must diffuse into the cell by a carrier substance. An example of facilitated diffusion is the transport of glucose into the cell.

### ACTIVE TRANSPORT

Active transport is similar to diffusion except that the substance moves from an area of low concentration to an area of greater concentration across a cell membrane. This process requires energy and depends on the availability of carrier substances. Examples of substances that move by active transport are sodium, potassium, and hydrogen.

### FILTRATION

Filtration is the movement of substances, both solutes and solvents, from an area of high hydrostatic pressure to an area of lower hydrostatic pressure. This process occurs most often in the intravascular compartment, especially in the kidneys, where almost 200 L of plasma is filtered each day.

### OSMOSIS

Osmosis is the movement of water across a cell membrane from an area of high solute concentration to an area of lower solute concentration. Osmosis is very important in forming concentrated urine in the kidneys.

## Concentration of Body Fluids

Two terms are commonly used to describe or quantify the concentration of body fluids: *osmolality* and *tonicity*.

### OSMOLALITY

Osmolality is the number of particles or amount of substance in fluid and is measured in milliosmoles per kilogram (mOsm/kg). *Osmolarity* is a related term and refers to the number of particles or amount of substance in a liter of solution. Therefore, it is measured in milliosmoles per liter (mOsm/L).

Osmolality of the extracellular fluid (ECF) can be determined by measuring the serum osmolality, or solute concentration of the blood. The normal value is 280 to 300 mOsm/kg. Sodium is primarily responsible for ECF osmolality and helps to hold water in that compartment. In addition to sodium, plasma proteins help to maintain the volume of fluid in the intravascular system. Potassium helps to maintain the volume of intracellular fluid (ICF).

### TONICITY

Some solutes such as urea move readily across cell membranes but have no real effect on the movement of fluid. Therefore, urea is an ineffective osmole. Sodium and glucose, however, are effective osmoles in that they affect the movement of fluids, especially across a permeable or semipermeable membrane. *Tonicity* is another term for effective osmolality. Fluids may be classified as isotonic, hypertonic, or hypotonic.

A fluid into which cells can be placed without changing the size of the cells is considered *isotonic* with the cells (Guyton, 1991). A 0.9% normal saline solution (NSS) or a 5% glucose (dextrose) in water solution (D5W) is isotonic. If NSS is added to the ECF compartment, no osmosis occurs and the ECF osmolality remains the same. Isotonic solutions for infusion are widely used because they do not upset the osmolality of body fluids.

A solution that can cause cells to shrink is called *hypertonic*. If a hypertonic solution of greater than 0.9% saline (such as 3% saline) is added to the ECF, the osmolality of the ECF *increases,* causing water to leave the cells and enter the ECF compartment.

Conversely, a solution that can cause cells to swell is called *hypotonic*. If a hypotonic solution of less than 0.9% saline (such as 0.45% saline) is added to the ECF, the osmolality *decreases,* causing water to leave the ECF and enter the cells.

Infusions are prescribed for a client to increase or decrease the client's ECF volume. Table 13–2 lists some common solutions given by infusion and classifies them according to their tonicity and common use.

## Life Span Considerations

The amount of fluid in the body decreases with age. As much as 80% of an infant's body weight is water, whereas a person over 70 years of age may have as little as 45% to 50%.

The ability of body systems and mechanisms to compensate for fluid and electrolyte changes also decreases as a person ages. For example, after age 65 years the kidneys lose nephrons and therefore are not as able to concentrate urine.

**TABLE 13–2**
**Characteristics of Common Intravenous Therapy Solutions**

| Solution | Osmolarity (mOsm/L) | pH | Calories* (kcal) | Tonicity |
|---|---|---|---|---|
| 0.9% saline | 308 | 5 | 0 | Isotonic |
| 0.45% saline | 154 | 5 | 0 | Hypotonic |
| 5% dextrose in water (D5W) | 272 | 3.5–6.5 | 170 | Isotonic |
| 10% dextrose in water (D10W) | 500 | 3.5–6.5 | 340 | Hypertonic |
| 5% dextrose in 0.9% saline | 560 | 3.5–6.5 | 170 | Hypertonic |
| 5% dextrose in 0.45% saline | 406 | 4 | 170 | Hypertonic |
| 5% dextrose in 0.225% saline | 321 | 4 | 170 | Isotonic |
| Ringer's lactate | 273 | 6.5 | 9 | Isotonic |
| 5% dextrose in Ringer's lactate | 525 | 4.0–6.5 | 179 | Hypertonic |

From Ignatavicius, D. D., Workman, M. L., & Mishler, M. A. (1995). *Medical-surgical nursing: A nursing process approach* (2nd ed., p. 272). Philadelphia: W. B. Saunders.

The atrophy of adrenal glands results in poor regulation of sodium and potassium, predisposing the client to sodium and potassium imbalances.

### Transcultural Variations

Fat cells contain little water. Since women typically have more body fat than men, they have proportionately less body water. African-Americans often have increased fat cells, and therefore have less body water than other groups (Giger et al., 1991).

## FLUID AND ELECTROLYTE IMBALANCE

Under healthy conditions the human body is able to maintain fluid and electrolyte imbalance by one or more of the body's compensatory mechanisms. When illness or other stressor, such as surgery or extreme environmental changes, occurs, fluid and electrolyte imbalances, which are often potentially life threatening, result. The nurse's primary responsibility is to assess for early signs and symptoms of imbalance so that it can be corrected before it worsens.

### Fluid Imbalances

Two broad categories of fluid imbalance can occur: fluid deficit and fluid excess. Both of these problems are often accompanied by electrolyte and acid-base imbalances but are discussed separately for a better understanding of each type of imbalance.

## FLUID DEFICIT

Depletion of ECF in the body is also called hypovolemia and dehydration. Fluid either may be actually lost from the body (e.g., diuresis, bleeding, excessive diaphoresis, or inadequate fluid intake) or may shift in excess from the IVF compartment to the ISF compartment (called third spacing). Dehydration, then, is a clinical condition resulting from a number of factors rather than a specific disease. Dehydration may be categorized as either isotonic, hypotonic, or hypertonic. The major causes for each type are summarized in Table 13–3.

- *Isotonic dehydration:* Isotonic dehydration is the most common type and involves a fluid deficit in both the intravascular and interstitial space. Serum osmolality remains in the normal range.
- *Hypotonic dehydration:* Hypotonic dehydration involves the loss of solutes from the ECF in excess of fluid loss. The result is a decreased serum osmolality.

**TABLE 13–3**
**Common Causes of Dehydration**

| Isotonic Dehydration | Hypertonic Dehydration |
|---|---|
| Hemorrhage | Hyperventilation |
| Vomiting | Watery diarrhea |
| Diarrhea | Renal failure |
| Profuse salivation | Ketoacidosis |
| Fistulas | Diabetes insipidus |
| Abscesses | Excessive fluid replacement (hypertonic) |
| Ileostomy | Excessive sodium bicarbonate administration |
| Cecostomy | Tube feedings |
| Frequent enemas | Dysphagia |
| Profuse diaphoresis | Impaired thirst |
| Burns | Unconsciousness |
| Severe wounds | Fever |
| Long-term NPO (nothing by mouth) | Impaired motor function |
| Diuretic therapy | Systemic infection |
| Gastrointestinal suction | |
| **Hypotonic Dehydration** | |
| Chronic illness | |
| Excessive fluid replacement (hypotonic) | |
| Renal failure | |
| Chronic or severe malnutrition | |

From Ignatavicius, D. D., Workman, M. L., & Mishler, M. A. (1995). *Medical-surgical nursing: A nursing process approach* (2nd ed., p. 266). Philadelphia: W. B. Saunders.

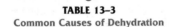

- *Hypertonic dehydration:* Hypertonic dehydration involves the loss of fluid from the ECF in excess of solute loss. This type of dehydration increases serum osmolality.

**Physical Assessment of Dehydration.** Although the signs and symptoms of each type of dehydration are sometimes different, common assessment findings are present:

- *Skin and mucous membranes:* dry skin; dry, sticky mucous membranes; poor skin turgor (tenting of skin) (Note: Test the skin over the sternum or forehead in the elderly client); pitting edema (hypertonic dehydration [third spacing]); pale skin; elevated temperature
- *Cardiovascular:* increased heart rate; decreased peripheral pulse quality; decreased blood pressure, especially orthostatic (postural) hypotension; flat neck and hand veins in dependent position; decreased pulmonary artery pressure (PAP), cardiac output (CO), central venous pressure (CVP), and mean arterial pressure (MAP); increased systemic vascular resistance (SVR)
- *Respiratory:* increased respiratory rate and depth
- *Neuromuscular:* lethargy; skeletal muscle weakness (hypotonic dehydration); thirst
- *Renal:* decreased urinary output, dark concentrated urine (in isotonic and hypertonic dehydration)
- *Gastrointestinal:* decreased motility; diminished bowel sounds; constipation (unless diarrhea is cause of dehydration); weight loss (except for third spacing)

**Diagnostic Findings in Dehydration.** Table 13–4 lists the changes in common laboratory tests that are associated with each of the three types of dehydration.

**Management of Dehydration.** The management of dehydration depends on the specific type of dehydration present and the cardiovascular status of the client. Fluid replacement is the primary treatment. In some cases the fluids can be replaced orally by encouraging the client to increase fluid intake. In many cases, intravenous (IV) fluids are needed, especially if the client is going into or is in hypovolemic shock. In general, isotonic dehydration is treated with isotonic fluids. Hypotonic dehydration is treated with hypertonic fluids, and hypertonic dehydration is treated with hypotonic fluids (see Table 13–2). In addition, for clients who have lost blood or serum proteins, blood transfusions, plasma expanders, and albumin replacement may be administered to expand the intravascular, or circulating, blood volume.

If electrolyte imbalances occur, these problems are also addressed. For example, if the serum sodium level is increased (as in hypertonic dehydration), sodium restriction is

**TABLE 13–4**
**Dehydration Reflected in Laboratory Test Results**

| Values* | Isotonic Dehydration | Hypotonic Dehydration | Hypertonic Dehydration |
|---|---|---|---|
| **Blood Values** | | | |
| Blood urea nitrogen | Normal or increased | Increased | Increased |
| Creatinine | Normal or increased | Increased | Increased |
| Sodium | Normal | <120 mEq/L (mmol) | >150 mEq/L (mmol) |
| Osmolarity | Normal | Decreased | Increased |
| Hematocrit | Increased | Increased | Normal or decreased |
| Hemoglobin | Increased | Increased | Normal or decreased |
| White blood cell count | Increased | Increased | Normal or decreased |
| Protein | Increased | Increased | Increased |
| **Urine Values** | | | |
| Specific gravity | >1.010 | <1.010 | >1.010 |
| Osmolarity | Increased | Decreased | Increased |
| Volume | Decreased | Increased | Decreased |

*All values reflect dehydration states alone and not the underlying pathologic changes or disease states contributing to the dehydration.
From Ignatavicius, D. D., Workman, M. L., & Mishler, M. A. (1995). *Medical-surgical nursing: A nursing process approach* (2nd ed., p. 270). Philadelphia: W. B. Saunders.

implemented. If the client has lost excessive potassium from diarrhea, potassium replacement, usually intravenously, is initiated. Correction of fluid and electrolyte imbalances usually corrects any accompanying acid-base imbalance.

**Nursing Interventions for Clients with Dehydration.** The following nursing interventions are essential for the client with dehydration:

- Monitor intake and output accurately. (NOTE: Report to the physician if urine output is less than 30 mL/h.) Measure and record urine specific gravity at least every 8 hours.
- Monitor daily weight using the same balanced scale and weigh before breakfast each day.
- Monitor vital signs with special attention to the possibility of orthostatic hypotension.
- If orthostatic hypotension is present, assist the client to slowly change positions and be alert for dizziness or weakness; protect the client from falling.
- For clients in critical care units, monitor hemodynamic measurements. (NOTE: Usual goals: PAP = 20 to 30/8 to 15 mm Hg; CVP = 2 to 7 mm Hg; CO = 4 to 7 L/min; MAP = 70 to 105 mm Hg).

- Administer IV fluids as ordered and document client response through improved assessment findings, e.g., increased urinary output, less dry skin, increased weight. (NOTE: Also monitor for signs of too much fluid replacement [fluid overload] such as dyspnea, bounding pulse, edema, neck vein distension, and abnormally increased CVP and PAP.)

## FLUID EXCESS (OVERLOAD)

When the body experiences increased fluid intake or retention relative to fluid loss, a state of fluid overload, or overhydration, occurs. Fluid may actually be gained or may shift from the ISF compartment to the IVF compartment. The primary causes of fluid overload are impaired kidney function and cardiovascular dysfunction. The two common types of overhydration are isotonic and hypotonic.

- *Isotonic overhydration:* Isotonic overhydration, often called hypervolemia, is the most common type of fluid overload. In this condition, fluid and solutes (especially sodium) are increased proportionately in the ECF compartments to keep the serum osmolality within normal range. The client with hypervolemia experiences circulatory overload and interstitial edema.
- *Hypotonic overhydration:* Hypotonic overhydration is less common and is sometimes referred to as water intoxication. In this condition the ECF becomes hypotonic and the serum osmolality decreases. As a result, excess ECF moves into the cells and causes expansion of all body fluid compartments. The client experiences circulatory overload, interstitial edema, cellular edema, and electrolyte dilution (e.g., hypokalemia).

**Physical Assessment of Overhydration.** Although the signs and symptoms of the two types of overhydration are somewhat different, common physical assessment findings are present:

- Decreased hematocrit (as a result of hemodilution)
- Decreased sodium and potassium as a result of electrolyte dilution; increased values if the overload is the result of renal failure
- Decreased urine specific gravity

**Management of Overhydration.** Treatment of overhydration is directed at eliminating the cause of the condition, removing excess fluid to restore fluid and electrolyte balance, and preventing or treating complications such as pulmonary edema. If renal function is intact, the physician prescribes diuretics to help the kidneys eliminate excess fluid from the body. Osmotic diurectics such as mannitol (✤Osmitrol) and urea are preferred over loop diuretics such as furosemide (Lasix, ✱Furoside) to prevent further electrolyte imbalance.

Other drug therapy is aimed at treating complications of the fluid imbalance. For example, dexamethasone (Decadron, ✱Dexasone) may be given to reduce cerebral edema in clients with hypotonic overhydration. Digoxin (Lanoxin) may be administered to strengthen the heart to improve cardiac output. Electrolytes are usually not replaced because they are present in the body in sufficient amounts but diluted.

**Nursing Interventions for Clients with Overhydration.** Nursing care for clients with overhydration includes the following:

- Monitor intake and output accurately. (NOTE: Unless the client has end-stage renal failure, the output should be greater than 30 to 60 mL/h.)
- Restrict fluids and sodium as ordered.
- Monitor daily weight using the same balanced scale and weigh before breakfast each day.
- Monitor vital signs frequently (at least every 4 hours).
- Observe the client for signs of edema; monitor the type and location of edema and progression.
- Listen to breath sounds at least every 8 hours.
- Document response to treatment, including diuretic therapy.
- Observe for signs of too much fluid loss or restriction, i.e., dehydration and electrolyte imbalances.
- Keep client in semi- or high-Fowler's position to facilitate breathing.
- Monitor arterial blood gas values. (NOTE: Goal: $PaO_2 >$ 80 mm Hg, pH=7.35 to 7.45, $Paco_2 >$ 35 mm Hg.)

## Electrolyte Imbalances

Electrolyte levels need to remain within a narrow range. The body can tolerate some electrolyte changes better than others. Age and general health condition are important factors in the body's ability to compensate for electrolyte imbalances. Older people are generally less able to tolerate electrolyte changes.

Only the most common imbalances for which infusion therapy is used are included here.

### HYPOKALEMIA

Hypokalemia is a decrease in serum potassium ($K^+$) below 3.5 mEq/L. This imbalance is very common and can result from a number of factors, such as those summarized in Table 13–5. Hypokalemia may occur as a result of actual loss of potassium from the ECF or as a result of abnormal movement of potassium from the ECF to the ICF compartment, as in metabolic alkalosis. The severity of the clinical manifesta-

**TABLE 13–5**
**Common Causes of Hypokalemia**

**Actual Potassium Deficits**
***Excessive Loss of Potassium***
Inappropriate or excessive use of drugs
Diuretics
Digitalis
Corticosteroids
Increased secretion of aldosterone
Cushing's syndrome
Diarrhea
Vomiting
Wound drainage (especially gastrointestinal)
Prolonged nasogastric suction
Heat-induced excessive diaphoresis
Renal disease impairing reabsorption of potassium

***Inadequate Potassium Intake***
Nothing by mouth (NPO)

**Relative Potassium Deficits**
***Movement of Potassium from Extracellular Fluid to Intracellular Fluid***
Alkalosis
Hyperinsulinism
Hyperalimentation
Total parenteral nutrition

***Dilution of Serum Potassium***
Water intoxication
Intravenous therapy with potassium-poor solutions

From Ignatavicius, D. D., Workman, M. L., & Mishler, M. A. (1995). *Medical-surgical nursing: A nursing process approach* (2nd ed., p. 292). Philadelphia: W. B. Saunders.

tions that result from hypokalemia depends on how quickly the condition occurs.

**Physical Assessment of Hypokalemia.** The nurse identifies the client at risk for hypokalemia to observe for early signs and symptoms of this imbalance. Any or all of the following may be present:

- Carefully monitor the client's heart rate, including quality. (NOTE: The client with severe hypokalemia is assessed by continuous cardiac monitoring in a critical care or telemetry unit.)
- Administer potassium supplements as ordered. For IV potassium, observe the IV insertion site for irritation or phlebitis, which commonly results from IV administration; change the IV site if these problems occur. Do not infuse more than 10 mEq of IV potassium per hour unless a cardiac monitor is being used; in some cases a "K run" is ordered to infuse a large amount of potassium as a bolus.

- Administer oral potassium, if ordered, with a full glass of water or juice to prevent gastric irritation. Do not give oral potassium on an empty stomach; do not interchange potassium supplements without a physician's order.
- Encourage high-potassium foods (see Table 13–6).
- Monitor intake and output. If output is below 30 mL/h, withhold potassium until the physician is informed.
- Carefully observe clients who are receiving digitalis preparations for signs of digitalis toxicity. (Hypokalemia increases the effect of these drugs.)

**TABLE 13–6**
**Common Food Sources of Potassium***

| Food Source | Amount (mg) |
|---|---|
| Corn flakes (1 1/4 c) | 26 |
| Cooked oatmeal (3/4 c) | 99 |
| Egg (1 large) | 66 |
| Codfish, raw (4 oz) | 400 |
| Salmon, pink, raw (3 1/2 oz) | 306 |
| Tuna fish (4 oz) | 375 |
| Apple, raw with skin (1 medium) | 159 |
| Banana (1 medium) | 451 |
| Cantaloupe (1 c pieces) | 494 |
| Grapefruit (1/2 medium) | 175 |
| Orange (1 medium) | 250 |
| Raisins (1/2 c) | 700 |
| Strawberries, raw (1 c) | 247 |
| Watermelon (1 c pieces) | 186 |
| White bread (1 slice) | 27 |
| Whole-wheat bread (1 slice) | 44 |
| Beef (4 oz) | 480 |
| Beef liver (3 1/2 oz) | 281 |
| Pork, fresh (4 oz) | 525 |
| Pork, cured (4 oz) | 325 |
| Chicken (4 oz) | 225 |
| Veal cutlet (3 1/2 oz) | 448 |
| Whole milk (8 oz) | 370 |
| Skim milk (8 oz) | 406 |
| Avocado (1 medium) | 1097 |
| Carrot (1 large) | 341 |
| Corn (4-inch ear) | 196 |
| Cauliflower (1 c pieces) | 295 |
| Celery (1 stalk) | 170 |
| Green beans (1 c) | 189 |
| Mushrooms (10 small) | 410 |
| Onion (1 medium) | 157 |
| Peas (3/4 c) | 316 |
| Potato, white (1 medium) | 407 |
| Spinach, raw (3 1/2 oz) | 470 |
| Tomato (1 medium) | 366 |

*U.S. Department of Agriculture recommended daily allowance for adults: 1875–5625 mg.

From Ignatavicius, D. D., Workman, M. L., & Mishler, M. A. (1995). *Medical-surgical nursing: A nursing process approach* (2nd ed. p. 256). Philadelphia: W. B. Saunders.

- Assist client with activities of daily living and mobility as needed because of weakness and lethargy; protect client from falls.
- Provide high-fiber foods and laxatives as ordered for constipation. (NOTE: Clients with paralytic ileus may need decompression with nasogastric suctioning until bowel sounds return.)

## HYPERKALEMIA

Hyperkalemia is an increase in serum potassium ($K^+$) above 5 mEq/L. Even slight increases above the normal range can have serious adverse effects on the function of excitable tissues, espe-cially the myocardium. Hyperkalemia typically occurs as a result of renal impairment, Addison's disease, adrenalectomy, or overuse of potassium-sparing diuretics or potassium supplements.

**Physical Assessment of Hyperkalemia.** The nurse assesses the client for signs and symptoms of hyperkalemia. Any or all of the following may be present:

- Discontinue supplemental potassium, both oral and IV.
- Collaborate with the dietitian to ensure the client's adherence to a potassium-restricted diet, if ordered.
- Provide oral and IV fluids for the client with dehydration; monitor intake and output carefully.
- Administer drugs to increase potassium excretion, as ordered.
- Administer IV regular insulin (a hypertonic solution given through a central line) to promote the movement of serum potassium back into the cells.
- Carefully monitor the client's heart rate. (NOTE: The client with severe hyperkalemia is assessed by continuous cardiac monitoring in a critical care or telemetry unit.)

## HYPONATREMIA

Hyponatremia is a serum sodium ($Na^+$) level less than 135 mEq/L. Imbalances of sodium are usually associated with fluid imbalances. Hyponatremia may be the result of loss of total body sodium, movement of sodium from the serum to other fluid spaces, or dilution of serum sodium when there is excessive water in the plasma. Specific causes are listed in Table 13–7.

**Physical Assessment of Hyponatremia.** The nurse identifies the client at risk for early signs and symptoms of hyponatremia. Any of the following may be present:

- Carefully monitor the IV fluid infusion rate.
- Monitor the client's response to sodium and fluid replacement.
- Measure intake and output, especially for clients receiving diuretics.

**TABLE 13–7**
**Common Causes of Hyponatremia**

**Actual Sodium Deficits**
***Increased Sodium Excretion***
Excessive diaphoresis
Diuretics (high-ceiling diuretics)
Wound drainage (especially gastrointestinal)
Decreased secretion of aldosterone
Hyperlipidemia
Renal disease (scarred distal convoluted tubule)

***Inadequate Sodium Intake***
Nothing by mouth (NPO)
Low-salt diet

**Relative Sodium Deficits**
***Dilution of Serum Sodium***
Excessive ingestion of hypotonic fluids
Psychogenic polydipsia
Freshwater drowning
Renal failure (nephrotic syndrome)
Irrigation with hypotonic fluids
Syndrome of inappropriate antidiuretic hormone secretion (SIADH)
Hyperglycemia
Congestive heart failure

From Ignatavicius, D. D., Workman, M. L., & Mishler, M. A. (1995). *Medical-surgical nursing: A nursing process approach* (2nd ed., p. 301). Philadelphia: W. B. Saunders.

- Collaborate with the dietitian to teach the client which foods are high in sodium.
- Administer drug therapy as ordered.
- Assess the client for changes in mental status.

## HYPERNATREMIA

Hypernatremia is a serum sodium ($Na^+$) level greater than 145 mEq/L. Common causes of hypernatremia include decreased sodium excretion, as in renal failure or hyperaldosteronism; increased sodium intake, as in excessive IV administration of sodium; decreased water intake; and increased water loss, as in fever, excessive diaphoresis, dehydration, infection, and diarrhea.

**Physical Assessment of Hypernatremia.** Gradual increases in sodium may not cause any observable physical changes. However, rapid sodium increases affect many body systems. The nurse assesses the following systems for clinical manifestations of acute sodium excess:

- Carefully monitor intake and output, including the rate of IV infusions.
- Monitor the client's response to diuretic therapy.
- Collaborate with the dietitian to teach the client how to restrict sodium intake in the diet.

- Monitor mental status carefully, reporting any significant changes.

## HYPOCALCEMIA

Calcium is essential for proper functioning of skeletal and cardiac muscle. It is also a critical cofactor in the blood-clotting process. Therefore, even small increases or decreases in serum calcium can have major effects on the body.

Hypocalcemia is a serum calcium ($Ca^{2+}$) level less than 9 mg/dL or 4.5 mEq/L. Common causes of this imbalance include decreased calcium absorption from the intestinal tract, increased calcium excretion, acute pancreatitis, hyperphosphatemia, and removal or destruction of the parathyroid glands.

**Physical Assessment of Hypocalcemia.** The primary findings associated with decreased calcium involve the neuromuscular and cardiovascular systems.

- Keep the environment as quiet as possible to avoid further overstimulation.
- Place the client in a relatively dark private room if possible and restrict activity (bed rest).
- Initiate seizure precautions per facility policy.
- Have emergency equipment available in case the client experiences respiratory problems.
- Monitor the client's cardiac pattern via monitor.
- Move the client gently to prevent bone fracture.
- Give oral calcium supplements 1 to 2 hours after meals to promote maximal absorption.

## HYPERCALCEMIA

Hypercalcemia is a serum calcium ($Ca^{2+}$) level greater than 11 mg/dL or 5.5 mEq/L. Even small increases in serum calcium can have severe effects on the body. Causes of hypercalcemia include decreased renal excretion of calcium, hyperparathyroidism, cancer, immobility, overuse of thiazide diuretics, and excessive oral calcium or vitamin D intake.

**Physical Assessment of Hypercalcemia.** The most life-threatening clinical manifestations of hypercalcemia are cardiovascular. Any or all of the following may be present:

- Monitor the client's response to fluid and diuretic therapy.
- Maintain meticulous intake and output records.
- Assess the client for changes in level of consciousness.
- Initiate measures, such as a high-fiber diet and intake of adequate fluids, to prevent or treat constipation.
- Monitor the abdomen for distention.
- Assess the lower extremities for signs and symptoms of thrombosis.

Chapter 14

# Parenteral Nutrition

*Marilyn Ferreri Booker*



Parenteral nutrition is a therapy that provides nourishment to the client via the venous system. Parenteral nutrition is also known as total parenteral nutrition (TPN), hyperalimentation, intravenous hyperalimentation (IVH), or intravenous (IV) feedings. No matter what the name, parenteral nutrition solutions are designed to meet the client's basal or maintenance requirements and in some cases the demands of growth and development, nutritional repletion, and stress states. These stress states may include critical illness or injury.

## INDICATIONS FOR PARENTERAL NUTRITION

There is essentially no difference in the clinical benefits derived from parenteral nutrition versus oral or enteral feedings. But when possible, the use of oral and enteral feedings is preferable to parenteral nutrition. When nutrition is provided orally or enterally, the body absorbs and digests the food naturally. Oral and enteral nutrition are also less invasive and less expensive than parenteral nutrition. However, in some cases the clients may have a condition in which oral or enteral nutrition is inadequate, inadvisable, or contraindicated (Fig. 14–1). Some examples of these conditions include pancreatitis, peritonitis, intestinal obstruction, paralytic ileus, gastrointestinal hemorrhage, intractable vomiting or diarrhea, intestinal fistulae, malabsorption, and short bowel syndrome. In each case the client is at risk for nutritional deficits.

## NUTRITIONAL DEFICIENCIES

Food provides the body with protein, carbohydrates, and fat. As these nutrients are metabolized, they produce energy measured in calories (also known as kilocalories). A normal healthy adult requires about 2000 to 3000 kcal/d, depending on activity patterns. Increases in metabolic activity such as seen in strenuous exercise or burns, trauma, or disease increase the number of calories required to maintain normal functioning.

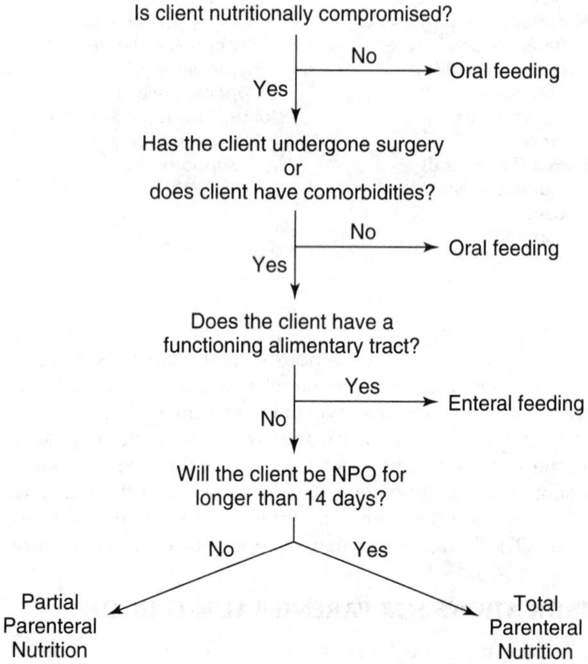


**FIGURE 14–1.** Algorithm for assessing need for total parenteral nutrition (TPN).

Protein and calorie deficits are the most commonly seen nutritional deficiencies. When the body perceives these deficiencies, it turns to its reserve stores to provide energy for bodily functions. First, through gluconeogenesis the body mobilizes and converts glycogen to glucose and urea. When glycogen stores are depleted, the body next turns to fat stored in adipose tissue. Finally, essential plasma proteins (serum albumin and transferrin) and somatic body proteins (skeletal, smooth muscle, and tissue proteins) are converted to carbohydrates for energy. The breaking down of these essential body proteins places the body in a catabolic state. Clients who have the potential to become catabolic and who cannot ingest and absorb food orally or enterally require parenteral nutrition.

## Protein-Calorie Malnutrition

When clients are deprived of protein and calories for a period of time they may exhibit protein-energy, or protein-calorie, malnutrition (PCM). PCM may occur in three forms: iatrogenic PCM, kwashiorkor, and marasmus.

### IATROGENIC PCM

Iatrogenic PCM is most often seen in hospitalized clients who for one reason or another do not receive adequate intake of protein or calories (energy). Blackburn and Bistrian in two studies (1974, 1976) involving surgical and medical hospitalized clients found that 50% and 40%, respectively, had PCM. Since these two classic studies, there has been little improvement in the nutritional status of hospitalized clients. As many as 50% were found to have moderate malnutrition, and 5% to 10% are classified as severely malnourished (the American Society of Parenteral and Enteral Nutrition [ASPEN], 1993). Nurses are well aware of clients who experience days of NPO (nothing by mouth) preparation for tests and procedures or who are severely ill postoperatively and cannot eat.

As the trend toward earlier discharges continues, some clients may be released from the hospital before they have resumed adequate oral intake. Fortunately, some of these clients receive home health care after discharge. In these cases the home care nurse can follow the client's nutritional intake and alert the physician if the client's dietary intake does not progress as it should. If there is no home care follow-up, other clients may be at risk for undetected malnutrition.

### KWASHIORKOR

In kwashiorkor the client has adequate calorie intake but the ingestion of protein is severely deficient. This type of malnutrition is most often seen in children between the ages of 1 and 3 years who reside in third world countries. In the United States this type of malnutrition may be secondary to malabsorption disorders, cancer and cancer therapies, kidney disease, hypermetabolic illness, and iatrogenic causes.

## MARASMUS

A prolonged and inadequate intake of protein, calories, and other nutrients leads to marasmus. This gradual wasting of muscle mass and subcutaneous fat occurs most frequently in infants between the ages of 6 to 18 months and in clients with postgastrectomy "dumping syndrome." Other common scenarios in which marasmus is seen include clients with carcinomas of the mouth and esophagus.

## EFFECTS OF PCM

The clinical manifestations of PCM are varied, but the following highlights the adverse effects that nutritional deprivation has on the structure and function of most organs and systems of the body. These adverse effects themselves may cause disease. In the presence of an underlying illness, without the intervention of parenteral nutrition, the effects of nutritional deprivation can be devastating to the client. The severity of PCM is dependent on the amount of deprivation and its length. Table 14–1 outlines the major effects of PCM on the structure and its effect on the function of the body's organs.

Most of the body's systems and processes are affected by PCM as well. Some of these systems and processes include the hematologic and immunologic processes, the client's susceptibility to infection, and the ability of the client to heal wounds and metabolize drugs.

**Hematologic System.** Clients with malnutrition exhibit anemia (insufficient numbers of red blood cells), leukopenia (insufficient numbers of white blood cells), and thrombocytopenia (insufficient numbers of platelets). As with most of these symptoms the extent is dependent on the length and severity of the calorie deprivation.

**Immunity.** Essentially every aspect of the immune system is compromised by malnutrition. This includes cellular immunity, immunoglobulin levels, specific antibody production, complement function, and secretory and mucosal immunity.

**Susceptibility to Infection.** Aside from the impairment to immunologic functions described above, severe PCM is associated with changes in the body's anatomic barriers such as the skin. These changes may facilitate the invasion and proliferation of infectious organisms.

**Wound Healing.** In mild PCM there is generally no change in the rate of wound healing. This is because the

**TABLE 14–1**
**Major Effects of Protein-Calorie Malnutrition (PCM)**

| Organ | Structure | Effects of Function |
|---|---|---|
| Body weight | Loss of fat and lean body weight; increase in extracellular water compartment | |
| Cardiovascular | Decrease in cardiac organ volume | Bradycardia; hypotension; decreased venous pressure, decreased oxygen consumption, stroke volume, and cardiac output |
| Pulmonary | | Decreased tidal volume, minute volume, and respiratory rate |
| Gastrointestinal | Mucous membranes become congested and edematous; intestinal mass reduced; enteric mucosa flattens | Decrease in gastric acid secretion; slowed gastric motility |
| Pancreas | | Pancreatic insufficiency and disaccharide intolerance lead to malabsorption syndrome and diarrhea |
| Liver | Initially an accumulation of fat in liver; if PCM severe, liver becomes smaller | |
| Kidney | | Impaired urine concentrating ability |
| Musculoskeletal | Decrease in muscle mass; some loss of bone and an osteoporotic effect | Increased muscle fatigue; altered pattern of muscle contraction and relaxation |

Data from Keys, A., Brozek, J., Henschel, A., Michelsen, O., & Taylor, H. L. (1950). *The Biology of Human Starvation.* Minneapolis: University of Minneapolis Press.

body places the healing of the wound as a priority and shunts its internal stores to the synthesis of collagen and other wound-healing factors to complete the healing process.

Clients who suffer from severe PCM exhibit delays in most aspects of wound healing, including the vascularization of the site and collagen synthesis. In addition, if the client's serum albumin level decreases, the ability to maintain oncotic pressure is compromised. Fluid then moves from the intravascular space to the interstitial spaces, resulting in edema. Edema in the area of a wound impairs healing.

**Drug Metabolism**. Conjugation is a part of normal drug metabolism. It is the process by which endogenous (within the body) molecules are added to the functional groups of the drug or its metabolites for use in the body. If dietary intake is inadequate, protein catabolism occurs, which causes a decrease in drug-metabolizing enzymes and the amino acids and peptides that participate in the conjugation reaction. This reduced drug metabolism may lead to enhanced pharmacologic activity and increased toxicity. In addition to impaired drug metabolism, malnutrition may also alter drug absorption, protein binding, and drug clearance.

## Vitamin Deficiency

Vitamins cannot be manufactured by the body. They function as essential cofactors in a number of important enzymatic processes in the body.

There are two types of vitamins: water-soluble and fat-soluble. The water-soluble vitamins include vitamin C, folate, and the B complex vitamins—thiamine, riboflavin, niacin, pyridoxine, cobalamin, and biotin. Vitamins A, D, E, and K make up the fat-soluble vitamins. Table 14–2 lists the function of some of these vitamins and the conditions associated with their deficiency.

## Macronutrient Deficiency

The body requires minerals such as sodium, chloride, potassium, calcium, magnesium, and phosphate in quantities greater than 200 mg/d. Consequently, such minerals are known as macronutrients. These minerals are essential for the maintenance of water balance; cardiac function; mineral-

**TABLE 14–2**
**Six Vitamin Functions and Conditions Associated with Their Deficiency**

| Vitamin | Function | Deficiency |
|---|---|---|
| Vitamin A | Important for proper retinal function and bone metabolism | Night blindness; difficulty with reproduction |
| B complex | Assists with the absorption of carbohydrates and proteins; cofactor for many enzymes | Enzymatic dysfunction; anemia |
| Vitamin C | Wound healing | Scurvy |
| Vitamin D | Used for bone metabolism and the maintenance of serum calcium levels | Rickets |
| Vitamin E | Protects the cell's membrane and prevents the oxidation of vitamins A and C | Possible hemolytic anemia and liver necrosis |
| Vitamin K | Assists with prothrombin production | Increased clotting times; bleeding |

Data from Mahan, L. K., & Arlin, M. (1992). *Krause's Food, Nutrition and Diet Therapy*. Philadelphia: W. B. Saunders.

ization of the skeleton; function of nerve, muscle, and enzyme systems; and energy transformation.

## Essential Fatty Acid Deficiency

Polyunsaturated fatty acids that cannot be synthesized in the body and are necessary for normal growth and maintenance and proper functioning are known as essential fatty acids (EFAs). These substances have a role in the regulation of cholesterol metabolism and are important for maintaining the function and integrity of cellular and subcellular membranes. Linoleic acid is the principal EFA for humans because it cannot be synthesized in vivo and it prevents or cures the clinical syndrome of EFA deficiency. Some of the clinical manifestations of EFA deficiency include eczematous desquamative dermatitis, hepatic dysfunction, anemia, thrombocytopenia, hair loss, and possible impaired wound healing. Infants may suffer growth retardation from EFA deficiency.

## Trace Element Deficiency

Like vitamins, trace elements cannot be manufactured by the body. Also like vitamins, trace elements function as cofactors in enzymatic processes. Fifteen trace elements have been identified, but the minimal daily requirement for each is unknown. Table 14–3 lists three of the trace elements thought to be essential, their functions, and the conditions associated with their deficiency.

**TABLE 14–3**
**Three Essential Trace Elements, Their Functions, and Conditions Associated with Their Deficiency**

| Trace Element | Function | Deficiency |
|---|---|---|
| Zinc | Essential to approximately 70 enzymes, metabolism of DNA, lipids, proteins, and carbohydrates | Anorexia, alopecia, impaired wound healing, inability to taste, hypogonadism, diarrhea, and vesicular dermatitis |
| Copper | Proper utilization of iron in production of hemoglobin; bone and elastic tissue development and normal function of central nervous system | Anemia |
| Chromium | Cofactor for insulin | Glucose intolerance |

Data from Mahan, L. K., & Arlin, M. (1992). *Krause's Food, Nutrition and Diet Therapy*. Philadelphia: W. B. Saunders.

## NUTRITIONAL ASSESSMENT

Assessment of nutritional status is an important step in providing optimal nutrition care to clients. Although not all clients require a complete nutritional assessment, clients who need parenteral nutrition require a complete nutritional assessment as a baseline. This assessment provides vital information needed to devise the appropriate formula and to use as a baseline against which to monitor the client's progress to maintaining nutritional stability.

Many health care facilities have nutritional support teams (NST) who work with clients who are at risk for nutritional deficits. These teams usually consist of dietitians, nurses, pharmacists, and physicians. The American Society of Parenteral and Enteral Nutrition (ASPEN) has developed standards of practice and certifying examinations for each of these disciplines. Each member of the team is responsible for assessing the client's nutritional status, planning the intervention, implementing the plan, and evaluating the client to provide proper nutritional and metabolic support.

### Initial Nutritional Assessment

Data for initial screening vary among health care agencies, but the following is a list of parameters that the nurse can easily obtain during the admission process as part of the client's nursing assessment. Through interview the nurse can obtain a weight history and information about any recent changes in appetite and oral intake. By completing a head-to-toe assessment, including inspection, palpation, percussion, and auscultation, the nurse can discern if the client has any conditions that cause nutrient loss. Some of these conditions include malabsorption syndromes, draining abscesses, wounds, fistulae, or protracted diarrhea. Table 14–4 outlines some clinical signs and symptoms of nutrient deficiencies.

Based on the findings of the nurse's initial nutritional assessment, the NST determines if a more in-depth nutritional assessment is warranted. If so, the NST completes an assessment of the client's body composition and biochemical indicators of nutritional well-being.

### Body Composition Analysis

The client in a catabolic state may draw energy from his or her body's adipose tissue (fat), skeletal muscle, or plasma proteins. Measurement of these factors is valuable in assessing the client's overall nutritional status. The adipose tissue and some skeletal muscle determinations are evaluated using anthropometric measurements. Other skeletal muscle and plasma protein determinations require biochemical evaluation.

**TABLE 14–4**
**Various Signs and Symptoms of Nutrient Deficiencies**

| Parameter | Sign/Symptom | Potential Nutritional Deficiency |
|---|---|---|
| Hair | Alopecia | Zinc, essential fatty acids |
| | Easy pluckability | Protein, essential fatty acids |
| | Lackluster | Protein, zinc |
| | "Corkscrew" hair | Vitamins C, A |
| | Decreased pigmentation | Protein, copper |
| Eyes | Xerosis of conjunctiva | Vitamin A |
| | Corneal vascularization | Riboflavin |
| | Keratomalacia | Vitamin A |
| | Bitot's spots | Vitamin A |
| Gastrointestinal tract | Nausea, vomiting | Pyridoxine |
| | Diarrhea | Zinc, niacin |
| | Stomatitis | Pyridoxine, riboflavin, iron |
| | Cheilosis | Pyridoxine, iron |
| | Glossitis | Pyridoxine, zinc, niacin, folic acid, vitamin $B_{12}$ |
| Skin | Dry and scaling | Vitamin A, essential fatty acids |
| | Petechiae/ecchymoses | Vitamins C, K |
| | Follicular hyperkeratosis | Vitamin A, essential fatty acids |
| | Nasolabial seborrhea | Niacin, pyridoxine, riboflavin |
| | Bilateral dermatitis | Niacin, zinc |
| Extremities | Subcutaneous fat loss | Calories |
| | Muscle wasting | Calories, protein |
| | Edema | Protein |
| | Osteomalacia, bone pain, rickets | Vitamin D |
| | Arthralgia | Vitamin C |
| Hematologic | Anemia | Vitamin $B_{12}$, iron, folic acid, copper, vitamin E |
| | Leukopenia, neutropenia | Copper |
| | Low prothrombin, prolonged clotting time | Vitamin K, manganese |
| Neurologic | Disorientation | Niacin, thiamine |
| | Confabulation | Thiamine |
| | Neuropathy, paresthesia | Thiamine, pyridoxine, chromium |
| Cardiovascular | Congestive heart failure, cardiomegaly, tachycardia | Thiamine |
| | Cardiomyopathy | Selenium |

Adapted from Nutritional Assessment Kit, Ross Laboratories, Columbuis, Ohio.

## ANTHROPOMETRIC MEASUREMENTS

Height, weight, triceps skinfold, and midarm muscle circumference are the anthropometric measurements typically evaluated.

**Height and Weight.** Height and weight reflect the client's body fat, the skeletal muscle mass, and hydration status. The client's body weight may be compared to accepted tables of "ideal weight" such as the Metropolitan Height and Weight Table (Table 14–5) or to the client's usual body weight.

Comparison to the client's usual body weight may be more appropriate, as the client serves as the reference for the comparison. This is of particular importance in the elderly. An elderly woman who is 5 feet 3 inches tall and presents with a weight of 95 lb may have weighed 110 lb her entire

**TABLE 14–5**
**Height and Weight Tables for Men and Women According to Frame, Ages 25–59**

| Height* | | Weight† | | |
|---|---|---|---|---|
| **Feet** | **Inches** | **Small Frame** | **Medium Frame** | **Large Frame** |
| **Men** | | | | |
| 5 | 2 | 128–134 | 131–134 | 138–150 |
| 5 | 3 | 130–136 | 133–143 | 140–153 |
| 5 | 4 | 132–138 | 135–145 | 142–156 |
| 5 | 5 | 134–140 | 137–148 | 144–160 |
| 5 | 6 | 136–142 | 139–151 | 146–164 |
| 5 | 7 | 138–145 | 142–154 | 149–168 |
| 5 | 8 | 140–148 | 145–157 | 152–172 |
| 5 | 9 | 142–151 | 148–160 | 155–176 |
| 5 | 10 | 144–154 | 151–163 | 158–180 |
| 5 | 11 | 146–157 | 154–166 | 161–184 |
| 6 | 0 | 149–160 | 157–170 | 164–188 |
| 6 | 1 | 152–164 | 160–174 | 168–192 |
| 6 | 2 | 155–168 | 164–178 | 172–197 |
| 6 | 3 | 158–172 | 167–182 | 176–202 |
| 6 | 4 | 162–176 | 171–187 | 181–207 |
| **Women** | | | | |
| 4 | 10 | 102–111 | 109–121 | 118–131 |
| 4 | 11 | 103–113 | 111–123 | 120–134 |
| 5 | 0 | 104–115 | 113–126 | 122–137 |
| 5 | 1 | 106–118 | 115–129 | 125–140 |
| 5 | 2 | 108–121 | 118–132 | 128–143 |
| 5 | 3 | 111–124 | 121–135 | 131–147 |
| 5 | 4 | 114–127 | 124–138 | 134–151 |
| 5 | 5 | 117–130 | 127–141 | 137–155 |
| 5 | 6 | 120–133 | 130–144 | 140–159 |
| 5 | 7 | 123–136 | 133–147 | 143–163 |
| 5 | 8 | 126–139 | 136–150 | 146–167 |
| 5 | 9 | 129–142 | 139–153 | 149–170 |
| 5 | 10 | 132–145 | 142–156 | 152–173 |
| 5 | 11 | 135–148 | 145–159 | 155–176 |
| 6 | 0 | 138–151 | 148–162 | 158–179 |

*Shoes with 1-inch heels.

†Weight in pounds. Men: allow 5 lb of clothing. Women: allow 3 lb of clothing.

Courtesy of Metropolitan Life Insurance Company, 1983.

life. For this client, it would not be appropriate to expect or suggest that she increase her body weight to the 130 to 152 lb listed in Table 14–5. For this client, comparison to her own usual body weight is more appropriate. The following formula would be used to determine the percentage of usual body weight:

$$\frac{95 \text{ lb (Present weight)}}{110 \text{ lb (Usual body weight)}} \times 100 = 86.36\%$$

The period over which the client sustained the weight loss should also be noted. An involuntary weight loss of 10% of usual weight over 6 months is an indicator of malnutrition.

**Skinfold Measurements.** In the hospital setting, clinical dietitians usually perform skinfold measurements, but in home care the nurse may complete these measurements. Skinfold measurements provide an estimate of body fat. During periods of inadequate intake the body uses stored fat to meet energy requirements. Using body fat as an energy source results in weight loss, but this fact may not be evident if the client has increases in body fluid or changes in other body compartments. Therefore, a measurement of body fat is important when assessing the overall status of the client's condition.

Measuring a variety of sites gives the most accurate picture of the client's overall body fat, but in practice the triceps and subscapular skinfold measurements are the most widely taken measurements. These baseline results can be compared to reference data and the client's future measurements (Fig. 14–2).

**Midarm Muscle Circumference.** Like adipose tissue, skeletal muscle can be used an an energy source in clients who receive an inadequate intake of calories. However, skeletal muscle is not intended to provide a source of energy for the body. But when caloric intake is less than required, both fat and skeletal muscle provide the body with sources for energy.

Assessing skeletal muscle mass is accomplished using both anthropometric and biochemical measurements. The nurse measures skeletal muscle mass anthropometrically using the midarm circumference (MAC) (Fig. 14–3). The midarm muscle circumference (MAMC) is a function of the MAC and the triceps skinfold. The following formula would be used to calculate the MAMC:

$$\text{MAC (cm)} - (3.14 \times \text{Triceps skinfold [cm]})$$

This calculation is then compared to reference standards to estimate skeletal muscle mass. Serial anthropometric measurements are valuable in assessing the client's progression toward nutritional stability.

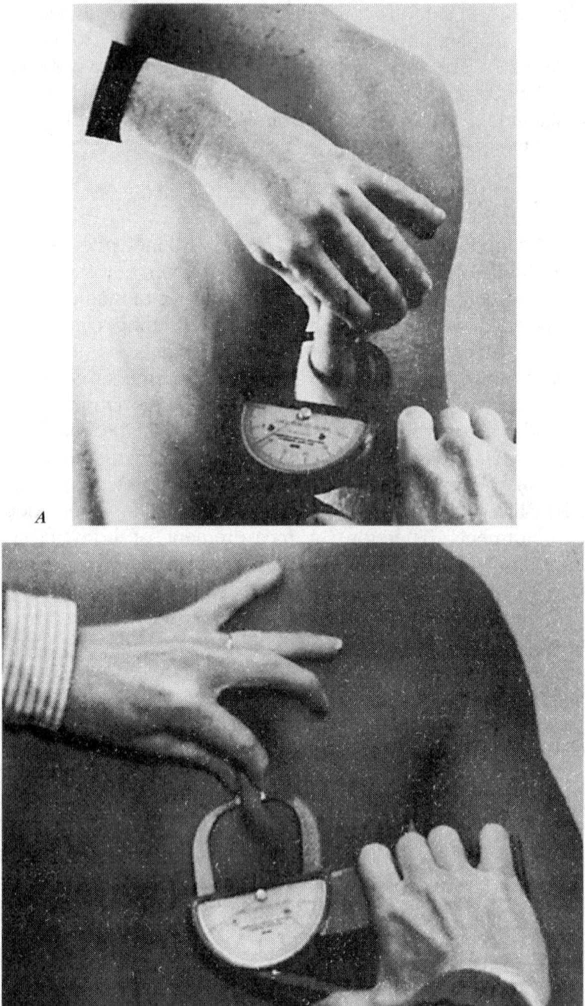

*A*

*B*

**FIGURE 14–2.** Measurement of triceps skinfold thickness **(A)** and subscapular skinfold thickness **(B).** (From Mahan L. K., Arlin M. [1992]. *Krause's food, nutrition and diet therapy,* [8th ed.]. Philadelphia: W. B. Saunders.

**Body Mass Index**. The body mass index (BMI) is useful as an indicator of body fat in cases when the nurse cannot obtain skinfold measurements. The index correlates weight and height to estimate overall fat stores. The client's hydration status may affect BMI. BMI is useful when used in conjunction with skinfold measurements to estimate body

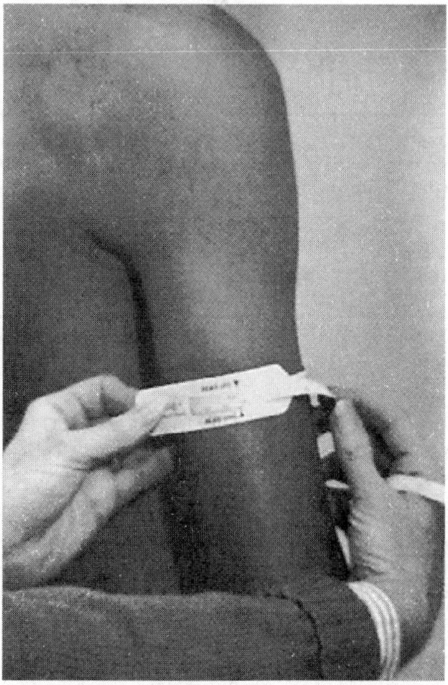

**FIGURE 14–3.** Measurement of the arm circumference at the midpoint. (From Mahan, L. K., Arlin, M. [1992]. *Krause's food, nutrition and diet therapy* [8th ed., p. 310]. Philadelphia: W. B. Saunders.

fat. The following formula is most commonly used to calculate the BMI:

$$\frac{\text{Present weight (kg)}}{\text{Height (cm}^2\text{)}} \times 100$$

## Biochemical Analysis

### PLASMA PROTEINS

The plasma proteins are vital for maintaining tissue function, oncotic pressure, enzymatic processes, and immune function. The presence of the plasma proteins (prealbumin, albumin, and transferrin) in the serum is the result of hepatic synthesis. Because the ability of the liver to make these proteins and, consequently, their circulating level depend on the availability of nutrients, plasma proteins are another indicator of the level of the client's nutritional well-being.

**Albumin.** Circulating albumin has a half-life of 20 days. Because of this, serum albumin does not indicate immediate changes in nutritional status and therefore is not valuable as a tool to monitor short-term nutritional changes. However, serum albumin is an appropriate biochemical screening tool

**TABLE 14–6**
**Serum Albumin Level and Corresponding Level of Plasma Protein Depletion**

| Serum Albumin | Level of Plasma Protein Depletion |
|---|---|
| **Normal Serum Albumin 3.5–5 mg/dL** | |
| > 3.5 | None |
| 2.8–3.5 | Mild |
| 2.1–2.7 | Moderate |
| < 2.1 | Severe |

Adapted from Nutritional Assessment Kit, Ross Laboratories, Columbus, Ohio.

for initial nutritional evaluation because it does reflect the client's nutritional status in the recent past. Table 14–6 lists the level of albumin and the corresponding level of plasma protein depletion it represents.

**Transferrin.** Serum transferrin is a more sensitive and earlier indicator of nutritional status because this plasma protein has a half-life of only 8 to 10 days. Serum transferrin may either be measured in the laboratory or calculated as a function of total iron-binding capacity (TIBC). Because analysis of serum transferrin is not a routine procedure for most laboratories, the calculated version is less expensive and more readily available albeit not as accurate.

$$\text{Calculated transferrin} = (0.68 \times \text{TIBC}) + 21$$

Table 14–7 lists the level of transferrin and the corresponding level of plasma protein depletion it represents.

**Prealbumin.** Prealbumin is a plasma protein with a shorter half-life than albumin or transferrin. The half-life of prealbumin is 2 to 3 days, making it very sensitive to short-term changes in plasma protein stores. Normal prealbumin levels range between 15.7 and 29.6 mg/dL.

**Creatinine Height Index.** Creatinine height index (CHI) is a biochemical measurement of skeletal muscle mass. Creati-

**TABLE 14–7**
**Serum Transferrin Level and Corresponding Level of Visceral Protein Depletion**

| Serum Transferrin | Level of Visceral Protein Depletion |
|---|---|
| **Normal Serum Transferrin 250–300 mg/dL** | |
| > 200 | None |
| 151–200 | Mild |
| 100–150 | Moderate |
| < 100 | Severe |

Adapted from Nutritional Assessment Kit, Ross Laboratories, Columbus, Ohio.

nine is a by-product of muscle metabolism that the body excretes in the urine. CHI is the ratio between the client's 24-hour urinary creatinine excretion and the ideal urinary creatinine excretion of an individual of the same height. Ideal creatinine excretion must be calculated and is the product of ideal body weight (kg) multiplied by 23 mg of creatinine for men or 18 mg of creatinine for women. The following formula would be used to calculate CHI:

$$\frac{\text{Measured 24-h urinary creatinine}}{\text{Ideal urinary creatinine}} \times 100$$

CHI is an indicator of the level of skeletal muscle mass depletion. A CHI at 60% to 80% of ideal indicates moderate muscle mass depletion. A CHI of less than 60% of ideal indicates severe depletion.

## IMMUNE FUNCTION

Immune function is influenced by many factors, including nutrition. Measuring immune function, therefore, is another valuable biochemical determination of the client's nutritional status. Total lymphocyte count (TLC) and anergy (the reactivity to specific antigens) are the immune functions most commonly measured in the clinical setting. The nurse may also see *delayed cutaneous hypersensitivity, reactivity to recall skin test antigens,* or *delayed-type hypersensitivity* (DTH) as some of the other terms for anergy testing.

**Total Lymphocyte Count.** TLC is a readily available and inexpensive biochemical indicator. This is a calculated indicator using the results obtained from a complete blood count with differential (CBC w/diff).

$$\text{TLC} = \frac{\text{\% of Lymphocytes}}{\text{(From the differential)}} \times \frac{\text{White blood cell count}}{100}$$

When interpreting TLC, the nurse must be aware that drug therapy, acute illness, stress, infection, and neoplastic disease can influence this value. Table 14–8 lists the level of TLC and the associated level of immunoincompetence.

**TABLE 14–8**
**Total Lymphocyte Count and Associated Level of Immunocompetence**

| Total Lymphocyte Count ($mm^3$) | Level of Immunoincompetence |
|---|---|
| > 2000 | None |
| 1200–2000 | Mild |
| 800–1199 | Moderate |
| < 800 | Severe |

Adapted from Nutritional Assessment Kit, Ross Laboratories, Columbus, Ohio.

**Anergy Testing.** Although not as popular as it once was, anergy testing is another method of determining nutritional health. By intradermally injecting the client with antigens to which he or she would normally have been exposed in a particular geographic area, the NST can determine the client's immune function and, consequently, nutritional status. It is expected that if the client had been previously exposed to particular antigens, he or she will react on reexposure if the immune system is intact. Candida, mumps, Trichophyton, purified protein derivative (PPD), tetanus toxoid, diphtheria toxoid, Streptococcus, and Proteus are the antigens commonly injected for evaluation. The test is usually completed by intradermally injecting three to five of these antigens at different sites on the inner aspect of the client's forearm. The nurse observes the response at 24 and 48 hours. Induration of 2 to 5 mm or more at the sites of any two tests indicates a normal response or immunocompetence. As with a TLC, factors such as disease, stress, drugs, and antineoplastic therapies affect the accuracy of the test.

## NUTRITIONAL REQUIREMENTS

After assessing the client's nutritional status the nutritional support team (NST) determines the number of calories necessary to meet the client's needs. These needs are based on the client's age, sex, activity, and nutritional depletion status and the presence and level of disease or injury. There are a number of methods the NST uses to determine the client's needs. Some are based on calculations, whereas others use sophisticated equipment.

### Basal Metabolic Rate

The basal metabolic rate (BMR) is the minimal amount of energy the body requires in a resting, fasting state to sustain life processes. The dietician usually calculates the client's BMR using the Harris-Benedict equation or indirect calorimetry.

## PARENTERAL NUTRITION SOLUTIONS

### Components

There are a variety of formulas for parenteral nutrition. These formulas may include carbohydrate, protein, fat, minerals, vitamins, and trace elements, as would an oral or enteral diet. Some formulas are incomplete, whereas others offer the client a complete diet. The volume of fluid and concentration of nutrients prescribed in the formula depend on the client's needs and the goals of therapy.

## DEXTROSE

Dextrose, or more appropriately glucose, usually provides the carbohydrate source in parenteral nutrition solutions. Glucose is the carbohydrate source of choice because it is a normal physiologic substrate occurring naturally in the blood. Commercially available concentrations vary from 2.5% to 70%. Each gram of IV dextrose provides the client with 3.4 kcal. Glucose may be the exclusive nonprotein calorie source in the parenteral nutrition solution, or it may be administered in varying proportions with lipids.

## LIPIDS

The major source of calories in an oral diet is lipids or fat, usually providing about 40% of the total caloric intake. In addition to mimicking the composition of an oral diet, the use of lipids in parenteral nutrition solutions provides the client with 9 kcal/g. This isotonic solution allows the infusion of a large number of calories for energy without the need for large volumes of solution. Lipid emulsions also provide the client with EFAs. When the nurse first sees a container of lipid emulsion, he or she may be surprised because rather than appearing clear, lipid emulsions appear white and "milky."

## CRYSTALLINE AMINO ACIDS

Crystalline amino acids are the protein and, consequently, the nitrogen source in parenteral nutrition solutions. Providing 4 kcal/g, crystalline amino acids have both the essential and nonessential amino acids generally thought necessary for clients receiving parenteral nutrition. They are available in several concentrations that give the same amounts and proportions of the different amino acids to the client in varying volumes of fluid. Modified amino acid solutions formulated for conditions of organ dysfunction and stress are available for use in clients with renal or hepatic disease or other requirements.

## ELECTROLYTES

The addition of electrolytes is based on the evaluation of the client's needs. Sodium is added in the form of an acetate, lactate, chloride, or bicarbonate. Potassium may be an acetate, lactate, chloride, or acid phosphate. Magnesium sulfate and calcium gluconate are also added based on the client's needs.

## VITAMINS

Clients require daily vitamins for normal body function and optimal utilization of nutrient substrates. The nurse or pharmacist adds commercially available preparations of both the fat- and water-soluble vitamins (MVI-12 or MVC 9 1 3) to the client's parenteral nutrition solution daily. The addition of vitamin preparations may give a yellow cast to the appearance of the parenteral nutrition solution. Most commercially prepared vitamin preparations do not provide vitamin K because it can interfere with coagulation therapy. Vitamin K is added to the parenteral nutrition solution individually, or the nurse gives the necessary amount in an intramuscular injection. Vitamins are not stable when exposed to temperature changes and light. For this reason, some agencies add vitamins just before hanging the parenteral solution. Then the solution should be protected from direct sunlight.

#### TRACE ELEMENTS

The body needs trace elements in small amounts. These micronutrients are available in commercial preparations in combination or individually. Chromium, copper, zinc, and manganese are the trace elements typical of commercial preparations. Some may also contain iodine and selenium. Iron is not routinely added to parenteral solutions because iron can cause anaphylaxis when administered intravenously. The client's laboratory data indicate which trace elements and the amounts the client requires.

### Preparation

Using strict aseptic technique, a clinical pharmacist or a trained pharmacy technician under the supervision of a pharmacist mixes the parenteral nutrition solution in the pharmacy under a laminar air flow hood. The pharmacist or technician wears a gown, mask, cap, and sterile gloves while mixing the solutions (Fig. 14–4).

## PARTIAL (PERIPHERAL) PARENTERAL NUTRITION

Partial (peripheral) parenteral nutrition (PPN) solutions offer nutrients that partially meet the client's nutritional requirements. PPN solutions infuse through peripheral access devices.

### Uses

PPN solutions are administered to the client whose nutritional assessment does not indicate that he or she is malnourished. These clients generally require some nutritional support for a limited period of time (2 to 3 weeks) when they may not be able to meet all their nutritional requirements orally or enterally. PPN solutions can maintain or restore fluid and electrolyte balance and help the client maintain a positive nitrogen balance during periods of nothing by mouth (NPO) before or after surgery. PPN solutions assist the client with meeting minimum calorie and protein requirements.

**FIGURE 14–4.** Pharmacist or technician mixing the solutions.

PPN is sometimes an adjunctive therapy for clients receiving oral or enteral nutrition. The PPN assists with boosting the client's calorie and protein intake to acceptable levels as needed.

## Formula

PPN solutions usually consist of 5% to 10% dextrose and 2.75% to 4.25% crystalline amino acids mixed in one infusion container. The pharmacy adds electrolytes, trace elements, and vitamins as prescribed. If the physician orders lipids, the lipid emulsion is either added to the glucose–amino acid solution or piggybacked through a Y-site on the administration set. PPN solutions provide approximately 1400 to 2000 kcal/d. Because PPN is administered through the peripheral veins, consideration for osmolarity limits the concentration of the solution. PPN solutions usually have an osmolarity no greater than 600 mOsm/L. Peripheral administration of solutions with higher osmolarities can cause venous irritation, resulting in sclerosis (Table 13–2).

## Administration

Clients can receive PPN through a peripheral vein. An electronic infusion device is necessary to control the rate of administration. Some agency policies require that the solution be filtered. If the solution consists of glucose and amino acids with additives, a 0.22-μm filter is recommended. If the

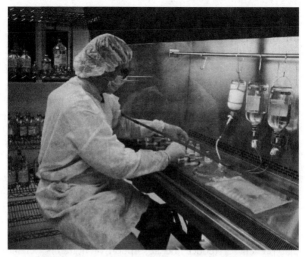

solution contains lipids, a 0.22-μm filter is too small and can damage the fat emulsion. In these cases the nurse uses a 1.2-μm filter. This filter is large enough to allow passage of the lipid molecules without damage.

## TOTAL PARENTERAL NUTRITION

TPN provides the client with complete nutritional support. Unlike PPN solutions, TPN infuses via a central venous catheter. Clients who are malnourished receive enough nutrients to restore a positive nitrogen balance, as well as needed vitamins, electrolytes, trace elements, and minerals.

### Uses

TPN is given to clients with severe illnesses lasting greater than 2 weeks. Clients with multiple trauma or severe burns receive TPN. Clients with illnesses of the gastrointestinal tract that prevent or reduce the absorption of nutrients benefit from TPN. Some of these illnesses are short bowel syndrome, bowel fistulae or obstruction, and inflammatory bowel disease. Other uses of TPN include the client with cancer whose cachectic state makes further chemotherapy dangerous or the burned client whose hypermetabolic state requires high calorie and protein intake. Clients with acute hepatic or renal failure tolerate TPN well, using amino acid solutions altered for the specific disease state.

### Formula

TPN solutions usually consist of 20% to 25% dextrose and 2.5% to 8.5% crystalline amino acids. The pharmacy adds electrolytes, vitamins, and trace elements. The lipid emulsion of 10% or 20% is administered peripherally, piggybacked through a Y-site on the administration set, or added into the infusion container with the glucose–amino acid solution. If the lipids are added to the glucose–amino acid container, the solution is known as a 3-in-1 solution or total nutrient admixture (TNA).

### Administration

Because TPN solutions are hypertonic, they must be administered through a central venous catheter. (Chapter 7 discusses the various types of central venous catheters and their care.) As with PPN, some agencies require that the nurse filter the TPN solution. In these cases, solutions that include the lipids with the glucose–amino acid solution must be filtered through a 1.2-μm filter. A 0.22-μm filter is sufficient for TPN solutions without lipids.

## INITIATION OF TPN THERAPY

After it is determined that the client requires TPN, the formula and the rate of administration are considerations for the NST.

### FORMULA

Usually in the beginning of a client's TPN therapy the prescription is written to provide for the glucose–amino acid solution to be administered daily, and the client's lipid requirements are provided two to three times per week as a piggyback administration. By not including the lipids in these early admixtures, the physician has more flexibility to adjust the additives in the base glucose–amino acid solution. The physician uses the assessment of the client's clinical tolerance of the initial formula and laboratory determination of the client's electrolytes to make these adjustments. After a base formula to meet the goals of therapy is determined, the pharmacy may add a portion of the client's weekly lipid allotment to each day's formula.

### RATE

The initial TPN schedule is usually a consistent rate over 24 hours. The total daily TPN volume is divided by 24 and administered at this rate per hour.

$$\frac{3000 \text{ mL}}{24\text{h}} = 125 \text{ mL/h}$$

The nurse assures this rate using an electronic control device. At the end of the twenty-fourth hour the nurse may notice that some TPN is left in the container. This is not unusual, as most IV solutions have some overfill. The nurse discards this amount and administers the next container of TPN.

Some agencies use a numbering system to order the administration of the TPN containers, since the additives prescribed may vary from TPN container to TPN container. It is important for the nurse to follow the numbers and hang the containers of TPN in numeric order to avoid administration errors and the wasting of expensive expired solutions.

### MONITORING

During this initiation phase of TPN therapy, the nurse, pharmacist, dietitian, and physician monitor the client's clinical status and laboratory results carefully. Intake and output measurements and daily weights measurements are taken to monitor fluid balance. Laboratory tests are drawn to monitor electrolyte balance. Because some TPN solutions have a high concentration of glucose, the nurse may monitor the client's blood sugar using fingersticks. Some agencies use electronic glucose monitoring equipment, whereas others depend on visual analysis of the glucose strip. Still others use urine glucose determination.

## CYCLING

After the client is stabilized in terms of fluid, electrolyte, and glucose tolerance of the TPN prescription, the physician may cycle the TPN solution. This means that the client receives a 24-hour volume of TPN over a shorter period of time; some cycles run over a 10- to 14- or 16-hour period. The rest of the day, the client receives no TPN.

Some physicians begin the cycling process by decreasing the number of hours the client receives the TPN by 2 hours every few days, depending on the client's tolerance. The same volume of TPN is administered over a shorter period of time. This means that the hourly rate of administration increases as the amount of time decreases. To decrease the amount of time over which the client receives the TPN volume, the physician usually orders a ramping schedule. A ramping schedule calls for the administration rate to begin slowly, reach a peak rate and sustain that rate over a period of time and then ramp back down to zero. At this point the nurse discontinues the TPN until the next cycle. Slowly ramping the TPN solution rate up to the steady-state rate allows the body's endogenous insulin production to increase to the level capable of handling the extra glucose load the solution provides. Tapering the TPN solution rate allows the body's feedback mechanisms to alert the pancreas to decrease the heightened production of insulin so that the client does not experience hypoglycemia when the TPN is discontinued.

Some electronic infusion devices are capable of "straight-line ramping," whereas others perform "step ramping."

**Straight-line Ramping.** With straight-line ramping the nurse programs the electronic infusion device to deliver the total volume of the TPN prescription, the number of hours for the ramp up, the number of hours for the ramp down, and the total number of hours for the infusion. After programming, the electronic infusion device ramps the infusion rate up from 0 mL/h to a steady-state rate for a specified period of time. At the end of that steady-state rate the device decreases the rate of infusion from the steady-state rate down to 0 mL/h. The electronic infusion device calculates the rate of the steady-state infusion automatically. A typical program for a straight-line ramp may read, "Infuse 3000 mL TPN over 14 hours, ramp up over 2 hours and ramp down over 2 hours."

**Step Ramping.** To perform step ramping the nurse either programs the electonic infusion device to automatically complete the ramping schedule, or the nurse must reset the rate on the pump for each period. A typical order for step ramping may read, "Infuse 3000 mL TPN over 14 hours, infuse 50 mL during the first hour; 100 mL during the second hour; 270 mL during hours 3 through 12; 100 mL during hour 13; and 50 mL during hour 14." Figure 14–5 graphically depicts step ramping.

## SPECIAL ADMINISTRATION CONSIDERATIONS

1. The nurse must use strict aseptic technique when handling TPN and the client's catheter.
2. To decrease the potential for infection the single-lumen central venous catheter should only be used for administration of TPN. Under ideal situations the catheter will have been placed for the purpose of the TPN administration and therefore have never been used for other administrations. In the case of multilumen catheters, one lumen should be isolated for the TPN administration. The TPN lumen is not appropriate for drawing blood or determining central venous pressure measurements.
3. Before hanging the TNA, the nurse should observe the solution for any changes in color, gray tinge, or "oily" appearance (Fig. 14–6). This may signal problems with the integrity of the solution. In this case if another container of TPN is not immediately available to hang, the nurse notifies the pharmacy and hangs 1 L of 10% dextrose in water (D10W) at the prescribed rate until a new container of TPN is available. Hanging the D10W keeps the client from experiencing hypoglycemia.

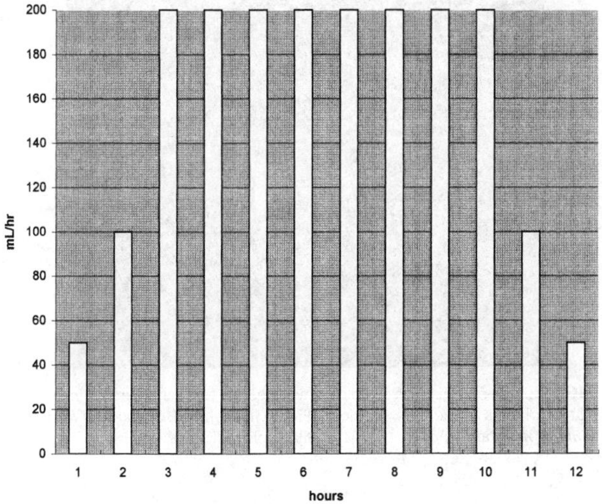


**FIGURE 14–5.** Step ramping.

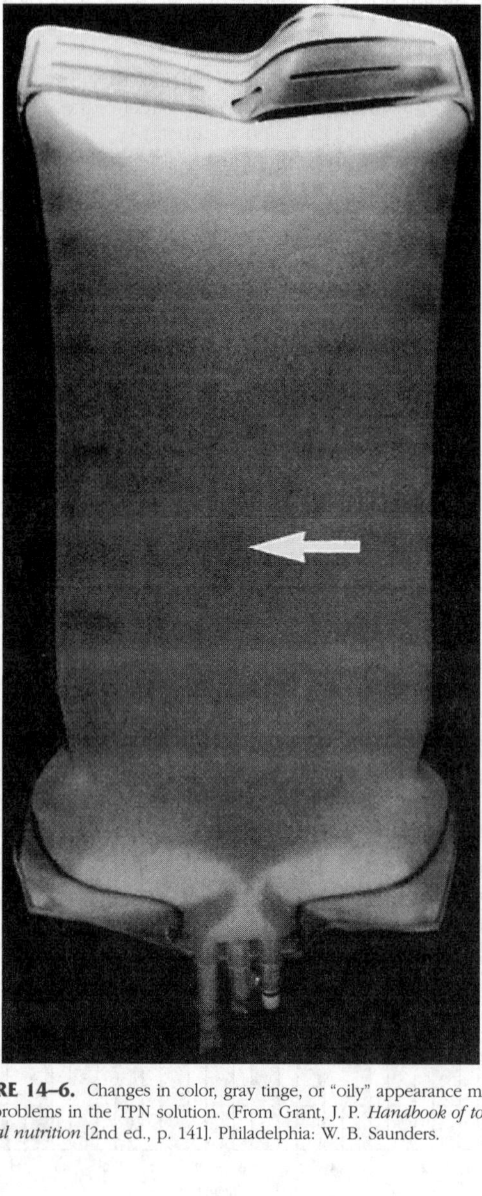

**FIGURE 14–6.** Changes in color, gray tinge, or "oily" appearance may indicate problems in the TPN solution. (From Grant, J. P. *Handbook of total parenteral nutrition* [2nd ed., p. 141]. Philadelphia: W. B. Saunders.

4. When the client is in the hospital, the pharmacy should make all additions to the TPN solution container in the laminar air flow hood to prevent contamination. Some additions outside of a laminar air flow hood such as vitamins may be necessary for home care clients.
5. No TPN solution may hang for longer than 24 hours.
6. During the administration if the rate falls behind schedule, the nurse should not attempt to catch up the infusion. The appropriate action is to readjust the infusion to the prescribed rate.
7. If the client spikes a temperature, the physician should be notified and the client evaluated for sepsis. Clients who have been stabilized on a TPN formula for a few weeks and suddenly have high blood glucose determinations should be evaluated for infection.
8. Clients whose TPN is cycled require glucose monitoring 1 hour after the TPN is discontinued to observe for reactive hypoglycemia.

## COMPLICATIONS

Clients receiving parenteral nutrition are at risk for a variety of complications. Some of these complications are due to the presence of the client's venous access device. For a discussion of these, see Chapters 6 and 7. Other complications are metabolic and are usually due to the parenteral nutrition solution itself.

### Hyperglycemia

**Causes.** Glucose concentration in formula is excessive; infusion rate is too rapid; or glucose tolerance is compromised by diabetes, stress, or sepsis.

**Signs and Symptoms.** Polyuria, dehydration, elevated blood and urine glucose levels.

**Treatment.** Decrease TPN infusion rate or dextrose concentration. Add insulin to TPN or initiate sliding scale insulin.

**Documentation.** Include all observations in the client's medical record. A flow sheet, including the client's intake and output, weight, vital signs, and fingerstick or urine glucose determinations, assists the NST in determining the cause of hyperglycemia and in preventing future occurrences.

### Hypoglycemia

**Cause.** Sudden interruption of TPN administration or excessive insulin administration.

**Signs and Symptoms.** Sweating, shaking, or irritability, particularly when the infusion is discontinued; low serum-glucose levels.

**Treatment.** If the next TPN container is unavailable, hang D10W at the same rate as the TPN solution. If the hypoglycemia is severe, the client may require a bolus of D50W. Reevaluate supplemental insulin requirements.

**Documentation.** The nurse documents all observations, including times of occurrence in relation to the discontinuation of the infusion.

## Hyperosmolar, Hyperglycemic, Nonketotic Coma

**Cause.** Hyperosmolar diuresis due to untreated hyperglycemia, which leads to electrolyte disturbances and eventual coma.

**Signs and Symptoms.** Confusion, lethargy, seizures, coma, hyperglycemia, dehydration, glycosuria.

**Treatment.** Stop any infusion containing dextrose. Administer 0.45% normal saline solution (NSS) to rehydrate the client and insulin to treat the hyperglycemia. Correct electrolyte imbalances.

**Documentation.** Document all signs and symptoms, including the client's level of consciousness. Maintain strict intake and output records.

## Hyperkalemia

**Causes.** Too much potassium in the TPN formula, renal disease, hyponatremia. Clients who have suffered severe trauma leak potassium from damaged cells.

**Signs and Symptoms.** Cardiac arrhythmias and rate disturbances, neuromuscular weakness or paralysis, mental confusion and paresthesias.

**Treatment.** Stop or decrease potassium administration. Correct electrolyte imbalances. If the hyperkalemia is severe, the client may require dialysis.

**Documentation.** Monitor and document the client's cardiac rate and rhythm. Maintain complete and accurate intake and output records.

## Hypokalemia

**Causes.** Excessive potassium losses secondary to gastrointestinal (GI) tract disturbances (diarrhea) or diuretic therapy; administration of large doses of insulin; insufficient potassium in the TPN formula.

**Signs and Symptoms.** Muscle weakness, paralysis, paresthesias, lethargy, drowsiness, irritability, apathy, confusion, hallucinations.

**Treatment.** Add or increase the amount of potassium in TPN formula. Determine if the hypokalemia is drug induced and discontinue or adjust medications as practical.

**Documentation.** Record accurate intake and output measurements, including any losses from diarrhea.

## Hypernatremia

**Causes.** Dehydration, diarrhea, diabetes insipidus, too much sodium in the TPN formula.

**Signs and Symptoms.** Lethargy (which may proceed to coma and convulsions), muscle tremors and rigidity, hyperactive reflexes.

**Treatment.** Decrease or eliminate sodium in the TPN formula; increase the amount of free water in the TPN formula. Treat the cause of the dehydration and adjust medications that may cause sodium retention, such as steroids.

**Documentation.** Maintain accurate intake and output measurements. Document the client's level of consciousness.

## Hyponatremia

**Causes.** Diuretics, vomiting, fistulas, renal failure, cirrhosis.

**Signs and Symptoms.** Muscle cramps, weakness, fatigue, confusion; convulsions and coma if the onset of hyponatremia is rapid and severe.

**Treatment.** Add sodium to the TPN formula. If the hyponatremia is severe, administer 3% to 5% NSS intravenously. Measure and replace GI tract losses. Alter the medications that caused the hyponatremia and administer antiemetics for vomiting.

**Documentation.** Note the client's sensorium and any somatic complaints. Measure and accurately document any GI tract losses.

## Hyperphosphatemia

**Causes.** Renal insufficiency, too much phosphate in the TPN formula.

**Signs and Symptoms.** Hypocalcemia, nausea, vomiting, anorexia.

**Treatment.** Decrease or omit phosphate in the TPN formula. Treat nausea and vomiting with antiemetics. Administer TPN formulated for clients with renal insufficiency.

**Documentation.** Measure and document intake and output accurately. Measure and document urine specific gravity.

## Hypophosphatemia

**Causes.** Insulin therapy, alcoholism, use of phosphate-binding antacids, hypocalcemia, renal insufficiency, diarrhea.

**Signs and Symptoms.** Irritability, weakness, paresthesias, coma, respiratory arrest.

**Treatment.** Add phosphate to the TPN formula and replace calcium. Treat diarrhea. Adjust medications as appropriate.

**Documentation.** Record the client's complaints of weakness. Maintain accurate intake and output documentation.

### Hypercalcemia

**Causes.** Pancreatitis, excessive replacement of calcium in clients who are bedridden.

**Signs and Symptoms.** Personality disorders, confusion, coma, muscle weakness, fatigue, nausea, vomiting.

**Treatment.** Decrease or omit calcium in the TPN formula.

**Documentation.** Monitor and document the client's level of consciousness and orientation.

### Hypocalcemia

**Causes.** Vitamin D deficiency, too little calcium added to the TPN formula, pancreatitis, hypomagnesemia, hypophosphatemia.

**Signs and Symptoms.** Paresthesias, twitching, positive Chvostek's sign (a spasm of the facial muscles elicited by tapping the facial nerve in the region of the parotid gland).

**Treatment.** Add calcium to the TPN formula. If the hypocalcemia is secondary to hypomagnesemia or hypophosphatemia, the latter disorders must also be corrected to adequately treat the hypocalcemia.

## HOME NUTRITIONAL SUPPORT

Some clients require parenteral nutrition administration of periods longer than their hospitalization. These clients may receive parenteral nutrition at home. The NST refers the client to a home infusion therapy company. This company generally employs home infusion nurses who instruct the client and caregiver(s) in the procedures associated with home nutritional support. These home infusion nurses assist the client in achieving and maintaining independence at home. The home infusion therapy company also has clinical pharmacists who mix the parenteral nutrition solution. The home infusion therapy nurse and clinical pharmacist work as a team to monitor the client's clinical status and laboratory data. They keep the physician informed of the client's status throughout the therapy. The home infusion therapy company also provides the client with the supplies and equipment necessary to infuse the parenteral nutrition and maintain the client's venous access device.

## Client and Caregiver Support

Disruption of oral intake and the activities associated with maintaining a client via home nutritional support can be a burden to the client and the caregiver. So much of our culture and social activities are designed around eating that the client may feel left out. Administration of the parenteral nutrition is also a burden on the caregiver and may interrupt the family's schedule. The nurse can assist the client and caregiver by listening to their fears and concerns. Discussions of other social activities or alternative methods to participate in activities that include food may assist the client with accepting his or her inability to eat. The nurse can work with the family to design a schedule that is least disruptive to the family activities.

The client may complain that his or her mouth feels dry and not fresh. The nurse can encourage frequent mouth care to include mouth rinses and teeth brushing. The use of lip gloss keeps the client's lips from cracking.

Clients who may eat should be encouraged to take small, frequent feedings. Some of these feedings should be scheduled at times when the rest of the family is at the table.

CHAPTER 15

# Blood Transfusion Therapy

*Marilyn Ferreri Booker*



Although the transfusion of blood and blood products is safer today than previously, transfusion therapy can be a dangerous procedure. In all cases the health care team (clients, physicians, and nurses) must weigh the potential risks (and there are many) against the benefits. In a study reported in *Transfusion,* the Journal of the American Association of Blood Banks, of 256 transfusion-related deaths over a 10-year period, 62% were secondary to acute hemolysis; 16% from hepatitis C (non-A, non-B hepatitis); 12% from acute pulmonary edema; and 10% each from hepatitis B, delayed hemolysis, and bacterial contamination (Sazama, 1990). These statistics are sobering when one realizes that a number of these deaths were avoidable. Clerical errors, misidentification, and nonadherence to sterile technique can lead to hemolysis and bacterial contamination. Vigilant observation of the client during the transfusion can ameliorate the consequences of pulmonary edema. It should be evident that well-informed, careful practitioners can provide transfusion therapy safely.

There are a number of roles that the nurse may play in assuring a safe transfusion for the client. A few of these are drawing and correctly labeling the typing and cross-matching specimen, positively identifying the recipient before hanging the blood product, and carefully monitoring the client for any reactions or side effects during and after the transfusion. Discussions of these and other nursing responsibilities are included in this chapter.

## HISTORY

Denis, a physician in the court of Louis XIV, performed the first blood transfusion in 1658, when he transfused a lamb's blood into a youth. This first procedure was successful, but Dr. Denis, or rather his patients, were not as fortunate in subsequent attempts.

Knowledge associated with the transfusion of blood remained stagnant until 1818. In that year Blundell, a physician in London, successfully transfused a moribund woman suffering with puerperal hemorrhage. The identification of blood types took place in 1900, and within 10 years, blood transfusions occurred frequently.

Before World War I, blood was transfused directly from donor to recipient. With the discovery of sodium citrate, an anticoagulant that prevents clotting ex vivo, health care providers could draw blood and store it for future use. This innovation marked the inception of blood banking.

## INDICATIONS

Indications for transfusion therapy include the treatment of decreased blood volume, the correction of insufficient oxygen-carrying capacity, or the replacement of coagulation components. The client may be suffering from trauma, cancer, sickle cell disease, hemorrhage, hepatic failure, immune system alterations, or hemophilia. Newborns suffering from hemolytic anemia require transfusions for blood exchange. Priming the oxygenating pump and maintaining circulation in cardiac surgery requires blood.

## COMPOSITION OF BLOOD

Blood consists of two components: cells and plasma.

### Blood Cells

The cellular components represent about 45% of the total volume of blood and consist of erythrocytes (red blood cells [RBCs]), leukocytes (white blood cells [WBCs]), and thrombocytes (platelets).

### Blood Plasma

Plasma, the liquid part of blood, is responsible for the other 55% of the volume. Plasma consists of 90% water and 10% solutes. Some of the solutes present in blood plasma are true solutes or crystalloids. Crystalloids are solute particles less than 1 nm in diameter (e.g., ions or glucose). Other solutes in plasma are colloids. Colloids are particles from 1 to about 100 nm (nanometer) in diameter (e.g., proteins of all types). Proteins represent the largest quantity of all the solutes. Other solutes include food substances, glucose, amino acids, and lipids; products of metabolism such as urea, uric acid, creatinine, and lactic acid; respiratory gases, oxygen, and carbon dioxide; and regulatory substances, hormones, and enzymes; and other substances.

Current technologies allow the separation of whole blood into a variety of products; RBCs, fresh frozen plasma, platelet concentrates, granulocytes, immune globulin, albumin, and coagulation factors including cryoprecipitate. To appreciate the way in which blood banks harvest these products and the circumstances dictating their use, the nurse requires a basic knowledge of immunohematology.

## IMMUNOHEMATOLOGY

Immunohematology is the study of blood's antigens and their corresponding antibodies. These antigens and antibodies play an important role in blood transfusion therapy because they determine blood compatibilities.

### Antigens

An antigen is a substance capable of stimulating the formation of an antibody. Some antigens occur naturally in the body, whereas others are acquired. When specific antigens and antibodies combine, they can cause agglutination or clumping of the blood. Antigens in the different blood typing systems are hereditary and located on the surface of the RBC.

Two of the most important antigens associated with blood compatibility are found in the ABO system. These antigens are antigen A and antigen B. The presence or absence of these two antigens determines an individual's blood group. People with antigen A have blood type A; with antigen B have blood type B; with both antigens A and B have blood type AB; and those with neither antigen on the RBC have blood group O. It may be helpful for the nurse to consider blood group O to be blood group 0 (zero) because this better describes the antigens present—none!

## Antibodies

An antibody is a protein substance present in the plasma. Like antigens, some antibodies occur naturally in the body. Others develop in response to stimulation by an antigen. The antibodies that make up the ABO antibody system for plasma are naturally occurring. Their names derive from the antigen with which they will react. Anti-A and anti-B react with antigen A and antigen B, respectively. RBC antigens and their corresponding antibodies do not exist naturally in the same person. An individual with type A blood, that is a person with antigen A on the RBC will not have anti-A antibody in the plasma.

### COMPLETE ANTIBODIES

The classification of antibodies is either complete or incomplete. A complete antibody is one that can agglutinate cells in a saline media without the presence of other proteins. This process is very direct and occurs in the vascular system; thus, the name intravascular hemolysis.

### INCOMPLETE ANTIBODIES

An incomplete antibody cannot cause agglutination by itself. The incomplete antibody coats the RBC. The body then recognizes the cell as defective and hides it away in either the liver or the spleen until the reticuloendothelial system destroys it. Because this process takes place outside of the vascular system, it is called extravascular hemolysis. In the ABO system, A and B are complete antibodies. Incomplete antibodies, such as those found in the Rh system, are also known as alloantigens.

Because the transfusion of incompatible blood can trigger life-threatening reactions in the body, it is important for the nurse to understand the basics of RBC and plasma compatibilities. Table 15–1 outlines the antibodies present in the plasma.

**TABLE 15–1**
**Plasma and RBC Compatibilities**

| Blood Group Recipient | Antibodies Present in Plasma | Compatible RBCs | Compatible Plasma |
|---|---|---|---|
| O | Anti-A and anti-B | O | O, A, B, and AB |
| A | Anti-B | O and A | A and AB |
| B | Anti-A | O and B | B and AB |
| AB | None | AB, A, B, and O | AB |

RBC = red blood cell.

## Rhesus System

Another group of antigens is important in the understanding of immunohematology. These are the Rhesus or Rh system antigens. The Rh system consists of antigens D, C, E, c, and e. These, too, are located on the RBC and are inherited. The most important of these antigens is D. The presence or absence of antigen D is one of the factors that determines if a person is Rh positive or Rh negative, which is an important factor in determining the compatibility of RBCs. The Rh antigen is very immunogenic (capable of initiating the body's immune responses). Therefore, it is more likely to stimulate antibody formation. A person with Rh positive blood does not have anti-Rh antibodies in the serum, or they would destroy his or her RBCs. A person with Rh negative blood transfused with Rh positive blood will develop anti-Rh antibodies after the exposure to the Rh (D) antigen. The reaction generally does not occur on the initial exposure because the Rh antibodies develop slowly. Once sensitized, this person will probably react with a transfusion reaction and hemolysis of the RBCs with the next exposure.

Transfusion is not the only opportunity for exposure. An Rh negative woman pregnant with an Rh positive fetus is essentially "exposed" to the Rh antigen during her pregnancy. Until about 25 years ago, subsequent pregnancies with Rh positive fetuses precipitated the development of anti-Rh antibodies that attacked the fetus. This phenomenon is known as erythroblastosis fetalis. Giving Rh immune globulin (RhoGam) by intramuscular injection within 72 hours of delivery, miscarriage, or abortion prevents the formation of anti-Rh antibodies and prevents hemolytic disease of newborns. This injection reduces the formation of anti-Rh (anti-D) to 1% to 2%. There is evidence that the formation of anti-Rh can be decreased to 0.1% by administering two doses of RhoGam; one at 28 weeks' gestation and the other at 72 hours after delivery. While the development of this drug was to treat erythroblastosis fetalis, it is now also given after transfusion of positive blood product to Rh negative recipients.

The blood bank performs an indirect Coombs' test to determine if the client has any antibodies in his or her serum that may react with the RBCs in the transfusion. Sometimes this test identifies some weak variants of the Rh (D) factor. This antigen is less immunogenic than Rh (D). Blood banks test donor blood for the D and $D^u$ antigen before determining Rh status. Individuals with these subantigens, called $D^u$, are Rh positive donors but are Rh negative recipients.

Other Rh antigens are clinically significant in special cases. They are less immunogenic and therefore less likely to produce hemolytic reactions. These antigens are important in establishing paternity.

### Human Leukocyte Antigens

Human leukocyte antigens (HLAs) are on the surface of lymphocytes and other nucleated cells. They are important to immunity and at times compatibility. HLAs determine the rate of histocompatibility between transplant recipients and donors. Clients receiving large or multiple transfusions over the course of their diseases require HLA testing and matching to donor cells. The frequency of exposure may cause these clients to develop antibodies to the donor platelets or RBCs. Other indications for HLA matching include clients receiving WBC transfusions, clients with a history of refractory febrile transfusion reactions, and clients preparing for organ transplantation.

## BLOOD DONATIONS

Blood donations fall into two categories: homologous or autologous.

### Homologous Blood

#### DEFINITION

Blood collections from human donors for use in human recipients are homologous.

#### TYPES OF HOMOLOGOUS DONATIONS

There are a few different types of homologous donors. The donor may be from the community at large, a community donor; or from parent to child, a parentologous donor. A directed donation occurs when the recipient selects the donor. This is generally a family member with a compatible blood grouping.

#### SCREENING HOMOLOGOUS DONORS

It is frequently the nurse at the donation center who advises donors of acquired immunodeficiency syndrome (AIDS) high-risk behavior and the practices and circumstances that should make them refrain from donating. The nurse assists donors with completion of a health assessment that includes a questionnaire on past and present illnesses. Certain illnesses such as hepatitis or malaria render the donor's blood unacceptable whether the disease is active or not. These, as well as physiologic and demographic criteria, are standards set by the American Association of Blood

Banks or the American Red Cross Blood Services. Donors must be a minimum of 17 years old, weigh at least 110 lbs (50 kg), and have a baseline hemoglobin of 12.5 g/dL for women and 13.5 g/dL for men. The nurse takes the donor's vital signs, which must be within normal limits. The nurse determines that the donor has not given blood within the last 56 days. The donor must have the opportunity to confidentially exclude his or her donation from transfusion. Honest and accurate information gathered from donors during the donation process is important in excluding blood from donors that may transmit diseases to recipients. It is important that the nurse's manner during this process encourage the donor to provide this information as accurately as possible.

## SPECIMEN TESTING

The blood bank tests a sample of the donor blood before making it available for routine transfusion. The label on the blood container states the donor's ABO group and, as necessary, Rh type. Blood noted as Rh negative has been tested for the D and the $D^u$ antigen.

Requests for blood transfusions require the blood bank to perform a typing and cross-matching test. This test includes an ABO and Rh determination, antibody screening, and cross-matching with donor blood. This test does not prevent sensitization to RBC antigens because it does not detect all incompatibilities, but it does minimize the potential for hemolytic reactions, which can be fatal. The nurse may draw the typing and matching specimen from the recipient, or the phlebotomy team may obtain the specimen. In either case the person performing the phlebotomy must take every possible precaution to assure that the blood in the vial belongs to the client for whom it is labeled. Clerical errors and misidentification are the leading causes of mismatching blood. The infusion of mismatched blood may cause the client to have an acute hemolytic reaction that can lead to death.

The blood bank also tests samples of donations intended for homologous use. This list of tests performed by most blood banks currently includes:

| | | |
|---|---|---|
| ABO | Rh | RBC antibodies |
| HbsAg | Anti-HBc | Anti-HCV (second generation) |
| ALT | RPR (syphilis) | |
| Anti-HTLV I/II | Anti-CMV (for certain recipients) | Anti-HIV 1/2 (AIDS) |

These tests are Food and Drug Administration (FDA)–licensed, and blood banks must meet all the standards set forth by this agency. In the future it is proposed that tests to detect

HTLV I/II, anti-HCV (third generation), Chagas' disease carriers, and donors with bacteremia be added to the list.

### PHERESIS

In some cases the blood bank draws the blood and keeps the entire unit. This blood may be given as whole blood; or the collection may be broken down into its components, and these may be given as separate products. In other cases the blood bank draws the blood and removes one or more of its components for use in transfusion. The blood bank returns the RBCs and the balance of the unit to the donor. This is hemapheresis or plasmapheresis. Frequently, blood banks use this process to harvest platelets or leukocytes. At times, platelet donors are HLA matched to a recipient with a chronic disease process. These HLA-matched donors are called to donate on a scheduled basis to provide platelets for the chronically ill client.

## Autologous Blood

### DEFINITION

An autologous donation, also known as autotransfusion, means that the blood donor and the blood recipient are the same person. This method of transfusion is gaining popularity for a variety of reasons.

### BENEFITS OF AUTOLOGOUS BLOOD

Autotransfusion virtually eliminates the possibility of fatal transfusion reactions or the transmission of blood-borne diseases. Autologous blood is immediately available without typing or cross-matching, thus saving time and money. Clients with certain religious objections to banked blood may find the infusion of their own blood more acceptable. Blood carefully salvaged from surgical sites is of higher quality than banked blood because this process usually maintains the integrity of platelets and clotting factors. The pH of the salvaged product is the same as the client's. This blood also retains its 2,3-diphosphoglycerate (DPG) level, thus enhancing oxygenation by increasing the hemoglobin's affinity for oxygen.

Autologous transfusion is an approach to obtaining compatible transfusion products rather than a procedure unto itself. The autologous blood product donation may be a predeposit donation, an intraoperative donation, intraoperative cell salvage, or a postoperative or posttraumatic salvage.

### PREDEPOSIT DONATION

Clients who know that they are going to have surgery requiring transfusions or who know that at some point they will require blood products may donate blood for their use in the future. The blood bank draws the unit and banks the product until the client needs it. Autologous blood has a 42-day shelf life, but if the blood bank has the capacity, freezing the donation extends this time. The client may donate weekly up to three days before the scheduled surgery. This cut off time decreases the probability of the client developing hypovolemia during the procedure. The client has a blood count before each donation. Most blood banks require that the client's hemoglobin be at least 11 g/dL and the hematocrit 33% before each donation. The nurse at the donation center may instruct the client to replenish bone marrow iron reserves with oral iron supplementation. In some cases, clients with antibodies to multiple antigens use this method to ensure that there is safe compatible blood available to them should they require it. Units donated and stored for undefined medical needs such as these are called speculative deposits.

### INTRAOPERATIVE DONATION (HEMODILUTION)

Clients who can tolerate the rapid withdrawal of blood immediately before surgery may be candidates for intraoperative hemodilution. This procedure involves the withdrawal of 1 to 2 U of blood either immediately before or after anesthesia induction. The withdrawal volume depends on the client's size, hematocrit, and estimated blood loss. Infusions of crystalline or colloid solutions replace the client's circulating volume. Intraoperative hemodilution improves blood flow in the microcirculation. Another benefit is a decreased loss of RBCs during the surgery because the client's hematocrit is reduced due to the infusion of the volume expanders. Reinfusion of the client's previously withdrawn blood takes place immediately after surgery or sooner if indicated.

Both predeposit and intraoperative donations are beneficial for the client having an elective surgery in which the surgeon knows that there is a need for blood transfusion therapy. In situations when these methods are impossible or the volumes collected are inadequate, intraoperative cell salvage may provide the client with an autologous source of blood.

### INTRAOPERATIVE CELL SALVAGE

Intraoperative cell salvage may supplement scheduled autologous blood collections or provide a source for autologous blood in emergency surgery. This technique involves salvaging blood from a clean surgical wound. Some of the procedures that lend themselves to this technique are open heart and vascular surgery, total joint replacement, ruptured ectopic pregnancy, and some neurosurgical procedures.

There are a number of processes available for intraoperative cell salvage. Each involves different equipment and processing of the salvaged blood. In general, the process involves collecting the client's blood lost during the surgery with a suction device. Filters remove clots, tissue, and sometimes bone fragments. Depending on the surgery and type of collection system used, a member of the operating team may wash and rinse the collection and spin it down to isolate the RBCs. The client then receives his or her own cells by infusion through a microaggregate filter. Microaggregate filters are between 20 and 40 $\mu$m, and their purpose is to retain small clots or particles.

## POSTOPERATIVE OR POSTTRAUMATIC SALVAGE

Postoperative or posttraumatic salvage may occur after cardiac or orthopedic surgeries or after a penetrating wound to the chest. Some of the same equipment used for intraoperative cell salvage is employed in these situations. Anticoagulation and washing of the collected blood depends on a variety of factors such as the rate of bleeding and the type of salvage system used.

Although autologous collections are safer than homologous donations, they are not without potential complications (see Table 15–2).

**TABLE 15–2**
**Autologous Transfusions with Potential Problems**

| Type | Potential Difficulties |
|---|---|
| Predeposit | • The client may experience anemia and hypovolemia after the donation.<br>• Scheduling around personal responsibilities may present a problem.<br>• Potential clerical errors in labeling exist.<br>• The blood product may be lost if the surgery is cancelled or delayed or during the thawing or washing process to deglycerolize the cells.<br>• The client may experience difficulty during the donation.<br>• If speculative, the blood may not be available in an emergency.<br>• The process is costly. |
| Intraoperative Donation | • Procedure may lead to intraoperative hypoxemia.<br>• Incorrect processing may cause damage to blood. |
| Intraoperative, Postoperative, or Posttraumatic Cell salvage | • Product is void of coagulation factors and platelets.<br>• Procedure may seed tumor cells throughout body.<br>• A contaminated wound may cause sepsis.<br>• Incorrect processing may cause damage to blood. |

## BLOOD PRODUCTS

In any situation in which treatment of a client with transfusion therapy is contemplated, the American Red Cross and the American Association of Blood Banks recommend that physicians consider treatment with pharmaceuticals or commercially prepared solutions if the client's condition will allow rather than transfusion therapy. Table 15–3 is a summary of blood components including their indications, actions, and nursing tips. Below is a complete guide to blood components.

### Whole Blood

**Description.** Whole blood consists of the RBCs and plasma components. Processing removes most of the plate-

**TABLE 15–3**
**Summary of Blood Components**

| Product | Indications/Actions | Nursing Tips |
|---|---|---|
| Whole blood | Symptomatic anemia with large volume deficit; restores oxygen-carrying capacity of blood and blood volume | Must be ABO identical; observe for volume overload in the elderly and children; infuse as rapidly as tolerated. |
| RBCs | Symptomatic anemia; restores oxygen-carrying capacity of blood | Must be ABO compatible; infuse as rapidly as tolerated but complete in 4 hours. |
| Leukocyte-poor RBCs | Restores oxygen-carrying capacity for clients with febrile reactions from leukocyte antibodies | Must be ABO compatible; infuse as rapidly as tolerated but complete in 4 hours. |
| Fresh frozen plasma | Deficit of labile and stable plasma coagulation factors and ITTP | Should be ABO compatible; infuse as rapidly as tolerated but complete in 4 hours. |
| Cryoprecipitated AHF | Hemophilia A, von Willebrand's disease, hypofibrinogenemia, factor XIII deficiency | Frequent repeated doses may be necessary; infuse as rapidly as tolerated but within 4 hours. |
| Platelets | Bleeding from thrombocytopenia or platelet function abnormality | Do not use some microaggregate filters (see manufacturers instructions); infuse in less than 4 hours. |
| Granulocytes | Neutropenia with infection | Must be ABO compatible; do not use some depthtype microaggregate filters; observe carefully for reactions. |

RBC = red blood cell, ITTP = idiopathic thrombotic thrombocytopenic purpura.

lets or WBCs. Any of these components remaining in stored blood are not viable after a few days. Usually, a unit of whole blood contains about 500 mL of blood anticoagulated with citrate having a hematocrit of 30% to 40%.

**Actions/Indications.** Whole blood provides RBCs to carry oxygen to tissues. It is also a blood volume expander and a source of proteins with oncotic and active coagulation properties. The indications for the use of whole blood include clients who have lost 25% to 30% or more of their blood volume from mass hemorrhage or neonates, infants, or adults who require exchange transfusions. In a nonbleeding adult, each unit of whole blood will raise an anemic adult's hemoglobin by 1 g/dL and hematocrit by three percentage points.

**Contraindications.** Clients should not receive whole blood if the anemia is treatable with medications such as iron, vitamin $B_{12}$, recombinant erythropoietin, or folic acid and if the client's condition permits sufficient time for these measures to promote erythropoiesis. Because of the risks of disease and the limited blood supply, whole blood is not the first treatment to expand blood volume. Crystalline solutions (0.9% normal saline solution [NSS] or Ringer's lactate) or colloids (albumin or plasma protein fraction) are the treatments of choice, as they provide safer alternatives. The appropriate coagulation products and derivatives are superior to whole blood in the treatment of coagulation deficiencies.

**Dosage and Administration.** Donor and recipient must be ABO identical. The blood bank tests for serologic incompatibility before releasing the unit for transfusion unless withholding blood might result in loss of life. The client's clinical situation dictates the volume of the transfusion. The administration rate of whole blood begins with a slow drip and then proceeds as rapidly as the client will tolerate it (see "Administering the Transfusion"). If the client requires a slow transfusion rate due to some cardiopulmonary weakness, it may be beneficial to administer a transfusion of RBCs rather than whole blood because the client receives the same oxygen-carrying capacity with RBCs as with whole blood without the extra volume.

## Red Blood Cells

### CELLS

**Description.** Preparation of a unit of RBCs involves the isolation of the red cells from the plasma by centrifugal or gravitational separation. This usually results in a 300-mL unit with a hematocrit of 65% to 80%. This process may remove some platelets or WBCs. In some cases the blood bank may add an adenine and saline product or other preservatives to increase the shelf life of the RBC unit. Some of these products have mannitol, an osmotic diuretic, as an RBC-stabilizing agent in them. The amount of mannitol is much lower than the approved dose to stimulate a diuretic effect in adults. Therefore, side effects from the mannitol are unlikely.

**Actions/Indications.** RBCs increase the oxygen-carrying capacity of the blood. Indications include the treatment of all clients with symptomatic deficit of oxygen-carrying capacity. Other indications include exchange transfusions and restoration of blood volume following significant hemorrhage. In a nonbleeding adult each unit of RBCs will raise an anemic adult's hemoglobin by 1 g/dL and hematocrit by three percentage points.

**Contraindications.** RBCs are not the treatment of choice when anemia is correctable with medications. See "Whole Blood, Contraindications."

**Dosage and Administration.** Administration of RBCs is similar to whole blood (see "Administering the Transfusion"). Because of the minimal amounts of plasma and hence ABO antibodies, it is possible to administer RBCs that are compatible but not ABO identical (see Table 15–1). RBCs with adenine and saline added require the same flow rate as whole blood because of the expanded volume. Therefore, for clients at risk for circulatory overload, concentrated RBCs are the preparation of choice.

## RED BLOOD CELL MODIFICATIONS

**Leukocyte Poor.** Clients who have had nonhemolytic febrile reactions may require a different preparation of RBCs. The cause of these reactions generally involves the WBCs present in the RBC units. Removing the leukocytes can make the transfusion less uncomfortable for these clients. Centrifugation, filtration, addition of sedimenting agents such as dextran or hydroxyethyl starch (HES), or any combination of these procedures removes leukocytes from units of RBCs. If the blood bank uses any of these agents in the preparation of the RBCs, the label lists them. Because small amounts of the agents may remain in the RBC unit, allergic reactions are possible, and the nurse must monitor the client closely for them. Some agencies use leukocyte removal filters to make the product leukocyte poor during the transfusion instead of treating the unit with additives.

Another method of leukocyte removal is washing. This is an expensive and less effective method to remove leukocytes. Washing, however, removes about 99% of the plasma. For this reason units prepared in this fashion may be indicated for use in clients with paroxysmal nocturnal hemoglobinuria (PNH) or other conditions that require transfusion of RBCs with minimal amounts of plasma. These units are appropriate for use in clients with antibodies to immunoglobulin A (IgA) or immunoglobulin E (IgE), although the preference is deglycerolized RBCs.

**Frozen Deglycerolized RBCs.** RBCs are frequently frozen until needed. To prevent damage to the cells during freezing, the blood bank adds glycerol to the unit. The glycerol coats the cells and acts as a protective agent. To use these cells the blood bank thaws them and washes them to remove the glycerol. The washed, deglycerolized cells are similar in function and posttransfusion survival to liquid RBCs. Washing removes virtually all the plasma, anticoagulant, residual platelets, and leukocytes. It is not unusual for some free hemoglobin to remain in the bags. A pink-tinged supernatant is acceptable for transfusion. However, if the supernatant is dark red or cloudy, the nurse returns the unit to the blood bank for evaluation.

Because these units contain no plasma or leukocytes, they are the preferred component for clients with clinically significant antibodies to IgA. These units also provide a reduced risk of febrile nonhemolytic reactions. Washing generally removes all the glycerol; but if the removal was not adequate, there is a risk of intravascular hemolysis, and the nurse must be alert to this.

## Plasma Components

The product known as plasma may be plasma, liquid plasma, or fresh frozen plasma.

### PLASMA OR LIQUID PLASMA

**Description.** Plasma and liquid plasma are the anticoagulated clear portion of blood separated by centrifugation or sedimentation. Plasma refers to the product that the blood bank stores frozen, whereas liquid plasma is refrigerated. The volumes of either type of unit are about 180 to 300 mL. Stable coagulation factors such as fibrinogen and factor IX are present, as well as some of the other coagulation factors.

**Actions/Indications.** Plasma is a volume expander. Because it is isotonic, plasma increases the client's circulating blood volume by its own volume. The fibrinogen and other coagulation factors in plasma are indicated for the treatment of stable clotting factor deficiencies for which no concentrates are available.

**Contraindications.** Plasma and liquid plasma are not appropriate for the replacement of labile coagulation factors such as factor V and VIII. The use of plasma or liquid plasma as a volume expander is contraindicated if volume can be replaced safely with other methods such as 0.9% NSS, Ringer's lactate, albumin, and plasma protein fraction.

**Dosage and Administration.** Plasma should be ABO compatible with the recipient's red cells; Rh is not a consideration.

### FRESH FROZEN PLASMA

**Description.** Fresh frozen plasma (FFP) is so named because the plasma is separated and frozen within 8 hours after the collection of whole blood. FFP contains about 200 U of factor VIII plus the other labile plasma coagulation factor, factor V.

**Actions/Indications.** Indications for FFP include the control of bleeding in clients who require labile plasma coagulation factors and blood volume expansion. FFP is essential in the treatment of idiopathic thrombotic thrombocytopenic purpura (ITTP).

**Contraindications.** FFP is not the treatment of choice when coagulopathy can be corrected more effectively with specific therapy such as vitamin K, cryoprecipitated antihemophilic factor (AHF) or AHF (factor VIII) concentrates. The use of FFP as a volume expander is contraindicated if volume can be replaced safely with other methods such as 0.9% NSS, Ringer's lactate, albumin, and plasma protein fraction.

**Dosage and Administration.** Plasma should be ABO compatible with the recipient's red cells; Rh is not a consideration. To use as a source of labile coagulation factors, use FFP as soon as possible but within 24 hours after thawing.

## Cryoprecipitate Components

**Description.** To prepare cryoprecipitated AHF, the blood bank thaws FFP to between 1° and 6° C and recovers the precipitate. Each bag of cryoprecipitated AHF contains on the average 80 or more factor VIII units and at least 150 mg of fibrinogen in less than 15 mL of plasma. If the bag label reads "cryoprecipitated AHF, pooled," the nurse can assume that several bags of cryoprecipitated AHF have been pooled and that different individuals were the donors for the cryoprecipitate in the pool.

**Actions/Indications.** Cryoprecipitated AHF provides a source of coagulation factor VIII, factor XIII fibrinogen, and von Willebrand's factor (AHF-VWF). This component controls bleeding in conditions associated with factor VIII deficiency such as hemophilia A. It is also the treatment indicated for von Willebrand's disease and for replacement of fibrinogen or factor XIII, such as with disseminated intravascular coagulation (DIC).

**Contraindication.** Use of cryoprecipitate components is limited to replacement of specific coagulation factors.

**Dosage and Administration.** While compatibility testing is unnecessary, it is preferable to use ABO-compatible material.

The blood bank keeps cryoprecipitated AHF, once thawed, at room temperature and releases it for transfusion as soon as possible but no more than 6 hours after thawing.

When treating bleeding in hemophilia A, rapid infusions (10 mL/min) of a loading dose produces the desired level of factor VIII:C. The nurse can expect to administer smaller maintenance doses every 8 to 12 hours. To maintain hemostasis after surgery a regimen of therapy for 10 days or longer may be required.

For treatment of von Willebrand's disease, smaller amounts of cryoprecipitated AHF correct the bleeding time. The frequency of administration is monitored by laboratory studies.

Clients requiring fibrinogen replacement should be monitored with fibrinogen assays, a blood test that measures the amount of fibrinogen in the client's blood.

## Platelet Components

Platelet components may include platelets, pooled platelets, or pheresed platelets.

### PLATELETS OR POOLED PLATELETS

**Description.** A unit of platelets is a concentrate of platelets separated from a single unit of whole blood and suspended in a small amount of the original plasma. Pooled platelets are from a number of units of whole blood from various donors. This is indicated on the bag label.

**Actions/Indications.** Normal hemostasis requires platelets. Platelets provide a source of phospholipids, a requirement for coagulation. The administration of platelets arrests bleeding in a thrombocytopenic client, corrects prolonged bleeding time, and increases the client's platelet count.

Platelets contain platelet-bound factors V and VIII. These may contribute to achieving hemostasis in clients who have received massive transfusions, have DIC, or are deficient in factor V.

Clients may receive platelets because of decreased numbers of platelets in their own blood. This may be secondary to inadequate production or to the production of functionally abnormal platelets. Platelets may be useful if given prophylactically to clients with rapidly falling or low platelet counts (10,000 to 20,000/mcL [microliters]) secondary to cancer or chemotherapy. In some clients with postoperative bleeding and platelet counts below 50,000/mcL, platelet administration is necessary.

**Contraindications.** Platelets are not the treatment of choice if the bleeding is unrelated to decreased numbers of or abnormally functioning platelets.

**Dosage and Administration.** Compatibility testing is not necessary for use of platelets or pooled platelets, although the donor plasma in platelets should be ABO compatible with the recipient's RBCs, especially when transfusing this component to neonatal recipients.

The clinical situation of each client determines the number of platelet concentrates to be administered. One bag of platelets increases the platelet count of a 154-lb (70-kg) adult by 5000 to 10,000/mcL and increases the count of a 40-lb (18-kg) child by 20,000/mcL. However, the client may require a repeat infusion in 1 to 3 days because of the short life span of transfused platelets. The expected response will not occur if the transfused platelets are destroyed rapidly, which may occur when the client has sepsis, a fever, or idiopathic thrombocytopenic purpura (ITP); when the client is alloimmunized by previous transfusions; when platelets are consumed, as with DIC; or when platelets are sequestered, as with splenomegaly. Some clients may also be refractory to platelet transfusions from unmatched donors. If 1 to 2 hours after the infusion the client exhibits no changes in hemostasis or a rise in platelet count of at least $2.5 \times 10^9$ per L/m$^2$, (2500/mcL/m$^2$), the client may be refractory. This is an indication for the blood bank to obtain HLA-matched platelets for the client to decrease the potential for the client's antibodies to react with the WBCs in the donor's platelets.

Transfusions of platelets proceed as rapidly as tolerated but take less than 4 hours. The nurse gently agitates the bag periodically to assure the infusion rate. The nurse flushes the container and filter with 0.9% NSS to be sure of administering all the platelets.

## PHERESED PLATELETS

**Description.** Hemapheresis is an effective way to harvest a therapeutic adult dose of platelets from an individual donor. These units contain more than 300,000/mcL of platelets. Some lymphocytes may be present in these units. At times, this component has been prepared from a combined platelet and granulocyte collection and may contain a sedimenting agent such as HES. This is listed on the label.

**Actions/Indications.** Pheresed platelets are indicated for clients requiring platelet transfusion. They are especially useful if they are HLA matched for clients refractory to platelets from unmatched donors. Pheresed platelets can be expected to increase the platelet count of a 154-lb (70-kg) adult by 30,000 to 60,000/mcL.

**Contraindications.** Same as for platelets.

**Dosage and Administration.** Similar to platelets. Platelet transfusions may be required every second or third day during a period of severe bone marrow depression. RBC compatibility testing must be performed before the transfusion if it is apparent that the component contains a significant number of RBCs. In these cases the nurse may notice that the plasma appears red or "bloody."

### Granulocyte Components

#### GRANULOCYTES BY PHERESIS

**Description.** Granulocytes by pheresis are most commonly collected from a single donor by a centrifugation hemapheresis technique. Granulocytes by pheresis usually contain a large number of other leukocytes and platelets, as well as 20 to 50 mL of RBCs. The product is usually suspended in 200 to 300 mL of anticoagulant and plasma. This is indicated on the label.

**Actions/Indications.** Granulocytes migrate toward, phagocytize, and kill bacteria. The nurse should not expect to notice a rise in the client's granulocyte count. This may be due to the sequestration of granulocytes that results from prior immunization to leukocyte antigens or due to consumption in the infection process.

The primary indication for granulocytes by pheresis is as supportive therapy for clients with neutropenia who have infections documented by culture, especially gram-negative bacteria, not responding to antibiotics or other modalities of therapy.

**Contraindications.** The use of granulocytes by pheresis as prophylaxis for infection is not recommended.

**Dosage and Administration.** Granulocytes by pheresis contain a significant number of RBCs, and serologic compatibility testing is necessary. When granulocyte transfusion therapy is indicated, support should continue at least daily until the infection is cured, the absolute granulocyte count returns to at least 500/mcL, or the physician decides to halt the therapy.

Granulocytes by pheresis should be transfused as soon as possible after collection, using a standard infusion set. Depthtype microaggregate filters and leukocyte depletion filters remove granulocytes and should not be used to transfuse this component.

## ADMINISTERING THE TRANSFUSION

The actual transfusion of the blood product includes three important phases: pretransfusion, transfusion, and posttransfusion. In each of these phases the nurse plays a critical role.

### Preparing for the Transfusion

Preparing for the transfusion involves a series of activities to ensure a safe transfusion for the client. The nurse prepares the client, draws the typing and matching specimen, and gathers the appropriate supplies.

## CLIENT PREPARATION

The physician has probably discussed the need for the transfusion with the client. If this has not occurred, the nurse may need to explain this. The nurse explains the reason the client requires the transfusion and the risks and benefits associated with it. The nurse outlines the procedure and describes any special equipment that may be necessary for the administration. The nurse obtains the client's medical history focusing on any previous transfusion experiences. Rather than ask the client "Have you ever had a transfusion reaction?" the nurse asks the client to describe his or her experience. It is important for the nurse to notify the physician and the blood bank for any positive history regarding previous transfusions and reactions. Some agencies require a consent form for transfusions. Follow the agency's policy.

## DRAWING THE TYPING AND MATCHING SPECIMEN

The nurse verifies the physician's order for the particular blood product, including the date for the transfusion. Agency policies differ in the types of paperwork and the specimen tubes required for the typing and cross-matching specimen. Consult the specific policy for this information. The nurse takes special care when labeling the specimen to ensure that it identifies the correct client. Some agencies use a special identification system along with the client's regular identification bracelet. This system includes an armband for the client and stickers, which the nurse places on the specimen, the type and cross-match requisition form, and the product requisition forms. The blood bank affixes other stickers from this set on the actual blood product bag. Each of these pieces has the same number to provide for positive identification.

No matter what system the agency uses, the nurse positively identifies the client. This can be done using the client's armband. Outpatient centers may use a driver's license. The nurse asks the client to state his or her name. Do not ask "Are you John (Jane) Doe?" Some clients who are medicated or confused may answer to any name. Only after the nurse is certain that the client being addressed is the correct person, the nurse draws the specimen for typing and cross-matching. The nurse labels the specimen with the client name and agency identification number before leaving the client's side.

The nurse arranges a time with the blood bank for the blood products to be available. Remember to consider any procedures, therapies, or tests for which the client may be scheduled. Clients should not be sent off the unit or out of the nurse's range while blood products are infusing.

Before the scheduled transfusion, establish a venous access device for the transfusion if one is not in place. Consider the size of the vein selected and the catheter's size. Remember, blood is a viscous solution and requires a large vein and at least a 20-gauge catheter to maintain the appropriate infusion rate for most adults.

## GATHERING THE SUPPLIES

The nurse considers the type and numsber of units ordered when preparing the supplies. Arrange to obtain an intravenous (IV) pole and a container of 0.9% NSS in the amount ordered or indicated in agency policy. The nurse never uses any other IV solution when infusing blood products. Dextrose-containing solutions cause cells to agglutinate. Hypotonic solutions cause fluid to enter the cells and rupture, causing hemolysis. Hypertonic solutions draw fluid from the cells, causing them to shrink or crenate.

**Filters.** Depending on the type and size, blood filters (Fig. 15–1) remove particulate matter, products of degradation, and unwanted components of blood such as WBCs from the blood product. The rating for filters depends on pore size or efficiency. Standard blood filters and microaggregate filters are rated on pore size; leukocyte removal filters on efficiency.

Standard blood filters have pore sizes ranging from 170 to 260 μm. (Manufacturers rate filters so that the larger the number on the rating, the larger the pore size.)

In general, a 170-μm filter especially designed for blood administration is acceptable for any blood product. The Intravenous Nurses Society (INS) states that the filter should be "an integral part of the administration set." INS recommends that the filter be "in-line" and not an added on device.

Blood stored for more than 5 days and some salvaged blood are more likely to form tiny clots. Some salvaged blood may have bone fragments suspended in it. Microaggregate blood filters have a pore size of 20 to 40 μm. These

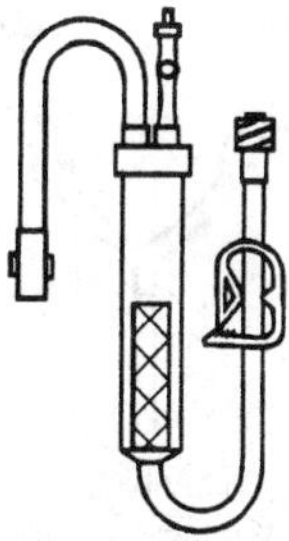

**FIGURE 15–1.** Blood filter. (Courtesy of Alton Dean Medical, Inc., Woods Cross, Utah.)

filters catch clots or bone fragments before they infuse into the client.

Leukocyte-poor filters remove WBCs from the infusion. This is important for clients who have a history of febrile nonhemolytic reactions to blood transfusions. The packaging for these filters indicates their rating by stating the efficiency with which they remove leukocytes. The nurse may see filters with ratings to 99%. This indicates that these filters remove 99% of all leukocytes in the transfusion.

**Blood Tubing.** Blood tubing usually has a drip factor of 10 drops (gtt)/mL. The tubing package indicates the drip factor. Some blood tubings have a Y above the filter. The tubing bifurcates above the filter making a Y (Fig. 15–2). At this point the tubing becomes two separate tubings, each with its own bag spike. Other blood tubings are straight line. When using a straight line tubing, a stopcock with Luer lock connections provides a secure closed system to connect the blood tubing and the 0.9% NSS flush tubing. Use gloves to avoid exposing yourself to any blood spills.

**Blood Warmers.** Some clinical situations require that the nurse consider the use of a blood warmer (Fig. 15–3). When the client requires large volumes of blood administered rapidly or when neonates and children receive blood for exchange transfusions or through a central line, it may be necessary to warm the blood to normal body temperature to avoid cardiac arrhythmias. Some clients have cold agglutinins, which are antibodies that react at temperatures below 20° C and cause agglutination of blood.

For a blood warmer to be effective it should maintain the transfusion temperature between 32° and 37° C and provide flow rates to 150 mL/min. Blood warmers may use a warm bath or a dry incubator. Some safety features include thermostats and alarms for temperature monitoring. The nurse

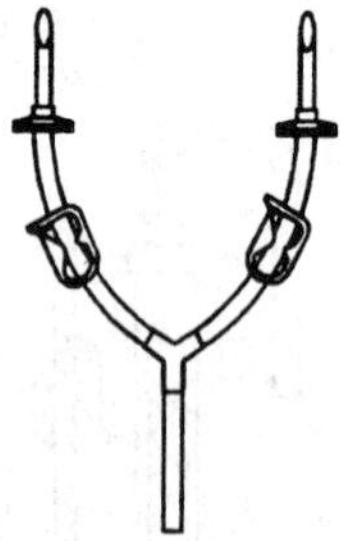

**FIGURE 15–2.** Blood tubing with Y bifurcation. Each of the separate tubing ends has its own bag spike. (Courtesy of Alton Dean Medical, Inc., Woods Cross, Utah.)

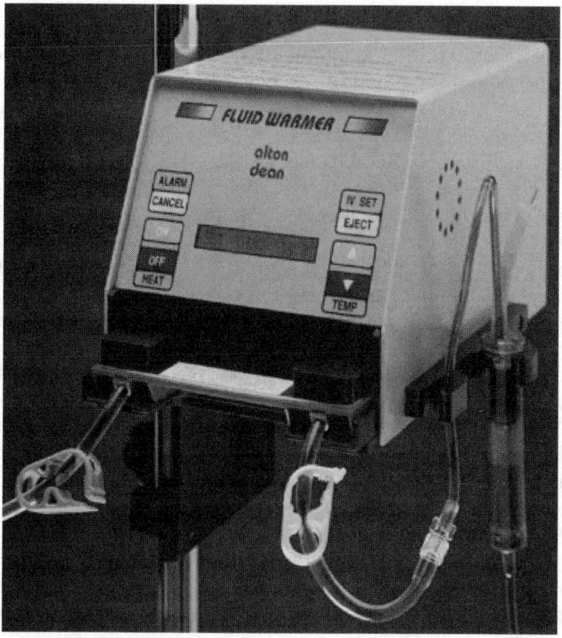


**FIGURE 15–3.** Blood warmer. This model includes an LCD screen that indicates operating instructions during the warming process. (Courtesy of Alton Dean Medical, Inc., Woods Cross, Utah.)

follows the manufacturer's instructions for use of the blood warmer and any special supplies such as tubing.

**Pressure Cuff.** A pressure cuff is one method the nurse may use to provide a rapid transfusion. The pressure cuff has a sleeve; a manometer, calibrated in mm Hg; and a pressure bulb, similar to a blood pressure cuff. The nurse places the sleeve around the blood bag and inflates the cuff by squeezing and releasing the bulb as though it were a blood pressure cuff. As the bag empties, the manometer decreases and the nurse must reinflate the cuff by pumping the bulb. Careful observation of the site is necessary to avoid infiltration.

**Positive Pressure Set.** A positive pressure set is another method of rapidly infusing blood. This set appears similar to straight line blood tubing. However, between the filter and the client is a bulb that collects blood. The nurse squeezes the bulb, which forces the blood into the client at a rate faster than gravity. The nurse allows the bulb to refill before squeezing the bulb again. The nurse must observe the site carefully for any signs of infiltration, which may develop rapidly.

## Transfusion

The administration of the transfusion requires that the nurse obtain the blood product, assess the client, and initiate the transfusion.

### OBTAINING THE BLOOD PRODUCT

The nurse follows agency policy when obtaining the blood product. Many agencies require that a nurse or physician pick up the blood product from the blood bank. Together, the nurse or physician and the blood bank technician check the unit against the requisition slip before the product leaves the blood bank. The client's name, identification number, and ABO and Rh types should match unless otherwise indicated by type of product (Table 15–4). The blood bank identification number on the unit must match the requisition slip. The nurse assures that the unit is within the expiration date and inspects the unit, making certain that the container has not been violated in any way and that there are no leaks. Some agencies require that the nurse sign for receipt of the product at the blood bank.

The nurse must initiate the transfusion within 30 minutes of removing the unit from the blood bank. If this is not possible, the nurse returns the unit to the blood bank. Under no

**TABLE 15–4**
**Labeling of Blood and Components**

Labels on blood products contain a wealth of information for the nurse. Some of the information (such as the volume of the unit) assists the nurse with record keeping, whereas other information alerts the nurse to monitor for potential problems with the transfusion. The nurse can find the following information on the blood and blood component bag:

- The proper name, whole blood or component, including an indication of any qualification or modification
- The method by which the component was prepared (e.g., from whole blood or by hemapheresis)
- The temperature range in which the component is to be stored
- The preservatives and the anticoagulant used in the preparation of the blood or components when appropriate
- The contents or volume
- The number of units in pooled components and any sedimenting agent used during cytopheresis
- The name, address, and registration number of the collection and processing location
- The expiration date and time if applicable: This varies with the method of preparation (open or closed system) and the preservatives and anticoagulant used. When the expiration time is not indicated, the product expires at midnight.
- The donation identification number
- The donor category (paid or volunteer, and autologous if applicable)
- Blood group and special handling information as required
- Statements regarding recipient identification

circumstances are blood products stored in the nursing unit or any other refrigerator.

## ASSESSING THE CLIENT

The nurse takes the client's vital signs. The nurse carefully inspects the client's skin, observing for moisture, rashes, and flushing. A good baseline assists the nurse in observing any changes the client may exhibit during the infusion. When observing clients receiving blood products, the nurse remembers that the earlier the signs and symptoms of a blood transfusion reaction are recognized and response made, the more successful the treatment of the reaction will be (see "Transfusion Reactions").

## CHECKING THE PRODUCT

To initiate the transfusion the nurse asks another nurse or a physician to check the unit against the client's identification band. There is usually a place on the product requisition slip for both parties to sign. Again ask the client to state his or her name if possible. If there is any discrepancy, no matter how slight, during this process, DO NOT administer the blood product. Notify the blood bank immediately.

## PREPARING THE SUPPLIES

**Priming Y Tubing.** If using a tubing with a Y site, close all three roller clamps before spiking the 0.9% NSS. Open the roller clamp on the arm to the 0.9% NSS and gently squeeze the drip chamber. The filter is at the bottom of the drip chamber. Squeeze the drip chamber until the filter is completely covered by fluid. This prevents blood from falling onto a dry filter and damaging the cells. Open the main roller clamp, the one below the filter, and allow the fluid to fill the rest of the tubing distal to the drip chamber. Carefully spike the blood product bag with the other bag spike. Keep this arm's roller clamp closed.

**Priming Straight Line Tubing.** If using straight line tubing, prime the blood set with 0.9% NSS as though it were any infusion set, making sure that the filter is covered with fluid. Close the roller clamp on this tubing. Carefully remove the 0.9% NSS container from the spike and spike the blood bag with it. Take the other infusion set and spike the 0.9% NSS container. Prime this tubing. Attach the end of each tubing to the stopcock. Attach the stopcock to the client's venous access device. Depending on agency policy, the nurse may wish to use an extension set between the stopcock and the client's venous access device.

## BEGINNING THE TRANSFUSION

Begin the infusion slowly with the 0.9% NSS. As a general rule drugs and blood products should not be the first solutions infused through a newly inserted catheter. Always test patency with an isotonic solution such as 0.9% NSS. If another solution was infusing through the catheter, infuse a small amount of the NSS to flush the line.

After infusing the amount of 0.9% NSS ordered by the physician or indicated in agency policy, stop the infusion by closing the roller clamp on that arm of the Y or by turning the stopcock so the "off" position is toward the 0.9% NSS infusion if using straight line tubing. Begin the blood product administration by opening the roller clamp on the arm of the Y tubing, which is spiked into the blood product. Regulate the infusion to about 20 gtt/min with the main roller clamp below the filter. If using a stopcock, position it so it is open between the blood tubing and the client's catheter and regulate the infusion to run at about 20 gtt/min during the first 15 minutes. Stay with the client and carefully observe for any changes in status that may indicate a transfusion reaction.

At the end of 15 minutes, take the client's vital signs. If there is no change in the client's condition, adjust the infusion to the rate prescribed by the physician. In general, transfusions are run as rapidly as tolerated by the client, but in all cases they should be completed within 4 hours of initiation (Table 15–5).

**NOTE:** If the client will not tolerate the volume of the infusion within 4 hours, request that the blood bank split the unit. In doing this, the blood bank retains half the unit at a controlled temperature while the nurse infuses the other half. When the first infusion is complete, the nurse obtains the second half of the unit from the blood bank and infuses it.

## MONITORING THE CLIENT

Consult the agency policy on monitoring during a transfusion. Most agencies require that the nurse monitor vital signs every 15 minutes for at least the first hour and then

**TABLE 15–5**
**Troubleshooting Tips**

If the infusion stops or runs sluggishly, nursing actions include the following:

- Check the administration set for kinks.
- Verify that the bottom of the bag is 3 ft (1 m) above the IV site.
- Make sure that the filter is completely covered with blood.
- Recall the gauge of the catheter used for the IV site. In adults it should be at least 20 gauge.
- Determine that the IV site is taped in a manner that does not cut off the flow.
- Gently agitate the blood container to redistribute the cells.
- Close the blood line and flush the catheter with the 0.9% NSS flush fluid.

IV = intravenous, NSS = normal saline solution.

every 30 minutes until the end of the transfusion. The nurse considers the client's transfusion history and maintains vigilant surveillance of those clients with positive histories. If there is any significant change in the client's vital signs or condition, stop the transfusion immediately and reestablish the infusion with the NSS. If using a Y set, *do not* establish the NSS drip by opening the clamp on the arm attached to the NSS bag. To do so delivers more of the causative agent of the reaction to the client. Instead, hang a new bag of NSS with new tubing (see "Transfusion Reactions").

When the blood product has finished, infuse another 10 to 15 mL of the 0.9% NSS or whatever amount the physician has ordered.

## Post Transfusion

### DISCONTINUING THE TRANSFUSION

If the client is to receive an infusion of another IV fluid or medication or if the client's venous access device is to be converted to a heparin lock, the nurse has the supplies ready at this time. After donning a pair of gloves, the nurse closes the roller clamp on the 0.9% NSS infusion and takes down the used blood bag, NSS container, and tubing. Dispose of these per agency policy keeping in mind that they are hazardous waste. The nurse completes the care of the client and the venous access device. Continue to monitor the client closely.

### DOCUMENTATION

After completing the infusion the nurse completes the documentation on the product requisition slip as required by agency policy.

In the client's record the nurse documents the following:

- Date and time of the transfusion
- The amount and type of blood product, as well as the blood bank unit number
- The amount of 0.9% NSS infused
- Status of the venous access device
- The client's tolerance of the procedure
- The name and title of the person performing the procedure

## TRANSFUSION REACTIONS

Transfusions can result in fatal reactions, but this is rare. By law, when complications from the transfusion of blood or blood components result in death, the blood bank notifies the FDA by phone within 24 hours and files a written report of the investigation of the reaction with the FDA within 7 days. The nurse assists the collection of data by thorough documentation of all actions and treatment.

## Hemolytic Transfusion Reactions

**Definition.** Hemolytic transfusion reactions are usually antigen-antibody reactions of varying seriousness. The client's blood cell antibodies react with the donor's plasma antigens, causing hemolysis, a lysing of blood cells. Some hemolytic transfusion reactions are not immunologically mediated and tend to have less severe consequences for the client. Hemolytic transfusion reactions may be intravascular or extravascular (see "Immunohematology").

### ACUTE HEMOLYTIC REACTION

**Cause.** Acute hemolytic reactions are secondary to an incompatibility between the recipient's plasma and the donor's RBCs. Practically all these reactions involve the ABO antigen-antibody system, and because of this the hemolysis is intravascular. Most acute hemolytic reactions are the direct result of either clerical errors or misidentification. These avoidable errors lead to an ABO mismatch and in turn can lead to client death.

**Signs and Symptoms.** Acute hemolytic reactions usually occur early in the transfusion. The client may complain of headache, chest pain, chills, facial flushing, pain or burning along the vein in which the blood is transfusing, and back pain. The nurse may discover the client is in shock and has fever and dyspnea. Surgical clients may have abnormal bleeding during the procedure or from the surgical site postoperatively. A late sign is hemoglobinemia (free hemoglobin in the circulation). Very severe reactions may lead to renal failure. *This reaction may be fatal.*

**Treatment.** The earlier the nurse discovers the symptoms and begins treatment, the better the chances are for success. The nurse immediately stops the infusion and maintains a KVO (keep vein open) infusion of 0.9% NSS. If the blood is running through Y tubing, *do not* infuse the 0.9% NSS through this tubing, as this practice administers more blood to the client. Hang a new bottle of 0.9% NSS with new tubing. Carefully monitor the client's vital signs and notify the physician and the blood bank.

The client's shock will be treated aggressively with fluids and possibly dopamine (Intropin). At low doses this sympathomimetic agent dilates the renal arteries and increases cardiac output. The nurse remembers that clients receiving drugs in this classification require careful monitoring of cardiac and renal functions. One of the goals of therapy is to infuse sufficient fluid to encourage diuresis while avoiding cardiopulmonary complications. For this reason the physician may order furosemide (Lasix). In the presence of renal failure, the client may receive intermittent peritoneal dialysis or hemodialysis.

Some blood banks require that the nurse save the blood bag and return it for evaluation. Refer to agency policy regarding this.

**Documentation.** The nurse carefully documents the incident in the client's record, including the type of product, the blood bank identification number on the unit, and the treatment, including any drugs. Most agencies require the nurse or physician, or both, complete a Transfusion Reaction Form. This form usually accompanies the blood bag and a freshly drawn blood specimen and urine specimen to the laboratory.

**Prevention.** Prevention of an acute hemolytic reaction includes care on the part of all health care personnel to avoid clerical and misidentification errors.

## DELAYED HEMOLYTIC REACTION

**Cause.** The cause of delayed hemolytic reaction is usually antibodies that are undetectable at the time of transfusion. Clients having this reaction have usually been sensitized to the antigen through a previous transfusion.

**Signs and Symptoms.** Clients with delayed hemolytic reaction may display a continued fall in hemoglobin 4 to 14 days after transfusion or continued anemia even after transfusion therapy. The client may have fever, hemoglobinuria, or hyperbilirubinemia (higher than normal levels of bilirubin in the blood with no other pathology).

**Treatment.** The nurse monitors the client for any signs and symptoms of cardiopulmonary compromise due to the anemia. Antipyretics are given for the fever. The course of this reaction is usually benign. Only in very rare cases is the outcome serious or fatal.

**Documentation.** The nurse documents the client's signs and symptoms with particular attention to cardiopulmonary status.

**Prevention.** These reactions are rarely preventable. A complete and accurate transfusion history may assist the blood bank in identifying clients at risk for this problem.

## ACUTE NONIMMUNOLOGICALLY MEDIATED HEMOLYSIS

**Cause.** Acute nonimmunologically mediated hemolysis reactions are not common and may be caused by administration of a hypotonic fluid with the transfusion product, bacterial infection of the client or contamination of the donor's blood, acute hemolytic anemia from any cause, or improper handling of the blood product by the blood bank, including overheating or freezing.

**Signs and Symptoms.** The client may experience chills, hemoglobinuria, and fever. In very rare severe cases, DIC and renal failure may occur.

**Treatment.** For mild reactions the client receives symptomatic treatment. In those rare cases of severe reactions the client's care is the same as that outlined for acute hemolytic transfusion reactions.

**Documentation.** The nurse records the client's signs and symptoms, as well as any treatment given.

**Prevention.** Prevention is dependent on cause. All health care personnel must comply with standards and procedures for safe blood transfusions.

## Nonhemolytic Transfusion Reactions

### FEBRILE REACTIONS

**Cause.** Febrile reactions are usually the result of the client's anti-HLA antibodies reacting with antigens on the donor's WBCs or platelets. These reactions occur in clients who have been previously sensitized by prior transfusions or pregnancy. This may lead to a phenomenon known as noncardiogenic pulmonary edema.

**Signs and Symptoms.** Febrile reactions generally occur toward the end of the transfusion or after it is completed. The client may or may not complain of chills. The client may report palpitations, chest tightness, lower back pain, general malaise, and headache. The nurse notes a temperature, flushed face, and fever that may be as high as 104° F. In severe cases the client may exhibit signs of pulmonary edema, including increased blood pressure, tachycardia, and dyspnea.

**Treatment.** The nurse reports the findings to the physician who will generally prescribe symptomatic treatment such as antipyretics for mild reactions. In the presence of noncardiac pulmonary edema the treatment is more aggressive and includes oxygen and diuretics.

**Documentation.** The nurse carefully documents the signs and symptoms and any treatment prescribed, as well as the client's response to the treatment.

**Prevention.** Febrile reaction occurs in approximately 1% of all transfusions. In general, tests for these antibodies are not useful in deciding which clients will benefit from leukocyte-poor transfusions. The nurse's instructions to the client about the cause of this reaction and the importance of the client informing future health care providers of his or her transfusion history may prevent future reactions of this type. HLA-matched products prevent complications of this nature in groups with a known risk. Leukocyte-poor products or the use of leukocyte-poor filters are also indicated.

## GRAFT-VERSUS-HOST DISEASE

**Cause**. Graft-versus-host disease (GVHD) is a complication of serious consequences and is secondary to active transfused lymphocytes present in blood products. At risk are children and adults with either underdeveloped or compromised immune systems. This is an immunologically mediated event. The client's immune system is unable to recognize the transfused lymphocytes as foreign. Instead, the transfused lymphocytes recognize the host as foreign, take over, and attack the host.

**Signs and Symptoms**. The client presents with fever, skin rash, diarrhea, and possibly jaundice. The symptoms are due to the graft lymphocytes attacking the client's skin, the gastrointestinal tract, and the liver. Unless interrupted, this cascade of events can lead to the client's death.

**Treatment**. Clients receive symptomatic treatment and supportive care based on the body systems exhibiting destruction. Strict aseptic technique and infection control precautions are necessary to protect the client. Immunosuppressing agents are given carefully to inhibit the attack on the host while maintaining the viability of the lymphocytes.

**Documentation**. The nurse records the client's symptoms, any palliative treatment, and the response to that treatment.

**Prevention**. Irradiation of RBCs is useful in preventing GVHD. However, this process may cause destruction of some cells and subsequent leakage of potassium ions into the product. Removal of all plasma from the RBC product may prove beneficial.

## ALLERGIC REACTIONS

**Cause**. Some of these reactions have unknown causes. Other, more severe reactions, occur in clients who have antibodies to IgA. These antibodies react with the donor's IgA. At times, an allergic reaction may occur if the donor is allergic to a particular drug and has developed antibodies to it. When the donor's blood is transfused into a client who is receiving the drug, the client experiences a reaction.

**Signs and Symptoms**. Mild reactions are manifested by urticaria, wheezing, and at times chills and fever. Severe or anaphylactic reactions produce bronchospasm, dyspnea, and pulmonary edema.

**Treatment**. Symptomatic treatment with antihistamines provides comfort to clients with mild reactions. More severe reactions necessitate the immediate administration of adrenaline and corticosteroids.

**Documentation**. The client's record indicates the signs and symptoms and the treatment the client receives, as well as the client's response to that treatment.

**Prevention**. Methods to prevent this reaction are dependent on cause. Donors with allergies should be eliminated from the donor pool. The nurse or other health care provider at the donation center may assist by obtaining this information from perspective donors. Clients whose reactions are secondary to IgA antibodies are instructed to provide this information to all future health care providers. These clients will require frozen or washed RBCs and IgA-deficient plasma for future transfusions.

### CIRCULATORY OVERLOAD

**Cause.** Circulatory overload occurs when the client receives excessive volume. This occurs more frequently in the elderly and clients with chronic severe anemia when there is low blood cell volume and increased plasma volume.

**Signs and Symptoms.** The client may complain of a pounding headache, chest tightness, flushed feeling, back pain, chills, fever, and dyspnea. The client likely has an increased blood pressure and a rapid, bounding pulse.

**Treatment.** On recognition of these symptoms the nurse stops the infusion, raises the client's head, and notifies the physician. The nurse prepares to initiate oxygen therapy and possibly administer diuretics. Careful monitoring of vital signs and intake and output is necessary.

**Documentation.** The nurse records the client's signs and symptoms and any medications administered. A record of vital signs and the client's response to treatment are reflected in the client's record.

**Prevention.** Frequent and careful monitoring of the client's vital signs during the transfusion alert the nurse to the onset of this problem. In the population at risk for circulatory overload, consideration is given to the use of packed RBCs instead of whole blood. The sodium content of a unit of whole blood is 56 mEq, whereas a unit of RBCs contains between 8 and 20 mEq. Some preservatives add sodium to the blood product and this should be considered.

## Metabolic Complications

In general, most metabolic complications occur when the client receives large quantities of blood in a short period of time.

### HYPOTHERMIA

**Cause.** Hypothermia occurs when large quantities of cold blood products are administered to a client or when cold blood is administered through a central line.

**Signs and Symptoms.** The nurse observes that the client has shaking chills, hypotension, and cardiac arrhythmias. If untreated, the client's condition may proceed to cardiac arrest.

**Treatment.** The nurse stops the transfusion, warms the client with blankets, and encourages warm liquids if tolerated. The nurse monitors the client's vital signs. The physician will order an electrocardiogram (ECG) to detect any arrhythmias.

**Documentation.** The nurse documents the client's symptoms and all treatments provided.

**Prevention.** Warming blood with automatic blood warmers to 35° C for massive, rapid transfusions prevents this complication.

## CITRATE TOXICITY OR HYPOCALCEMIA

**Cause.** Although rare, citrate toxicity can occur, particularly in clients with severe liver disease receiving rapid massive transfusions. In these clients the liver is unable to metabolize the large quantities of citrate present in the circulation from the transfusion. Citrate, the anticoagulant found in most blood products, binds to ionized calcium, causing a fall in serum calcium levels.

**Signs and Symptoms.** The client may state that he or she feels tingling in the fingertips or muscular cramping. If left untreated, the client may experience seizures, hypotension, and cardiac arrest.

**Treatment.** Unless the client is experiencing severe symptoms from the hypocalcemia, treatment consists of slowing or discontinuing the transfusion. This situation eventually corrects itself without further intervention. If the client is experiencing severe symptoms, the physician may order a slow infusion of calcium chloride. Consult the agency policy regarding the nurse's role in this infusion. Generally, this is a physician responsibility, since there are serious risks associated with this infusion.

**Documentation.** The nurse maintains a record of the client's symptoms and treatment.

**Prevention.** Careful screening and monitoring of clients at risk is the only prevention of citrate toxicity.

## HYPERKALEMIA

**Cause.** Some cells in stored RBCs break down and leak potassium into the plasma. This is not normally a problem for clients receiving 1 to 2 U of product. However, if large quantities of RBC preparations are given, the client may exhibit signs and symptoms of hyperkalemia.

**Signs and Symptoms.** Clients may complain of intestinal cramping, muscle twitching, decreased urine output, and possible renal failure. Laboratory data show a high serum potassium level and ECGs exhibit high, peaked T waves and wide QRS complexes. Untreated, the client's cardiac status can deteriorate to bradycardia and asystole.

**Treatment.** To decrease potassium levels the physician may order sodium polystyrene sulfonate (Kayexalate). Dependent on client condition, this may be administered orally or per rectum in a retention enema. The nurse monitors the client for any cardiac difficulty.

**Documentation.** The nurse records the client's signs and symptoms. The treatment regimen and the client's response are recorded in the client's record.

**Prevention.** In cases when large quantities of blood are necessary, the nurse notifies the blood bank and requests that fresh blood be available.

## Transmission of Infectious Disease

The following diseases are delayed transfusion complications. For treatment information, refer to a medical-surgical text such as *Medical-Surgical Nursing: A Nursing Process Approach* (Ignatavicius, Workman, and Mishler, 1995).

### VIRAL HEPATITIS

Viral hepatitis was a common complication for clients receiving blood transfusions until recently. Now, the blood bank screens all donated blood with tests specific for hepatitis B and C (previously known as non-A, non-B hepatitis). These tests do not identify units contaminated with these diseases 100% of the time. Recent figures estimate that risk of contracting hepatitis B is 1 in 200,000 for each screened unit and hepatitis C is 1 in 3300 (Dodd, 1992).

### HUMAN RETROVIRUSES

HIV and other retroviruses can be transmitted via blood transfusion. These viruses are the causative agents in AIDS. Donor selection criteria are designed to eliminate those who are potential carriers. Further, each blood sample is tested for antibodies to these diseases. Because the incubation period of these viruses is uncertain, this screening is not perfect and therefore does not totally eliminate the risk of disease transmission.

### CYTOMEGALOVIRUS

Cytomegalovirus (CMV) is present in about 50% of donors as indicated by positive antibody titers. This indicates that they have either a current infection or have previously had one. For the general public this virus is of no concern. However, for clients who are immunocompromised and premature infants weighing less than 1200 g who have antibody-negative mothers, this infection can be serious. These clients require blood from antibody-negative donors. Leukocyte-poor components may also reduce the risk of infection in this population.

## LIFE SPAN CONSIDERATIONS

### Neonates

#### EXCHANGE TRANSFUSIONS

Neonates who suffer from hemolytic disease in the newborn require exchange transfusions. This disease occurs when there is Rh incompatibility between the fetus and the mother. Left untreated, hemolytic disease may lead to kernicterus, a serious neurologic syndrome manifested by high levels of unconjugated bilirubin in the neonate's brain cells. The effects of kernicterus range from mental retardation with deficits in motor ability to seizures, choreoathetosis, and impaired speech, hearing, and vision.

The procedure for the exchange transfusion involves removing 5 to 15 mL of the infant's blood through the umbilical vein and replacing it with blood that has been cross-matched to the mother's blood. The mother's blood is used because her blood contains the same antibodies present in the infant at birth.

This procedure requires advanced training and skill. The nurse is referred to pediatric and neonatal specialty texts for further information on this procedure.

### Infants and Children

Some distinct differences exist between transfusing adults and transfusing children. The following is an outline of the most common.

- The nurse explains the procedure to the parents and the child (dependent on age), outlining the risks and the benefits of the transfusion as it relates to the child. The nurse obtains consent as outlined in agency policy and a complete and accurate transfusion history and notifies the physician and the blood bank for any positive history.
- The nurse uses a 22- to 24-gauge catheter for venous access (see Chapter 6).
- The amount of blood for the transfusion is calculated in milliliters per kilogram (mL/kg) of weight. The average volume for infants and children older than 1 month is 75 mL/kg.
- The blood bank prepares units for this group of clients in half unit packs or Pedipacks. The volume is approximately half the usual unit. The nurse checks the volume listed on the unit.
- For children, the nurse calculates 5% to 10% of the total volume of the transfusion and administers this during the first 15 minutes of the infusion. This assists with early detection of any signs of transfusion

reaction. The nurse remains with the child during this time.

- Most agencies use microaggregate filters for all routine blood and blood product transfusions in this group of clients.
- Blood warmers prevent hypothermia and are recommended for all transfusions in this population but are particularly recommended for transfusions through a central vascular line.
- Electronic infusion devices assist with maintaining the appropriate rate for the transfusion. The nurse checks the device to assure the manufacturer's recommendation regarding the use of its product for blood products. Not all devices are appropriate for the transfusion of blood.

## The Elderly

The elderly client with a history of cardiac disease requires careful monitoring by the nurse. These clients may not tolerate a full unit of blood without developing cardiopulmonary complications. The nurse alerts the blood bank and requests split units. While the first half of the unit infuses, the blood bank maintains the second half. This allows a slower infusion without risking bacterial proliferation in a unit that hangs too long at room temperature.

Decreased immune responses in the elderly may delay the signs of transfusion reaction. A large volume of blood may have infused before the client's condition indicates any danger. Confusion or an increase in the level of confusion may be the first signs of a reaction in this group of clients. The delay of symptoms of immunologically mediated reactions may complicate treatment or make the reaction more severe.

PART

# IV

# INFUSION MEDICATION

CHAPTER 16

# Antiinfectives

*Elaine Kennedy*

**Definition**
**Classifications**
  By Mechanism
  By Activity (Spectrum)
**Selection**
**Laboratory Tests**
**Empirical Treatment**
**Resistance**
  Causes
  Nosocomial Infections
  Suprainfections
  Delaying the Development of Resistance
**Aminoglycosides**
  Amikacin Sulfate
  Gentamicin Sulfate
  Kanamycin Sulfate
  Netilmicin Sulfate
  Tobramycin
**Cephalosporins**
***First-Generation Cephalosporins***
  Cefazolin Sodium
***Second-Generation Cephalosporins***
  Cefonicid
  Cefotetan Disodium
  Cefoxitin
  Cefuroxime Sodium
***Third-Generation Cephalosporins***
  Cefoperazone
  Cefotaxime
  Ceftazidime
  Ceftriaxone Sodium
**Chloramphenicols**
  Chloramphenicol
**Erythromycins**
  Erythromycin Lactobionate
**Penicillins**
  Penicillin G Potassium
***Penicillinase-Resistant Penicillins***
  Methicillin
  Nafcillin
  Oxacillin
***Ampicillins***
  Ampicillin Sodium
  Ampicillin Sodium and Sulbactam Sodium
***Extended-Spectrum Penicillins***
  Mezlocillin Sodium
  Piperacillin
  Ticarcillin Disodium
  Ticarcillin Disodium and Clavulanate Potassium
**Quinolones (Fluoroquinolones)**
  Ciprofloxacin
  Ofloxacin
**Tetracyclines**
  Doxycycline Hyclate
  Minocycline Hydrochloride
  Oxytetracycline Hydrochloride
**Unclassified Antibiotics**
  Aztreonam
  Imipenem and Cilastatin Sodium
**Antifungals**
  Amphotericin B
  Fluconazole
  Miconazole
**Antituberculars**
  Rifampin
**Antivirals**
  Acyclovir
  Foscarnet Sodium
  Ganciclovir
  Vidarabine
  Zidovudine
**Miscellaneous Antiinfectives**
  Clindamycin Phosphate
  Metronidazole
  Pentamidine
  Trimethoprim-Sulfamethoxazole
  Vancomycin

## DEFINITION

Antiinfectives, also known as antimicrobials, are any agents, natural or synthetic, that destroy or suppress the growth or reproduction of microorganisms. The ability of these drugs to kill or suppress the invading microorganisms without injuring the host cells is called selective toxicity.

## CLASSIFICATIONS

### By Mechanism

Antiinfectives can be classified in a number of ways. One classification system is based on the drug's mechanism of action; how it accomplishes its task. There are seven types of mechanisms:

- The first group of drugs inhibits cell wall synthesis or activates enzymes that cause a disruption of the cell wall's integrity. The penicillins and cephalosporins are examples of this group of drugs.They weaken the bacteria's cell wall, causing the cell to lyse and be destroyed. These agents are bactericidal.
- The next group are drugs that increase the permeability of the cell wall. Drugs such as amphotericin B and polymyxins change the permeability of the bacteria's cell wall, causing cellular material to leak. This action has bactericidal effects.
- Some drugs such as the aminoglycosides inhibit the ability of the bacteria to make proteins. This inability to synthesize proteins is lethal (bactericidal) to the bacteria.
- In similar fashion, chloramphenicol and the tetracyclines inhibit the ability of the bacteria to make proteins. In this case the interference is not lethal but slows growth. For this reason these agents are considered bacteriostatic.
- The drugs rifampin and nalidixic acid prevent the synthesis of nucleic acids, and thereby the production of DNA and RNA, by binding with the nucleic acids or by interfering with nucleic acid synthesis. This prevents the cell from replicating or translating genetic material. These drugs are bacteriostatic.
- Antimetabolites such as trimethoprim and the sulfonamides disrupt specific biochemical reactions in the cell, causing either a decrease in the manufacture of essential cellular components or the synthesis of nonfunctional components. This is a bacteriostatic effect.
- The last group is viral DNA inhibitors. They prevent the cell from synthesizing DNA, which precludes the cell's ability to replicate. These drugs are bacteriostatic.

### By Activity (Spectrum)

The second way in which antiinfective drugs are classified is on the basis of the drug's activity. Antimicrobial agents vary in their activity. Narrow-spectrum drugs are active against only a few organisms, while broad-spectrum agents are active against a wide variety of organisms.

## SELECTION

When treating infections the therapeutic objective is to achieve maximal antimicrobial effect while causing minimal harm to the client. Meeting this objective requires the selection of the drug(s) that is(are) most appropriate for the individual client. Three factors guide the physician in this choice: (1) the identity of the infecting organism, (2) the sensitivity of the infecting organism, and (3) client factors such as the site of infection and the status of the client's defenses.

In the treatment of an infection, several drugs may provide effective treatment, but for most infections one drug is usually superior to the others. This first choice may be preferred for several reasons such as greater efficacy (ability to achieve the desired result), lower toxicity, or more narrow spectrum. When possible, the physician prescribes the first-choice drug. There are, however, situations that preclude the use of the first-choice drug: (1) The client may be allergic to this drug; (2) the drug may not be able to penetrate the site of infection; or (3) the client may be particularly susceptible to a toxicity of the agent.

## LABORATORY TESTS

To identify the infecting organism and determine its sensitivity to a particular drug requires laboratory evaluation, known as a culture and sensitivity. Completion of this test requires at least 72 hours. Microscopic identification of a gram-stained preparation is a quick and simple technique for identification of infecting microorganisms. Pus, sputum, urine, blood, and other body fluids are appropriate specimens for cultures, sensitivities, and Gram's stains.

It is important for the nurse to remember that any specimens for laboratory analyses must be obtained before beginning the therapy. Initiating therapy before obtaining specimens can impede the identification of the organism(s) causing the infection by suppressing microbial growth. In addition, collection of specimens for culture must be completed in a manner to minimize contamination with normal body flora. To facilitate identification of the organism(s) the nurse avoids exposing the specimen to low temperatures, antiseptics, or oxygen.

## EMPIRICAL TREATMENT

Frequently, the client's condition does not permit the physician to delay treatment until definitive laboratory data are available. For this reason the physician selects a drug empirically (based on the evaluation of the client's clinical condition and the physician's knowledge of which organisms are most likely to cause infection at a particular site in a given client). It is in these cases that broad-spectrum antimicrobials are employed. When laboratory information is available, the physician may prescribe a drug that is more selective for the organism and its sensitivity.

Table 16–1 is a simplified table of classifications of antibacterial agents and susceptible organisms. Some of these drugs such as the polymyxins cannot be given parenterally but are included here to illustrate the bactericidal (ability to kill) and bacteriostatic (ability to slow microbial growth) actions of antimicrobials. Bacteriostatic drugs require assistance of the host's immune defenses (the immune system and the phagocytic cells) to ultimately complete the task of eliminating infection.

**TABLE 16–1**
**Narrow Spectrum and Broad-Spectrum Antibacterial Agents and Susceptible Organisms**

| Susceptible Organisms | Antibacterial Agents |
|---|---|
| | **Narrow-Spectrum Agents** |
| Gram-positive cocci | Penicillin G |
| Gram-positive bacilli | Penicillinase-resistant penicillin |
| | Erythromycin |
| | Clindamycin |
| | Vancomycin |
| | Bacitracin |
| Primarily gram-negative aerobes | Aminoglycosides |
| | Cephalosporins (first and second generation) |
| Mycobacteria | Isoniazid |
| | Rifampin |
| | Ethambutol |
| | Pyrazinamide |
| | Dapsone |
| | **Broad-Spectrum Agents** |
| Gram-positive cocci and gram-negative bacilli | Broad-spectrum penicillins |
| | Cephalosporins (third generation) |
| | Tetracyclines |
| | Chloramphenicol |
| | Trimethoprim |
| | Sulfonamides |
| | Imipenem |
| | Ciprofloxacin |

## RESISTANCE

At times, an organism that was once very sensitive to a particular drug may become less susceptible or lose sensitivity to the drug. This phenomenon, known as "acquired resistance," is of concern to clinicians because it can mean that drugs currently available are of no value in treating infections and requires that new antimicrobials be developed. Acquired resistance refers to the organism's becoming resistant to the drug because of alterations in the organism's function or structure. It does not mean that the client has become resistant.

### CAUSES

**Conditions.** Antimicrobial use promotes drug resistance in a microorganism, but antimicrobials are not the cause of an organism's change in function or structure. Antimicrobial use only makes conditions favorable for overgrowth of organisms that possess drug resistance.

**Drug Spectrum.** Although all drugs have the potential to promote resistance, some are more likely than others to cause resistance. By virtue of their action, broad-spectrum drugs kill off more competing organisms than narrow-spectrum drugs. Therefore, drugs with a broad antimicrobial spectrum are more likely to potentiate resistance.

**Drug Use.** The amount of antimicrobial use influences the emergence of resistance in microorganisms. The more often the client receives antimicrobials, the faster resistant pathogens develop. Further, these drugs promote overgrowth of normal flora that have mechanisms for resistance. These mechanisms for resistance can be transferred to pathogens. Therefore, indiscriminate use of antibiotics in clients who do not really need them can be more harmful than helpful.

### NOSOCOMIAL INFECTIONS

Hospitals are the sites of intense antimicrobial use. For this reason organisms found in these institutions can be extremely resistant. This makes nosocomial infections (health care agency–acquired infections) among the most difficult to treat.

### SUPRAINFECTIONS

Suprainfections (superinfections) are another example of problems associated with drug resistance. A suprainfection is a new infection that develops during the treatment of the primary infection. Proliferation of these new infections is due to the elimination of the body's normal flora that usually inhibits their development. Again, because broad-spectrum agents destroy more normal flora than narrow-spectrum agents, they are more likely to be associated with the development of suprainfections.

### DELAYING THE DEVELOPMENT OF RESISTANCE

There are three ways in which the medical community can delay the development of microbial resistance to drugs. First, antimicrobials should be used only when actually necessary; second, narrow-spectrum drugs should be employed whenever possible; third, newer antimicrobials should be prescribed only in cases when older drugs are no longer effective.

The major classes and subclasses of antiinfectives administered parenterally are listed in Table 16–2.

## AMINOGLYCOSIDES

### THERAPEUTIC EFFECTS

Aminoglycosides are usually bactericidal. The exact mechanism of action is not known but appears to inhibit protein synthesis in certain bacteria. Aminoglycosides are effective against many aerobic gram-negative bacteria such as *Escherichia coli* and *Klebsiella* and some aerobic gram-positive bacteria such as *Staphylococcus aureus* and *Staphylococcus epidermidis*.

### PHARMACOKINETICS

**Distribution.** Aminoglycosides are easily distributed throughout the body but poorly diffused into the cerebral spinal fluid (CSF). Therefore, to obtain therapeutic effects in the central nervous system (CNS), intrathecal administration is required.

**Excretion.** The half-life is usually 2 to 4 hours in adults with normal renal function. Aminoglycosides are not metabolized and are excreted unchanged in the urine. Because a small amount of each dose accumulates in body tissues, complete recovery takes 10 to 20 days in adults with normal renal function.

### CAUTIONS

**Side/Adverse Effects.** Clients with renal impairment or preexisting eighth cranial nerve damage are most likely to experience side/toxic effects. Further, clients receiving aminoglycosides or other renal or ototoxic drugs for long periods of time or in high doses are also likely to experience side/toxic effects.

#### Contraindications

***Pregnancy and Lactation.*** Aminoglycosides cross the placental barrier and can cause fetal harm. Small amounts

**TABLE 16–2**
**Antiinfective Parenteral Drugs**

***Aminoglycosides***
- Amikacin sulfate
- Gentamicin sulfate
- Kanamycin sulfate
- Netilmicin sulfate
- Tobramycin

***Cephalosporins***
- First Generation
  - Cefazolin sodium
  - Cephalothin sodium*
  - Cepharine*
  - Cephapirin sodium*
- Second Generation
  - Cefamandole*
  - Cefmetazole sodium*
  - Cefonicid sodium
  - Ceforanide for injection*
  - Cefotetan disodium
  - Cefoxitin
  - Cefuroxime sodium
- Third Generation
  - Cefoperazone
  - Cefotaxime
  - Ceftazidime
  - Ceftriaxone sodium
  - Ceftizoxime sodium*
  - Moxalactam disodium for injection*

***Chloramphenicols***
- Chloramphenicol

***Erythromycins***
- Erythromycin lactobionate for injection
- Erythromycin gluceptate*

***Penicillins***
- Penicillin G potassium
- Penicillin G sodium*
- Penicillinase-resistant
  - Methicillin
  - Nafcillin
  - Oxacillin
- Ampicillins
  - Ampicillin*
  - Ampicillin sodium
  - Ampicillin sodium and sulbactam sodium
- Extended Spectrum
  - Mezlocillin sodium
  - Piperacillin
  - Ticarcillin disodium
  - Ticarcillin disodium and clavulanate potassium

***Quinolones***
- Ciprofloxacin
- Ofloxacin

***Tetracyclines***
- Doxycycline hydate
- Minocycline hydrochloride
- Oxytetracycline hydrochloride

***Unclassified Antibiotics***
- Aztreonam
- Imipenem and cilastatin sodium

**Antifungals**
- Amphotericin B
- Fluconazole
- Miconazole

**Antituberculars**
- Rifampin

**Antivirals**
- Acyclovir
- Foscarnet sodium
- Didanosine*
- Ganciclovir
- Vidarabine
- Zalcitabine*
- Zidovudine

**Miscellaneous Antiinfectives**
- Clindamycin phosphate
- Colistimethate sodium*
- Lincomycin*
- Polymixin B*
- Metronidazole
- Pentamidine
- Trimethoprim-sulfamethoxazole
- Vancomycin

*Not discussed in this chapter.

can be distributed into breast milk. For this reason the client must decide whether to continue with breast-feeding or the drug.

*Pediatrics.* Aminoglycosides should be used with caution and in reduced dosage in premature and full-term neonates younger than 6 weeks due to renal immaturity.

*Geriatrics.* The most serious side/toxic effects are likely to occur in the elderly, particularly those who are dehydrated.

## TOXICITY

See Table 16–3 for aminoglycoside toxicities.

## POTENTIAL DRUG/FOOD INTERACTIONS

Concurrent use of aminoglycosides with general anesthetics or neuromuscular blocking agents may potentiate neuromuscular blockade and cause respiratory paralysis.

# AMIKACIN SULFATE

*Trade Name:* Amikin
*Canadian Availability:* Not specified
*Pregnancy Risk:* Category D
*pH:* 3.5–5.5
*Storage/Stability:* Store solution between 15° and 30° C. Stable in solution at room temperature for 24 hours. Commercially available solutions may become a very pale yellow, but this does not indicate loss of potency.

### ASSESSMENT: DRUG CHARACTERISTICS

#### ACTION

Usually bactericidal. Exact mechanism of action not known, but appears to inhibit protein synthesis in certain bacteria.

#### INDICATIONS

Used for infections of the gastrointestinal, genitourinary, and respiratory tracts. Also used for septicemia and infections of the bones and joints, skin, and soft tissues.

#### CAUTIONS

ADVERSE EFFECTS. Hearing loss (temporary or permanent), tinnitus, dizziness, nystagmus, vertigo, and ataxia; neuromuscular manifestations such as peripheral neuropathy, seizures, headache, blurred vision, rash, urticaria, respiratory depression, stomatitis, pruritus, fever, and eosinophilia; nausea, vomiting, bone marrow depression, decreased liver function. Cross allergenicity among aminoglycosides may occur.

CONTRAINDICATIONS. Myasthenia gravis, Parkinson's disease, eighth cranial nerve damage, renal impairment, or known sensitivity to amikacin or other aminoglycosides.

#### POTENTIAL DRUG/FOOD INTERACTIONS

Do not mix with any other drug. Use with another aminoglycoside or capreomycin may increase the incidence of ototoxicity. Use with methoxyflurane polymyxins, nephrotoxic drugs, or ototoxic drugs may increase the incidence of nephrotoxicity and ototoxicity. Use with neuromuscular blocking agents may result in respiratory depression or apnea. Incompatible with or inactivated by heparin, dopamine, cephalosporins, amphotericin B, phenytoin, penicillins, and calcium gluconate.

▼

**TABLE 16–3**
**Aminoglycoside Toxicities**

| Body System | Side/Toxic Effects | Physical Assessment Indicators | Laboratory Indicators | Nursing Interventions |
|---|---|---|---|---|
| Neurologic | Neuromuscular blockade | Numbness, tingling, seizures, muscle twitching, headache | N/A | Observe the client for seizures; assist with ADLs and mobility; protect from falls. |
| Respiratory | Respiratory depression | Decreased respiratory rate and diminished breath sounds | N/A | Auscultate breath sounds. |
| Renal | Nephrotoxicity | Oliguria (rare) | Elevated BUN and serum creatinine; serum drug concentration > 12 mcg/mL; decreased urine specific gravity and creatinine clearance, proteinuria | Monitor BUN and serum creatinine, urine specific gravity and creatinine clearance; measure and record intake and output; encourage fluid intake to at least 2000 mL/d unless contraindicated. |
| Gastrointestinal | Gastrointestinal disturbance | Nausea, vomiting (rare) | Transient increases in serum AST, ALT, LDH, alkaline phosphatase, and bilirubin | Monitor laboratory values and report abnormal findings. |
| Hematologic | Blood dyscrasias | Fatigue, shortness of breath, bruising, diminished wound-healing capacity | Decreased RBC, Hgb, Hct, WBC, platelets | Observe for bruising; monitor laboratory values and report abnormal findings. |
| Dermatologic | Hypersensitivity | Rash, urticaria, pruritus | N/A | Be prepared to administer epinephrine or corticosteroids for allergic response. |
| Sensory | Ototoxicity | Tinnitus, roaring in the ears, loss of high-frequency sounds, dizziness, ataxia | N/A | Assess baseline auditory acuity before first dose and monitor during course of therapy; question client about presence of tinnitus, fullness in ears, vertigo, blurred vision. |
| Other | Systemic effects | Pain, sterile abscess, thrombophlebitis, nerve root pain, burning at the injection site | N/A | Question client for pain; observe for evidence of thrombophlebitis. |

ADLs = activities of daily living, ALT = alanine aminotransferase, AST = aspartate aminotransferase, BUN = blood urea nitrogen, Hct = hematocrit, Hgb = hemoglobin, LDH = lactate dehydrogenase, N/A = not applicable, RBC = red blood cell count, WBC = white blood cell count.

**INTERVENTIONS: ADMINISTRATION**

For intravenous (IV) use, 500 mg diluted in 100–200 mL 5% dextrose in water (D5W) or 0.9% normal saline solution (NSS).

**MODE/RATE OF ADMINISTRATION**

IV push not recommended. May be given by intermittent IV infusion over at least 30 min.

INTRAVENOUS USE (WITH NORMAL RENAL FUNCTION)

**Adults:** A loading dose of 5–7.5 mg/kg lean body weight (LBW) followed by up to 15 mg/kg LBW in divided doses daily administered q8–12h (depends on severity of infection). Maximum daily dose should not exceed 1.5 g in 24 h.

**Children > 1 year:** Same as adult dosage.

**Infants/Neonates:** Safe use has not been established, and amikacin should only be given if the organism is resistant to other aminoglycosides. When given, administer a loading dose of 10 mg/kg followed by 7.5 mg/kg q12h.

**Geriatrics:** Clients are more likely to have age-related diminished renal function that may require a lesser dose.

INTRATHECAL USE OR OTHER INFUSION ROUTES AS INDICATED. Intrathecal administration should be carefully monitored. Intrathecal administration has caused nerve root pain, burning, paraplegia, radiculitis, transverse myelitis, and changes in renal and eighth cranial nerve function.

**POTENTIAL PROBLEMS IN ADMINISTRATION**

Thrombophlebitis with IV administration; space administration of amikacin and IV penicillins at least 1 h apart in medication regimen; do not mix with other drugs. If signs of side/toxic effects (renal and otic) occur, stop the infusion and report them immediately to the physician. If overdose occurs, client may need hemodialysis. Complexation (inactivation) with ticarcillin or carbenicillin may be as effective as hemodialysis. Exchange transfusions may be done in the newborn.

**INDEPENDENT NURSING ACTIONS**

Encourage fluids/maintain hydration (unless client has renal disease). Monitor laboratory reports and report abnormal findings.

**ADMINISTRATION IN ALTERNATE SETTINGS**

Administer amikacin to infants and neonates only in settings where they can be carefully monitored for negative outcomes.

**EVALUATION: OUTCOMES OF DRUG THERAPY**

**EXPECTED OUTCOMES**

PHYSICAL ASSESSMENT. Temperature usually returns to baseline within 3 days. Decrease in erythema or purulent discharge or other evidence of infection. Client reports decreased pain.

LABORATORY. Client maintains therapeutic level between

8 and 15 mcg/mL. During therapy serum peak concentration levels remain below 35 mcg/mL and trough levels below 10 mcg/mL. As therapy continues, cultures report a decreasing colony count. Aspartate aminotransferase (AST) remains between 7 and 27 U/L. Alanine aminotransferase (ALT) remains between 1 and 21 U/L. Blood urea nitrogen (BUN) remains between 8 and 25 mg/dL. Serum creatine remains between 0.6 and 1.5 mg/dL. Specific gravity remains between 1.003 and 1.035. No proteinuria.

#### NEGATIVE OUTCOMES

Temperature more than 37.5° C. Pulse more than 100 beats per minute (bpm) and irregular. Client complains of headache, abdominal pain, muscle aches, malaise, lethargy, or ringing or roaring noise in ears. Hot, flushed skin. Rashes. Diaphoresis. Client may have neck rigidity or discharge or drainage from wounds. Nausea, vomiting, diarrhea, or joint pain.

## GENTAMICIN SULFATE

*Trade Names:* Garamycin, G-Myticin, Jenamicin
*Canadian Availability:* Cidomycin, Garamycin
*Pregnancy Risk:* Category C
*pH:* 3–5.5
*Storage/Stability:* Store solution between 15° and 30° C. Stable in solution at room temperature for 24 hours.

### ASSESSMENT: DRUG CHARACTERISTICS

#### ACTION

Usually bactericidal. Exact mechanism of action not known, but appears to inhibit protein synthesis in certain bacteria.

#### INDICATIONS

Used for infections of the gastrointestinal, genitourinary, and respiratory tracts. Also used for septicemia and infections of the bones and joints, CNS (intrathecal or intraventricular administration), skin, and soft tissue.

#### CAUTIONS

ADVERSE EFFECTS. Hearing loss (temporary or permanent), tinnitus, dizziness, nystagmus, vertigo, and ataxia; neuromuscular manifestations such as peripheral neuropathy, seizures, headache, blurred vision, rash, urticaria, stomatitis, pruritus, fever, and eosinophilia; nausea, vomiting, bone marrow depression, decreased liver function. Cross allergenicity among aminoglycosides may occur.

CONTRAINDICATIONS. Myasthenia gravis, Parkinson's disease, eighth cranial nerve damage, renal impairment, or known sensitivity to gentamicin or other aminoglycosides.

#### POTENTIAL DRUG/FOOD INTERACTIONS

Do not mix with any other drug. Use with another aminoglycoside or capreo-

▼

mycin may increase the incidence of ototoxicity. Use with methoxyflurane polymyxins, nephrotoxic drugs, or ototoxic drugs may increase the incidence of nephrotoxicity and ototoxicity. Use with neuromuscular blocking agents may result in respiratory depression or apnea. Incompatible with or inactivated by heparin, dopamine, cephalosporins, amphotericin B, phenytoin, penicillins, and calcium gluconate.

**INTERVENTIONS: ADMINISTRATION**

For IV use, 1 mg/mL dilution in 50–200 mL D5W or 0.9% NSS. For intrathecal use a quantity of CSF is mixed with the drug just prior to administration. If the CSF is grossly purulent or unobtainable, the drug may be diluted with 0.9% preservative-free NSS for injection.

**MODE/RATE OF ADMINISTRATION**

IV push not recommended. May be given by intermittent IV infusion over at least 30 min. May be given by intrathecal/intraventricular administration over 3–5 min with the bevel of the needle upward; intraventricular administration is preferred over intrathecal administration to ensure adequate drug concentration throughout the CSF. When used with intramuscular or IV administration, intrathecal or intraventricular therapy should be continued for at least 1 d after CSF cultures or Gram's stain becomes negative.

INTRAVENOUS USE (WITH NORMAL RENAL FUNCTION)

**Adults:** A loading dose of 1.5–2 mg/kg LBW followed by 1–1.5 mg/kg LBW q6–8h (depends on severity of infection).

For prevention of bacterial endocarditis from surgery or invasive procedures, 1.5 mg/kg 30–60 min before procedure, then q8h after procedure for up to two doses.

**Children > 1 year:** The usual dosage is 2–2.5 mg/kg of body weight q8h.

**Infants:** The usual dosage is 2–2.5 mg/kg of body weight q8h.

**Neonates < 1 week/Premature Infants:** The usual dosage is 2.5 mg/kg of body weight q12h.

**Geriatrics:** Elderly clients are more likely to have age-related decreases in renal function and are thus at greater risk for ototoxicity and nephrotoxicity.

INTRATHECAL USE OR OTHER INFUSION ROUTES AS INDICATED. May be given by intrathecal or intraventricular administration; the usual dosage for adults is 4–8 mg daily. For intrathecal or intraventricular use. The usual dosage for children >1 year is 1–2 mg/d.

**POTENTIAL PROBLEMS IN ADMINISTRATION**

Thrombophlebitis with IV administration; space administration of gentamicin and IV penicillins at least 1 h apart in medication regimen; do not mix with other drugs. If signs of side/toxic effects (renal and otic) occur, stop the infusion and report them immediately to the physician. If overdose occurs, client may need hemodialysis. Complexation (inactivation) with ticarcillin or carbenicillin may be as effective as hemodialysis. Exchange transfusions may be done in the newborn.

**INDEPENDENT NURSING ACTIONS**

Encourage fluids/maintain hydration (unless client has renal disease). Monitor laboratory reports and report abnormal findings. Check temperature.

**ADMINISTRATION IN ALTERNATE SETTINGS**

Administer gentamicin to infants and neonates only in settings where they can be carefully monitored for negative outcomes.

**EVALUATION: OUTCOMES OF DRUG THERAPY**

**EXPECTED OUTCOMES**

PHYSICAL ASSESSMENT. Temperature usually returns to baseline within 3 days. Pulse between 60 and 100 bpm and regular. Skin warm, pink, and dry. No rashes, no flushing, no drainage. Breath sounds clear. Clear yellow urine. Clear CSF. Decrease in erythema or purulent discharge. Client reports decreased pain.

LABORATORY. Client maintains therapeutic level between 4 and 8 mcg/mL. During therapy serum peak concentration levels remain below 10 mcg/mL and trough levels below 2 mcg/mL. As therapy continues, cultures report a decreasing colony count. AST remains between 7 and 27 U/L. ALT remains between 1 and 21 U/L. BUN remains between 8 and 25 mg/dL. Serum creatinine remains between 0.6 and 1.5 mg/dL. Specific gravity remains between 1.003 and 1.035. No proteinuria.

**NEGATIVE OUTCOMES**

Temperature more than 37.5° C. Pulse more than 100 bpm and irregular. Client complains of headache, abdominal pain, muscle aches, malaise, lethargy, or ringing or roaring noise in ears. Hot, flushed skin. Rashes. Diaphoresis. Client may have neck rigidity or discharge or drainage from wounds.

LABORATORY. Client maintains therapeutic level between 4 and 8 mcg/mL. During therapy serum peak concentration levels remain below 10 mcg/mL and trough levels below 2 mcg/mL. As therapy continues, cultures report a decreasing colony count. AST remains between 7 and 27 U/L. ALT remains between 1 and 21 U/L. BUN remains between 8 and 25 mg/dL. Serum creatinine remains between 0.6 and 1.5 mg/dL. Specific gravity remains between 1.003 and 1.035. No proteinuria.

**NEGATIVE OUTCOMES**

Temperature more than 37.5° C. Pulse more than 100 bpm and irregular. Client complains of headache, abdominal pain, muscle aches, malaise, lethargy, or ringing or roaring noise in ears. Hot, flushed skin. Rashes. Diaphoresis. Client may have neck rigidity or discharge or drainage from wounds.

## Kanamycin Sulfate

*Trade Name:* Kantrex
*Canadian Availability:* Not specified
*Pregnancy Risk:* Category D
*pH:* 4.5
*Storage/Stability:* Store solution between 15° and 30° C. Stable in solution at room temperature for 24 hours.

### ASSESSMENT: DRUG CHARACTERISTICS

#### ACTION

Usually bactericidal. Exact mechanism of action not known, but appears to inhibit protein synthesis in certain bacteria.

#### INDICATIONS

Used for infections of the gastrointestinal, genitourinary, and respiratory tracts. Also used for septicemia and infections of the bones and joints, skin, and soft tissues.

#### CAUTIONS

ADVERSE EFFECTS. Hearing loss (temporary or permanent), tinnitus, dizziness, nystagmus, vertigo, and ataxia; neuromuscular manifestations such as peripheral neuropathy, seizures, headache, blurred vision, rash, urticaria, stomatitis, pruritus, fever, and eosinophilia; nausea, vomiting, bone marrow depression, decreased liver function. Cross allergenicity among aminogycosides may occur.

CONTRAINDICATIONS. Myasthenia gravis, Parkinson's disease, eighth cranial nerve damage, renal impairment, or known sensitivity to gentamicin or other aminoglycosides.

#### POTENTIAL DRUG/FOOD INTERACTIONS

Do not mix with any other drug. Use with another aminoglycoside or capreomycin may increase the incidence of ototoxicity. Use with methoxyflurane polymyxins, nephrotoxic drugs, or ototoxic drugs may increase the incidence of nephrotoxicity and ototoxicity. Use with neuromuscular blocking agents may result in respiratory depression or apnea. Incompatible with or inactivated by heparin, dopamine, cephalosporins, amphotericin B, phenytoin, penicillins, and calcium gluconate.

### INTERVENTIONS: ADMINISTRATION

For IV use, 500 mg diluted in 100–200 mL of D5W or 0.9% NSS.

#### MODE/RATE OF ADMINISTRATION

IV push not recommended. May be given by intermittent IV infusion over at least 30 min.

INTRAVENOUS USE (WITH NORMAL RENAL FUNCTION)

**Adults:** A loading dose of 5–7.5 mg/kg LBW followed by up to 5–7.5 mg/kg LBW in divided doses administered q8–12h (depends on severity of infection). Maximum daily dose should not exceed 1.5 g in 24 h.

**Children > 1 year:** The usual dosage is 5–7.5 mg/kg q8–12h.

**Infants/Neonates:** The usual dosage is 5–7.5 mg/kg q8–12h.

**Neonates < 1 week/Premature Infants < 2 kg:** The usual dosage is 7.5 mg/kg q12h.

**Neonates >1 week/Premature Infants > 2 kg:** The usual dosage is 10 mg/kg q12h.

**Geriatrics:** Elderly clients are more likely to have age-related decreases in renal function and are thus at greater risk for ototoxicity and nephrotoxicity.

INTRATHECAL USE OR OTHER INFUSION ROUTES AS INDICATED. May be given by intraperitoneal administration. The usual dose is 500 mg in 20 mL of sterile water injected into an intraperitoneal access device.

### POTENTIAL PROBLEMS IN ADMINISTRATION

Thrombophlebitis with IV administration; space administration of kanamycin and IV penicillins at least 1 h apart in medication regimen; do not mix with other drugs. If signs of side/toxic effects (renal and otic) occur, stop the infusion and report them immediately to the physician. If overdose occurs, client may need hemodialysis. Complexation (inactivation) with ticarcillin or carbenicillin may be as effective as hemodialysis. Exchange transfusions may be done in the newborn.

### INDEPENDENT NURSING ACTIONS

Encourage fluids/maintain hydration (unless client has renal disease). Monitor laboratory reports and report abnormal findings. Check temperature.

### ADMINISTRATION IN ALTERNATE SETTINGS

No additional considerations.

### EVALUATION: OUTCOMES OF DRUG THERAPY

#### EXPECTED OUTCOMES

PHYSICAL ASSESSMENT. Temperature usually returns to baseline within 3 days. Pulse between 60 and 100 bpm and regular. Skin warm, pink, and dry. No rashes, no flushing, no drainage. Breath sounds clear. Clear yellow urine. Clear CSF. Decrease in erythema or purulent discharge. Client reports decreased pain.

LABORATORY. Client maintains therapeutic level between 8 and 15 mcg/mL. During therapy serum peak concentration levels remain below 30 mcg/mL and trough levels below 10 mcg/mL. As therapy continues, cultures report a decreasing colony count. AST remains between 7 and 27 U/L. ALT remains between 1 and 21 U/L. BUN remains between 8 and 25 mg/100 mL/ Serum creatinine remains between 0.6 and 1.5 mg/dL. Specific gravity remains between 1.003 and 1.035. No proteinuria.

#### NEGATIVE OUTCOMES

Temperature more than 37.5° C. Pulse more than 100 bpm and irregular. Client complains of headache, abdominal pain, muscle aches,

▼

malaise, lethargy, or ringing or roaring noise in ears. Hot, flushed skin. Rashes. Diaphoresis. Client may have neck rigidity or discharge or drainage from wounds.

## Netilmicin Sulfate

*Trade Name:* Netromycin
*Canadian Availability:* Not specified
*Pregnancy Risk:* Category D
*pH:* 3.5–6
*Storage/Stability:* Store solution between 15° and 30° C. Stable in solution at room temperature for 72 hours.

### ASSESSMENT: DRUG CHARACTERISTICS

#### ACTION

Usually bactericidal. Exact mechanism of action not known, but appears to inhibit protein synthesis in certain bacteria. Usual half-life is 2 to 2.5 hours; however, this can be prolonged in infants; postpartum females; clients with liver disease and ascites, spinal cord injury, cystic fibrosis; and the elderly. Excreted through the kidneys.

#### INDICATIONS

Used for infections of the gastrointestinal, genitourinary, and respiratory tracts. Also used for septicemia and infections of the bones and joints, CNS (intrathecal or intraventricular administration), skin, and soft tissue.

#### CAUTIONS

ADVERSE EFFECTS. Hearing loss (temporary or permanent), tinnitus, dizziness, nystagmus, vertigo, and ataxia; neuromuscular manifestations such as peripheral neuropathy, seizures, headache, blurred vision, rash, urticaria, stomatitis, pruritus, fever, and eosinophilia; nausea, vomiting, bone marrow depression, decreased liver function. Cross allergenicity among aminoglycosides may occur.

CONTRAINDICATIONS. Known sensitivity to netilmicin or other aminoglycosides.

#### POTENTIAL DRUG/FOOD INTERACTIONS

Do not mix with any other drug. Incompatible with or inactivated by heparin, dopamine, cephalosporins, phenytoin, amphotericin B, penicillins, and calcium gluconate.

### INTERVENTIONS: ADMINISTRATION

For IV use, 2.1–3 mg/mL dilution in 50–200 mL of D5W or 0.9 NSS.

#### MODE/RATE OF ADMINISTRATION

IV push not recommended. May be given by intermittent IV infusion over at least 30 min.

INTRAVENOUS USE (WITH NORMAL RENAL FUNCTION)

**Adults:** Usual dosage is 4–6.5 mg/kg of LBW daily in equally divided doses q8–12h (depends on severity of infection).

**Children > 1 year:** Usual dosage is 5.5–8 mg/kg LBW q8–12h.

**Infants/Neonates:** Usual dosage is 5.5–8 mg/kg LBW q8–12h.

**Neonates < 6 weeks/ Premature Infants:** Usual dosage is 4–6.5 mg/kg LBW q12h.

**Geriatrics:** Elderly clients are more likely to have age-related decreases in renal function and are thus at greater risk for ototoxicity and nephrotoxicity.

INTRATHECAL USE OR OTHER INFUSION ROUTES AS INDICATED. Intrathecal administration should be carefully monitored. Intrathecal administration has caused nerve root pain, burning, paraplegia, radiculitis, transverse myelitis, and changes in renal and eighth cranial nerve function.

**POTENTIAL PROBLEMS IN ADMINISTRATION**

Thrombophlebitis with IV administration; space administration of netilmicin and IV penicillins at least 1 h apart in medication regimen; do not mix with other drugs. If signs of side/toxic effects (renal and otic) occur, stop the infusion and report them immediately to the physician. If overdose occurs, client may need hemodialysis. Complexation (inactivation) with ticarcillin or carbenicillin may be as effective as hemodialysis. Exchange transfusions may be done in the newborn.

**INDEPENDENT NURSING ACTIONS**

Encourage fluids/maintain hydration (unless client has renal disease). Monitor laboratory reports and report abnormal findings. Check temperature.

**ADMINISTRATION IN ALTERNATE SETTINGS**

No additional considerations.

**EVALUATION: OUTCOMES OF DRUG THERAPY**

**EXPECTED OUTCOMES**

PHYSICAL ASSESSMENT. Temperature usually returns to baseline within 3 days. Pulse between 60 and 100 bpm and regular. Skin warm, pink, and dry. No rashes, no flushing, no drainage. Breath sounds clear. Clear yellow urine. Clear CSF. Decrease in erythema or purulent discharge. Client reports decreased pain.

LABORATORY. Client maintains therapeutic level between 4 and 8 mcg/mL. During therapy serum peak concentration levels remain between 6 and 12 mcg/mL and trough levels below 0.5 and 2 mcg/mL. As therapy continues, cultures report a decreasing colony count. BUN remains between 8 and 25 mg/dL. Serum creatinine remains between 0.6 and 1.5 mg/dL. Specific gravity remains between 1.003 and 1.035. No proteinuria.

**NEGATIVE OUTCOMES**

Temperature more than 37.5° C. Pulse more than 100 bpm and irregular. Client complains of headache, ab-

▼

dominal pain, muscle aches, malaise, or lethargy. Hot, flushed skin. Rashes. Diaphoresis. Client may have neck rigidity or discharge or drainage from wounds.

## TOBRAMYCIN

*Trade Name:* Nebcin
*Canadian Availability:* Not specified
*Pregnancy Risk:* Category D
*pH:* 3.3–6.5
*Storage/Stability:* Store solution between 15° and 30° C. Stable in solution at room temperature for 24 hours.

### ASSESSMENT: DRUG CHARACTERISTICS

#### ACTION

Usually bactericidal. Exact mechanism of action not known, but appears to inhibit protein synthesis in susceptible bacteria such as *E. coli, Klebsiella, Proteus,* and *Pseudomonas*. Unlike most aminoglycosides, tobramycin is ineffective against mycobacterium.

#### INDICATIONS

Used for infections of the gastrointestinal, genitourinary, and respiratory tracts. Also used for septicemia and infections of the bones and joints, CNS (intrathecal or intraventricular administration), skin, and soft tissue.

#### CAUTIONS

ADVERSE EFFECTS. Hearing loss (temporary or permanent), tinnitus, dizziness, nystagmus, vertigo, and ataxia; neuromuscular manifestations such as peripheral neuropathy, seizures, headache, blurred vision, rash, urticaria, stomatitis, pruritus, fever, and eosinophilia; nausea, vomiting, bone marrow depression, decreased liver function. Cross allergenicity among aminoglycosides may occur.

CONTRAINDICATIONS. Myasthenia gravis, Parkinson's disease, eighth cranial nerve damage, renal impairment, or known sensitivity to tobramycin or other aminoglycosides.

#### POTENTIAL DRUG/FOOD INTERACTIONS

Do not mix with any other drug. Use with another aminoglycoside or capreomycin may increase the incidence of ototoxicity. Use with methoxyflurane polymyxins, nephrotoxic drugs, or ototoxic drugs may increase the incidence of nephrotoxicity and ototoxicity. Use with neuromuscular blocking agents may result in respiratory depression or apnea. Incompatible with or inactivated by heparin, dopamine, cephalosporins, amphotericin B, phenytoin, penicillins (when given within 1 hour of each other), and calcium gluconate. Use with loop diuretics (e.g., ethacrynic acid) may potentiate ototoxicity. Less synergistic than other aminoglycosides when used with penicillins.

#### INTERVENTIONS: ADMINISTRATION

For IV use, 1 mg/mL dilution in 50–200 mL of D5W or 0.9% NSS. For intrathecal use a quantity of CSF is mixed with the drug just prior to administration. If the CSF is grossly purulent or unobtainable, the drug may be diluted with 0.9% preservative-free NSS for injection.

#### MODE/RATE OF ADMINISTRATION

IV push not recommended. May be given by intermittent IV infusion over at least 20 min. May be given by intrathecal/intraventricular administration over 3–5 min with the bevel of the needle upward; intraventricular administration is preferred over intrathecal administration to ensure adequate drug concentration throughout the CSF. When used with intramuscular or IV administration, intrathecal or intraventricular therapy should be continued for at least 1 d after CSF cultures or Gram's stain becomes negative.

#### INTRAVENOUS USE (WITH NORMAL RENAL FUNCTION)

**Adults:** A loading dose of 1.5–2 mg/kg LBW followed by 1–1.5 mg/kg LBW q6–8h (depends on severity of infection).

For prevention of bacterial endocarditis from surgery or invasive procedures, 1.5 mg/kg 30–60 min before procedure, then q8h after procedure for up to two doses.

**Children > 1 year:** The usual dosage is 2–2.5 mg/kg of body weight q8h.

**Infants:** The usual dosage is 2–2.5 mg/kg of body weight q8h.

**Neonates < 1 week/Premature Infants:** The usual dosage is 2 mg/kg of body weight q12h.

**Geriatrics:** Elderly clients are more likely to have age-related decreases in renal function and are thus at greater risk for ototoxicity and nephrotoxicity. Reductions in dosage or increase in dosing interval may be necessary to avoid these toxicities.

#### INTRATHECAL USE OR OTHER INFUSION ROUTES AS INDICATED.

May be given intrathecally or intraventricularly. The usual dosage for adults is 4–8 mg daily. The usual dosage for children > 1 year is 1–2 mg daily.

#### POTENTIAL PROBLEMS IN ADMINISTRATION

Thrombophlebitis with IV administration; space administration of tobramycin and IV penicillins at least 1 h apart in medication regimen; do not mix with other drugs. If signs of side/toxic effects (renal and otic) occur, stop the infusion and report them immediately to the physician. If overdose occurs, client may need hemodialysis. Complexation (inactivation) with ticarcillin or carbenicillin may be as effective as hemodialysis. Exchange transfusions may be done in the newborn.

▼

**INDEPENDENT NURSING ACTIONS**

Encourage fluids/maintain hydration (unless client has renal disease). Monitor laboratory reports and report abnormal findings. Check temperature

**ADMINISTRATION IN ALTERNATE SETTINGS**

Administer tobramycin to infants and neonates only in settings where they can be carefully monitored for negative outcomes.

**EVALUATION: OUTCOMES OF DRUG THERAPY**

**EXPECTED OUTCOMES**

PHYSICAL ASSESSMENT. Temperature usually returns to baseline within 3 days. Pulse between 60 and 100 bpm and regular. Skin warm, pink, and dry. No rashes, no flushing, no drainage. Breath sounds clear. Clear yellow urine. Clear CSF. Decrease in erythema or purulent discharge. Client reports decreased pain.

LABORATORY. Client maintains therapeutic level between 4 and 8 mcg/mL. During therapy serum peak concentration levels remain below 10 mcg/mL and trough levels below 2 mcg/mL. As therapy continues, cultures report a decreasing colony count. AST remains between 7 and 27 U/L. ALT remains between 1 and 21 U/L. BUN remains between 8 and 25 mg/dL. Serum creatinine remains between 0.6 and 1.5 mg/dL. Specific gravity remains between 1.003 and 1.035. No proteinuria.

**NEGATIVE OUTCOMES**

Temperature more than 37.5° C. Pulse more than 100 bpm and irregular. Client complains of headache, abdominal pain, muscle aches, malaise, lethargy, or ringing or roaring noise in ears. Hot, flushed skin. Rashes. Diaphoresis. Client may have neck rigidity or discharge or drainage from wounds. Client reports episodes of ataxia or dizziness.

## CEPHALOSPORINS

### THERAPEUTIC EFFECTS

Cephalosporins are usually bactericidal. They inhibit cell wall synthesis and cell division and growth. Cephalosporins may cause lysis in susceptible bacteria; rapidly dividing bacteria are most susceptible. The decision of which cephalosporin to use rests on what type of organism is present, what site is affected, resistance, side effects, and cost. First- and second-generation cephalosporins are very effective against gram-negative anaerobes. Third-generation cephalosporins are effective against gram-positive cocci and gram-negative bacilli.

## PHARMACOKINETICS

**Distribution.** Cephalosporins are widely distributed throughout the body, and most body tissues and body fluids reach therapeutic levels. Cephalosporins readily cross the placental barrier and enter breast milk. Some cephalosporins enter the CSF.

**Excretion.** The half-life is usually 0.5 to 1.5 hours in adults with normal renal function. The drugs are metabolized in the liver, kidneys, and other body tissues. Cephalosporins are excreted by the kidneys and may be removed by hemodialysis or peritoneal dialysis.

## CAUTIONS

Clients with reduced kidney function are more likely to experience side/toxic effects.

**Side/Adverse Effects.** Clients receiving other nephrotoxic drugs, or are using these drugs for long periods of time or in high doses, are likely to experience side/toxic effects.

### Contraindications

***Pregnancy and Lactation.*** Cephalosporins cross the placental barrier. Studies have not shown fetal harm. Small amounts can be distributed into breast milk. For this reason the client must decide whether to continue with breast-feeding or the drug.

***Pediatrics.*** Cephalosporins should be used with caution and in reduced dosage in premature and full-term neonates younger than 6 weeks due to renal immaturity.

***Geriatrics.*** Studies have not documented specific age-related problems. However, the elderly are more likely to have diminished renal function, which increases the risk of side/toxic effects. The most serious side/toxic effects are likely to occur if the client is dehydrated.

## TOXICITY

See Table 16–4 for cephalosporin toxicities.

## POTENTIAL DRUG/FOOD INTERACTIONS

Cephalosporins may interact with aminoglycosides to increase the risk of nephrotoxicity. Chloramphenicol may inhibit bactericidal activity. Probenecid may delay renal clearance and cause an increased plasma level of the agent. Cephalosporins may interact with alcohol to cause a disulfiram-like reaction (flushing, pounding headache, nausea, vomiting, tachycardia). If cephalosporins are used with oral anticoagulants, or other agents affecting clotting, there is an increased risk of bleeding or bruising.

**TABLE 16–4**
**Cephalosporin Toxicities**

| Body System | Side/Toxic Effects | Physical Assessment Indicators | Laboratory Indicators | Nursing Interventions |
|---|---|---|---|---|
| Neurologic | Neurotoxicity | Seizures | N/A | Observe the client for seizures; assist with ADLs and mobility; protect from falls. |
| Renal | Nephrotoxicity | Oliguria, decreased urine concentration | Elevated BUN and serum creatinine; decreased urine specific gravity and creatinine clearance | Monitor BUN and serum creatinine, urine specific gravity, and creatinine clearance; measure and record intake and output; encourage fluid intake to at least 2000 mL/d unless contraindicated. |
| Gastrointestinal | Pseudomembranous colitis | Mild nausea, vomiting (rare), abdominal pain, cramping, tenderness, diarrhea | N/A | Monitor laboratory values and report abnormal findings. |
| Hematologic | Hypoprothrombinemia | Bruising, diminished wound-healing capacity | Decreased RBC, Hgb, Hct, WBC, platelets | Observe for bruising; monitor laboratory values and report abnormal findings. |
| | Serum sickness reaction | Joint pain, skin rash, fever | | |
| Dermatologic | Hypersensitivity | Rash, urticaria, pruritus | N/A | Be prepared to administer epinephrine or corticosteroids for allergic response. |
| | Stevens-Johnson syndrome | Blistering, peeling of skin, or mucous membranes of eyes or other organs | | |
| Other | Secondary infections, oral or vaginal candidiasis | Pain, burning, itching, white patches on mucous membranes | N/A | Question client for pain; observe for evidence of thrombophlebitis. |

ADLs = activities of daily living, BUN = blood urea nitrogen, Hct = hematocrit, Hgb = hemoglobin, N/A = not applicable, RBC = red blood cell count, WBC = white blood cell count.

# First-Generation Cephalosporins

## CEFAZOLIN SODIUM

*Trade Names:* Ancef, Kefzol, Zolicef
*Canadian Availability:* Ancef, Kefzol
*Pregnancy Risk:* Category B
*pH:* 4.8–5.5
*Storage/Stability:* Do not store above −10° C. May be stored for 48 hours after thawing at room temperature. May be stored up to 10 days if refrigerated. Should not be refrozen. Do not use if solution is cloudy or has a precipitate.

### ASSESSMENT: DRUG CHARACTERISTICS

#### ACTION

A broad-spectrum, β-lactam antibiotic, first-generation cephalosporin whose bactericidal properties depend on attaching to penicillin-binding proteins in bacterial cell membranes. Inhibits bacterial cell wall synthesis, causing weakness and lack of rigidity. Bacterial cell division and growth are inhibited, and bacteria that rapidly divide are the most susceptible.

#### INDICATIONS

Used to treat most gram-positive bacteria and gram-negative *E. coli, Klebsiella,* and *Proteus mirabilis.* Is more effective against *E. coli* and *Klebsiella* than other first-generation cephalosporins, but may be less stable against staphylococcal penicillinases. Indicated for perioperative prophylaxis and treatment of severe systemic infections, bone and joint infections, otitis media, pneumonia, skin and soft tissue infections, and urinary tract infections.

#### CAUTIONS

ADVERSE EFFECTS. Allergic reactions, severe abdominal pain or cramping, abdominal tenderness, diarrhea, fever, oral candidiasis, vaginitis, and thrombophlebitis.

CONTRAINDICATIONS. History of bleeding disorders, gastrointestinal diseases such as ulcerative colitis, impaired renal or hepatic functioning, or history of hypersensitivity to cefazolin.

#### POTENTIAL DRUG/FOOD INTERACTIONS

May interact with aminoglycosides to increase the risk of nephrotoxicity. Chloramphenicol may inhibit cefazolin's bactericidal activity. Probenecid may delay renal clearance and cause an increased plasma level of cefazolin.

### INTERVENTIONS: ADMINISTRATION

Thaw container at room temperature. Inspect for unthawed ice crystals before use.

#### MODE/RATE OF ADMINISTRATION

May be given by IV push at a rate of 500 mg–1 g over 3–5 min. May be given by intermittent infusion. Not

▼

recommended for continuous infusion.

INTRAVENOUS USE (WITH NORMAL RENAL FUNCTION)

**Adults:** For perioperative prophylaxis the usual dosage is 500 mg–1 g 1 h before surgery, 500 mg–1 g during surgery, and 500 mg–1 g q8h for 24 h after surgery.

For active infection the usual dosage is 500 mg–1 g q8–12h for 10 d. Usual maximum dosage is 6 g/24 h.

**Children:** The usual dosage is 6.25–25 mg/kg of body weight q6h or 8.3–33.3 mg/kg of body weight q8h.

**Infants/Neonates:** Dose not established for neonates up to 1 month.

**Geriatrics:** Elderly clients are more likely to have age-related diminished renal function that may require a lesser dose.

INTRATHECAL USE OR OTHER INFUSION ROUTES AS INDICATED. Not recommended.

**POTENTIAL PROBLEMS IN ADMINISTRATION**

If allergic reactions or seizures occur, the infusion should be discontinued immediately. Severe allergic symptoms should be treated with the usual agents such as antihistamines, adrenocorticoids, or epinephrine. Anticonvulsants may be needed for seizures.

**INDEPENDENT NURSING ACTIONS**

Monitor vital signs and laboratory values, especially BUN, serum creatinine, and prothrombin time (PT). Collect specimens as required. Keep skin clean and dry. Change dressings as needed. Use appropriate aseptic techniques and isolation precautions. Teach risk factors for infection.

**ADMINISTRATION IN ALTERNATE SETTINGS**

May be given in a variety of clinical settings and in the home by a qualified IV nurse.

**EVALUATION: OUTCOMES OF DRUG THERAPY**

**EXPECTED OUTCOMES**

PHYSICAL ASSESSMENT. Temperature less than 37.5° C. Pulse between 60 and 100 bpm and regular. Skin warm, pink, and dry. No rashes, no flushing, no drainage. Breath sounds clear. Clear yellow urine. Clear CSF. No complaints of headache or abdominal pain, chills, malaise, or lethargy.

LABORATORY. BUN between 10 and 20 mg/dL. Serum creatinine between 0.7 and 1.4 mg/dL. White blood count 5000 to 10,000/mm$^3$. Neutrophils 60% to 70%. Erythrocyte sedimentation rate below 20 mm/h. No abnormal findings from cultures of urine, blood, or CSF. PT 9.5 to 12 seconds.

**NEGATIVE OUTCOMES**

Temperature more than 37.5° C. Pulse more than 100 bpm and irregular. Client complains of headache, abdominal pain, muscle aches, malaise, or lethargy. Hot, flushed skin. Rashes. Diaphoresis. Client may have neck rigidity or discharge or drainage from wounds.

# Second-Generation Cephalosporins

## CEFONICID

*Trade Name:* Monocid
*Canadian Availability:* Monocid
*Pregnancy Risk:* Category B
*pH:* 3.5–6.5
*Storage/Stability:* Store below 8° C. Protect from light. May be stored for 24 hours at room temperature or up to 72 hours if refrigerated after reconstituting. Solution should be clear but may be used if slightly yellow in appearance.

### ASSESSMENT: DRUG CHARACTERISTICS

#### ACTION

A broad-spectrum, β-lactam antibiotic, second-generation cephalosporin whose bactericidal properties depend on attaching to penicillin-binding proteins in bacterial cell membranes. Inhibits bacterial cell wall synthesis, causing weakness and lack of rigidity. Bacterial cell division and growth are inhibited, and bacteria that rapidly divide are the most susceptible.

#### INDICATIONS

Has a greater effectiveness than first-generation cephalosporins against gram-negative bacteria such as *E. coli, Klebsiella,* and *Proteus mirabilis.* Is slightly less effective than first-generation cephalosporins against gram-positive bacteria. Indicated for perioperative prophylaxis and treatment of severe systemic infections, bone and joint infections, otitis media, pneumonia, skin and soft tissue infections, and urinary tract infections.

#### CAUTIONS

ADVERSE EFFECTS. Allergic reactions, severe abdominal pain or cramping, abdominal tenderness, diarrhea, fever, oral candidiasis, vaginitis, and thrombophlebitis.

CONTRAINDICATIONS. History of bleeding disorders, gastrointestinal diseases such as ulcerative colitis, impaired renal or hepatic functioning, or history of hypersensitivity to cefonicid.

#### POTENTIAL DRUG/FOOD INTERACTIONS

May interact with aminoglycosides to increase the risk of nephrotoxicity. Chloramphenicol may inhibit cefonicid's bactericidal activity. Probenecid may delay renal clearance and cause an increased plasma level of cefonicid.

### INTERVENTIONS: ADMINISTRATION

To reconstitute, add 2 mL of sterile water for injection to each 500-mg vial for a concentration of 220 mg/mL or 2.5 mL to each 1-g vial. The solution may be further diluted in 50–100 mL of D5W or 0.9% NSS for injection.

▼

**MODE/RATE OF ADMINISTRATION**

May be given by IV push over 3–5 min. May be given by intermittent infusion over 20–30 min.

INTRAVENOUS USE (WITH NORMAL RENAL FUNCTION)

**Adults:** For perioperative prophylaxis the usual dose is 1 g 1 h before surgery.

For an active infection the usual dosage is 500 mg–1 g q24h for 10 d. If the infection is severe, the dosage may be as high as 2 g q24h.

**Children:** Dose not established.

**Infants/Neonates:** Dose not established.

**Geriatrics:** Elderly clients are more likely to have age-related diminished renal function that may require a lesser dose.

INTRATHECAL USE OR OTHER INFUSION ROUTES AS INDICATED. Not recommended.

**POTENTIAL PROBLEMS IN ADMINISTRATION**

If allergic reactions or seizures occur, the infusion should be discontinued immediately. Severe allergic symptoms should be treated with the usual agents such as antihistamines, adrenocorticoids, or epinephrine. Anticonvulsants may be needed for seizures.

**INDEPENDENT NURSING ACTIONS**

Monitor vital signs and laboratory values, especially BUN, serum creatinine, and PT. Collect specimens as required. Keep skin clean and dry. Change dressings as needed. Use appropriate aseptic techniques and isolation precautions. Teach risk factors for infection.

**ADMINISTRATION IN ALTERNATE SETTINGS**

May be given in a variety of clinical settings and in the home by a qualified IV nurse.

**EVALUATION: OUTCOMES OF DRUG THERAPY**

**EXPECTED OUTCOMES**

PHYSICAL ASSESSMENT. Temperature less than 37.5° C. Pulse between 60 and 100 bpm and regular. Skin warm, pink, and dry. No rashes, no flushing, no drainage. Breath sounds clear. Clear yellow urine. Clear CSF. No complaints of headache or abdominal pain, chills, malaise, or lethargy.

LABORATORY. BUN between 10 and 20 mg/dL. Serum creatinine between 0.7 and 1.4 mg/dL. White blood count 5000 to 10,000/mm$^3$. Neutrophils 60% to 70%. Erythrocyte sedimentation rate below 20 mm/h. No abnormal findings from cultures of urine, blood, or CSF. PT 9.5 to 12 seconds.

**NEGATIVE OUTCOMES**

Temperature more than 37.5° C. Pulse more than 100 bpm and irregular. Client complains of headache, abdominal pain, muscle aches, malaise, or lethargy. Hot, flushed skin. Rashes. Diaphoresis. Client may have neck rigidity or discharge or drainage from wounds.

## Cefotetan Disodium

*Trade Name:* Cefotan
*Canadian Availability:* Cefotan
*Pregnancy Risk:* Category B
*pH:* 4.5–6.5
*Storage/Stability:* Do not store above 22° C. Protect from light. May be stored for 24 hours at room temperature or 96 hours if refrigerated at 5° C or 1 week if frozen. Should not be refrozen. Do not use if solution is darker than light yellow.

### ASSESSMENT: DRUG CHARACTERISTICS

**ACTION**

A broad-spectrum, *β*-lactam antibiotic, second-generation cephalosporin whose bactericidal properties depend on attaching to penicillin-binding proteins in bacterial cell membranes. Inhibits bacterial cell wall synthesis, causing weakness and lack of rigidity. Bacterial cell division and growth are inhibited, and bacteria that rapidly divide are the most susceptible.

**INDICATIONS**

Used to treat most gram-positive bacteria and gram-negative *E. coli, Klebsiella,* and *Proteus mirabilis.* Is more effective against *E. coli, Klebsiella,* and a wider range of gram-negative organisms than first-generation cephalosporins are. Indicated for perioperative prophylaxis and treatment of severe systemic infections, bone and joint infections, otitis media, pneumonia, skin and soft tissue infections, and urinary tract infections.

**CAUTIONS**

ADVERSE EFFECTS. Allergic reactions, unusual bleeding or bruising, severe abdominal pain or cramping, abdominal tenderness, diarrhea, fever, oral candidiasis, vaginitis, and thrombophlebitis.

CONTRAINDICATIONS. History of bleeding disorders, gastrointestinal diseases such as ulcerative colitis, impaired renal or hepatic functioning, or history of hypersensitivity to cefotetan.

**POTENTIAL DRUG/FOOD INTERACTIONS**

May interact with alcohol to cause a disulfiram-like reaction. If used with aminoglycosides, may increase the risk of nephrotoxicity. If used with oral anticoagulants, or other agents affecting clotting, there is an increased risk of bleeding or bruising. Chloramphenicol may inhibit cefotetan's bactericidal activity. Probenecid may delay renal clearance and cause an increased plasma level of cefotetan.

### INTERVENTIONS: ADMINISTRATION

Add 10 mL of sterile water for injection to each 1-g vial to achieve a concentration of 95 mg/mL. May be further diluted in 50–100 mL of D5W or 0.9% NSS.

▼

**MODE/RATE OF ADMINISTRATION**

May be given by IV push at a rate of 95–182 mg/mL over 3–5 min. May be given by intermittent IV infusion over 20–30 min.

INTRAVENOUS USE (WITH NORMAL RENAL FUNCTION)

**Adults:** For perioperative prophylaxis the usual dosage is 1–2 g 1 h before surgery, 500 mg–1 g during surgery, and 500 mg–1 g q8h for 24 h after surgery.

For mild to moderate infections the usual dosage is 1–2 g q12h for 5–10 d.

For severe infections the usual dosage is 2 g q12h.

For life-threatening infections the usual dosage is 3 g q12h.

Usual maximum dosage is 6 g/24 h.

**Children:** Dose not established.

**Infants/Neonates:** Dose not established.

**Geriatrics:** Elderly clients are more likely to have age-related diminished renal function that may require a lesser dose.

INTRATHECAL USE OR OTHER INFUSION ROUTES AS INDICATED. Not recommended.

**POTENTIAL PROBLEMS IN ADMINISTRATION**

If allergic reactions or seizures occur, the infusion should be discontinued immediately. Severe allergic symptoms should be treated with the usual agents such as antihistamines, adrenocorticoids, or epinephrine. Anticonvulsants may be needed for seizures.

**INDEPENDENT NURSING ACTIONS**

Monitor vital signs and laboratory values, especially BUN, serum creatinine, and PT. Collect specimens as required. Keep skin clean and dry. Change dressings as needed. Use appropriate aseptic techniques and isolation precautions. Teach risk factors for infection.

**ADMINISTRATION IN ALTERNATE SETTINGS**

May be given in a variety of clinical settings and in the home by a qualified IV nurse.

**EVALUATION: OUTCOMES OF DRUG THERAPY**

**EXPECTED OUTCOMES**

PHYSICAL ASSESSMENT. Temperature less than 37.5° C. Pulse between 60 and 100 bpm and regular. Skin warm, pink, and dry. No rashes, no flushing, no drainage. Breath sounds clear. Clear yellow urine. Clear CSF. No complaints of headache or abdominal pain, chills, malaise, or lethargy.

LABORATORY. BUN between 10 and 20 mg/dL. Serum creatinine between 0.7 and 1.4 mg/dL. White blood count 5000 to 10,000/mm$^3$. Neutrophils 60% to 70%. Erythrocyte sedimentation rate below 20 mm/h. No abnormal findings from cultures of urine, blood, or CSF. PT 9.5 to 12 seconds.

**NEGATIVE OUTCOMES**

Temperature more than 37.5% C. Pulse more than 100 bpm and irregular. Client complains of headache, abdominal pain, muscle aches, malaise, or lethargy. Hot, flushed skin. Rashes. Diaphoresis. Client may have neck rigidity or discharge or drainage from wounds.

---

## CEFOXITIN

*Trade Name:* Mefoxin
*Canadian Availability:* Mefoxin
*Pregnancy Risk:* Category B
*pH:* 4.2–7
*Storage/Stability:* Do not store above −20° C. May be stored for 24 hours after thawing at room temperature. May be stored up to 5 days if refrigerated. Should not be refrozen. Do not use if solution is cloudy or has a precipitate.

### ASSESSMENT: DRUG CHARACTERISTICS

#### ACTION

A broad-spectrum, β-lactam antibiotic, a second-generation cephalosporin whose bactericidal properties depend on attaching to penicillin-binding proteins in bacterial cell membranes. Inhibits bacterial cell wall synthesis, causing weakness and lack of rigidity. Bacterial cell division and growth are inhibited, and bacteria that rapidly divide are the most susceptible.

#### INDICATIONS

Used to treat most gram-positive bacteria and gram-negative *E. coli, Klebsiella,* and *Proteus mirabilis.* Is more effective against *E. coli, Klebsiella,* and a wider range of gram-negative organisms than first-generation cephalosporins. Is particularly useful against anaerobic organisms. Indicated for perioperative prophylaxis and treatment of severe systemic infections, bone and joint infections, otitis media, pneumonia, skin and soft tissue infections, and urinary tract infections.

#### CAUTIONS

ADVERSE EFFECTS. Allergic reactions, unusual bleeding or bruising, severe abdominal pain or cramping, abdominal tenderness, diarrhea, fever, oral candidiasis, vaginitis, and thrombophlebitis.

CONTRAINDICATIONS. History of bleeding disorders, gastrointestinal diseases such as ulcerative colitis, impaired renal or hepatic functioning, or history of hypersensitivity to cefoxitin.

#### POTENTIAL DRUG/FOOD INTERACTIONS

If used with aminoglycosides, may increase the risk of nephrotoxicity. Chloramphenicol may inhibit cefoxitin's bactericidal activity. Probenecid may delay renal clearance and cause an increased plasma level of cefoxitin.

▼

**INTERVENTIONS: ADMINISTRATION**

Thaw container at room temperature. Inspect for unthawed ice crystals before use.

**MODE/RATE OF ADMINISTRATION**

May be given by IV push at a rate of 500 mg–1 g over 3–5 min. May be given by intermittent infusion and continuous infusion if an infusion pump is used.

INTRAVENOUS USE (WITH NORMAL RENAL FUNCTION)

**Adults:** For perioperative prophylaxis the usual dosage is 2 g 1 h before surgery and 2 g q6h for 24 h after surgery.

For mild to moderate infections the usual dosage is 1 g q6–8h for 5–10 d.

For severe infections the usual dosage is 1 g q4h or 2 g q6–8h.

For life-threatening infections the usual dosage is 2 g q4h or 3 g q6h.

Usual maximum dosage is 12 g/24 h.

**Children > 12 years:** Follow adult dosing schedule.

**Infants ≤ 3 months:** Dose not established.

**Infants > 3 months:** The usual dosage is 13.3–26.7 mg/kg of body weight q4h or 20–40 mg/kg of body weight q6h.

**Geriatrics:** Elderly clients are more likely to have age-related diminished renal function that may require a lesser dose.

INTRATHECAL USE OR OTHER INFUSION ROUTES AS INDICATED. Not recommended.

**POTENTIAL PROBLEMS IN ADMINISTRATION**

If allergic reactions or seizures occur, the infusion should be discontinued immediately. Severe allergic symptoms should be treated with the usual agents such as antihistamines, adrenocorticoids, or epinephrine. Anticonvulsants may be needed for seizures.

**INDEPENDENT NURSING ACTIONS**

Monitor vital signs and laboratory values, especially BUN, serum creatinine, and PT. Collect specimens as required. Keep skin clean and dry. Change dressings as needed. Use appropriate aseptic techniques and isolation precautions. Teach risk factors for infection.

**ADMINISTRATION IN ALTERNATE SETTINGS**

May be given in a variety of clinical settings and in the home by a qualified IV nurse.

**EVALUATION: OUTCOMES OF DRUG THERAPY**

**EXPECTED OUTCOMES**

PHYSICAL ASSESSMENT. Temperature less than 37.5° C. Pulse between 60 and 100 bpm and regular. Skin warm, pink, and dry. No rashes, no flushing, no drainage. Breath sounds clear. Clear yellow urine. Clear CSF. No complaints of headache or abdominal pain, chills, malaise, or lethargy.

LABORATORY. BUN between 10 and 20 mg/dL. Serum creatinine between 0.7 and 1.4 mg/dL. White blood count 5000 to 10,000/mm$^3$. Neutrophils 60% to 70%. Erythrocyte sedimentation rate below 20 mm/h. No abnormal findings from cultures of urine, blood, or CSF. PT 9.5 to 12 seconds.

**NEGATIVE OUTCOMES**

Temperature more than 37.5° C. Pulse more than 100 bpm and irregular. Client complains of headache, abdominal pain, muscle aches, malaise, or lethargy. Hot, flushed skin. Rashes. Diaphoresis. Client may have neck rigidity or discharge or drainage from wounds.

## CEFUROXIME SODIUM

*Trade Name:* Zinacef
*Canadian Availability:* Not specified
*Pregnancy Risk:* Category B
*pH:* 6–8.5
*Storage/Stability:* Store below −20° C. May be stored for 6 months if frozen. May be stored for 24 hours at room temperature after thawing or up to 7 days if refrigerated. Do not use if solution is cloudy or has a precipitate.

**ASSESSMENT: DRUG CHARACTERISTICS**

**ACTION**

A broad-spectrum, β-lactam antibiotic, second-generation cephalosporin whose bactericidal properties depend on attaching to penicillin-binding proteins in bacterial cell membranes. Inhibits bacterial cell wall synthesis, causing weakness and lack of rigidity. Bacterial cell division and growth are inhibited, and bacteria that rapidly divide are the most susceptible.

**INDICATIONS**

Has a greater effectiveness than first-generation cephalosporins against gram-negative bacteria such as *E. coli, Klebsiella,* and *Proteus mirabilis*. Is slightly less effective than first-generation cephalosporins against gram-positive bacteria. Is the only second-generation cephalosporin to adequately cross into CSF. Indicated for perioperative prophylaxis and treatment of severe systemic infections, bone and joint infections, otitis media, pneumonia, skin and soft tissue infections, and urinary tract infections.

**INDICATIONS**

ADVERSE EFFECTS. Allergic reactions, severe abdominal pain or cramping, abdominal tenderness, diarrhea, fever, oral candidiasis, vaginitis, and thrombophlebitis.

CONTRAINDICATIONS. History of bleeding disorders, gastrointestinal diseases such as ulcerative colitis, impaired renal or hepatic functioning, or history of hypersensitivity to cefuroxime.

**POTENTIAL DRUG/FOOD INTERACTIONS**

May interact with aminoglycosides to increase the risk of nephrotoxicity. Chloramphenicol may inhibit cefuroximes bactericidal activity. Probenecid may delay renal clearance and cause an increased plasma level of cefuroxime.

**INTERVENTIONS: ADMINISTRATION**

Thaw container at room temperature. Inspect for unthawed ice crystals before use.

**MODE/RATE OF ADMINISTRATION**

May be given by IV push over 3–5 min. May be given by intermittent infusion over 20–30 min. May also be given as a continuous infusion.

INTRAVENOUS USE (WITH NORMAL RENAL FUNCTION)

**Adults:** For an active infection the usual dosage is 750 mg–1.5 g q8h.

For bacterial meningitis the usual dosage is up to 3 g q8h.

For perioperative prophylaxis the usual dose is 1.5 g ½–1h before surgery, 750 mg during surgery, and q8h for 24 h after surgery.

**Infants and Children ≥ 3 months:** The usual dosage is 16.7–33.3 mg/kg of body weight q8h.

**Children:** For meningitis the usual dosage is 50–60 mg/kg of body weight q6h or 66.7–80 mg/kg of body weight q12h.

**Infants/Neonates:** For neonates the usual dosage is 10–33.3 mg/kg of body weight q8h or 15–50 mg/kg of body weight q12h.

For meningitis the usual dosage is 33.3 mg/kg of body weight q8h or 50 mg/kg of body weight q12h.

**Geriatrics:** Elderly clients are more likely to have age-related diminished renal function that may require a lesser dose.

INTRATHECAL USE OR OTHER INFUSION ROUTES AS INDICATED. Not recommended.

**POTENTIAL PROBLEMS IN ADMINISTRATION**

If allergic reactions or seizures occur, the infusion should be discontinued immediately. Severe allergic symptoms should be treated with the usual agents such as antihistamines, adrenocorticoids, or epinephrine. Anticonvulsants may be needed for seizures.

**INDEPENDENT NURSING ACTIONS**

Monitor vital signs and laboratory values, especially BUN, serum creatinine, and PT. Collect specimens as required. Keep skin clean and dry. Change dressings as needed. Use appropriate aseptic techniques and isolation precautions. Teach risk factors for infection.

**ADMINISTRATION IN ALTERNATE SETTINGS**

May be given in a variety of clinical settings and in the home by a qualified IV nurse.

**EVALUATION: OUTCOMES OF DRUG THERAPY**

**EXPECTED OUTCOMES**

PHYSICAL ASSESSMENT. Temperature less than 37.5° C. Pulse between 60 and 100 bpm and regular. Skin warm, pink, and dry. No rashes, no flushing, no drainage. Breath sounds clear. Clear yellow urine. Clear CSF. No complaints of headache or abdominal pain, chills, malaise, or lethargy.

LABORATORY. BUN between 10 and 20 mg/dL. Serum creatinine between 0.7 and 1.4 mg/dL. White blood count 5000 to 0,000/mm³. Neutrophils 60% to 70%. Erythrocyte edimentation rate below 20 mm/h. No abnormal findings from cultures of urine, blood, or CSF. PT 9.5 to 12 seconds.

**NEGATIVE OUTCOMES**

Temperature more than 37.5° C. Pulse more than 100 bpm and irregular. Client complains of headache, abdominal pain, muscle aches, malaise, or lethargy. Hot, flushed skin. Rashes. Diaphoresis. Client may have neck rigidity or discharge or drainage from wounds.

# Third-Generation Cephalosporins

## CEFOPERAZONE

*Trade Name:* Cefobid
*Canadian Availability:* Cefobid
*Pregnancy Risk:* Category B
*pH:* 4.5–6.5
*Storage/Stability:* Store between 15° and 30° C. Solutions that have been reconstituted, have a concentration of 2 to 300 mg/mL, and are mixed with D5W, 0.9% NSS, or combinations of dextrose and sodium chloride, and Ringer's lactated solution may be stored at room temperature for 24 hours or up to 5 days if refrigerated at 2° to 8° C. Solutions that have been reconstituted, have a concentration of 2 and 50 mg/mL, and are mixed with D5W, 0.9% NSS, or combinations of dextrose and sodium chloride may be frozen and stored for 3 weeks. Some concentrations and solutions may be frozen and stored for up to 5 weeks. Once thawed, solutions should not be refrozen.

### ASSESSMENT: DRUG CHARACTERISTICS

**ACTION**

A broad-spectrum, β-lactam antibiotic, third-generation cephalosporin whose bactericidal properties depend on attaching to penicillin-binding proteins in bacterial cell membranes. Inhibits bacterial cell wall synthesis, causing weakness and lack of rigidity. Bacterial cell division and growth are inhibited, and bacteria that rapidly divide are the most susceptible.

**INDICATIONS**

Used to treat a wide range of gram-positive bacteria and most gram-negative bacteria. Has slightly less effect against *Enterobacteriaceae* than other third-generation cephalosporins. Used to treat severe gram-negative ▼

infections including systemic infections, bone and joint infections, female pelvic infections, intraabdominal infections, gram-negative pneumonia, skin and soft tissue infections including burn wounds, and urinary tract infections.

#### CAUTIONS

ADVERSE EFFECTS. Allergic reactions, severe abdominal pain or cramping, abdominal tenderness, diarrhea, fever, oral candidiasis, vaginitis, and thrombophlebitis.

CONTRAINDICATIONS. History of bleeding disorders, gastrointestinal diseases such as ulcerative colitis, impaired renal or hepatic functioning, or history of hypersensitivity to cefoperazone.

#### POTENTIAL DRUG/FOOD INTERACTIONS

May interact with aminoglycosides to increase the risk of nephrotoxicity. Chloramphenicol may inhibit cefoperazone's bactericidal activity. Probenecid may delay renal clearance and cause an increased plasma level of cefoperazone.

#### INTERVENTIONS: ADMINISTRATION

Reconstituted solutions should be thoroughly thawed before using. Check for ice crystals.

#### MODE/RATE OF ADMINISTRATION

May be administered by intermittent IV infusion over 15–30 min or by continuous infusion. Not recommended for IV push.

INTRAVENOUS USE (WITH NORMAL RENAL FUNCTION)

**Adults:** For mild to moderate infections the usual dosage is 2 g q12h.

For severe infections the usual dosage is 2–4 g q8h or 3–6 g q12h.

Maximum daily dose should not exceed 12 g. On occasion, as much as 16 g/d has been given.

**Children ≥ 12 years:** Follow adult dosing schedule.

**Infants/Neonates:** Dose not established.

**Geriatrics:** Elderly clients are more likely to have age-related diminished renal function that may require a lesser dose.

INTRATHECAL USE OR OTHER INFUSION ROUTES AS INDICATED. Not recommended.

#### POTENTIAL PROBLEMS IN ADMINISTRATION

If allergic reactions or seizures occur, the infusion should be discontinued immediately. Severe allergic symptoms should be treated with the usual agents such as antihistamines, adrenocorticoids, or epinephrine. Anticonvulsants may be needed for seizures.

#### INDEPENDENT NURSING ACTIONS

Monitor vital signs and laboratory values, especially BUN, serum creatinine, and PT. Collect specimens as required. Keep skin clean and dry. Change dressings as needed. Use appropriate aseptic techniques and isolation precautions. Teach risk factors for infection.

**ADMINISTRATION IN ALTERNATE SETTINGS**

May be given in a variety of clinical settings and in the home by a qualified IV nurse.

**EVALUATION: OUTCOMES OF DRUG THERAPY**

**EXPECTED OUTCOMES**

PHYSICAL ASSESSMENT. Temperature less than 37.5° C. Pulse between 60 and 100 bpm and regular. Skin warm, pink, and dry. No rashes, no flushing, no drainage. Breath sounds clear. Clear yellow urine. Clear CSF. No complaints of headache or abdominal pain, chills, malaise, or lethargy.

LABORATORY. BUN between 10 and 20 mg/dL. Serum creatinine between 0.7 and 1.4 mg/dL. White blood count 5000 to 10,000/mm³. Neutrophils 60% to 70%. Erythrocyte sedimentation rate below 20 mm/h. No abnormal findings from cultures of urine, blood, or CSF. PT 9.5 to 12 seconds.

**NEGATIVE OUTCOMES**

Temperature more than 37.5° C. Pulse more than 100 bpm and irregular. Client complains of headache, abdominal pain, muscle aches, malaise, or lethargy. Hot, flushed skin. Rashes. Diaphoresis. Client may have neck rigidity or discharge or drainage from wounds.

## CEFOTAXIME

*Trade Name:* Claforan
*Canadian Availability:* Claforan
*Pregnancy Risk:* Category B
*pH:* 5–7.5
*Storage/Stability:* Store below 30° C. May store for 24 hours at room temperature, 10 days if refrigerated, or up to 13 weeks if frozen after reconstituting. Do not refreeze solutions.

**ASSESSMENT: DRUG CHARACTERISTICS**

**ACTION**

A broad-spectrum, $\beta$-lactam antibiotic, third-generation cephalosporin whose bactericidal properties depend on attaching to penicillin-binding proteins in bacterial cell membranes. Inhibits bacterial cell wall synthesis, causing weakness and lack of rigidity. Bacterial cell division and growth are inhibited, and bacteria that rapidly divide are the most susceptible.

**INDICATIONS**

Used to treat a wide range of gram-positive bacteria and most gram-negative bacteria. Used to treat severe gram-negative infections including meningitis, systemic infections, bone and joint infections, female pelvic infections, intraabdominal infections, gram-negative pneumonia, skin and soft tissue infections including burn wounds, and urinary tract infections.

▼

**CAUTIONS**

ADVERSE EFFECTS. Allergic reactions, severe abdominal pain or cramping, abdominal tenderness, diarrhea, fever, oral candidiasis, vaginitis, and thrombophlebitis.

CONTRAINDICATIONS. History of bleeding disorders, gastrointestinal diseases such as ulcerative colitis, impaired renal or hepatic functioning, or history of hypersensitivity to cefotaxime.

**POTENTIAL DRUG/FOOD INTERACTIONS**

May interact with aminoglycosides to increase the risk of nephrotoxicity. Chloramphenicol may inhibit cefotaxime's bactericidal activity. Probenecid may delay renal clearance and cause an increased plasma level of cefotaxime.

**INTERVENTIONS: ADMINISTRATION**

Add 2 mL to each 500-mg vial, 3 mL to each 1-g vial, or 5 mL to each 2-g vial. Add 10 mL of sterile water for injection to further dilute for IV push. May be added to 50–100 mL of 0.9% NSS or D5W solution for intermittent IV infusion or to larger volumes for constant IV infusions.

**MODE/RATE OF ADMINISTRATION**

May be given by IV push over 3–10 min. May be given by intermittent IV infusions over 30 min.

INTRAVENOUS USE (WITH NORMAL RENAL FUNCTION)

**Adults:** For infections the usual doage is 1 g q4–12h.

For moderate to severe infections the usual dosage is 1–2 g q6–8h.

For life-threatening infections the usual dosage is 2 g q4h.

Maximum daily dose should not exceed 12 g.

**Children >12 years:** Follow adult dosing schedule.

**Infants/Neonates:** For infants and children under 50 kg the usual dosage is 8.3–30 mg/kg of body weight q4h or 12.5–45 mg/kg of body weight q6h.

**Neonates 1–4 weeks:** The usual dosage is 50 mg/kg of body weight q8h.

**Neonates ≤1 week:** The usual dosage is 50 mg/kg of body weight q12h.

Maximum daily dose should not exceed 12 g.

**Geriatrics:** Elderly clients are more likely to have age-related diminished renal function that may require a lesser dose.

INTRATHECAL USE OR OTHER INFUSION ROUTES AS INDICATED. Not recommended.

**POTENTIAL PROBLEMS IN ADMINISTRATION**

If allergic reactions or seizures occur, the infusion should be discontinued immediately. Severe allergic symptoms should be treated with the usual agents such as antihistamines, adrenocorticoids, or epinephrine. Anticonvulsants may be needed for seizures.

**INDEPENDENT NURSING ACTIONS**

Monitor vital signs and laboratory values, especially BUN, serum creatinine, and PT. Collect specimens as required. Keep skin clean and dry. Change dressings as needed. Use appropriate aseptic techniques and isolation precautions. Teach risk factors for infection.

**ADMINISTRATION IN ALTERNATE SETTINGS**

May be given in a variety of clinical settings and in the home by a qualified IV nurse.

**EVALUATION: OUTCOMES OF DRUG THERAPY**

**EXPECTED OUTCOMES**

PHYSICAL ASSESSMENT. Temperature less than 37.5° C. Pulse between 60 and 100 bpm and regular. Skin warm, pink, and dry. No rashes, no flushing, no drainage. Breath sounds clear. Clear yellow urine. Clear CSF. No complaints of headache or abdominal pain, chills, malaise, or lethargy.

LABORATORY. BUN between 10 and 20 mg/dL. Serum creatinine between 0.7 and 1.4 mg/dL. White blood count 5000 to 10,000/mm³. Neutrophils 60% to 70%. Erythrocyte sedimentation rate below 20 mm/h. No abnormal findings from cultures of urine, blood, or CSF. PT 9.5 to 12 seconds.

**NEGATIVE OUTCOMES**

Temperature more than 37.5° C. Pulse more than 100 bpm and irregular. Client complains of headache, abdominal pain, muscle aches, malaise, or lethargy. Hot, flushed skin. Rashes. Diaphoresis. Client may have neck rigidity or discharge or drainage from wounds.

## CEFTAZIDIME

*Trade Names:* Ceptaz, Fortaz, Tazicef

*Canadian Availability:* Ceptax, Fortaz

*Pregnancy Risk:* Category B

*pH:* 5–8

*Storage/Stability:* Do not store above −20° C. After thawing, solutions may be stored at room temperature for 24 hours or up to 10 days if refrigerated at 5° C. Do not refreeze. Do not use if the solution is cloudy or has a precipitate.

**ASSESSMENT: DRUG CHARACTERISTICS**

**ACTION**

A broad-spectrum, β-lactam antibiotic, third-generation cephalosporin whose bactericidal properties depend on attaching to penicillin-binding proteins in bacterial cell membranes. Inhibits bacterial cell wall synthesis, causing weakness and lack of rigidity. Bacterial cell division and growth are inhibited, and bacteria that rapidly divide are the most susceptible.

**INDICATIONS**

Used to treat a wide range of gram-positive bacteria and most gram-negative bacteria. Good action against *Pseudomonas aeruginosa*. Used to treat severe gram-negative infections, including systemic infections, meningitis in both children and adults, bone and joint infections, female pelvic infections, intraabdominal infections, gram-negative pneumonia, skin and soft tissue infections including burn wounds, and urinary tract infections.

**CAUTIONS**

ADVERSE EFFECTS. Allergic reactions, bleeding or bruising, severe abdominal pain or cramping, abdominal tenderness, diarrhea, fever, oral candidiasis, vaginitis, and thrombophlebitis.

CONTRAINDICATIONS. Should not be used in clients with a history of bleeding disorders, gastrointestinal diseases such as ulcerative colitis, impaired renal or hepatic functioning, or history of hypersensitivity to ceftazidime.

**POTENTIAL DRUG/FOOD INTERACTIONS**

May interact with aminoglycosides to increase the risk of nephrotoxicity. Chloramphenicol may inhibit ceftazidime's bactericidal activity. Probenecid may delay renal clearance and cause an increased plasma level of ceftazidime.

**INTERVENTIONS: ADMINISTRATION**

Reconstituted solutions should be thoroughly thawed before using. Check for ice crystals.

**MODE/RATE OF ADMINISTRATION**

May be administered by intermittent IV infusion over 15–30 min or by continuous infusion. Not recommended for IV push.

INTRAVENOUS USE (WITH NORMAL RENAL FUNCTION)

**Adults:** For infections the usual dosage is 500 mg–1 g q8–12h.

For bone or joint infections the usual dosage is 2 g q12h.

For urinary tract infections the usual dosage is 500 mg q8–12h.

For pneumonia the usual dosage is 500 mg–1 g q8h.

For life-threatening infections the usual dosage is 2 g q8h. Maximum dose is 12 g/24 h.

**Children > 12 years:** Follow adult dosing schedule.

**Neonates ≤ 4 weeks:** The usual dosage is 30 mg/kg of body weight q8h.

**Infants and children ≤ 12 years:** The usual dosage is 30–50 mg/kg of body weight q8h. Maximum dose should not exceed 6 g in 24h.

**Geriatrics:** Elderly clients are more likely to have age-related diminished renal function that may require a lesser dose.

INTRATHECAL USE OR OTHER INFUSION ROUTES AS INDICATED. NOT RECOMMENDED.

**POTENTIAL PROBLEMS IN ADMINISTRATION**

If allergic reactions or seizures occur, the infusion should be discontinued immediately. Severe allergic symptoms should be treated with the usual agents such as antihistamines, adrenocorticoids, or epinephrine.

Anticonvulsants may be needed for seizures.

**INDEPENDENT NURSING ACTIONS**

Monitor vital signs and laboratory values, especially BUN, serum creatinine, and PT. Collect specimens as required. Keep skin clean and dry. Change dressings as needed. Use appropriate aseptic techniques and isolation precautions. Teach risk factors for infection.

**ADMINISTRATION IN ALTERNATE SETTINGS**

May be given in a variety of clinical settings and in the home by a qualified IV nurse.

**EVALUATION: OUTCOMES OF DRUG THERAPY**

**EXPECTED OUTCOMES**

PHYSICAL ASSESSMENT. Temperature less than 37.5° C. Pulse between 60 and 100 bpm and regular. Skin warm, pink, and dry. No rashes, no flushing, no drainage. Breath sounds clear. Clear yellow urine. Clear CSF. No complaints of headache or abdominal pain, chills, malaise, or lethargy.

LABORATORY. BUN between 10 and 20 mg/dL. Serum creatinine between 0.7 and 1.4 mg/dL. White blood count 5000 to 10,000/mm$^3$. Neutrophils 60% to 70%. Erythrocyte sedimentation rate below 20 mm/h. No abnormal findings from cultures of urine, blood, or CSF. PT 9.5 to 12 seconds.

**NEGATIVE OUTCOMES**

Temperature more than 37.5° C. Pulse more than 100 bpm and irregular. Client complains of headache, abdominal pain, muscle aches, malaise, or lethargy. Hot, flushed skin. Rashes. Diaphoresis. Client may have neck rigidity or discharge or drainage from wounds.

## CEFTRIAXONE SODIUM

*Trade Name:* Rocephin
*Canadian Availability:* Rocephin
*Pregnancy Risk:* Category B
*pH:* 6.7
*Storage/Stability:* Do not store above −20° C. After thawing, solutions may be stored at room temperature for 24 hours or up to 10 days if refrigerated at 5° C. Do not refreeze. Do not use if the solution is cloudy or has a precipitate.

**ASSESSMENT: DRUG CHARACTERISTICS**

**ACTION**

A broad-spectrum, β-lactam antibiotic, third-generation cephalosporin whose bactericidal properties depend on attaching to penicillin-binding proteins in bacterial cell membranes. Inhibits bacterial cell wall synthesis, causing weakness and lack of rigidity. Bacterial cell division and growth are in-

▼

hibited, and bacteria that rapidly divide arez the most susceptible.

**INDICATIONS**

Used to treat a wide range of gram-positive bacteria and most gram-negative bacteria. Used to treat severe gram-negative infections, including systemic infections, meningitis in both children and adults, bone and joint infections, female pelvic infections such as gonorrhea, intraabdominal infections, gram-negative pneumonia, skin and soft tissue infections including burn wounds, urinary tract infections, and late stages of Lyme disease.

**CAUTIONS**

ADVERSE EFFECTS. Allergic reactions, severe abdominal pain or cramping, abdominal tenderness, diarrhea, fever, oral candidiasis, vaginitis, and thrombophlebitis.

CONTRAINDICATIONS. History of bleeding disorders, gastrointestinal diseases such as ulcerative colitis, impaired renal or hepatic functioning, or history of hypersensitivity to ceftriaxone.

**POTENTIAL DRUG/FOOD INTERACTIONS**

May interact with aminoglycosides to increase the risk of nephrotoxicity. Chloramphenicol may inhibit ceftriaxone's bactericidal activity. Probenecid may delay renal clearance and cause an increased plasma level of ceftriaxone.

**INTERVENTIONS: ADMINISTRATION**

Reconstituted solutions should be thoroughly thawed before using. Check for ice crystals.

**MODE/RATE OF ADMINISTRATION**

May be administered by intermittent IV infusion over 15–30 min or by continuous infusion. Not recommended for IV push.

INTRAVENOUS USE (WITH NORMAL RENAL FUNCTION)

**Adults:** For infections the usual dosage is 500 mg–2 g q8–12h.

For bone or joint infections the usual dosage is 2 g q12h.

For uncomplicated urinary tract infections the usual dosage is 250 mg q8–12h.

For complicated urinary tract infections the usual dosage is 500 mg q8–12h.

For pneumonia the usual dosage is 500 mg–1 g q8h.

For life-threatening infections the usual dosage is 2 g q8h.

**Children $>$12 years:** Follow adult dosing schedule.

**Neonates $\leq$4 weeks:** The usual dosage is 30 mg/kg of body weight q8h.

**Infants and Children $\leq$12 years:** The usual dosage is 50–75 mg/kg of body weight q8h. Maximum dose should not exceed 6 g in 24h.

**Geriatrics:** Elderly clients are more likely to have age-related diminished renal function that may require a lesser dose.

INTRATHECAL USE OR OTHER INFUSION ROUTES AS INDICATED. Not recommended.

**POTENTIAL PROBLEMS IN ADMINISTRATION**

If allergic reactions or seizures occur, the infusion should be discontinued immediately. Severe allergic symptoms should be treated with the usual agents such as antihistamines, adrenocorticoids, or epinephrine. Anticonvulsants may be needed for seizures.

**INDEPENDENT NURSING ACTIONS**

Monitor vital signs and laboratory values, especially BUN, serum creatinine, and PT. Collect specimens as required. Keep skin clean and dry. Change dressings as needed. Use appropriate aseptic techniques and isolation precautions. Teach risk factors for infection.

**ADMINISTRATION IN ALTERNATE SETTINGS**

May be given in a variety of clinical settings and in the home by a qualified IV nurse.

**EVALUATION: OUTCOMES OF DRUG THERAPY**

**EXPECTED OUTCOMES**

PHYSICAL ASSESSMENT. Temperature less than 37.5° C. Pulse between 60 and 100 bpm and regular. Skin warm, pink, and dry. No rashes, no flushing, no drainage. Breath sounds clear. Clear yellow urine. Clear CSF. No complaints of headache or abdominal pain, chills, malaise, or lethargy.

LABORATORY. BUN between 10 and 20 mg/dL. Serum creatinine between 0.7 and 1.4 mg/dL. White blood count 5000 to 10,000/mm$^3$ Neutrophils 60% to 70%. Erythrocyte sedimentation rate below 20 mm/h. No abnormal findings from cultures of urine, blood, or CSF. PT 9.5 to 12 seconds.

**NEGATIVE OUTCOMES**

Temperature more than 37.5° C. Pulse more than 100 bpm and irregular. Client complains of headache, abdominal pain, muscle aches, malaise, or lethargy. Hot, flushed skin. Rashes. Diaphoresis. Client may have neck rigidity or discharge or drainage from wounds.

## Chloramphenicols

### CHLORAMPHENICOL

*Trade Name:* Chloromycetin
*Canadian Availability:* Chloromycetin
*Pregnancy Risk:* Category C
*pH:* 8.5–9.5
*Storage/Stability:* Store between 15° and 30° C. May be stored at room temperature for 2 to 30 days after being reconstituted to 100 mg/mL. Diluted solutions may be stored at room temperature for 1 to 2 days.

**ASSESSMENT: DRUG CHARACTERISTICS**

**ACTION**

A broad-spectrum antibiotic that acts by inhibiting protein synthesis.

▼

**INDICATIONS**

Used to treat severe infections caused by a large number of gram-positive, gram-negative, and anaerobic bacteria when other less toxic antimicrobials are not effective or are contraindicated. Used to treat meningitis (especially those caused by *Haemophilus influenzae, Streptococcus pneumoniae,* and *Neisseria meningitidis*) acute typhoid fever, paratyphoid fever, and brain abscesses. May also be used to treat common rickettsial infections (such as Rocky Mountain spotted fever and Q fever, and typhus), spirochetes, and *Chlamydia*.

**CAUTIONS**

ADVERSE EFFECTS. Blood dyscrasias; allergic reactions; neurotoxic reactions such as confusion, headache, or delirium; gray syndrome in neonates characterized by blue-gray skin, abdominal distention, hypothermia, and cardiovascular collapse; optic neuritis, nausea, vomiting, or diarrhea.

CONTRAINDICATIONS. History of allergic reaction to chloramphenicol, history of chemotherapy or radiation therapy, or bone marrow depression or impaired hepatic functioning.

**POTENTIAL DRUG/FOOD INTERACTIONS**

May interact with alfentanil to prolong the action of alfentanil. May interact with bone marrow depressants or radiation therapy to cause further depression. May potentiate the effects of some oral hypoglycemic agents. Use with clindamycin, erythromycin, or lincomycin may mutually inhibit the effectiveness of all agents. May interact with phenobarbital, phenytoin, or warfarin to delay the metabolism of chloramphenicol.

**INTERVENTIONS: ADMINISTRATION**

Add 10 mL of sterile water for injection or D5W solution to a 1-g vial to achieve a concentration of 100 mg/mL. May be further diluted in 50–100 mL of D5W solution.

**MODE/RATE OF ADMINISTRATION**

May be given by IV push over at least 1 min. May be given by intermittent IV infusion. Not recommended for continuous infusion.

INTRAVENOUS USE (WITH NORMAL RENAL FUNCTION)

**Adults:** Usual IV dosage is 12.5 mg/kg of body weight q6h. Maximum dosage is 4 g q24h.

**Children > 12 years:** Follow adult dosing schedule.

**Neonates ≤ 2 weeks:** The usual dosage is 6.25 mg/kg of body weight q6h.

**Infants > 2 weeks:** The usual dosage is 12.5 mg/kg of body weight q6h or 25 mg/kg of body weight q12h.

**Infants/Neonates:** For meningitis or severe infections, dosages of 75–100 mg/kg of body weight q24h may be used.

**Geriatrics:** Follow adult dosing schedule.

INTRATHECAL USE OR OTHER INFUSION ROUTES AS INDICATED. Not recommended.

**POTENTIAL PROBLEMS IN ADMINISTRATION**

Clients with impaired hepatic functioning should be closely monitored for serum chloramphenicol levels. Levels should remain below 30 mcg/mL to avoid blood dyscrasias.

**INDEPENDENT NURSING ACTIONS**

Monitor vital signs and laboratory values, especially BUN, serum creatinine, and liver enzymes. Collect specimens as required. Keep skin clean and dry. Change dressings as needed. Use appropriate aseptic techniques and isolation precautions. Teach risk factors for infection.

**ADMINISTRATION IN ALTERNATE SETTINGS**

Should be given in acute care settings by a qualified IV nurse. Not recommended for home infusion therapy.

**EVALUATION: OUTCOMES OF DRUG THERAPY**

**EXPECTED OUTCOMES**

PHYSICAL ASSESSMENT. Temperature less than 37.5° C. Pulse between 60 and 100 bpm and regular. Skin warm, pink, and dry. No rashes, no flushing, no drainage, no bleeding or bruises. Breath sounds clear. Clear yellow urine. Clear CSF. No complaints of headache or abdominal pain, chills, malaise, or lethargy.

LABORATORY. Liver enzymes lactate dehydrogenase (LDH) 100 to 225 mU/mL, AST 7 to 40 U/mL, ALT between 10 and 40 U/mL, BUN between 10 and 20 mg/dL. Serum creatinine between 0.7 and 1.4 mg/dL. White blood count 5000 to 10,000/mm$^3$. Neutrophils 60% to 70%. Erythrocyte sedimentation rate below 20 mm/h. No abnormal findings from cultures of urine, blood, or CSF. PT 9.5 to 12 seconds.

**NEGATIVE OUTCOMES**

Temperature more than 37.5° C. Pulse more than 100 bpm and irregular. Client complains of headache, abdominal pain, muscle aches, malaise, or lethargy. Hot, flushed skin. Rashes. Diaphoresis. Client may have neck rigidity.

## Erythromycins

### ERYTHROMYCIN LACTOBIONATE

*Trade Names:* Erythrocin
*Canadian Availability:* Erythrocin
*Pregnancy Risk:* Category B
*pH:* 6.5–7.5
*Storage/Stability:* Store below 40° C. May be stored at room temperature for 24 hours or 14 days if refrigerated after reconstituting to 50 mg/mL. If further diluted, may be stored for 8 hours at room temperature, 24 hours if refrigerated, or 30 days if frozen.

▼

## ASSESSMENT: DRUG CHARACTERISTICS

### ACTION

A broad-spectrum antibiotic that acts by preventing cell synthesis.

### INDICATIONS

Used to treat infections caused by a number of gram-negative and many gram-positive organisms and may be used as a substitute for penicilin or tetracycline preparations. May be used to treat chlamydial conjunctivitis, genitourinary tract infections, diphtheria, bacterial endocarditis, gonorrhea, legionnaires' disease, acute otitis media, pertussis, pneumonia, rheumatic fever, syphilis, and nongonococcal urethritis.

### CAUTIONS

ADVERSE EFFECTS. Allergic reactions, jaundice, irritation at the injection site, nausea, vomiting, diarrhea, candidiasis, or hearing loss.

CONTRAINDICATIONS. History of hypersensitivity to erythromycin or hepatic impairment.

### POTENTIAL DRUG/FOOD INTERACTIONS

May interact with alfentanil to prolong the action of alfentanil. May increase the incidence of carbamazepine toxicity. Mutual inhibition may occur if used with chloramphenicol or lincomycin. May increase hepatotoxicity if used with other hepatotoxic drugs. May increase the risk of cardiotoxicity if used with terfenadine. May increase PT if used with warfarin. May increase serum theophylline levels if used with xanthine drugs.

## INTERVENTIONS: ADMINISTRATION

Add 10 mL of sterile water for injection to a 500-mg vial or 20 mL to a 1-g vial. May be further diluted in 0.9% NSS or Ringer's lactate solution to a concentration of 1–5 mg/mL.

### MODE/RATE OF ADMINISTRATION

May be given by intermittent or continuous IV infusion.

INTRAVENOUS USE (WITH NORMAL RENAL FUNCTION)

**Adults:** The usual dosage is 250–500 mg q6h or 3.75–5 mg/kg q6h. Maximum daily dose is 4 gm.

**Children:** The usual dosage is 3.75–5 mg/kg of body weight q6h.

**Infants/Neonates:** Follow children's dosing schedule.

**Geriatrics:** Follow adult dosing schedule.

INTRATHECAL USE OR OTHER INFUSION ROUTES AS INDICATED. Not recommended.

### POTENTIAL PROBLEMS IN ADMINISTRATION

If administering the agent to neonates, use of diluents containing benzyl alcohol may precipitate a fatal toxic syndrome.

### INDEPENDENT NURSING ACTIONS

Monitor vital signs and laboratory values, especially BUN, serum creatinine, and PT. Collect specimens as required. Keep skin clean and dry. Change dressings as needed. Use appropriate aseptic techniques and isolation precautions. Teach risk factors for infection.

**ADMINISTRATION IN ALTERNATE SETTINGS**

May be given in a variety of clinical settings and in the home by a qualified IV nurse.

**EVALUATION: OUTCOMES OF DRUG THERAPY**

**EXPECTED OUTCOMES**

PHYSICAL ASSESSMENT. Temperature less than 37.5° C. Pulse between 60 and 100 bpm and regular. Skin warm, pink, and dry. No rashes, no flushing, no drainage. Breath sounds clear. Clear yellow urine. Clear CSF. No complaints of headache or abdominal pain, chills, malaise, or lethargy.

LABORATORY. BUN between 10 and 20 mg/dL. Serum creatinine between 0.7 and 1.4 mg/dL. White blood count 5000 to 10,000/mm$^3$. Neutrophils 60% to 70%. Erythrocyte sedimentation rate below 20 mm/h. No abnormal findings from cultures of urine, blood, or CSF.

**NEGATIVE OUTCOMES**

Temperature more than 37.5° C. Pulse more than 100 bpm and irregular. Client complains of headache, abdominal pain, muscle aches, malaise, or lethargy. Hot, flushed skin. Rashes. Diaphoresis. Client may have neck rigidity or discharge or drainage from wounds. Nausea, vomiting, diarrhea.

## PENICILLINS

### THERAPEUTIC EFFECTS

Penicillins are usually bactericidal. They bind with penicillin-binding receptor sites in the cytoplasmic membranes. They inhibit bacterial septal and cell wall synthesis, probably by causing protein chains to tangle. Penicillins also inhibit cell division and growth and cause lysis of susceptible bacteria. Rapidly dividing bacteria are most susceptible.

### PHARMACOKINETICS

**Distribution.** Penicillins are widely distributed throughout most body fluids and bone. They penetrate poorly into the eye and normal meninges. Inflammation of the meninges improves penetration of the blood-brain barrier.

**Excretion.** The half-life of penicilins in adults with normal renal function is usually between 0.5 and 1.5 hours. If renal function is impaired, the half-life of penicillins is extended as much as 10 to 15 times normal.

## CAUTIONS

Penicillins are one of the most common causes of drug allergy. Between 1% and 10% of clients who receive penicillin experience an allergic reaction. Further, cross allergy is common. Clients who are allergic to one penicillin should be considered to be allergic to all penicillins. In addition, between 5% and 10% of clients who are allergic to penicillins are allergic to cephalosporins.

**Side/Adverse Effects.** Penicillins may cause allergic reactions, rash, joint pain, fever, hives, itching, neutropenia, platelet dysfunction, seizures, pseudomembranous colitis with severe abdominal cramps, diarrhea, nausea, vomiting, or oral candidiasis.

### Contraindications

***Pregnancy and Lactation.*** Penicillins cross the placental barrier. Studies have not indicated that penicillins cause fetal harm. They are excreted in breast milk. They may cause allergic responses, rashes, diarrhea, and candidiasis in the infant.

***Pediatrics.*** Penicillins should be used with caution and in reduced doses in premature and full-term neonates younger than 6 weeks due to renal immaturity since excretion may be delayed.

***Geriatrics.*** Age does not appear to pose specific problems. However, the elderly are more at risk for age-related diminished renal function, which may require that doses be decreased.

## TOXICITY

Toxicities of penicillins are listed in Table 16–5.

## POTENTIAL DRUG/FOOD INTERACTIONS

Penicillins may interact with estrogen-based contraceptives to diminish their effectiveness. Probenecid may inhibit renal excretion of penicillin and prolong penicillin's half-life. Use of anticoagulants, heparin, nonsteroidal antiinflammatory drugs (NSAIDs), platelet aggregate inhibitors, sulfinpyrazone, or other thrombolytic agents with ticarcillin may increase the risk of hemorrhage. Use of captopril, potassium-sparing diuretics, enalapril, lisinopril, or potassium supplements may cause hyperkalemia.

---

## PENICILLIN G POTASSIUM

*Trade Name:* Pfizerpen
*Canadian Availability:* Ayercillin
*Pregnancy Risk:* Category B
*pH:* 6–7

*Storage/Stability:* Store below 40° C. May be stored at room temperature for 24 hours or for 7 days if refrigerated after reconstituting.

▼

**TABLE 16–5**
**Penicillin Toxicities**

| Body System | Side/Toxic Effects | Physical Assessment Indicators | Laboratory Indicators | Nursing Interventions |
|---|---|---|---|---|
| Renal | Interstitial nephritis | Fever, rash, decreased urine output, proteinuria, hematuria | Protein in urine, RBCs in urine | Encourage fluids to 2000 mL/24h unless contraindicated; measure and record intake and output; monitor laboratory values and report abnormal findings. |
| Gastrointestinal | Pseudomembranous colitis | Severe abdominal pain, stomach cramps, tenderness, severe diarrhea, fever | N/A | Auscultate bowel sounds; report diarrhea or pain. |
| | Oral candidiasis | Sore mouth and tongue | | |
| Hematologic | Neutropenia | Sore throat, fever | Decreased RBC, Hgb, Hct, WBC, platelets | Observe for unusual bleeding; monitor laboratory values and report abnormal values. |
| | Platelet dysfunction | Bruising, unusual bleeding | | |
| Other | Allergic reactions or anaphylactic shock | Bronchospasm, hypotension, rash, hives, itching, skin rash, joint pain, fever | N/A | Auscultate breath sounds. |
| | Serum sickness–like reaction | | | |

Hct = hematocrit, Hgb = hemoglobin, N/A = not applicable, RBC = red blood cell count, WBC = white blood cell count.

## ASSESSMENT: DRUG CHARACTERISTICS

### ACTION

A broad-spectrum antibiotic. Binds with penicillin-binding receptor sites in the cytoplasmic membranes. May also inhibit cell wall synthesis and cell division and growth and cause lysis of susceptible bacteria. Rapidly dividing bacteria are most susceptible.

### INDICATIONS

Used to treat a wide variety of gram-positive aerobic and anaerobic and gram-negative cocci and bacilli infections, including pneumococcal pneumonia, meningococcal meningitis, gonococcal arthritis, bacterial septicemias, syphilis, and Lyme disease.

### CAUTIONS

ADVERSE EFFECTS. Allergic reactions, rash, joint pain, fever, hives, itching, neutropenia, bleeding, seizures, severe abdominal cramps, diarrhea, nausea, vomiting, or oral candidiasis.

CONTRAINDICATIONS. History of hypersensitivity to penicillins, cephalosporins, cephamycins, or penicillamine. Should be used with caution in clients with a history of bleeding disorder, gastrointestinal disorders such as ulcerative colitis, infectious mononucleosis, or impaired renal function.

### POTENTIAL DRUG/FOOD INTERACTIONS

May interact with captopril, potassium-sparing diuretics, enalapril, lisinopril, or potassium supplements to cause hyperkalemia. Cholestyramine or colestipol may inhibit the absorption of penicillin G. Probenecid may inhibit renal excretion of penicillin G and prolong the half-life of penicillin G.

## INTERVENTIONS: ADMINISTRATION

Dilute with sterile water for injection. May be further diluted with 0.9% NSS.

### MODE/RATE OF ADMINISTRATION

May be given by intermittent or continuous IV infusion using an infusion pump.

#### INTRAVENOUS USE (WITH NORMAL RENAL FUNCTION)

**Adults:** For most infections the usual dosage is 10,000,000–20,000,000 U/d in divided doses q4–6h. Dosages as low as 1,000,000 to as high as 24,000,000 U/d are not unusual. Adult dosage limit should not exceed 100,000,000 U/d.

**Children > 12 years:** Follow adult dosing schedule.

**Infants/Neonates:** For premature infants and full-term neonates the usual dosage is 30,000 U/kg of body weight q12h.

**Older Infants/Children ≤12 years:** For older infants and children up to age 12 the usual dosage is 4167–16,667 U/kg of body weight q4h or 6250–25,000 U/kg of body weight q6h.

**Geriatrics:** Elderly clients may be more likely to have age-related diminished renal function that would require a lower dosing schedule.

INTRATHECAL USE OR OTHER INFUSION ROUTES AS INDICATED. Not recommended.

**POTENTIAL PROBLEMS IN ADMINISTRATION**

Penicillin G potassium is inactivated by solutions that are acid or alkaline or contain oxidizing agents or carbohydrates. Should be administered at least 1 hour after aminoglycosides. May cause mutual inactivation if given sooner.

**INDEPENDENT NURSING ACTIONS**

Monitor vital signs and laboratory values, especially BUN, and serum creatinine. Collect specimens as required. Keep skin clean and dry. Change dressings as needed. Use appropriate aseptic techniques and isolation precautions. Teach risk factors for infection.

**ADMINISTRATION IN ALTERNATE SETTINGS**

May be given in a variety of clinical settings and in the home by a qualified IV nurse.

**EVALUATION: OUTCOMES OF DRUG THERAPY**

**EXPECTED OUTCOMES**

PHYSICAL ASSESSMENT. Temperature less than 37.5° C. Pulse between 60 and 100 bpm and regular. Skin warm, pink, and dry. No rashes, no flushing, no drainage. Breath sounds clear. Clear yellow urine. Clear CSF. No complaints of headache or abdominal pain, chills, malaise, or lethargy.

LABORATORY. BUN between 10 and 20 mg/dL. Serum creatinine between 0.7 and 1.4 mg/dL. White blood count 5000 to 10,000/mm$^3$. Neutrophils 60% to 70%. Erythrocyte sedimentation rate below 20 mm/h. Negative cultures of urine, blood, or CSF.

**NEGATIVE OUTCOMES**

Temperature more than 37.5° C. Pulse more than 100 bpm and irregular. Client complains of headache, abdominal pain, muscle aches, malaise, or lethargy. Hot, flushed skin. Rashes. Diaphoresis. Client may have neck rigidity or discharge or drainage from wounds.

## Penicillinase-Resistant Penicillins

### METHICILLIN

*Trade Name:* Staphcillin
*Canadian Availability:* Not specified.
*Pregnancy Risk:* Category B
*pH:* 6–8.5
*Storage/Stability:* Store below 40° C. May be stored at room temperature for 4 hours for concentrations of 2 mg/mL or for 8 hours for concentrations of 10 to 30 mg/mL. If refrigerated, stable for up to 96 hours.

▼

## ASSESSMENT: DRUG CHARACTERISTICS

### ACTION

A broad-spectrum antibiotic with bactericidal action. Binds with penicillin-binding receptor sites in the cytoplasmic membranes. May also inhibit cell wall synthesis and cell division and growth and cause lysis of susceptible bacteria. Rapidly dividing bacteria are most susceptible.

### INDICATIONS

Used to treat a wide variety of gram-positive aerobic and anaerobic organisms, especially penicillinase-producing staphylococci. Used to treat infections due to susceptible strains of penicillinase-producing staphylococci causing infections of the respiratory tract, skin, bones, joints, urinary tract, endocarditis, septicemia, and meningitis.

### CAUTIONS

ADVERSE EFFECTS. Allergic reactions, rash, joint pain, fever, hives, and itching. Neutropenia, bleeding, seizures, anemia, glossitis, monilial (oral and rectal) infections, nephrotoxicity (interstitial nephritis), and stomatitis may occur. There have been reports of diarrhea, nausea, vomiting, and in some cases hepatitis. Hypersensitivity myocarditis can occur with the client exhibiting fever, eosinophilia, rash, sinus tachycardia, ST-T changes, and cardiomegaly.

CONTRAINDICATIONS. History of hypersensitivity to penicillins or cephalosporins.

### POTENTIAL DRUG/FOOD INTERACTIONS

Chloramphenicol, erythromycin, and tetracyclines inactivate methicillin's bactericidal action. Aminohippuric acid and probenecid each act to inhibit renal excretion of methicillin and prolong its half-life, thus possibly causing toxicities. As with other penicillins, administration within an hour of aminoglycosides yields both drugs inactivated. Use with clients who are receiving $\beta$-adrenergic blockers (propranolol) increases the risk of anaphylaxis. Anticoagulation effect of heparin is increased in the presence of methicillin. Client must be observed for bleeding. Clients taking oral contraceptive agents should be advised that methicillin inhibits the effectiveness of these drugs and the client may experience breakthrough bleeding or become pregnant.

## INTERVENTIONS: ADMINISTRATION

Dilute with 1.8 mL of sterile water for injection for each 1-g vial (5.7 mL for each 4-g vial; 8.6 mL for each 6-g vial) for a concentration of 500 mg/mL. May be further diluted with 25 mL for each 500 mg (1 mL) of 0.9% NSS for injection.

### MODE/RATE OF ADMINISTRATION

Administer each 10 mL of solution over 1 min or longer. More rapid administration may cause vein irritation. May be given by IV infusion over 30 min or over a period of up to 8h.

INTRAVENOUS USE (WITH NORMAL RENAL FUNCTION)

**Adults:** For most infections the usual dosage is 4–12 g/24 h in equally divided doses q4–6h. Dose should not exceed 2 g/12 h for clients with a creatinine clearance of less than 10 mL/min.

**Children > 12 years:** Follow adult dosing schedule.

**Children < 12 years:** Administer 100–300 mg/kg of body weight in 24 h in equally divided doses q4–6h.

**Neonates < 2000 g and < 7 days:** 50 mg/kg of body weight per 24 h in equally divided doses q12h (for meningitis—100 mg/kg/24h).

**Neonates < 2000 g and > 7 days:** 75 mg/kg/24h in equally divided doses q8h (for meningitis—150 mg/kg/24 h).

**Neonates > 2000 g and < 7 days:** 75 mg/kg/24h in equaly divided doses q8h (for meningitis—150 mg/kg/24h).

**Neonates > 2000 g and > 7 days:** 100 mg/kg/24h in equally divided doses q6h (for meningitis—150–200 mg/kg/24h).

**Geriatrics:** Elderly clients may be more likely to have age-related diminished renal function that would require a lower dosing schedule.

INTRATHECAL USE OR OTHER INFUSION ROUTES AS INDICATED. Not recommended.

**POTENTIAL PROBLEMS IN ADMINISTRATION**

Should be administered at least 1 hour after aminoglycosides. May cause mutual inactivation if given sooner.

**INDEPENDENT NURSING ACTIONS**

Monitor vital signs and laboratory values, especially BUN, serum creatinine, and PT. Collect specimens as required. Keep skin clean and dry. Change dressings as needed. Use appropriate aseptic techniques and isolation precautions. Teach risk factors for infection and signs and symptoms of suprainfections.

**ADMINISTRATION IN ALTERNATE SETTINGS**

May be given in a variety of clinical settings and in the home by a qualified IV nurse.

**EVALUATION: OUTCOMES OF DRUG THERAPY**

**EXPECTED OUTCOMES**

PHYSICAL ASSESSMENT. Temperature less than 37.5° C. Pulse between 60 and 100 bpm and regular. Skin warm, pink, and dry. No rashes, no flushing, no drainage. Breath sounds clear. Clear yellow urine. Clear CSF. No complaints of headache or abdominal pain, chills, malaise, or lethargy.

LABORATORY. BUN between 10 and 20 mg/dL. Serum creatinine between 0.7 and 1.4 mg/dL. White blood count 5000 to 10,000/mm$^3$. Neutrophils 60% to 70%. Erythrocyte sedimentation rate below 20 mm/h. No abnormal findings from cultures of urine, blood, or CSF.

**NEGATIVE OUTCOMES**

Temperature more than 37.5° C. Pulse more than 100

▼

bpm and irregular. Client complains of headache, abdominal pain, muscle aches, malaise, or lethargy. Hot, flushed skin. Rashes. Diaphoresis. Client may have neck rigidity or discharge or drainage from wounds.

## NAFCILLIN

*Trade Names:* Nafcil, Unipen
*Canadian Availability:* Unipen
*Pregnancy Risk:* Category B
*pH:* 6–6.5
*Storage/Stability:* Store below 40° C. May be stored at room temperature for 24 hours or for 96 hours if refrigerated after reconstituting to a concentration of 2 to 40 mg/mL. Do not use if darker than very pale yellow.

### ASSESSMENT: DRUG CHARACTERISTICS

#### ACTION

A broad-spectrum antibiotic. Binds with penicillin-binding receptor sites in the cytoplasmic membranes. May also inhibit cell wall synthesis and cell division and growth and cause lysis of susceptible bacteria. Rapidly dividing bacteria are most susceptible.

#### INDICATIONS

Used to treat a wide variety of gram-positive aerobic and anaerobic and gram-negative cocci and bacilli infections, including staphylococcal pneumonia, bacterial septicemias, skin and soft tissue infections, and sinusitis.

#### CAUTIONS

ADVERSE EFFECTS. Allergic reactions, rash, joint pain, fever, hives, itching, neutropenia, bleeding, seizures, severe abdominal cramps, diarrhea, nausea, vomiting, or oral candidiasis.

CONTRAINDICATIONS. History of hypersensitivity to penicillins, cephalosporins, cephamycins, or penicillamine. Should be used with caution in clients with a history of bleeding disorder, gastrointestinal disorders such as ulcerative colitis, infectious mononucleosis, or impaired renal function.

#### POTENTIAL DRUG/FOOD INTERACTIONS

May interact with probenecid to inhibit renal excretion of nafcillin and prolong the half-life of nafcillin.

### INTERVENTIONS: ADMINISTRATION

Dilute with 1.7–1.8 mL of sterile water for injection, 0.9% NSS, or D5W solution for each 500-mg vial for a concentration of 250 mg/mL. For IV push, further dilute in 15–30 mL of 0.9% NSS.

#### MODE/RATE OF ADMINISTRATION

May be given by IV push at 500 mg over 5 min or by intermittent IV infusion over 30 min, using an infusion pump.

INTRAVENOUS USE (WITH NORMAL RENAL FUNCTION)

**Adults:** For most infections the usual dosage is 500 mg–1.5 g q4h. Maximum dose should not exceed 20 g/d.

**Children >12 years:** Follow adult dosing schedule.

**Neonates:** The usual dosage is 10–20 mg/kg of body weight q4h or 20–40 mg//kg of body weight q8h.

**Infants and Children 6 weeks–12 years:** The usual dosage is 25 mg/kg of body weight q4h or 20–40 mg/kg of body weight q8h.

**Geriatrics:** Elderly clients may be more likely to have age-related diminished renal function that would require a lower dosing schedule.

INTRATHECAL USE OR OTHER INFUSION ROUTES AS INDICATED. Not recommended.

**POTENTIAL PROBLEMS IN ADMINISTRATION**

Should be administered at least 1 hour after aminoglycosides. May cause mutual inactivation if given sooner.

**INDEPENDENT NURSING ACTIONS**

Monitor vital signs and laboratory values, especially BUN, serum creatinine, and PT. Collect specimens as required. Keep skin clean and dry. Change dressings as needed. Use appropriate aseptic techniques and isolation precautions. Teach risk factors for infection.

**ADMINISTRATION IN ALTERNATE SETTINGS**

May be given in a variety of clinical settings and in the home by a qualified IV nurse.

**EVALUATION: OUTCOMES OF DRUG THERAPY**

**EXPECTED OUTCOMES**

PHYSICAL ASSESSMENT. Temperature less than 37.5° C. Pulse between 60 and 100 bpm and regular. Skin warm, pink, and dry. No rashes, no flushing, no drainage. Breath sounds clear. Clear yellow urine. Clear CSF. No complaints of headache or abdominal pain, chills, malaise, or lethargy.

LABORATORY. BUN between 10 and 20 mg/dL. Serum creatinine between 0.7 and 1.4 mg/dL. White blood count 5000 to 10,000/mm$^3$. Neutrophils 60% to 70%. Erythrocyte sedimentation rate below 20 mm/h. No abnormal findings from cultures of urine, blood, or CSF.

**NEGATIVE OUTCOMES**

Temperature more than 37.5° C. Pulse more than 100 bpm and irregular. Client complains of headache, abdominal pain, muscle aches, malaise, or lethargy. Hot, flushed skin. Rashes. Diaphoresis. Client may have neck rigidity or discharge or drainage from wounds.

## OXACILLIN

*Trade Names:* Bactocill, Prostaphlin
*Canadian Availability:* Not specified
*Pregnancy Risk:* Category B
*pH:* 6–8.5
*Storage/Stability:* Store below 40° C. May be stored at room temperature for 3 days or 7 days if refrigerated after reconstituting to a concentration of 250 mg/1.5 mL.

### ASSESSMENT: DRUG CHARACTERISTICS

#### ACTION

Semisynthetic penicillin with bactericidal effect. Resistant to the action of penicillinase. Binds with penicillin-binding receptor sites in the cytoplasmic membranes. May also inhibit cell wall synthesis and cell division and growth and cause lysis of susceptible bacteria. Rapidly dividing bacteria are most susceptible.

#### INDICATIONS

Used to treat a wide variety of gram-positive aerobic and anaerobic and gram-negative cocci and bacilli infections, including staphylococcal pneumonia, bacterial septicemias, skin and soft tissue infections, bone and joint infections, urinary tract infections, endocarditis, and meningitis.

#### CAUTIONS

ADVERSE EFFECTS. Allergic reactions, rash, joint pain, fever, hives, itching, neutropenia, bleeding, seizures, severe abdominal cramps, diarrhea, nausea, vomiting, or suprainfections such as oral candidiasis. May cause neuromuscular excitability and seizures if given in higher than usual doses. Clients with cystic fibrosis experience a higher incidence of adverse effects.

CONTRAINDICATIONS. History of hypersensitivity to penicillins or cephalothin. Should be used with caution in clients with a history of bleeding disorders, gastrointestinal disorders such as ulcerative colitis, infectious mononucleosis, or impaired renal function.

#### POTENTIAL DRUG/FOOD INTERACTIONS

Chloramphenicol, erythromycin, and tetracyclines inactivate oxacillin's bactericidal action. Aminohippuric acid and probenecid each act to inhibit renal excretion of oxacillin and prolong its half-life, thus possibly causing toxicities. As with other penicillins, administration within an hour of aminoglycosides yields both drugs inactivated. Use with clients receiving $\beta$-adrenergic blockers (propranolol) increases the risk of anaphylaxis. Anticoagulation effect of heparin is increased in the presence of oxacillin. Client must be observed for bleeding. Clients taking oral contraceptive agents should be advised that oxacillin inhibits the effectiveness of these drugs and the client may experience break-through bleeding or become pregnant.

**INTERVENTIONS: ADMINISTRATION**

Dilute with 1.4 mL of sterile water for injection, 0.9% NSS, or D5W solution for each 250-mg vial (2.7–2.8 mL to each 500-mg vial, 5.7 mL to each 1-g vial). For IV push, further dilute in 5 mL of sterile water or 0.9% NSS.

**MODE/RATE OF ADMINISTRATION**

Each gram may be given by IV push over 10 min or by intermittent IV infusion over 30 min or over a period of up to 6 h.

INTRAVENOUS USE (WITH NORMAL RENAL FUNCTION)

**Adults:** For most infections the usual dosage is 1–2 g q4h. Maximum dosage should not exceed 20 g/d.

**Children > 12 years:** Follow adult dosing schedule.

**Children < 40 kg:** 250–1 g q4–6h. Maximum dose should not exceed 200 mg/kg/24 h.

**Infants/Neonates:** The usual dosage is 25 mg/kg of body weight in 24 h in equally divided doses q6h for premature infants and neonates.

**Geriatrics:** Elderly clients may be more likely to have age-related diminished renal function that would require a lower dosing schedule.

INTRATHECAL USE OR OTHER INFUSION ROUTES AS INDICATED. Not recommended.

**POTENTIAL PROBLEMS IN ADMINISTRATION**

Should be administered at least 1 hour after aminoglycosides. May cause mutual inactivation if given sooner.

**INDEPENDENT NURSING ACTIONS**

Monitor vital signs and laboratory values, especially BUN, serum creatinine, and PT. Collect specimens as required. Keep skin clean and dry. Change dressings as needed. Use appropriate aseptic techniques and isolation precautions. Teach risk factors for infection.

**ADMINISTRATION IN ALTERNATE SETTINGS**

May be given in a variety of clinical settings and in the home by a qualified IV nurse.

**EVALUATION: OUTCOMES OF DRUG THERAPY**

**EXPECTED OUTCOMES**

PHYSICAL ASSESSMENT. Temperature less than 37.5° C. Pulse between 60 and 100 bpm and regular. Skin warm, pink, and dry. No rashes, no flushing, no drainage. Breath sounds clear. Clear yellow urine. Clear CSF. No complaints of headache or abdominal pain, chills, malaise, or lethargy.

LABORATORY. BUN between 10 and 20 mg/dL. Serum creatinine between 0.7 and 1.4 mg/dL. White blood count 5000 to 10,000/mm$^3$. Neutrophils 60% to 70%. Erythrocyte sedimentation rate below 20 mm/h. No abnormal findings from cultures of urine, blood, or CSF.

**NEGATIVE OUTCOMES**

Temperature more than 37.5° C. Pulse more than

▼

100 bpm and irregular. Client complains of headache, abdominal pain, muscle aches, malaise, or lethargy. Hot, flushed skin. Rashes. Diaphoresis. Client may have neck rigidity or discharge or drainage from wounds.

## Ampicillins

### Ampicillin Sodium

*Trade Names:* Omnipen-N, Polycillin-N, Totacillin-N,
*Canadian Availability:* Ampicin, Ampilean, Penbritin
*Pregnancy Risk:* Category B
*pH:* 8.5–10
*Storage/Stability:* Store below 40° C. May be stored at room temperature for 24 hours or for 7 days if refrigerated after reconstituting.

**ASSESSMENT: DRUG CHARACTERISTICS**

**ACTION**

A broad-spectrum antibiotic. Binds with penicillin-binding receptor sites in the cytoplasmic membranes. May also inhibit cell wall synthesis and cell division and growth and cause lysis of susceptible bacteria. Rapidly dividing bacteria are most susceptible.

**INDICATIONS**

Used to treat a wide variety of gram-positive aerobic and anaerobic and gram-negative cocci and bacilli infections, including genitourinary tract infections, pneumonia, meningitis, otitis media, gonorrhea, some gastrointestinal tract infections, bacterial septicemias, skin and soft tissue disease, and sinusitis.

**CAUTIONS**

**ADVERSE EFFECTS.** Allergic reactions, rash, joint pain, fever, hives, itching, neutropenia, bleeding, seizures, severe abdominal cramps, diarrhea, nausea, vomiting, or oral candidiasis.

**CONTRAINDICATIONS.** History of hypersensitivity to penicillins, cephalosporins, cephamycins, or penicillamine. Should be used with caution in clients with a history of bleeding disorder, gastrointestinal disorders such as ulcerative colitis, infectious mononucleosis, or impaired renal function.

**POTENTIAL DRUG/FOOD INTERACTIONS**

May interact with estrogen-based contraceptives to diminish their effectiveness. Probenecid may inhibit renal excretion of ampicillin and prolong the half-life.

**INTERVENTIONS: ADMINISTRATION**

Dilute with 0.9–1.2 mL of sterile water for injection to each 125-mg vial. May further dilute with 0.9% NSS. Further dilute with 5 mL of sterile water for injection for IV push or 50 mL of 0.9%

NSS or D5W solution for intermittent infusion.

**MODE/RATE OF ADMINISTRATION**

May be given by IV push at a rate not to exceed 500 mg in 5 min or intermittent IV infusion over 30 min using an infusion pump.

INTRAVENOUS USE (WITH NORMAL RENAL FUNCTION)

**Adults:** For most infections the usual dosage is 250–500 mg q6h.

For bacterial meningitis the usual dosage is 1–2 g q3–4h or 18.75–25 mg/kg of body weight q3h or 25–33.3 mg/kg of body weight q4h.

For gonorrhea the usual dosage is 500 mg q8–12h for two doses.

Maximum dose should not exceed 16 g/d.

**Children > 12 years:** Follow adult dosing schedule.

**Children > 20 kg of body weight:** Follow adult dosing schedule.

**Children < 20 kg of body weight:** The usual dosage is 6.25–25 mg/kg of body weight q6h or 8.3–33.3 mg/kg of body weight q8h.

**Geriatrics:** Elderly clients may be more likely to have age-related diminished renal function that would require a lower dosing schedule.

INTRATHECAL USE OR OTHER INFUSION ROUTES AS INDICATED. Not recommended.

**POTENTIAL PROBLEMS IN ADMINISTRATION**

Should be administered at least 1 hour after aminoglycosides. May cause mutual inactivation if given sooner.

**INDEPENDENT NURSING ACTIONS**

Monitor vital signs and laboratory values, especially BUN, serum creatinine, and PT. Collect specimens as required. Keep skin clean and dry. Change dressings as needed. Use appropriate aseptic techniques and isolation precautions. Teach risk factors for infection.

**ADMINISTRATION IN ALTERNATE SETTINGS**

May be given in a variety of clinical settings and in the home by a qualified IV nurse.

**EVALUATION: OUTCOMES OF DRUG THERAPY**

**EXPECTED OUTCOMES**

PHYSICAL ASSESSMENT. Temperature less than 37.5° C. Pulse between 60 and 100 bpm and regular. Skin warm, pink, and dry. No rashes, no flushing, no drainage. Breath sounds clear. Clear yellow urine. Clear CSF. No complaints of headache or abdominal pain, chills, malaise, or lethargy.

LABORATORY. BUN between 10 and 20 mg/dL. Serum creatinine between 0.7 and 1.4 mg/dL. White blood count 5000 to 10,000/mm$^3$. Neutrophils 60% to 70%. Erythrocyte sedimentation rate below 20 mm/h. No abnormal findings from cultures of urine, blood, or CSF. PT 9.5 to 12 seconds.

**NEGATIVE OUTCOMES**

Temperature more than 37.5° C. Pulse more than

▼

100 bpm and irregular. Client complains of headache, abdominal pain, muscle aches, malaise, or lethargy. Hot, flushed skin. Rashes. Diaphoresis. Client may have neck rigidity or discharge or drainage from wounds.

## Ampicillin Sodium and Sulbactam Sodium

*Trade Name:* Unasyn
*Canadian Availability:* Not specified
*Pregnancy Risk:* Category C
*pH:* 8–10
*Storage/Stability:* Store below 40° C. Use within 1 hour after reconstituting with sterile water for injection. May be stored for up to 8 hours at a temperature below 25° C if reconstituted to a concentration of 45 mg/mL with 0.9% NSS or sterile water for injection. Dextrose solutions may cause inactivation and should not be used.

### ASSESSMENT: DRUG CHARACTERISTICS

#### ACTION

A broad-spectrum antiinfective that is bactericidal in action and is effective against a wide range of gram-positive and gram-negative agents. Ampicillin binds with penicillin-binding receptor sites in the cytoplasmic membranes. May also inhibit cell wall synthesis and cell division and growth and cause lysis of susceptible bacteria. Sulbactam has a strong affinity for and inhibits the β-lactamases. Jointly, ampicillin and sulbactam act synergistically against *Pseudomonas, Citrobacter, Enterobacter,* and *Serratia* but do not seem to cause type 1 chromosomally mediated cephalosporinases.

#### INDICATIONS

Generally used to treat skin, skin structure, and gynecologic infections caused by gram-positive aerobic cocci such as *Streptococcus pneumoniae, Staphylococcus aureus* (including methicillin-resistant strains), and *Enterococcus faecalis.* Also used to treat infections, including CNS infections, caused by gram-negative aerobic cocci such as *Neisseria* (including penicillin-resistant strains), *Haemophilus, Enterobacteriaceae,* and *Acinetobacter.* Has also been used to treat some anaerobic bacterial infections that may be resistant to other agents such as clindamycin, metronidazole, and other β-lactam antibiotics.

#### CAUTIONS

ADVERSE EFFECTS. Most commonly, pain at the injection site and diarrhea; nausea and vomiting and symptoms of pseudomembranous colitis such as abdominal pain, diarrhea, and bloody stools; pruritus, urticaria, dry skin, erythema, or other allergic reactions.

CONTRAINDICATIONS. History of hypersensitivity to penicillins, cephalosporins, cephamycins, or penicillamine. Should be used with caution in clients with a history of bleeding disorder, gastrointestinal disorders such as ulcerative colitis, infectious mononucleosis, or impaired renal function.

**POTENTIAL DRUG/FOOD INTERACTIONS**

May interact with aminoglycosides and cause inactivation of amikin, gentamicin, netilmicin, and tobramycin. Probenecid delays the renal excretion of sulbactam and will increase the half-life up to 45%. Use with allopurinol in clients with hyperuricemia may cause a rash.

**INTERVENTIONS: ADMINISTRATION**

Reconstitute with 0.9% NSS or sterile water for injection.

**MODE/RATE OF ADMINISTRATION**

May be given by IV push slowly over 10–15 min. May be given by intermittent IV infusion over 15–30 min.

INTRAVENOUS USE (WITH NORMAL RENAL FUNCTION)

**Adults:** The usual dosage for skin, skin structure, intra-abdominal, or gynecologic infections is 1.5 g (1 g ampicillin and 0.5 g sulbactam) to 3 g (2 g of ampicillin and 1 g sulbactam) q6h.

For clients with renal disease and creatinine clearance of 30 mL/min, the usual dosage is 1.5–3 g q6–8h. For clients with creatinine clearances of 15–29 mL/min or 5–14 mL/min the usual dosage is 1.5–3 g q12h or q24h, respectively.

**Children > 12 years:** Follow adult dosing schedule.

**Infants > 3 months:** The recommended dosage is 150 mg/kg of body weight in divided doses over 6–8 h.

**Infants < 3 months:** The recommended dosage is 150 mg/kg of body weight in divided doses over 12 h.

**Geriatrics:** For clients with normal renal function, follow the adult dosing schedule. For clients with renal impairment, dose adjustment should follow the recommendation for adult renal clients.

INTRATHECAL USE OR OTHER INFUSION ROUTES AS INDICATED. Not recommended.

**POTENTIAL PROBLEMS IN ADMINISTRATION**

May cause seizures if administered too rapidly. Should be administered at least 1 hour after aminoglycosides. May cause mutual inactivation if given sooner.

**INDEPENDENT NURSING ACTIONS**

Determine if client has a history of allergic reactions. Monitor vital signs and laboratory values, especially BUN, serum creatinine, and PT. Collect specimens as required. Keep skin clean and dry. Change dressings as needed. Use appropriate aseptic techniques and isolation precautions. Teach risk factors for infection.

▼

**ADMINISTRATION IN ALTERNATE SETTINGS**

May be given in a variety of clinical settings and in the home by a qualified IV nurse.

**EVALUATION: OUTCOMES OF DRUG THERAPY**

**EXPECTED OUTCOMES**

PHYSICAL ASSESSMENT. Temperature less than 37.5° C. Pulse between 60 and 100 bpm and regular. Skin warm, pink, and dry. No rashes, no flushing, no drainage. Breath sounds clear. Clear yellow urine. Clear CSF. No complaints of headache or abdominal pain, diarrhea, chills, malaise, or lethargy.

LABORATORY. BUN between 10 and 20 mg/dL. Serum creatinine between 0.7 and 1.4 mg/dL. White blood count 5000 to 10,000/mm$^3$. Neutrophils 60% to 70%. Erythrocyte sedimentation rate below 20 mm/h. No abnormal findings from cultures of urine, blood, or CSF. PT 9.5 to 12 seconds.

**NEGATIVE OUTCOMES**

Temperature more than 37.5° C. Pulse more than 100 bpm and irregular. Client complains of headache, abdominal pain, diarrhea, muscle aches, malaise, or lethargy. Hot, flushed skin, urticaria, or skin rashes. Diaphoresis. Client may have neck rigidity or discharge or drainage from wounds. Nausea, vomiting, diarrhea.

## Extended-Spectrum Penicillins

### Mezlocillin Sodium

*Trade Name:* Mezlin
Canadian Availability: Not specified.
*Pregnancy Risk:* Category B
*pH:* 4.5–8
*Storage/Stability:* Store below 40° C. May be stored at room temperature for 24 to 72 hours after reconstituting to a concentration of 10 and 100 mg/mL or for 1 to 7 days if refrigerated. Do not use if darker than very pale yellow.

**ASSESSMENT: DRUG CHARACTERISTICS**

**ACTION**

A broad-spectrum antibiotic. Binds with penicillin-binding receptor sites in the cytoplasmic membranes. May also inhibit cell wall synthesis and cell division and growth and cause lysis of susceptible bacteria. Rapidly dividing bacteria are most susceptible.

**INDICATIONS**

Used to treat a wide variety of gram-positive aerobic and anaerobic and gram-negative cocci and bacilli infections, including genitourinary tract infections, intraabdominal infections, staphylococcal pneumonia, bacterial septicemias, and skin and soft tissue infections.

**CAUTIONS**

ADVERSE EFFECTS. Allergic reactions, rash, joint pain, fever, hives, itching, neutropenia, bleeding, seizures, severe abdominal cramps, diarrhea, nausea, vomiting, or oral candidiasis.

CONTRAINDICATIONS. History of hypersensitivity to penicillins, cephalosporins, cephamycins, or penicillamine. Should be used with caution in clients with a history of bleeding disorder, gastrointestinal disorders such as ulcerative colitis, infectious mononucleosis, or impaired renal function.

**POTENTIAL DRUG/FOOD INTERACTIONS**

May interact with probenecid to inhibit renal excretion of mezlocillin and prolong the half-life of mezlocillin.

**INTERVENTIONS: ADMINISTRATION**

Dilute with at least 10 mL of sterile water for injection, 0.9% NSS, or D5W solution for each 1-g vial for a concentration of not more than 100 mg/mL. For intermittent IV infusion the concentration can be further diluted in 50–100 mL of 0.9% NSS or D5W solution.

**MODE/RATE OF ADMINISTRATION**

May be given by IV push over 3–5 min or by intermittent IV infusion.

INTRAVENOUS USE (WITH NORMAL RENAL FUNCTION)

**Adults:** For most infections the usual dosage is 33.3–58.3 mg/kg of body weight q4h or 50–87.5 mg/kg of body weight q6h or 3–4 g q4–6h. Maximum daily dose should not exceed 24 g.

**Children >12 years:** Follow adult dosing schedule.

**Children >1 month–12 years:** The usual dosage is 50 mg/kg of body weight q4h.

**Neonates 8 days–1 month:** The usual dosage is 75 mg/kg of body weight q6–8h.

**Neonates ≤ 7 days:** The usual dosage is 75 mg/kg of body weight q12h.

**Geriatrics:** Elderly clients may be more likely to have age-related diminished renal function that would require a lower dosing schedule.

INTRATHECAL USE OR OTHER INFUSION ROUTES AS INDICATED. Not recommended.

**POTENTIAL PROBLEMS IN ADMINISTRATION**

Should be administered at least 1 hour after aminoglycosides. May cause mutual inactivation if given sooner.

**INDEPENDENT NURSING ACTIONS**

Monitor vital signs and laboratory values, especially BUN, serum creatinine, and PT. Collect specimens as required. Keep skin clean and dry. Change dressings as needed. Use appropriate aseptic techniques and isolation precautions. Teach risk factors for infection.

**ADMINISTRATION IN ALTERNATE SETTINGS**

May be given in a variety of clinical settings and in the home by a qualified IV nurse.

▼

**EVALUATION: OUTCOMES OF DRUG THERAPY**

**EXPECTED OUTCOMES**

PHYSICAL ASSESSMENT. Temperature less than 37.5° C. Pulse between 60 and 100 bpm and regular. Skin warm, pink, and dry. No rashes, no flushing, no drainage. Breath sounds clear. Clear yellow urine. Clear CSF. No complaints of headache or abdominal pain, chills, malaise, or lethargy.

LABORATORY. BUN between 10 and 20 mg/dL. Serum creatinine between 0.7 and 1.4 mg/dL. White blood count 5000 to 10,000/mm³. Neutrophils 60% to 70%. Erythrocyte rate below 20 mm/h. No abnormal findings from cultures of urine, blood, or CSF. PT 9.5 to 12 seconds.

**NEGATIVE OUTCOMES**

Temperature more than 37.5° C. Pulse more than 100 bpm and irregular. Client complains of headache, abdominal pain, muscle aches, malaise, or lethargy. Hot, flushed skin. Rashes. Diaphoresis. Client may have neck rigidity or discharge or drainage from wounds.

## PIPERACILLIN

*Trade Name:* Pipracil
*Canadian Availability:* Pipracil
*Pregnancy Risk:* Category B
*pH:* 5.5–7.5
*Storage/Stability:* Store below 40° C. May be stored at room temperature for 24 hours, for 7 days if refrigerated, or for 1 month if frozen after reconstituting to a concentration of 1 g/2.5 mL. Do not use if darker than very pale yellow.

**ASSESSMENT: DRUG CHARACTERISTICS**

**ACTION**

A broad-spectrum antibiotic. Binds with penicillin-binding receptor sites in the cytoplasmic membranes. May also inhibit cell wall synthesis and cell division and growth and cause lysis of susceptible bacteria. Rapidly dividing bacteria are most susceptible.

**INDICATIONS**

Used to treat a wide variety of gram-positive aerobic and anaerobic and gram-negative cocci and bacilli infections, including bone and joint infections, genitourinary tract infections, intraabdominal infections, pneumonias, bacterial septicemias, and skin and soft tissue infections.

**CAUTIONS**

ADVERSE EFFECTS. Allergic reactions, rash, joint pain, fever, hives, itching, neutropenia, bleeding, seizures, severe abdominal cramps, diarrhea, nausea, vomiting, or oral candidiasis.

CONTRAINDICATIONS. History of hypersensitivity to penicillins, cephalosporins, cephamycins, or penicillamine. Should be used with caution in clients with a history of bleeding disorder, gastrointestinal disorders such as ulcerative colitis, infectious mononucleosis, or impaired renal function.

**POTENTIAL DRUG/FOOD INTERACTIONS**

May interact with probenecid to inhibit renal excretion of piperacillin and prolong the half-life of piperacillin.

**INTERVENTIONS: ADMINISTRATION**

Dilute with at least 5 mL of sterile water for injection, 0.9% NSS, or D5W solution for each 1-g vial for a concentration of 100 mg/mL. May be further diluted in 50–100 mL of solution.

**MODE/RATE OF ADMINISTRATION**

May be given reconstituted but undiluted by IV push over 3–5 min or by intermittent IV infusion over 30 min using an infusion pump.

INTRAVENOUS USE (WITH NORMAL RENAL FUNCTION)

**Adults:** For most infections the usual adult dosage is 4 g q4–6h.

For perioperative prophylaxis the usual adult dosage is 2 g 30 min–1 h prior to surgery, 2 g during surgery, and 2 g q6h for 24 h following surgery. Maximum dosage should not exceed 24 g daily.

**Children >12 years:** Follow adult dosing schedule.

**Infants/Neonates:** Dose not established.

**Geriatrics:** Elderly clients may be more likely to have age-related diminished renal function that would require a lower dosing schedule.

INTRATHECAL USE OR OTHER INFUSION ROUTES AS INDICATED. Not recommended.

**POTENTIAL PROBLEMS IN ADMINISTRATION**

Should be administered at least 1 hour after aminoglycosides. May cause mutual inactivation if given sooner.

**INDEPENDENT NURSING ACTIONS**

Monitor vital signs and laboratory values, especially BUN, and serum creatinine. Collect specimens as required. Keep skin clean and dry. Change dressings as needed. Use appropriate aseptic techniques and isolation precautions. Teach risk factors for infection.

**ADMINISTRATION IN ALTERNATE SETTINGS**

May be given in a variety of clinical settings and in the home by a qualified IV nurse.

**EVALUATION: OUTCOMES OF DRUG THERAPY**

**EXPECTED OUTCOMES**

PHYSICAL ASSESSMENT. Temperature less than 37.5° C. Pulse between 60 and 100 bpm and regular. Skin warm, pink, and dry. No rashes, no flushing, no drainage. Breath sounds clear. Clear yellow urine. Clear CSF. No complaints of headache, abdominal pain, chills, malaise, lethargy, nausea, vomiting, or diarrhea.

LABORATORY. BUN between 10 and 20 mg/dL. Serum creatinine between 0.7 and 1.4 mg/dL. White blood count 5000 to 10,000/mm$^3$. Neutrophils 60% to 70%. Eryth-

▼

rocyte sedimentation rate below 20 mm/h. No abnormal findings from cultures of urine, blood, or CSF. PT 9.5 to 12 seconds.

**NEGATIVE OUTCOMES**

Temperature more than 37.5° C. Pulse more than 100 bpm and irregular. Client complains of headache, abdominal pain, muscle aches, malaise, or lethargy. Hot, flushed skin. Rashes. Diaphoresis. May have neck rigidity or discharge or drainage from wounds.

---

## TICARCILLIN DISODIUM

*Trade Name:* Ticar
*Canadian Availability:* Ticar
*Pregnancy Risk:* Category B
*pH:* 6–8
*Storage/Stability:* Store below 40° C. May be stored at room temperature for 6 hours or for 72 hours if refrigerated after reconstituting to a concentration of 200 mg/mL. May be frozen for up to 30 days if reconstituted with sterile water, 0.9% NSS, or D5W solution to a concentration of 100 mg/mL. Do not use if darker than very pale yellow.

**ASSESSMENT: DRUG CHARACTERISTICS**

**ACTION**

A broad-spectrum antibiotic. Binds with penicillin-binding receptor sites in the cytoplasmic membranes. May also inhibit cell wall synthesis and cell division and growth and cause lysis of susceptible bacteria. Rapidly dividing bacteria are most susceptible. Drug is widely absorbed in all body fluids and tissues. Appears in CSF if inflammation is present.

**INDICATIONS**

Used to treat a wide variety of gram-positive aerobic and anaerobic and gram-negative cocci and bacilli infections, including bone and joint infections, pneumonias, intraabdominal or urinary tract infections, bacterial septicemias, and skin and soft tissue infections.

**CAUTIONS**

**ADVERSE EFFECTS.** Allergic reactions, rash, joint pain, fever, hives, itching, neutropenia, hypokalemia, hypernatremia, hematuria (in children), blood dyscrasias and bleeding, seizures (with high doses), severe abdominal cramps, diarrhea, nausea, vomiting, phlebitis, or oral candidiasis.

**CONTRAINDICATIONS.** History of hypersensitivity to penicillins, cephalosporins, cephamycins, or penicillamine. Should be used with caution in clients with a history of bleeding disorders, gastrointestinal disorders such as ulcerative colitis, infectious mononucleosis, or impaired renal function. Ticarcillin disodium has 5 mEq of sodium per gram and should be used with caution in clients with history of congestive heart failure (CHF).

**POTENTIAL DRUG/FOOD INTERACTIONS**

May interact with warfarin, heparin, thrombolytic agents, NSAIDs, or sulfinpyrazone to increase the risk of bleeding. May interact with probenecid to inhibit renal excretion of ticarcillin and prolong the half-life of ticarcillin. May inhibit the action of oral contraceptives. The client may experience breakthrough bleeding or become pregnant. Bactericidal effect is negated by chloramphenicol, erythromycin, and tetracyclines. Use with $\beta$-adrenergic blockers (propranolol) may increase risk of anaphylaxis. Administration within 1 hour of aminoglycosides causes mutual inactivation.

**INTERVENTIONS: ADMINISTRATION**

Dilute with at least 4 ml of sterile water for injection. For direct IV push, dilute with an additional 10–20 mL of sterile water for injection, D5W, or 0.9% NSS. May further dilute in 50–100 mL of 0.9% NSS, D5W, or Ringer's lactate solution for intermittent infusion.

**MODE/RATE OF ADMINISTRATION**

May be given reconstituted but undiluted in concentrations of 50 mg/mL by IV push over 3–5 min. Pain or irritation along vein is minimized by slowing the rate of administration. Intermittent IV infusion over 30 min, using an infusion pump. Rapid administration has been associated with irritability of the CNS and seizures.

INTRAVENOUS USE (WITH NORMAL RENAL FUNCTION)

**Adults:** Dosing depends on the severity of the infection and may range between 150–300 mg/kg of body weight per 24 h given in divided doses every 3, 4, or 6h.

**Children $< 40$ kg:** 50–300 mg/kg of body weight per 24 h in divided doses every 4, 6, or 8 h.

**Infants/Neonates $< 2$ g or $< 1$ week:** 75 mg/kg body weight q12h.

**Neonates $> 2$ g but $< 1$ week:** 75 mg q8h.

**Infants/Neonates $> 2$ g or $> 1$ week:** 100 mg/kg q8h.

**Geriatrics:** Elderly clients may be more likely to have age-related diminished renal function that would require a lower dosing schedule.

INTRATHECAL USE OR OTHER INFUSION ROUTES AS INDICATED. Not recommended.

**POTENTIAL PROBLEMS IN ADMINISTRATION**

Should be administered at least 1 hour after aminoglycosides. May cause mutual inactivation if given sooner. Dose or interval adjustments may be necessary for clients exhibiting renal impairment. Rapid administration is associated with seizures. Venous irritation during administration is rate related and should be treated by slowing infusion.

▼

**INDEPENDENT NURSING ACTIONS**

Monitor vital signs. Observe clients with history of CHF and arrythmias for recurrence during ticarcillin therapy. Monitor laboratory values, especially sodium, potassium, BUN, serum creatinine, and PT before and during therapy. Collect specimens as required. Keep skin clean and dry. Change dressings as needed. Use appropriate aseptic techniques and isolation precautions. Teach risk factors for infection. Teach client to observe for suprainfections.

**ADMINISTRATION IN ALTERNATE SETTINGS**

May be given in a variety of clinical settings and in the home by a qualified IV nurse.

**EVALUATION: OUTCOMES OF DRUG THERAPY**

**EXPECTED OUTCOMES**

PHYSICAL ASSESSMENT. Temperature less than 37.5° C. Pulse between 60 and 100 bpm and regular. Skin warm, pink, and dry. No rashes, no flushing, no drainage. Breath sounds clear. Clear yellow urine. Clear CSF. No complaints of headache, abdominal pain, chills, malaise, lethargy, nausea, vomiting, or diarrhea.

LABORATORY. BUN between 10 and 20 mg/dL. Serum creatinine between 0.7 and 1.4 mg/dL. White blood count 5000 to 10,000/mm$^3$. Neutrophils 60% to 70%. Erythrocyte sedimentation rate below 20 mm/h. No abnormal findings from cultures of urine, blood, or CSF. PT 9.5 to 12 seconds. Client may have false-positive urine protein testing.

**NEGATIVE OUTCOMES**

Temperature more than 37.5° C. Pulse more than 100 bpm and irregular. Client complains of headache, abdominal pain, muscle aches, malaise, or lethargy. Hot, flushed skin. Rashes. Diaphoresis. Client may have neck rigidity or discharge or drainage from wounds.

## TICARCILLIN DISODIUM AND CLAVULANATE POTASSIUM

*Trade Name:* Timentin
Canadian Availability: Not specified.
*Pregnancy Risk:* Category B
*pH:* 5.5–7.5
*Storage/Stability:* Store below 40° C. May be stored at room temperature for 6 hours or for 72 hours if refrigerated after reconstituting to a concentration of 200 mg/mL. Stability extended with further dilution. May be frozen for up to 30 days if reconstituted with sterile water. 0.9% NSS, or D5W solution to a concentration of 100 mg/mL. Do not use if darker than very pale yellow.

**ASSESSMENT: DRUG CHARACTERISTICS**

**ACTION**

A broad, extended-spectrum antibiotic. Binds with

penicillin-binding receptor sites in the cytoplasmic membranes. May also inhibit cell wall synthesis and cell division and growth and cause lysis of susceptible bacteria. The addition of clavulanate provides an enhanced resistance to β-lactamase–producing bacteria. Absorbed in all body fluids and tissues. Found in CSF if inflammation present. Rapidly dividing bacteria are most susceptible.

**INDICATIONS**

Used to treat a wide variety of gram-positive aerobic and anaerobic and gram-negative cocci and bacilli infections. The addition of clavulanate shields ticarcillin from degradation by β-lactamase enzymes unless produced by *Enterobacteriaceae*. Used in the treatment of bone and joint infections, pneumonias, intraabdominal or genitourinary tract infections, bacterial septicemias, and skin and soft tissue infections.

**CAUTIONS**

**ADVERSE EFFECTS.** Allergic reactions, rash, joint pain, fever, hives, itching, neutropenia, hypokalemia, hypernatremia, hematuria (in children), blood dyscrasias and bleeding, neuromuscular excitability or seizures (with high doses), severe abdominal cramps, diarrhea, nausea, vomiting, phlebitis, or oral candidiasis.

**CONTRAINDICATIONS.** History of hypersensitivity to penicillins, cephalosporins, cephamycins, or penicillamine. Should be used with caution in clients with a history of bleeding disorders, gastrointestinal disorders such as ulcerative colitis, infectious mononucleosis, or impaired renal function. Clients with cystic fibrosis may be more likely to exhibit side effects. Drug has 5 mEq of sodium per gram and should be used with caution in clients with history of CHF and arythmias.

**POTENTIAL DRUG/FOOD INTERACTIONS**

May interact with warfarin, heparin, thrombolytic agents, NSAIDs, or sulfinpyrazone to increase the risk of bleeding. May interact with probenecid to inhibit renal excretion of this agent and prolong the half-life. Alters excretion of amphotericin B, diuretics, and glucocorticoids. May inhibit the action of oral contraceptives. The client may experience breakthrough bleeding or become pregnant. Bactericidal effect is negated by chloramphenicol, erythromycin, and tetracyclines. Use with β-adrenergic blockers (propranolol) may increase risk of anaphylaxis. Administration within 1 hour of aminoglycosides causes mutual inactivation.

**INTERVENTIONS: ADMINISTRATION**

Dilute with at least 13 mL of sterile water for injection, 0.9% NSS, or D5W solution for each 3.1-g vial for a concentration of ticarcillin 200 mg/mL and clavulanic acid 6.7 mg/mL. May be further diluted in 50–100 mL of 0.9%

▼

NSS, D5W, or Ringer's lactate solution.

**MODE/RATE OF ADMINISTRATION**

May be given reconstituted but undiluted in concentrations of 50 mg/mL or less by IV push over 3–5 min or by intermittent IV infusion over 30 min using an infusion pump. Pain or irritation along vein is minimized by slowing the rate of administration. Rapid administration has been associated with irritability of the CNS and seizures.

INTRAVENOUS USE (WITH NORMAL RENAL FUNCTION)

**Adults < 60 kg of Body Weight:** The usual dosage is 33.3–50 mg/kg of body weight q4h or 50 mg/kg of body weight q6h.

**Adults > 60 kg of Body Weight:** The usual dosage is 3 g ticarcillin and 100 mg clavulanic acid q4–6h.

**Children > 12 years:** Follow adult dosing schedule.

**Infants/Neonates:** Dose not established.

**Geriatrics:** Elderly clients may be more likely to have age-related diminished renal function that would require a lower dosing schedule.

INTRATHECAL USE OR OTHER INFUSION ROUTES AS INDICATED. Not recommended.

**POTENTIAL PROBLEMS IN ADMINISTRATION**

Should be administered at least 1 hour after aminoglycosides. May cause mutual inactivation if given sooner. Rapid administration has been associated with seizures. Venous irritation during administration is rate related and should be treated by slowing infusion.

**INDEPENDENT NURSING ACTIONS**

Monitor vital signs and laboratory values, especially sodium, potassium, BUN, serum creatinine, and PT. Observe clients with history of CHF and arrhythmias for recurrence during therapy. Collect specimens as required. Keep skin clean and dry. Change dressings as needed. Use appropriate aseptic techniques and isolation precautions. Teach risk factors for infection. Teach client to observe for suprainfections.

**ADMINISTRATION IN ALTERNATE SETTINGS**

May be given in a variety of clinical settings and in the home by a qualified IV nurse.

**EVALUATION: OUTCOMES OF DRUG THERAPY**

**EXPECTED OUTCOMES**

PHYSICAL ASSESSMENT. Temperature less than 37.5° C. Pulse between 60 and 100 bpm and regular. Skin warm, pink, and dry. No rashes, no flushing, no drainage. Breath sounds clear. Clear yellow urine. Clear CSF. No complaints of headache or abdominal pain, chills, malaise, or lethargy.

LABORATORY. BUN between 10 and 20 mg/dL. Serum creatinine between 0.7 and 1.4 mg/dL. White blood count 5000 to 10,000/mm$^3$. Neu-

▼

trophils 60% to 70%. Erythrocyte sedimentation rate below 20 mm/h. No abnormal findings from cultures of urine, blood, or CSF. PT 9.5 to 12 seconds. Client may have false-positive protein in urine. Clavulanic acid is associated with false-positive Coombs' test.

**NEGATIVE OUTCOMES**

Temperature more than 37.5° C. Pulse more than 100 bpm and irregular. Client complains of headache, abdominal pain, muscle aches, malaise, or lethargy. Hot, flushed skin. Rashes. Diaphoresis. Client may have neck rigidity or discharge or drainage from wounds. Nausea, vomiting, or diarrhea.

## QUINOLONES (FLUOROQUINOLONES)

### THERAPEUTIC EFFECTS

Quinolones interfere with the action of the enzyme DNA gyrase. DNA gyrase is necessary for the synthesis of bacterial DNA. Quinolones are bactericidal and have a broad spectrum of activity on gram-positive and gram-negative organisms, including *Pseudomonas aeruginosa*. Quinolones may penetrate leukocytes and macrophages and can kill intraphagocytic organisms.

### PHARMACOKINETICS

**Distribution**. Quinolones are widely distributed throughout the body, including good distribution throughout extravascular tissue sites. Distribution to CSF and eye fluid is less than serum levels. Quinolones cross the placental barrier and are found in breast milk.

**Excretion**. The half-life is usually 4 hours in adults with normal renal function. The drugs are metabolized in the liver and the kidneys.

### CAUTIONS

Clients with reduced kidney/hepatic function are more likely to experience side/toxic effects. Quinolones are associated with phototoxicity, and the client may experience severe sunburn with exposure to excessive sunlight.

**Side/Adverse Effects**. Clients receiving other nephrotoxic or hepatotoxic drugs or using these drugs for long periods of time or in high doses are likely to experience side/toxic effects.

#### Contraindications

***Pregnancy and Lactation.*** Quinolones cross the placental barrier. Studies have shown fetal toxicity. Small amounts can be distributed into breask milk, and clients should be instructed to discontinue breast-feeding.

***Pediatrics.*** Safety in use with children under 18 years of ages is not established. Studies have shown arthropathy and osteochondrosis in juvenile animals.

***Geriatrics.*** Studies have documented a lengthening of this class of drugs' half-life in the elderly even with normal renal function.

## TOXICITY

Toxicities of quinolones are listed in Table 16–6.

## POTENTIAL DRUG/FOOD INTERACTIONS

Quinolones have been associated with serious or fatal reactions when administered with theophyllines. Cimetidine may increase quinolone serum levels. Serum levels of cyclosporine may be increased with concomitant quinolone use. Quinolones may potentiate oral anticoagulants. Probenecid may delay renal clearance of quinolones and cause an increased plasma level of quinolones.

---

# CIPROFLOXACIN

*Trade Name:* Cipro IV
Canadian Availability: Not specified.
*Pregnancy Risk:* Category C
*pH:* 3.3–4.6
*Storage/Stability:* Store between 5° and 25° C. Protect from light. Protect from freezing. Reconstituted solutions may be stored for up to 14 days at room temperature or if refrigerated.

## ASSESSMENT: DRUG CHARACTERISTICS

### ACTION

An antibacterial that seems to work by preventing DNA replication and by promoting breakage of the DNA strand.

### INDICATIONS

A broad-spectrum agent that is effective against a wide variety of aerobic gram-positive and gram-negative organisms. Is generally not effective against most anaerobic organisms. Used to treat bone and joint infections, bacterial diarrhea, gram-negative pneumonia, urinary tract infections, and skin and soft tissue infections.

### CAUTIONS

ADVERSE EFFECTS. Allergic reactions, confusion, agitation, tremors, interstitial nephritis, severe abdominal pain or cramping, abdominal tenderness, nausea, or vomiting.

CONTRAINDICATIONS. Known history of hypersensitivity to ciprofloxacin or renal impairment.

▼

## TABLE 16–6
### Quinolone Toxicities

| Body System | Side/Toxic Effects | Physical Assessment Indicators | Laboratory Indicators | Nursing Interventions |
|---|---|---|---|---|
| Neurologic | Neurostimulation | Seizures, tremors, dizziness or light-headedness; restlessness or toxic psychosis | N/A | Observe the client for tremors or seizures; assist with ADLs and mobility; protect from falls; advise client to avoid use of heavy equipment. |
| Renal | Nephrotoxicity | Oliguria, decreased urine concentration | Elevated BUN and serum creatinine; decreased urine specific gravity and creatinine clearance; possible crystalluria | Monitor BUN and serum creatinine, urine specific gravity, and creatinine clearance; measure and record intake and output; encourage fluid intake to at least 2000 mL/d unless contraindicated. |
| Gastrointestinal | Pseudomembranous enterocolitis | Mild nausea, vomiting (rare), abdominal pain, cramping, tenderness, diarrhea | N/A | Monitor laboratory values and report abnormal findings. |
| Hematologic | Hypoprothrombinemia | Bruising, diminished wound-healing capacity | Decreased RBC, Hgb, Hct, WBC, platelets | Observe for bruising; monitor laboratory values and report abnormal findings. |
| | Serum sickness reaction | Joint pain, skin rash, fever | | |
| Dermatologic | Hypersensitivity | Rash, urticaria, pruritus, blistering, peeling of skin, or mucous membranes of eyes or other organs | N/A | Be prepared to administer epinephrine or corticosteroids for allergic response. |
| | Photosensitivity | Sunburn | | |
| Other | Secondary infections, oral or vaginal candidiasis | Pain, burning, itching, white patches on mucous membranes | N/A | Question client for pain; observe for evidence of thrombophlebitis. |

ADLs = activities of daily living, BUN = blood urea nitrogen, Hct = hematocrit, Hgb = hemoglobin, N/A = not applicable, RBC = red blood cell count, WBC = white blood cell count.

**POTENTIAL DRUG/FOOD INTERACTIONS**

May interact with antacids, ferrous sulfate, magnesium-containing laxatives, sucralfate or zinc to lower the serum levels of ciprofloxacin. May delay the excretion of theophyllines and increase the risk of toxic reactions to theophyllines. May increase the anticoagulant effects of warfarin.

**INTERVENTIONS: ADMINISTRATION**

Dilute to a concentration of 1–2 mg/mL for IV infusion.

**MODE/RATE OF ADMINISTRATION**

May be given by intermittent IV infusion over 1 h. Not recommended for IV push.

INTRAVENOUS USE (WITH NORMAL RENAL FUNCTION)

**Adults:** For bone and joint, bacterial pneumonia, and skin and soft tissue infections, the usual dose is 400 mg q12h for 7–14 d.

**Children:** Not recommended. May cause arthropathy.

**Infants/Neonates:** Not recommended. May cause arthropathy.

**Geriatrics:** Elderly clients are more likely to have age-related diminished renal function that may require a lesser dose.

INTRATHECAL USE OR OTHER INFUSION ROUTES AS INDICATED. Not recommended.

**POTENTIAL PROBLEMS IN ADMINISTRATION**

Infusions should run over 1 h to minimize the risk of venous irritation. Crystalluria has been noted in clients with alkaline urine. Fluids to 1500 mL/d should be strongly encouraged.

**INDEPENDENT NURSING ACTIONS**

Monitor vital signs and laboratory values, especially BUN, serum creatinine, and PT. Collect specimens as required. Keep skin clean and dry. Change dressings as needed. Use appropriate aseptic techniques and isolation precautions. Teach risk factors for infection.

**ADMINISTRATION IN ALTERNATE SETTINGS**

May be given in a variety of clinical settings and in the home by a qualified IV nurse.

**EVALUATION: OUTCOMES OF DRUG THERAPY**

**EXPECTED OUTCOMES**

PHYSICAL ASSESSMENT. Temperature less than 37.5° C. Pulse between 60 and 100 bpm and regular. Skin warm, pink, and dry. No rashes, no flushing, no drainage. Breath sounds clear. Clear yellow urine. Clear CSF. No complaints of headache or abdominal pain, chills, malaise, or lethargy.

LABORATORY. BUN between 10 and 20 mg/dL. Serum creatinine between 0.7 and 1.4 mg/dL. White blood count 5000 to 10,000/mm$^3$. Neutrophils 60% to 70%. Erythrocyte sedimentation rate below 20 mm/h. No abnormal findings from cultures of urine, blood, or CSF. PT 9.5 to 12 seconds.

**NEGATIVE OUTCOMES**

Temperature more than 37.5° C. Pulse more than 100 bpm and irregular. Client complains of headache, abdominal pain, muscle aches, malaise, or lethargy. Hot, flushed skin. Rashes. Diaphoresis. Client may have neck rigidity or discharge or drainage from wounds. Unusual bleeding.

---

## OFLOXACIN

*Trade Name:* Floxin IV
*Canadian Availability:* Floxin IV
*Pregnancy Risk:* Category C
*pH:* 3.8–5.5
*Storage/Stability:* Store below 30° C. Protect from freezing and from light. Stable for 72 hours when stored at 24° C or below and for 14 days when stored at 5° C or below if reconstituted to a concentration of 0.4 to 4 mg/mL.

### ASSESSMENT: DRUG CHARACTERISTICS

**ACTION**

A broad-spectrum quinolone antibacterial agent effective against a number of gram-positive and gram-negative bacteria. Interferes with bacterial replication by preventing resealing of DNA double-strands.

**INDICATIONS**

Used to treat bacterial bronchitis, nongonococcal cervicitis, chlamydia infections, gonorrhea, pneumonia, prostatitis, skin and soft tissue infections, and urinary tract infections. Effective against most *Enterobacteriaceae, Enterobacter, E. coli, Klebsiella, Morganella, Proteus, Salmonella, Shigella, Yersinia,* some *Serratia, Neisseria, Haemophilus, Vibrio cholerae, Staphylococcus aureus,* including methicillin-resistant *S. aureus* (MRSA), and others.

**CAUTIONS**

ADVERSE EFFECTS. Hypersensitivity reactions; neuropsychiatric toxicity such as hallucinations, acute psychosis, agitation, confusion, phlebitis; CNS toxicity such as drowsiness, slurred speech, nausea, dizziness, or disorientation; or gastrointestinal symptoms of diarrhea, abdominal pain, nausea, or vomiting. Women may experience external genital pruritus, candidal vaginitis, and vaginal discharge. Chest or trunk pain has been reported.

CONTRAINDICATIONS. Should not be given to clients with known hypersensitivity to the agent. Should be used with caution in clients with hepatic or renal impairment.

**POTENTIAL DRUG/FOOD INTERACTIONS**

If used with theophylline, may inhibit hepatic metabolism of theophylline and thus increase the serum levels of that agent. May react with cimetidine and increase serum levels of ofloxacin.

▼

Serum cyclosporine levels increase with concomitant ofloxacin use. May potentiate oral anticoagulants, causing prolonged PTs. Probenecid may enhance ofloxacin levels.

#### INTERVENTIONS: ADMINISTRATION

Add the ordered amount of ofloxacin to 50–100 mL of 0.9% NSS or D5W to achieve a concentration of 4 mg/mL.

#### MODE/RATE OF ADMINISTRATION

Given by slow intermittent IV infusion over 1 h using an infusion control device.

#### INTRAVENOUS USE (WITH NORMAL RENAL FUNCTION)

**Adults:** For bacterial bronchitis or skin and soft tissue infections the usual dosage is 400 mg over 1 h q12h for at least 10 d.

For chlamydial infections the usual dosage is 300 mg over 1 h q12h for 7 d.

For gonorrhea the usual dosage is 400 mg over 60 min as a single dose.

For prostatitis, the usual dosage is 300 mg over 1 h q12h for 6 wk.

For urinary tract infections the usual dosage is 200 mg over 1 h q12h for 3–10 d, depending on the severity of the infection.

The dose must be altered for adults with impaired renal function, depending on the creatinine clearance values. Generally, if the creatinine clearance is more than 50 mL/min, the client receives 100% of the dose on a 12-h schedule. If the value is between 10–50 mL/min, the client receives 100% of the dose on a 24-h schedule. If the value is less than 10 mL/min, the client receives 50% of the dose on a 24-h schedule.

**Children:** Not recommended. May cause arthropathy.

**Infants/Neonates:** Not recommended. May cause arthropathy.

**Geriatrics:** For clients with normal renal function, follow the adult dosing schedule. For clients with renal impairment, dose adjustment should follow the recommendations for adult clients with renal disorders.

INTRATHECAL USE OR OTHER INFUSION ROUTES AS INDICATED. Not recommended.

#### POTENTIAL PROBLEMS IN ADMINISTRATION

IV push or bolus injection of ofloxacin may cause hypotension.

#### INDEPENDENT NURSING ACTIONS

Monitor vital signs and laboratory values, especially BUN, serum creatinine, and PT. Collect specimens as required. Keep skin clean and dry. Change dressings as needed. Use appropriate aseptic techniques and isolation precaution. Teach risk factors for infection. Observe for evidence of neuropsychiatric symptoms.

#### ADMINISTRATION IN ALTERNATE SETTINGS

May be given in a variety of clinical settings and in the home by a qualified IV nurse.

**EVALUATION: OUTCOMES OF DRUG THERAPY**

**EXPECTED OUTCOMES**

PHYSICAL ASSESSMENT. Temperature less than 37.5° C. Pulse between 60 and 100 bpm and regular. Skin warm, pink, and dry. No rashes, no flushing, no drainage. Breath sounds clear. Clear yellow urine. Clear CSF. No complaints of headache or abdominal pain, diarrhea, chills, malaise, or lethargy. No dizziness or light-headedness. No neuropsychiatric symptoms.

LABORATORY. BUN between 10 and 20 mg/dL. Serum creatinine between 0.7 and 1.4 mg/dL. White blood count 5000 to 10,000/mm$^3$. Neutrophils 60% to 70%. Erythrocyte sedimentation rate below 20 mm/h. No abnormal findings from cultures of urine, blood, or CSF. PT 9.5 to 12 seconds.

**NEGATIVE OUTCOMES**

Temperature more than 37.5° C. Pulse more than 100 bpm and irregular. Client complains of headache, abdominal pain, muscle aches, malaise, or lethargy. Hot, flushed skin, urticaria, or skin rashes. Diaphoresis. Client may have neck rigidity or discharge or drainage from wounds. Client experiences acute psychosis, hallucinations, agitation, or confusion. Decreased creatinine clearance.

## Tetracyclines

### DOXYCYCLINE HYCLATE

*Trade Names:* Doxy, Vibramycin
*Canadian Availability:* Vibramycin
*Pregnancy Risk:* Category D
*pH:* 2.8–4
*Storage/Stability:* Store below 40° C. Protect from light. May be stored at room temperature for 12 hours or for 72 hours if refrigerated after reconstituting to a concentration of 100 mcg/mL. May be frozen for up to 4 weeks if reconstituted using sterile water for injection to a concentration of 10 mg/mL.

**ASSESSMENT: DRUG CHARACTERISTICS**

**ACTION**

An antibacterial and antiprotozoal agent that inhibits protein synthesis by binding to specific sites on bacterial RNA.

**INDICATIONS**

Used to treat a wide variety of gram-negative and gram-positive infections, including acne, anthrax, bronchitis, brucellosis, genitourinary tract infections, granuloma inguinale, pneumonia, various rickettsial infections,

▼

syphilis, trachoma, non-gonococcal urethritis, yaws, and various mycobacterium infections.

**CAUTIONS**

ADVERSE EFFECTS. Discoloration of teeth in infants and children, photosensitivity, nephrogenic diabetes insipidus, hepatotoxicity, pancreatitis, abdominal cramps, diarrhea, nausea, vomiting, dizziness, or a benign increased intracranial pressure.

CONTRAINDICATIONS. History of nephrogenic diabetes insipidus or impaired renal or hepatic function.

**POTENTIAL DRUG/FOOD INTERACTIONS**

May interact with contraceptives to decrease their effectiveness. May interact with phenytoin to decrease the serum concentrations of doxycycline. If used with methoxyflurane, may increase the incidence of nephrotoxicity. May inhibit the activity of penicillins. If used with vitamin A, there may be an increased risk of benign intracranial hypertension.

**INTERVENTIONS: ADMINISTRATION**

Add 10 mL of sterile water for injection to each 100-mg vial. May be further diluted with 100–1000 mL of 0.9% NSS, D5W, or Ringer's lactate solution.

**MODE/RATE OF ADMINISTRATION**

May be given by intermittent IV infusion over 1–4 h or by continuous infusion, using an infusion pump. Should not be given by IV push.

INTRAVENOUS USE (WITH NORMAL RENAL FUNCTION)

**Adults:** For most infections the usual dosage is 200 mg qd or 100 mg q12h.

For syphilis the usual dosage is 150 mg q12h for at least 10 d. Maximum daily dose should not exceed 300 mg.

**Children:** Follow adult dosing schedule.

**Infants/Neonates <45 kg:** The usual dosage is 4.4 mg/kg of body weight q.d. or 1.1–2.2 mg/kg of body weight q12h.

**Geriatrics:** Follow adult dosing schedule.

INTRATHECAL USE OR OTHER INFUSION ROUTES AS INDICATED. Not recommended.

**POTENTIAL PROBLEMS IN ADMINISTRATION**

May cause a permanent yellow-brown or gray stain on teeth of children younger than 8 years of age. Should not be given unless no other suitable agent can be used.

**INDEPENDENT NURSING ACTIONS**

Monitor vital signs and laboratory values, especially liver enzymes, BUN, and serum creatinine. Collect specimens as required. Keep skin clean and dry. Change dressings as needed. Use appropriate aseptic techniques and isolation precautions. Teach risk factors for infection.

**ADMINISTRATION IN ALTERNATE SETTINGS**

May be given in a variety of clinical settings and in the home by a qualified IV nurse.

**EVALUATION: OUTCOMES OF DRUG THERAPY**

**EXPECTED OUTCOMES**

PHYSICAL ASSESSMENT. Temperature less than 37.5° C. Pulse between 60 and 100 bpm and regular. Skin warm, pink, and dry. No rashes, no flushing, no drainage. Breath sounds clear. Clear yellow urine. Clear CSF. No complaints of headache or abdominal pain, chills, malaise, or lethargy.

LABORATORY. AST between 7 and 40 U/mL. ALT between 10 and 40 U/mL. BUN between 10 and 20 mg/dL. Serum creatinine between 0.7 and 1.4 mg/dL. White blood count 5000 to 10,000/mm$^3$. Neutrophils 60% to 70%. Erythrocyte sedimentation rate below 20 mm/h. No abnormal findings from cultures of urine, blood, or CSF.

**NEGATIVE OUTCOMES**

Temperature more than 37.5° C. Pulse more than 100 bpm and irregular. Client complains of headache, abdominal pain, muscle aches, malaise, or lethargy. Hot, flushed skin. Rashes. Diaphoresis. Client may have neck rigidity or discharge or drainage from wounds.

## MINOCYCLINE HYDROCHLORIDE

*Trade Name:* Minocin
*Canadian Availability:* Minocin
*Pregnancy Risk:* Category D
*pH:* 2–2.8
*Storage/Stability:* Store below 40° C. Protect from light. May be stored at room temperature for 24 hours.

**ASSESSMENT: DRUG CHARACTERISTICS**

**ACTION**

An antibacterial and antiprotozoal agent that inhibits protein synthesis by binding to specific sites on bacterial RNA.

**INDICATIONS**

Used to treat a wide variety of gram-negative and gram-positive infections, including acne, anthrax, bronchitis, brucellosis, genitourinary tract infections, granuloma inguinale, pneumonia, various rickettsial infections, syphilis, trachoma, nongonococcal urethritis, yaws, and various mycobacterium infections.

**CAUTIONS**

ADVERSE EFFECTS. Discoloration of teeth in infants and children, photosensitivity, nephrogenic diabetes insipidus, hepatotoxicity, pancreatitis, abdominal cramps, diarrhea, nausea, vomiting, dizziness, or a benign increased intracranial pressure.

CONTRAINDICATIONS. History of nephrogenic diabetes insipidus or impaired renal or hepatic function.

**POTENTIAL DRUG/FOOD INTERACTIONS**

May interact with contraceptives to decrease their effectiveness. If used with

▼

methoxyflurane, may increase the incidence of nephrotoxicity. May inhibit the activity of penicillins. If used with vitamin A, there may be an increased risk of benign intracranial hypertension.

**INTERVENTIONS: ADMINISTRATION**

Add 5–10 mL of sterile water for injection to each 100-mg vial. May be further diluted with 0.9% NSS, D5W, Ringer's injection, or Ringer's lactate injection.

**MODE/RATE OF ADMINISTRATION**

May be given by intermittent IV infusion over 1–4 h or by continuous infusion, using an infusion pump. Should not be given by IV push.

INTRAVENOUS USE (WITH NORMAL RENAL FUNCTION)

**Adults:** For most infections the usual dosage is 200 mg q.d. or 100 mg q12h. Maximum daily dose should not exceed 400 mg.

**Children > 8 years:** The usual dosage is 4 mg/kg of body weight initially, then 2 mg/kg of body weight q12h.

**Infants/Neonates:** Not recommended.

**Geriatrics:** Follow adult dosing schedule.

INTRATHECAL USE OR OTHER INFUSION ROUTES AS INDICATED. Not recommended.

**POTENTIAL PROBLEMS IN ADMINISTRATION**

May cause a permanent yellow-brown or gray stain on teeth of children younger than 8 years of age. Should not be given unless no other suitable agent can be used.

**INDEPENDENT NURSING ACTIONS**

Monitor vital signs and laboratory values, especially liver enzymes, BUN, and serum creatinine. Collect specimens as required. Keep skin clean and dry. Change dressings as needed. Use appropriate aseptic techniques and isolation precautions. Teach risk factors for infection.

**ADMINISTRATION IN ALTERNATE SETTINGS**

May be given in a variety of clinical settings and in the home by a qualified IV nurse.

**EVALUATION: OUTCOMES OF DRUG THERAPY**

**EXPECTED OUTCOMES**

PHYSICAL ASSESSMENT. Temperature less than 37.5° C. Pulse between 60 and 100 bpm and regular. Skin warm, pink, and dry. No rashes, no flushing, no drainage. Breath sounds clear. Clear yellow urine. Clear CSF. No complaints of headache or abdominal pain, chills, malaise, or lethargy.

LABORATORY. AST between 7 and 40 U/mL. ALT between 10 and 40 U/mL. BUN between 10 and 20 mg/dL. Serum creatinine between 0.7 and 1.4 mg/dL. White blood count 5000 to 10,000/mm$^3$. Neutrophils 60% to 70%. Erythrocyte sedimentation rate below 20 mm/h. No abnormal findings from cultures of urine, blood, or CSF.

**NEGATIVE OUTCOMES**

Temperature more than 37.5° C. Pulse more than 100 bpm and irregular. Client complains of headache, abdominal pain, muscle aches, malaise, or lethargy. Hot, flushed skin. Rashes. Diaphoresis. Client may have neck rigidity or discharge or drainage from wounds.

## OXYTETRACYCLINE HYDROCHLORIDE

*Trade Name:* Terramycin
*Canadian Availability:* Terramycin
*Pregnancy Risk:* Category D
*pH:* 2–3
*Storage/Stability:* Store below 40° C. Protect from light. May be stored at room temperature for 6 to 24 hours or for 48 hours if refrigerated after reconstituting.

**ASSESSMENT: DRUG CHARACTERISTICS**

**ACTION**

An antibacterial and antiprotozoal agent that inhibits protein synthesis by binding to specific sites on bacterial RNA.

**INDICATIONS**

Used to treat a wide variety of gram-negative and gram-positive infections incuding acne, anthrax, bronchitis, brucellosis, genitourinary tract infections, granuloma inguinale, pneumonia, various rickettsial infections, syphilis, trachoma, nongonococcal urethritis, yaws, and various mycobacterium infections.

**CAUTIONS**

ADVERSE EFFECTS. Discoloration of teeth in infants and children, photosensitivity, nephrogenic diabetes insipidus, hepatotoxicity, pan creatitis, abdominal cramps, diarrhea, nausea, vomiting, dizziness, or a benign increased intracranial pressure.

CONTRAINDICATIONS. History of nephrogenic diabetes insipidus or impaired renal or hepatic function.

**POTENTIAL DRUG/FOOD INTERACTIONS**

May interact with contraceptives to decrease their effectiveness. If used with methoxyflurane, may increase the incidence of nephrotoxicity. May inhibit the activity of penicillins. If used with vitamin A, there may be an increased risk of benign intracranial hypertension.

**INTERVENTIONS: ADMINISTRATION**

Add 10 mL of sterile water for injection to each 250-mg vial. Should be further diluted with at least 100 mL of 0.9% NSS, D5W, or Ringer's solution.

**MODE/RATE OF ADMINISTRATION**

May be given by intermittent IV infusion over 1–4 h or by continuous infusion, using an infusion pump. Should not be given by IV push.

▼

INTRAVENOUS USE (WITH NORMAL RENAL FUNCTION)

**Adults:** For most infections the usual dosage is 250–500 mg q12h. Maximum daily dose should not exceed 2 g.

**Children > 8 years:** The usual dose is 5–10 mg/kg of body weight q12h.

**Infants/Neonates:** Not recommended.

**Geriatrics:** Follow adult dosing schedule.

INTRATHECAL USE OR OTHER INFUSION ROUTES AS INDICATED. Not recommended.

**POTENTIAL PROBLEMS IN ADMINISTRATION**

May cause a permanent yellow-brown or gray stain on teeth of children younger than 8 years of age. Should not be given unless no other suitable agent can be used.

**INDEPENDENT NURSING ACTIONS**

Monitor vital signs and laboratory values, especially liver enzymes, BUN, serum creatinine, and PT. Collect specimens as required. Keep skin clean and dry. Change dressings as needed. Use appropriate aseptic techniques and isolation precautions. Teach risk factors for infection.

**ADMINISTRATION IN ALTERNATE SETTINGS**

May be given in a variety of clinical settings and in the home by a qualified IV nurse.

**EVALUATION: OUTCOMES OF DRUG THERAPY**

**EXPECTED OUTCOMES**

PHYSICAL ASSESSMENT. Temperature less than 37.5° C. Pulse between 60 and 100 bpm and regular. Skin warm, pink, and dry. No rashes, no flushing, no drainage. Breath sounds clear. Clear yellow urine. Clear CSF. No complaints of headache or abdominal pain, chills, malaise, or lethargy.

LABORATORY. AST between 7 and 40 U/mL. ALT between 10 and 40 U/mL. BUN between 10 and 20 mg/dL. Serum creatinine between 0.7 and 1.4 mg/dL. White blood count 5000 to 10,000/mm$^3$. Neutrophils 60% to 70%. Erythrocyte sedimentation rate below 20 mm/h. No abnormal findings from cultures of urine, blood, or CSF.

**NEGATIVE OUTCOMES**

Temperature more than 37.5° C. Pulse more than 100 bpm and irregular. Client complains of headache, abdominal pain, muscle aches, malaise, or lethargy. Hot, flushed skin. Rashes. Diaphoresis. Client may have neck rigidity or discharge or drainage from wounds.

# Unclassified Antibiotics

## AZTREONAM

*Trade Name:* Azactam
*Canadian Availability:* Not specified.
*Pregnancy Risk:* Category B
*pH:* 4.5–7.5
*Storage/Stability:* Store below −20° C. May store at room temperature for 48 hours or 14 days if refrigerated after thawing.

### ASSESSMENT: DRUG CHARACTERISTICS

#### ACTION

A narrow-spectrum antibiotic that acts by inhibiting bacterial cell wall synthesis.

#### INDICATIONS

Is effective against aerobic, gram-negative organisms. Used to treat gram-negative pneumonia, urinary tract infections, intraabdominal infections, bacterial septicemias, skin and soft tissue infections, cystitis, and bronchitis.

#### CAUTIONS

ADVERSE EFFECTS. Allergic reaction, thrombophlebitis at IV site, or abdominal symptoms such as cramps, diarrhea, nausea, or vomiting.

CONTRAINDICATIONS. Known hypersensitivity to aztreonam or impaired renal or hepatic functioning.

#### POTENTIAL DRUG/FOOD INTERACTIONS

May interact with aminoglycosides to increase the risk of nephrotoxicity. Probenecid may increase serum levels of aztreonam.

### INTERVENTIONS: ADMINISTRATION

Thaw at room temperature before giving. Inspect solution to assure that no ice crystals are present before starting infusion. May be further diluted in 50–100 mL of 0.9% NSS, D5W, or Ringer's lactate solution.

#### MODE/RATE OF ADMINISTRATION

May be given by IV push over 3–5 min. May be given by intermittent infusion. Not recommended for continuous infusion.

INTRAVENOUS USE (WITH NORMAL RENAL FUNCTION)

**Adults:** For moderate infections the usual dosage is 1–2 g q8–12h for 10 d.

For severe infections the usual dosage is 2 g q6–8h.

Usual maximum dosage is 8 g/24 h.

**Children:** Dose not established.

**Infants/Neonates:** Dose not established.

**Geriatrics:** Elderly clients are more likely to have age-related diminished renal function that may require a lesser dose.

INTRATHECAL USE OR OTHER INFUSION ROUTES AS INDICATED. Not recommended.

#### POTENTIAL PROBLEMS IN ADMINISTRATION

If allergic reactions or seizures occur, the infusion should be discontinued immediately. Severe allergic

▼

symptoms should be treated with the usual agents such as antihistamines, adrenocorticoids, or epinephrine. Anticonvulsants may be needed for seizures.

**INDEPENDENT NURSING ACTIONS**

Monitor vital signs and laboratory values, especially BUN, and serum creatinine. Collect specimens as required. Keep skin clean and dry. Change dressings as needed. Use appropriate aseptic techniques and isolation precautions. Teach risk factors for infection.

**ADMINISTRATION IN ALTERNATE SETTINGS**

May be given in a variety of clinical settings and in the home by a qualified IV nurse.

**EVALUATION: OUTCOMES OF DRUG THERAPY**

**EXPECTED OUTCOMES**

PHYSICAL ASSESSMENT. Temperature less than 37.5° C. Pulse between 60 and 100 bpm and regular. Skin warm, pink, and dry. No rashes, no flushing, no drainage. Breath sounds clear. Clear yellow urine. Clear CSF. No complaints of headache or abdominal pain, chills, malaise, or lethargy.

LABORATORY. BUN between 10 and 20 mg/dL. Serum creatinine between 0.7 and 1.4 mg/dL. White blood count 5000 to 10,000/mm$^3$. Neutrophils 60% to 70%. Erythrocyte sedimentation rate below 20 mm/h. No abnormal findings from cultures of urine, blood, or CSF.

**NEGATIVE OUTCOMES**

Temperature more than 37.5° C. Pulse more than 100 bpm and irregular. Client complains of headache, abdominal pain, muscle aches, malaise, or lethargy. Hot, flushed skin. Rashes. Diaphoresis. Client may have neck rigidity or discharge or drainage from wounds.

## IMIPENEM AND CILASTATIN SODIUM

*Trade Name:* Primaxin IV
*Canadian Availability:* Primaxin
*Pregnancy Risk:* Category C
*pH:* 6.5–7.5
*Storage/Stability:* Store below 30° C. May be stored at room temperature for 8 hours or 48 hours if refrigerated at 4° C after reconstituting with sterile water for injection. May be stored at room temperature for 10 hours or 48 hours if refrigerated at 4° C after reconstituting with .9% NSS.

**ASSESSMENT: DRUG CHARACTERISTICS**

**ACTION**

A very broad-spectrum antibacterial. Imipenem acts by binding to penicillin-binding proteins on the cytoplasmic membranes, which causes inhibition of cell wall synthesis. Cilastatin acts by inhibiting tubular excretion of imipenem and prolonging the activity of imipenem.

**INDICATIONS**

Used to treat a wide variety of gram-positive and gram-negative organisms, both aerobic and anaerobic. Indicated for treatment of severe systemic infections, bone and joint infections, intraabdominal infections, female pelvic infections, pneumonia, skin and soft tissue infections, and urinary tract infections.

**CAUTIONS**

ADVERSE EFFECTS. Allergic reactions, dizziness, seizures, thrombophlebitis, and gastrointestinal distress such as diarrhea, nausea, or vomiting.

CONTRAINDICATIONS. History of hypersensitivity to the agent, seizures, or impaired renal functioning.

**POTENTIAL DRUG/FOOD INTERACTIONS**

May interact with probenecid to increase serum levels of imipenem.

**INTERVENTIONS: ADMINISTRATION**

Dilute with 10 mL diluent to each 250- to 500-mg vial. Shake well. Solution should be further diluted in at least 100 mL of 0.9% NSS or other suitable solutions.

**MODE/RATE OF ADMINISTRATION**

May be given by intermittent infusion over 20–30 min. Should not be given by IV push. Not recommended for continuous infusion.

INTRAVENOUS USE (WITH NORMAL RENAL FUNCTION)

**Adults:** For mild infections the usual dosage is 250–500 g q6h.

For moderate infections the usual dosage is 500 mg q6–8h to 1 g q8h.

For severe infections the usual dosage is 500 mg q6h to 1 g q6–8h.

Usual maximum dose is 50 mg/kg of body weight or not more than 4 g.

**Children >12 years:** Follow adult dosing schedule.

**Infants/Neonates:** Dose not established.

**Geriatrics:** Elderly clients are more likely to have age-related diminished renal function that may require a lesser dose.

INTRATHECAL USE OR OTHER INFUSION ROUTES AS INDICATED. Not recommended.

**POTENTIAL PROBLEMS IN ADMINISTRATION**

If imipenem with cilastatin is administered too rapidly, nausea, vomiting, or hypotension may result. Slow the rate of the infusion if this occurs. If allergic reactions or seizures occur, the infusion should be discontinued immediately. Severe allergic symptoms should be treated with the usual agents such as antihistamines, adrenocorticoids, or epinephrine. Anticonvulsants may be needed for seizures.

**INDEPENDENT NURSING ACTIONS**

Monitor vital signs and level of consciousness. Monitor laboratory values, especially BUN and serum creatinine. Collect specimens as required. Keep skin clean and dry. Change dressings as needed. Use appropriate aseptic techniques and isolation precautions. Teach risk factors for infection.

▼

**ADMINISTRATION IN ALTERNATE SETTINGS**

May be given in a variety of clinical settings and in the home by a qualified IV nurse.

**EVALUATION: OUTCOMES OF DRUG THERAPY**

**EXPECTED OUTCOMES**

PHYSICAL ASSESSMENT. Temperature less than 37.5° C. Pulse between 60 and 100 bpm and regular. Skin warm, pink, and dry. No rashes, no flushing, no drainage. Breath sounds clear. Clear yellow urine. Clear CSF. No seizures. No complaints of headache or abdominal pain, chills, malaise, or lethargy.

LABORATORY. BUN between 10 and 20 mg/dL. Serum creatinine between 0.7 and 1.4 mg/dL. White blood count 5000 to 10,000/mm$^3$. Neutrophils 60% to 70%. Erythrocyte sedimentation rate below 20 mm/h. No abnormal findings from cultures of urine, blood, or CSF. PT 9.5 to 12 seconds.

**NEGATIVE OUTCOMES**

Temperature more than 37.5° C. Pulse more than 100 bpm and irregular. Client complains of headache, abdominal pain, muscle aches, malaise, or lethargy. Hot, flushed skin. Rashes. Diaphoresis. Client may have neck rigidity, discharge or drainage from wounds, or dizziness or seizures.

# Antifungals

## AMPHOTERICIN-B

*Trade Name:* Fungizone Intravenous
*Canadian Availability:* Fungizone Intravenous
*Pregnancy Risk:* Category B
*pH:* 5.7
*Storage/Stability:* Store between 2° and 8° C. Protect from light. May be stored up to 24 hours at room temperature if protected from light after being reconstituted. May be stored up to 1 week if refrigerated. Do not use if solution is cloudy or has a precipitate.

**ASSESSMENT: DRUG CHARACTERISTICS**

**ACTION**

An antifungal agent that appears to bind to steroids in the fungal cell wall. The process changes cell wall permeability and permits potassium and other small molecules to leak out of the cell.

**INDICATIONS**

Used to treat aspergillosis, blastomycosis, candidiasis, coccidioidomycosis, cryptococcus, fungal endocarditis, fungal meningitis, cryptococcal meningitis, intraabdominal infections, histoplasmosis, mucormycosis, fungal septicemia, fungal urinary tract infections, and sporotrichosis.

**CAUTIONS**

ADVERSE EFFECTS. Allergic reactions, anemia, arrhythmias,

hypokalemia, leukopenia, polyneuropathy, thrombocytopenia, thrombophlebitis, impaired renal function, difficult urination, or visual changes.

CONTRAINDICATIONS. Impaired renal function or hypersensitivity to amphotericin B.

**POTENTIAL DRUG/FOOD INTERACTIONS**

May interact with adrenocorticoids, carbonic anhydrase inhibitors, or corticotropin to cause severe hypokalemia. May interact with bone marrow depressants or radiation therapy to increase anemia. May interact with digitalis glycosides to increase the incidence of digitalis toxicity. May interact with other nephrotoxic agents to increase the nephrotoxic effects of the agents. If used with diuretics, may increase the chance of hypokalemia.

**INTERVENTIONS: ADMINISTRATION**

To reconstitute, add 10 mL of sterile water for injection to 50 mg of amphotericin B for a concentration of 5 mg/mL. For intravenous infusion the solution may be further diluted to a concentration of 0.1 mg/mL by adding 1 mL (5 mg)–49 mL of D5W that has a pH above 4.2. For intrathecal infusion the solution may be further diluted to a concentration of 0.25 mg/mL by adding 1 mL (5 mg)–19 mL of D5W that has a pH above 4.2. Intrathecal doses are further diluted with 5–30 mL of CSF.

**MODE/RATE OF ADMINISTRATION**

Should not be given by IV push. Intermittent infusions should run over 4–6 h.

INTRAVENOUS USE (WITH NORMAL RENAL FUNCTION)

**Adults:** For intravenous infusion a test dose of 1 mg in 50 mL of D5W solution is given over 10–30 min. If the client tolerates the test dose, the dosage is gradually increased by 5–10 mg up to a maximum of 50 mg/d.

**Children:** For intravenous infusion the initial dosage is 0.25 mg/kg of body weight in D5W per day over 6 h. The dosage is gradually increased to a maximum of 1 mg/kg of body weight per day.

**Infants/Neonates:** Follow children's dosing schedule.

**Geriatrics:** Follow adult dosing schedule.

INTRATHECAL USE OR OTHER INFUSION ROUTES AS INDICATED. For intrathecal infusion the initial dosage is 0.025–0.1 mg/kg of body weight q48–72h. The dose is gradually increased to 0.5 mg/kg. Maximum total dose is 15 mg.

**POTENTIAL PROBLEMS IN ADMINISTRATION**

Extravasation may cause severe local irritation. Heparin may be added to the agent to decrease the incidence of thrombophlebitis at the injection site. Treatment

▼

that has been interrupted for more than 7 days should use the initial dose and progression to avoid severe responses to the agent.

**INDEPENDENT NURSING ACTIONS**

Monitor vital signs and laboratory values, especially BUN and serum creatinine. Collect specimens as required. Keep skin clean and dry. Change dressings as needed. Use appropriate aseptic techniques and isolation precautions. Teach risk factors for infection.

**ADMINISTRATION IN ALTERNATE SETTINGS**

May be given in a variety of clinical settings or in the home by a qualified IV nurse.

**EVALUATION: OUTCOMES OF DRUG THERAPY**

**EXPECTED OUTCOMES**

PHYSICAL ASSESSMENT. Temperature less than 37.5° C. Pulse between 60 and 100 bpm and regular. Skin warm, pink, and dry. No rashes, no flushing, no drainage. Breath sounds clear. Clear yellow urine. Clear CSF. No complaints of headache or pain, chills, malaise, or lethargy.

LABORATORY. BUN between 10 and 20 mg/dL. Serum creatinine between 0.7 and 1.4 mg/dL. White blood count 5000 to 10,000/mm$^3$. Neutrophils 60% to 70%. Erythrocyte sedimentation rate below 20 mm/h. No abnormal findings from cultures of urine, blood, or CSF.

**NEGATIVE OUTCOMES**

Temperature more than 37.5° C. Pulse more than 100 bpm and irregular. Client complains of pain, muscle aches, malaise, or lethargy. Hot, flushed skin. Rashes. Diaphoresis. Client may have neck rigidity or discharge or drainage from wounds.

## FLUCONAZOLE

*Trade Name:* Diflucan
Canadian Availability: Not specified.
*Pregnancy Risk:* Category C
*pH:* 3.5–8
*Storage/Stability:* Store below 30° C. Protect from freezing. Use immediately if viaflex overwrap is removed.

**ASSESSMENT: DRUG CHARACTERISTICS**

**ACTION**

An antifungal with fungistatic and fungicidal properties that interfere with fungal cell wall synthesis and repair. Also appears to metabolize to hydrogen peroxide within the fungal cell.

**INDICATIONS**

Used to treat cryptococcal meningitis, *Candida* infections of the esophagus, and systemic infections caused by *Candida*.

**CAUTIONS**

ADVERSE EFFECTS. Pruritus, exfoliative skin disorders, hepatotoxicity, leukopenia, thrombocytopenia, diarrhea, nausea, vomiting, abdominal pains, anorexia, or headache.

CONTRAINDICATIONS. Known hypersensitivity to fluconazole or impaired hepatic or renal function.

**POTENTIAL DRUG/FOOD INTERACTIONS**

May interact with oral antidiabetic agents to increase the serum level of these agents. Blood sugar levels should be monitored and doses lowered where appropriate. May inhibit the metabolism of phenytoin, cyclosporine, and warfarin, increasing the serum levels of those agents. Rifampin may increase the metabolism of fluconazole. Dose of fluconazole may need to be increased if used with rifampin.

**INTERVENTIONS: ADMINISTRATION**

Comes premixed in 200 mg/dL or 400 mg/2 dL containers. Open overwrap just before administration.

**MODE/RATE OF ADMINISTRATION**

Give by intermittent IV infusion. Rate should not exceed 200 mg/h.

INTRAVENOUS USE (WITH NORMAL RENAL FUNCTION)

**Adults:** For cryptococcal meningitis the usual dosage is 400 mg q.d. until the client responds, then 200–400 mg q.d. for 10–12 wk after negative results from a spinal fluid culture have been achieved.

For fungistatic (suppressive) therapy for cryptococcal meningitis the usual dosage is 200 mg q.d.

For oropharyngeal candidiasis the usual dosage is 200 mg the first day, then 100 mg/d for 2 wk.

For esophageal candidiasis the usual dose is 200 mg the first day, then 100 mg/d for 3 wks. Doses should continue for 2 weeks after symptoms resolve. Doses up to 400 mg/d may be given to achieve resolution of the infection.

For systemic fungal infections the usual dose is 400 mg the first day, then 200 mg/d for at least 4 wk or at least 2 wk after symptoms resolve.

For clients with renal impairment the dose is dependent on creatinine clearance values. If creatinine clearance is more than 50, the dose is 100% of recommended adult dose. If creatinine clearance is between 21–50, the dose should be 50% of recommended dose. If creatinine clearance is between 11–20, 25% of recommended dose is given. Clients receiving hemodialysis and continuous ambulatory peritoneal dialysis (CAPD) can receive 100% of the recom mended dose, depending on timing.

**Children > 12 years:** Follow adult dosing schedule.

**Children 3–12 years:** Some have been given doses of 3–6 mg/kg of body weight q.d.

**Infants/Neonates:** Dose has not been fully established.

▼

**Geriatrics:** Elderly clients are more likely to have age-related decreased renal function that may require dose adjustment.

INTRATHECAL USE OR OTHER INFUSION ROUTES AS INDICATED. Not recommended.

**POTENTIAL PROBLEMS IN ADMINISTRATION**

Extravasation may cause severe local irritation.

**INDEPENDENT NURSING ACTIONS**

Determine client history of hypersensitivity to fluconazole. Monitor vital signs and laboratory values, especially BUN, serum creatinine, AST, and ALT. Collect specimens as required. Keep skin clean and dry. Change dressings as needed. Use appropriate aseptic techniques and isolation precautions. Teach risk factors for infection.

**ADMINISTRATION IN ALTERNATE SETTINGS**

May be given in a variety of clinical settings or in the home by a qualified IV nurse.

**EVALUATION: OUTCOMES OF DRUG THERAPY**

**EXPECTED OUTCOMES**

PHYSICAL ASSESSMENT. Temperature less than 37.5° C. Pulse between 60 and 100 bpm and regular. Skin warm, pink, and dry. No white material in mouth, pharynx, or esophagus. No rashes, no flushing, no drainage. Breath sounds clear. Clear yellow urine. Clear CSF. No complaints of headache or pain, chills, malaise, or lethargy.

LABORATORY. BUN between 10 and 20 mg/dL. Serum creatinine between 0.7 and 1.4 mg/dL. White blood count 5000 to 10,000/mm$^3$. Neutrophils 60% to 70%. Erythrocyte sedimentation rate below 20 mm/h. No abnormal findings from cultures of urine, blood, or CSF.

**NEGATIVE OUTCOMES**

Temperature more than 37.5° C. Pulse more than 100 bpm and irregular. Client complains of pain, muscle aches, malaise, or lethargy. Hot, flushed skin. Rashes. Diaphoresis. Client may have neck rigidity or white material in mouth, pharynx, or esophagus. Client does not report relief of oropharyngeal pain.

## MICONAZOLE

*Trade Name:* Monistat IV
*Canadian Availability:* Not specified.
*Pregnancy Risk:* Category C
*pH:* 3.7–5.7
*Storage/Stability:* Store below 40° C. Protect from freezing. Stable for 24 hours at room temperature. Solution will be clear to slightly yellow.

**ASSESSMENT: DRUG CHARACTERISTICS**

**ACTION**

An antifungal with fungistatic and fungicidal properties that interfere with fungal cell wall synthesis and repair.

INDICATIONS

Used to treat cryptococcal meningitis, serious *Candida* infections of the esophagus, and systemic infections caused by *Candida* and *Cryptococcus*.

CAUTIONS

ADVERSE EFFECTS. Phlebitis and pruritus with or without skin eruptions are the most common adverse reaction to IV miconazole. Some clients require premedication with diphenhydramine. May cause exfoliative skin disorders, hepatotoxicity, leukopenia, thrombocytopenia, diarrhea, nausea, vomiting, abdominal pains, anorexia, or headache. Some transient adverse effects seen in early days of treatment include nausea, vomiting, febrile reactions, drowsiness, diarrhea, anorexia, flushing, dizziness, anxiety, increased libido, blurred vision, dryness of the eyes, headache, and bitter taste. Nausea and vomiting may be dose and infusion rate related.

CONTRAINDICATIONS. Should not be given to clients with a known hypersensitivity to fluconazole. Give with caution in clients who have impaired hepatic or renal function.

POTENTIAL DRUG/FOOD INTERACTIONS

Enhances the effect of coumarin drugs. Possible interaction with astemizole and terfenadine, resulting in cardiovascular effects that can include prolongation of QT interval, dysrhythmia, and palpitations. May interact with oral antidiabetic agents, increasing their effect and causing hypoglycemia. Because of its similarity to ketoconazole, there is a potential for ketoconazole-like interactions with rifampin, cyclosporine, and phenytoin.

INTERVENTIONS: ADMINISTRATION

Dilute each dose in at least 200 mL 0.9% NSS or D5W.

MODE/RATE OF ADMINISTRATION

May be given by intermittent IV infusion over 30–60 min so that the rate does not exceed 200 mg/h.

INTRAVENOUS USE (WITH NORMAL RENAL FUNCTION)

**Adults:** Initial dose of 200 mg then 200–3600 mg/d in equally divided doses q8h, depending on severity of infection.

**Children > 12 years:** Follow adult dosing schedule.

**Children 1–12 years:** 20–40 mg/kg/d in divided doses—not to exceed 15 mg/kg/per dose.

**Infants/Neonates < 1 year:** 15–30 mg/kg/d in divided doses q8h.

**Geriatrics:** Elderly clients are more likely to have age-related decreased renal function that may require dose adjustment.

INTRATHECAL USE OR OTHER INFUSION ROUTES AS INDICATED.

**Intrathecal:** 20-mg dose may be given q1–2d via

▼

subcutaneous reservoir or q3–7d if reservoir is not used. Both methods are to be in conjunction with IV administration.

**Bladder Instillation:** 200 mg of miconazole in a diluted solution 2–4 times per day or by continuous irrigation. Use in conjunction with IV miconazole.

#### POTENTIAL PROBLEMS IN ADMINISTRATION

Extravasation may cause severe local irritation.

#### INDEPENDENT NURSING ACTIONS

Determine client history of hypersensitivity to miconazole. Monitor vital signs and laboratory values, especially BUN, serum creatinine, AST, and ALT. Collect specimens as required. Keep skin clean and dry. Change dressings as needed. Use appropriate aseptic techniques and isolation precautions. Teach risk factors for infection. Encourage oral fluids to 2000 mL/d. Assess need for premedication.

#### ADMINISTRATION IN ALTERNATE SETTINGS

Therapy must be initiated in a controlled setting with a physician available for any untoward events. After initiation of therapy, may be given in a variety of clinical settings or in the home by a qualified IV nurse.

#### EVALUATION: OUTCOMES OF DRUG THERAPY

#### EXPECTED OUTCOMES

PHYSICAL ASSESSMENT. Temperature less than 37.5° C. Pulse between 60 and 100 bpm and regular. Skin warm, pink, and dry. No white material in mouth, pharynx, or esophagus. No rashes, no flushing, no drainage. Breath sounds clear. Clear yellow urine. Clear CSF. No complaints of headache or pain, chills, malaise, or lethargy.

LABORATORY. BUN between 10 and 20 mg/dL. Serum creatinine between 0.7 and 1.4 mg/dL. White blood count 5000 to 10,000/mm$^3$. Neutrophils 60% to 70%. Erythrocyte sedimentation rate below 20 mm/h. No abnormal findings from cultures of urine, blood, or CSF.

#### NEGATIVE OUTCOMES

Temperature more than 37.5° C. Pulse more than 100 bpm and irregular. Client complains of pain, muscle aches, malaise, or lethargy. Hot, flushed skin. Rashes. Diaphoresis. Client may have neck rigidity or white material in mouth, pharynx, or esophagus.

## Antituberculars

### RIFAMPIN

*Trade Name:* Rifadin IV
Canadian Availability: Not specified.

*Pregnancy Risk:* Category C
*pH:* Not specified

*Storage/Stability:* Store below 40° C. Protect from light. After reconstituting to a concentration of 60 mg/mL, solution is stable at room temperature for 24 hours.

## ASSESSMENT: DRUG CHARACTERISTICS

### ACTION

An antimycobacterial and antileprosy agent that acts by inhibiting RNA synthesis. Rifampin binds to RNA and prevents RNA from transcription.

### INDICATIONS

Used to treat tuberculosis and meningococcal carriers.

### CAUTIONS

ADVERSE EFFECTS. Flulike symptoms, blood dyscrasias, hepatitis, hypersensitivity reactions, nephritis, facial edema, pruritus, or a generalized red-orange discoloration of skin, mucous membranes, sclera, urine, feces, saliva, sputum, sweat, and tears; frequently, gastrointestinal symptoms of diarrhea and abdominal pain and fungal overgrowth in the mouth.

CONTRAINDICATIONS. History of alcoholism, hepatic impairment, or known hypersensitivity to rifampin.

### POTENTIAL DRUG/FOOD INTERACTIONS

Rafampin enhances the hepatic metabolism of a wide variety of drugs and requires careful monitoring of the serum levels of those drugs to keep serum levels high enough to achieve the desired therapeutic effects. Drugs to be monitored include corticosteroids, aminophylline, theophylline, warfarin, antidiabetic agents, chloramphenicol, digoxin, disopyramide, mexiletine, quinidine, tocainide, fluconazole, phenytoin, and verapamil. Rifampin may decrease the effectiveness of oral contraceptives, estrogens, and methadone. If given with other hepatotoxic drugs such as ketoconazole, miconazole, or isoniazid, the risk of hepatotoxicity is increased.

## INTERVENTIONS: ADMINISTRATION

Add 10 mL of sterile water for injection to each 600-mg vial. Rotate gently to dissolve rifampin. Add the ordered dose amount to 500 mL of D5W.

### MODE/RATE OF ADMINISTRATION

Given by intermittent IV infusion over 3 h, using an infusion pump. Occasionally, the desired dose may be mixed in 100 mL of solution and infused in 30 min.

INTRAVENOUS USE (WITH NORMAL RENAL FUNCTION)

**Adults:** For tuberculosis the usual dosage is 600 mg q.d.

For meningococccal carriers the usual dosage is 600 mg b.i.d. for 2 d.

Severely debilitated clients may have dosing of 10 mg/kg of body weight q.d. Adult dosage should not exceed 600 mg/d.

**Children $>$ 12 years:** Follow adult dosing schedule.

▼

**Children 1 month–12 years:** For tuberculosis the usual dosage is 10–20 mg/kg of body weight q.d. For meningococcal carriers the usual dosage is 10 mg/kg of body weight q12h for 2 d.

**Neonates ≤1 month:** For tuberculosis the usual dosage is 10–20 mg/kg of body weight q.d. For meningococcal carriers the usual dosage is 5 mg/kg of body weight q12h for 2 d. The maximum dosage should not exceed 600 mg/d.

**Geriatrics:** Dose should not exceed 10 mg/kg of body weight per day.

INTRATHECAL USE OR OTHER INFUSION ROUTES AS INDICATED. Not recommended.

#### POTENTIAL PROBLEMS IN ADMINISTRATION

No identified potential problems reported specific to rifampin.

#### INDEPENDENT NURSING ACTIONS

Determine client history of hypersensitivity to rifampin. Caution client to use appropriate dental hygiene in light of possible leukopenia or thrombocytopenia. Monitor vital signs and laboratory values, especially ALT, AST, and complete blood counts. Keep skin clean and dry. Use appropriate aseptic techniques. Teach risk factors for infection.

#### ADMINISTRATION IN ALTERNATE SETTINGS

May be given in a variety of clinical settings or in the home by a qualified IV nurse.

### EVALUATION: OUTCOMES OF DRUG THERAPY

#### EXPECTED OUTCOMES

PHYSICAL ASSESSMENT. Vital signs remain within 15% of client's baseline. Temperature less than 37.5° C. Skin warm, pink, and dry. No complaints of headache, chills, malaise, blurred vision, nausea, vomiting, diarrhea, or lethargy. No unusual bruising or bleeding. No jaundice, fatigue, anorexia, or weakness. No bloody or cloudy urine, facial edema, pruritus, or a generalized red-orange discoloration of skin, mucous membranes, and sclera.

LABORATORY. Serum potassium between 3.5 and 5 mEq/L. Serum calcium between 9 and 11 mg/dL. BUN between 10 and 20 mg/dL. Serum creatinine between 0.7 and 1.4 mg/dL. Red blood cell count 4.2 to 6.2 million/mm$^3$. White blood count 5000 to 10,000/mm$^3$. Lymphocytes 20% to 30%. Erythrocyte sedimentation rate below 20 mm/h.

#### NEGATIVE OUTCOMES

Vital signs are more than 15% from client's baseline. Temperature more than 37.5° C. Skin hot and dry or cold and clammy. Client complains of headache, chills, malaise, blurred vision, nausea, vomiting, diarrhea, or lethargy; demonstrates unusual bruising or bleeding; has jaundice, fatigue, anorexia, or weakness; has bloody or cloudy urine, facial edema, pruritus, or a generalized red-orange discoloration of skin, mucous membranes, and sclera.

## ANTIVIRALS

### THERAPEUTIC EFFECTS

Antivirals inhibit viral replication by suppressing DNA replication. Antivirals inhibit viral DNA polymerase, which is necessary to convert the antiviral agent into a compound that will inhibit DNA replication. Further, antivirals are incorporated into the viral DNA strand to block continued strand growth. Viruses develop resistance to these agents by decreasing production of enzymes needed to convert the antiviral agent to the compound directly responsible for inhibiting DNA replication.

### PHARMACOKINETICS

**Distribution.** Antivirals are widely distributed throughout body tissue and fluid. In general, levels in CSF are approximately 50% of the levels achieved in plasma.

**Excretion.** Antivirals are eliminated through the kidneys. The half-life of antivirals is between 1 and 5 hours, depending on the specific antiviral. Diminished renal function prolongs the half-life of the agent.

### CAUTIONS

**Side/Adverse Effects.** Antivirals may cause a phlebitis at the IV injection site; acute renal failure; neurologic disturbances such as dizziness, coma, confusion, hallucinations, or seizures; or gastrointestinal distress such as nausea, vomiting, or anorexia.

#### Contraindications

***Pregnancy and Lactation.*** Most agents cross the placental barrier. Studies have not revealed any increased incidence of fetal harm. Most agents are passed in breast milk, but studies have not found an association with harm to the infant.

***Pediatrics.*** Studies have not found specific problems associated with pediatric clients. Infants younger than 1 year should be monitored very closely because immature renal function may cause prolonged half-life of the agent.

***Geriatrics.*** Studies have not found specific problems associated with elderly clients. Elderly clients have a greater incidence of diminished renal function, which may require lower doses of these agents.

### TOXICITY

Toxicities of antivirals are listed in Table 16–7.

### POTENTIAL DRUG/FOOD INTERACTIONS

Antivirals may interact with other nephrotoxic drugs to increase the incidence of impaired renal function. Probenecid may cause a delay in excretion of the agent and may increase the incidence of toxicity.

**TABLE 16–7**
**Antiviral Toxicities**

| Body System | Side/Toxic Effects | Physical Assessment Indicators | Laboratory Indicators | Nursing Interventions |
|---|---|---|---|---|
| Neurologic | Encephalopathic changes | Coma, confusion, hallucinations, seizures, tremors, light-headedness, headache | N/A | Observe the client for seizures; assist with ADLs and mobility; protect from falls. |
| Renal | Acute renal failure | Abdominal pain, decreased urination, increased thirst, anorexia, nausea, vomiting, weakness, fatigue | Elevated BUN and serum creatinine; decreased urine specific gravity and creatinine clearance; proteinuria | Monitor BUN and serum creatinine, urine specific gravity and creatinine clearance; measure and record intake and output; encourage fluid intake to at least 2000 mL/d unless contraindicated. |
| Gastrointestinal | Gastrointestinal disturbances | Nausea, vomiting, diarrhea, abdominal pain | N/A | Observe the client for nausea or diarrhea; report abdominal pain and medicate as indicated. |
| Other | Phlebitis, inflammation at injection site | Pain, redness, swelling | N/A | Observe for signs of inflammation; rotate IV site frequently. |

ADLs = activities of daily living, BUN = blood urea nitrogen, IV = intravenous, N/A = not applicable.

## Acyclovir

*Trade Name:* Zovirax
*Canadian Availability:* Zovirax
*Pregnancy Risk:* Category C
*pH:* 11
*Storage/Stability:* Store between 15° and 30° C. May be stored for 12 hours after reconstituting with sterile water for injection to a concentration of 50 mg/mL. May be stored for 24 hours at room temperature if further diluted with standard IV infusion solutions. May form a precipitate if refrigerated. Allow solution to come to room temperature and precipitate should redissolve.

### ASSESSMENT: DRUG CHARACTERISTICS

#### ACTION

An antiviral that acts by interfering with viral DNA replication.

#### INDICATIONS

Used to treat herpes simplex, herpes genitalis, herpes zoster, and varicella.

#### CAUTIONS

ADVERSE EFFECTS. Phlebitis at the IV injection site, acute renal failure, dizziness, coma, confusion, hallucinations, seizures, or gastrointestinal distress such as nausea, vomiting, or anorexia.

CONTRAINDICATIONS. Dehydration or impaired renal function.

#### POTENTIAL DRUG/FOOD INTERACTIONS

May interact with other nephrotoxic drugs to increase the incidence of impaired renal function. Probenecid may cause a delay in excretion of acyclovir and may increase the incidence of toxicity. Incompatible with blood products or protein-containing solutions.

### INTERVENTIONS: ADMINISTRATION

Add 10–20 mL of sterile water for injection to each 500-mg to 1-g vial to achieve a concentration of 50 mg/mL. May further dilute in 0.9% NSS, D5W, combinations of sodium chloride and dextrose, and Ringer's lactate injection.

#### MODE/RATE OF ADMINISTRATION

Should be given by intermittent IV infusion at a constant rate over 1 h. Not recommended for IV push.

##### INTRAVENOUS USE (WITH NORMAL RENAL FUNCTION)

**Adults:** For herpes simplex the usual dosage is 5–10 mg/kg of body weight q8h for 7–10 d.

For herpes genitalis the usual dosage is 5 mg/kg of body weight q8h for 5 d.

For varicella in immunocompromised clients the usual dosage is 10 mg/kg of body weight q8h for 7 d.

Maximum daily dose should not exceed 30 mg/kg of body weight.

**Children $>$ 12 years:** Follow the adult dosing schedule.

**Children $\leq$ 12 years:** For herpes simplex the usual dosage is 250 mg/m² of body surface area (BSA) q8h for 7 d.

▼

**Infants/Neonates:** For herpes simplex encephalitis the usual dosage is 10 mg/kg of body weight q8h for 10 d.

For herpes genitalis the usual dosage is 250 mg/m$^2$ of BSA q8h for 5 d.

For varicella in immunocompromised clients the usual dosage is 500 mg/m$^2$ of BSA q8h for 7 d.

**Geriatrics:** Elderly clients are more likely to have age-related diminished renal functioning that may require a lower dose.

INTRATHECAL USE OR OTHER INFUSION ROUTES AS INDICATED. Not recommended.

**POTENTIAL PROBLEMS IN ADMINISTRATION**

Should be given at a constant rate over 1 h. Maximum serum levels are achieved within 2 h of infusion. Clients should be well hydrated during this period to decrease incidence of renal toxicity.

**INDEPENDENT NURSING ACTIONS**

Monitor vital signs and laboratory values, especially BUN and serum creatinine. Keep skin clean and dry. Use appropriate aseptic techniques and isolation precautions. Teach risk factors for infection.

**ADMINISTRATION IN ALTERNATE SETTINGS**

May be given in acute care settings or in the home by a qualified IV nurse.

**EVALUATION: OUTCOMES OF DRUG THERAPY**

**EXPECTED OUTCOMES**

PHYSICAL ASSESSMENT. Skin warm, pink, and dry. No blisters, no lesions, no drainage. Clear yellow urine. Able to void without discomfort. Clear CSF. No complaints of headache, chills, malaise, or lethargy.

LABORATORY. BUN between 10 and 20 mg/dL. Serum creatinine between 0.7 and 1.4 mg/dL. White blood count 5000 to 10,000/mm$^3$. Lymphocytes 20% to 30%. Erythrocyte sedimentation rate below 20 mm/h. No abnormal findings from cultures of urine, blood, or CSF.

**NEGATIVE OUTCOMES**

Temperature more than 37.5° C. Skin warm, pink, and moist. Evidence of blisters, lesions, or drainage. Unable to void without discomfort. Cloudy CSF. Client complains of headache, chills, malaise, or lethargy.

## FOSCARNET SODIUM

*Trade Name:* Foscavir
*Canadian Availability:* Not specified.
*Pregnancy Risk:* Category C
*pH:* Not specified.
*Storage/Stability:* Store below 40° C. Do not freeze. If diluted solution is refrigerated, solution may crystallize. Undiluted agent can be stored at 25° C for 24 months. If diluted, should be used within 24 hours.

### ASSESSMENT: DRUG CHARACTERISTICS

#### ACTION

An antiviral that has virustatic action by blocking viral replication by interfering with the viral DNA chain. Viral replication resumes as soon as foscarnet is discontinued.

#### INDICATIONS

Used to treat cytomegalovius retinitis in clients with acquired immunodeficiency syndrome (AIDS).

#### CAUTIONS

ADVERSE EFFECTS. Nephrotoxicity, anemia, granulocytopenia, or leukopenia; neurotoxicity such as dizziness, confusion, fatigue, headache, or anxiety; gastrointestinal symptoms such as abdominal pain, nausea, vomiting, and diarrhea.

CONTRAINDICATIONS. Anemia, dehydration, renal impairment, or known hypersensitivity to foscarnet.

#### POTENTIAL DRUG/FOOD INTERACTIONS

May interact with other nephrotoxic agents such as acyclovir, amphotericin B, or aminoglycosides to increase the risk of nephrotoxicity. May interact with pentamidine to cause severe hypocalcemia and nephrotoxicity. Use with zidovudine may increase the incidence of anemia.

### INTERVENTIONS: ADMINISTRATION

Dilute foscarnet 6000 mg in 250 mL (24 mg/mL) or 12,000 mg in 500 mL (24 mg/mL) with D5W or 0.9% NSS 1:1 to a concentration of 12 mg/mL. After calculating the correct dose, any amount of foscarnet over the calculated dose should be discarded to prevent accidental overdose.

#### MODE/RATE OF ADMINISTRATION

Given by intermittent IV infusion or by continuous IV infusion using an infusion pump at a rate not to exceed 60 mg/kg of body weight in 1 h. Higher doses should be infused over at least 2 h.

INTRAVENOUS USE (WITH NORMAL RENAL FUNCTION)

**Adults:** For cytomegalovirus retinitis, initially, the dosage is 60 mg/kg of body weight over 1 h q8h for 14–21 d.

For maintenance the usual dosage is 90–120 mg/kg of body weight over at least 2 h daily.

Clients with renal impairment require adjusted doses based on the creatinine clearance values.

**Children:** Follow adult dosing schedule.

**Infants/Neonates:** Follow adult dosing schedule.

**Geriatrics:** Elderly clients are more likely to have age-related decreases in renal function that may necessitate dose adjustment.

INTRATHECAL USE OR OTHER INFUSION ROUTES AS INDICATED. Not recommended.

#### POTENTIAL PROBLEMS IN ADMINISTRATION

Undiluted foscarnet can only be given through a central venous line because of

▼

its potential to cause venous irritation. May cause severe hypocalcemia if infused too rapidly. Clients should be well hydrated to prevent nephrotoxicity.

**INDEPENDENT NURSING ACTIONS**

Determine client history of hypersensitivity to foscarnet. Monitor vital signs, especially cardiac rate and rhythm. Monitor laboratory values, especially BUN, serum creatinine, ALT, AST, and complete blood counts. Keep skin clean and dry. Monitor bowel sounds. Use appropriate aseptic techniques and isolation precautions. Teach risk factors for infection.

**ADMINISTRATION IN ALTERNATE SETTINGS**

May be given in acute care settings or in the home by a qualified IV nurse.

**EVALUATION: OUTCOMES OF DRUG THERAPY**

**EXPECTED OUTCOMES**

PHYSICAL ASSESSMENT. Skin warm, pink, and dry. No complaints of eye pains, headache, chills, malaise, or lethargy.

LABORATORY. Serum potassium between 3.5 and 5 mEq/L. Serum calcium between 9 and 11 mg/dL. BUN between 10 and 20 mg/dL. Serum creatinine between 0.7 and 1.4 mg/dL. Red blood cell count 4.2 to 6.2 million/mm$^3$. White blood cell count returns to baseline.

**NEGATIVE OUTCOMES**

Temperature more than 37.5° C. Skin warm, pink, and moist. Client complains of eye pain, headache, chills, malaise, or lethargy.

## GANCICLOVIR

*Trade Name:* Cytovene
*Canadian Availability:* Cytovene
*Pregnancy Risk:* Category C
*pH:* 9–11
*Storage/Stability:* Store between 15° and 30° C. May be stored for 12 hours after reconstituting with sterile water for injection to a concentration of 50 mg/mL. If further diluted with standard IV infusion solutions, may be stored for up to 24 hours if refrigerated. Do not freeze.

**ASSESSMENT: DRUG CHARACTERISTICS**

**ACTION**

An antiviral that acts by interfering with viral DNA replication.

**INDICATIONS**

Used to treat cytomegalovirus retinitis in immunocompromised clients.

**CAUTIONS**

ADVERSE EFFECTS. Granulocytopenia, thrombocytopenia, anemia, CNS symptoms such as mood changes or tremor, allergic reactions, hepatic dysfunction, or gastrointestinal distress such as nausea, vomiting, or anorexia.

CONTRAINDICATIONS. Neutrophil count less than $500/mm^3$, platelet count less than $25{,}000/mm^3$, or impaired renal function.

**POTENTIAL DRUG/FOOD INTERACTIONS**

May interact with other bone marrow depressants or with radiation therapy to increase bone marrow depressant effects. If used with zidovudine, severe bone marrow depression may occur. Probenecid may cause a delay in excretion of the agent and may increase the incidence of toxicity. If used with imipenem and cilastatin, seizures may occur.

**INTERVENTIONS: ADMINISTRATION**

Add 10 mL of sterile water for injection to each 500-mg vial to achieve a concentration of 50 mg/mL. Shake until clear. May be further diluted in 100 mL of 0.9% NSS, D5W, Ringer's injection, and Ringer's lactate injection to achieve a concentration of 10 mg/mL.

**MODE/RATE OF ADMINISTRATION**

Should be given by intermittent IV infusion at a constant rate over 1 h. Not recommended for IV push.

INTRAVENOUS USE (WITH NORMAL RENAL FUNCTION)

**Adults:** For initial treatment the usual IV dosage is 5 mg/kg of body weight q12–14h for 21 d. The usual intravitreous injection dosage is 200 mcg twice a week for 3 wk.

For maintenance the usual IV dosage is 5 mg/kg of body weight per day 7 d/wk. The usual intravitreous injection dosage is 200 mcg once a week.

**Children:** Dose not established.

**Infants/Neonates:** Dose not established.

**Geriatrics:** Elderly clients are more likely to have age-related diminished renal functioning that may require a lower dose.

INTRATHECAL USE OR OTHER INFUSION ROUTES AS INDICATED. May be given by intravitreous injection.

**POTENTIAL PROBLEMS IN ADMINISTRATION**

Should be handled with the same precautions used when handling cytotoxic infusions. Should be given at a constant rate over 1 h. Maximum serum levels are achieved within 2 h of infusion. Clients should be well hydrated during this period to decrease incidence of renal toxicity.

**INDEPENDENT NURSING ACTIONS**

Monitor vital signs and laboratory values, especially BUN and serum creatinine. Keep skin clean and dry. Use appropriate aseptic techniques and isolation precautions. Teach risk factors for infection. Caution client that dental work may increase the risk of bleeding or microbial infection.

**ADMINISTRATION IN ALTERNATE SETTINGS**

May be given in acute care settings or in the home by a qualified IV nurse.

▼

### EVALUATION: OUTCOMES OF DRUG THERAPY

#### EXPECTED OUTCOMES

PHYSICAL ASSESSMENT. Temperature less than 37.5° C. Client's vision does not deteriorate. No complaints of headache, chills, malaise, or lethargy. No evidence of bleeding.

LABORATORY. Platelets more than 25,000/mm³. BUN between 10 and 20 mg/dL. Serum creatinine between 0.7 and 1.4 mg/dL. White blood cell count returns to baseline. No abnormal findings from cultures of urine, blood, or CSF. PT between 9.5 and 12 seconds.

#### NEGATIVE OUTCOMES

Temperature more than 37.5° C. Client's vision deteriorates to blindness. Client complains of headache, chills, malaise, or lethargy. Bleeding from gums or bruising.

## VIDARABINE

*Trade Name:* Vira-A
*Canadian Availability:* Vira-A
*Pregnancy Risk:* Category C
*pH:* 5–6.2
*Storage/Stability:* Store between 15° and 30° C. May be stored for 48 hours after reconstituting with sterile water for injection. Should not be refrigerated after reconstitution.

### ASSESSMENT: DRUG CHARACTERISTICS

#### ACTION

An antiviral nucleoside that acts by interfering with viral DNA replication.

#### INDICATIONS

Used to treat herpes simplex encephalitis, neonatal herpes simplex infections, herpes zoster, and viral infections such as varicella and cytomegalovirus in immunocompromised clients.

#### CAUTIONS

ADVERSE EFFECTS. Nausea, vomiting, anorexia, weight loss, phlebitis at the IV injection site, dizziness, ataxia, confusion, hallucinations, transient elevations in liver enzymes, and bone marrow depression.

CONTRAINDICATIONS. Dehydration, impaired renal or hepatic function, significant bone marrow depression, or history of hypersensitivity to vidarabine.

#### POTENTIAL DRUG/FOOD INTERACTIONS

Allopurinol may interfere with the metabolism of vidarabine and cause tremors, nausea, pain, or pruritus.

### INTERVENTIONS: ADMINISTRATION

Add 2.2 mL of infusate, either sterile water for injection or 0.9% NSS, for each 200-mg/mL vial. May further dilute in 0.9% NSS.

#### MODE/RATE OF ADMINISTRATION

Should be given by continuous IV infusion at a constant rate over 1 h. Not recommended for IV push.

INTRAVENOUS USE (WITH NORMAL RENAL FUNCTION)

**Adults:** For herpes simplex encephalitis the usual dosage is 15 mg/kg of body weight daily for 10 d.

For herpes zoster the usual dosage is 10 mg/kg of body weight q.d. for 5–10 d.

For varicella in immunocompromised clients the usual dosage is 10 mg/kg of body weight daily for 5–7 d.

**Children > 12 years:** Follow adult dosing schedule.

**Infants/Neonates:** For neonates, for herpes simplex virus (HSV) infections the usual dosage is 15–30 mg/kg of body weight daily for 10–14 d. In some cases, therapy may be continued for up to 21 d.

**Geriatrics:** Elderly clients are more likely to have age-related diminished renal functioning that may require a lower dose.

INTRATHECAL USE OR OTHER INFUSION ROUTES AS INDICATED. Not recommended.

**POTENTIAL PROBLEMS IN ADMINISTRATION**

Great caution should be exercised to ensure that vidarabine infusions run slowly in neonates to avoid toxic symptoms and fluid overload.

**INDEPENDENT NURSING ACTIONS**

Monitor vital signs and laboratory values, especially BUN and serum creatinine. Keep skin clean and dry. Use appropriate aseptic techniques and isolation precautions. Teach risk factors for infection.

**ADMINISTRATION IN ALTERNATE SETTINGS**

May be given in acute care settings or in the home by a qualified IV nurse.

**EVALUATION: OUTCOMES OF DRUG THERAPY**

**EXPECTED OUTCOMES**

PHYSICAL ASSESSMENT. Skin warm, pink, and dry. No blisters, no lesions, no drainage. Clear yellow urine. Able to void without discomfort. Clear CSF. No complaints of headache, chills, malaise, or lethargy.

LABORATORY. BUN between 10 and 20 mg/dL. Serum creatinine between 0.7 and 1.4 mg/dL. White blood cell count returns to baseline. No abnormal findings from cultures of urine, blood, or CSF.

**NEGATIVE OUTCOMES**

Temperature more than 37.5° C. Skin warm, pink, and moist. Evidence of blisters, lesions, or drainage. Unable to void without discomfort. Cloudy CSF. Client complains of headache, chills, malaise, or lethargy.

---

## ZIDOVUDINE

*Trade Name:* Retrovir
*Canadian Availability:* Retrovir

*Pregnancy Risk:* Category C
*pH:* 5.5

*Storage/Stability:* Store between 15° and 25° C. Protect from light. May store at room temperature for 24 hours or 48 hours if refrigerated after diluting. Solution should be clear. Do not use if discolored.

## ASSESSMENT: DRUG CHARACTERISTICS

### ACTION

An antiviral that acts by inhibiting viral DNA replication. Also has some inhibiting effects on hepatitis B, Epstein-Barr viruses, and some bacteria. Does not seem effective against hepatitis B in clients with human immunodeficiency virus (HIV), and bacteria quickly develop resistance to the agent.

### INDICATIONS

Used to treat HIV or AIDS.

### CAUTIONS

ADVERSE EFFECTS. Leukopenia, neutropenia, thrombocytopenia, anemia, CNS toxicity, bone marrow depression, hepatotoxicity, or gastrointestinal distress such as nausea, vomiting, or anorexia.

CONTRAINDICATIONS. Neutrophil count less than 500/mm³, or platelet count less than 25,000/mm³, impaired liver function, history of hypersensitivity to zidovudine.

### POTENTIAL DRUG/FOOD INTERACTIONS

May interact with other bone marrow depressants or with radiation therapy to increase bone marrow depressant effects. If used with ganciclovir, severe bone marrow depression may occur. Probenecid may cause a delay in excretion of the agent and may increase the incidence of toxicity. Clarithromycin may lower the serum levels of zidovudine.

## INTERVENTIONS: ADMINISTRATION

Must be diluted to a concentration of 4 mg/mL before administering. May be diluted in 0.9% NSS, D5W, combinations of sodium chloride and dextrose, and Ringer's lactate injection.

### MODE/RATE OF ADMINISTRATION

Should be given by intermittent IV infusion at a constant rate over 1 h. Not recommended for IV push.

INTRAVENOUS USE (WITH NORMAL RENAL FUNCTION)

**Adults:** For HIV infection the usual dosage is 1–2 mg/kg of body weight q4h until the client can be switched to oral therapy.

**Children > 12 years:** Follow adult dosing schedule.

**Infants/Neonates:** For HIV infection the usual dosage is 120 mg/m² of BSA q6h. Dose should not exceed 160 mg for any single dose.

**Geriatrics:** Dose not established. Elderly clients are more likely to have age-related diminished renal functioning that may require a lower dose.

INTRATHECAL USE OR OTHER INFUSION ROUTES AS INDICATED. Not recommended.

#### POTENTIAL PROBLEMS IN ADMINISTRATION

Should be given at a constant rate over 1 h. Maximum serum levels are achieved within 2 h of infusion. Clients should be well hydrated during this period to decrease incidence of renal toxicity.

#### INDEPENDENT NURSING ACTIONS

Monitor vital signs and laboratory values, especially BUN, serum creatinine, and liver enzymes. Keep skin clean and dry. Use appropriate aseptic techniques and isolation precautions. Teach risk factors for infection. Caution client that dental work may increase the risk of bleeding or microbial infection.

#### ADMINISTRATION IN ALTERNATE SETTINGS

May be given in acute care settings or in the home by a qualified IV nurse.

### EVALUATION: OUTCOMES OF DRUG THERAPY

#### EXPECTED OUTCOMES

PHYSICAL ASSESSMENT. Temperature less than 37.5° C. Skin warm, pink, and dry. No complaints of headache, chills, malaise, or lethargy. No bleeding. No jaundice. Able to void without difficulty. Urine clear and yellow.

LABORATORY. Platelets more than 25,000/mm³. BUN between 10 and 20 mg/dL. Serum creatinine between 0.7 and 1.4 mg/dL. AST between 7 and 40 U/mL. ALT between 10 and 40 U/mL. White blood cell count returns to baseline. PT between 9.5 and 12 seconds.

#### NEGATIVE OUTCOMES

Temperature more than 37.5° C. Skin warm, pink, and moist. Unable to void without discomfort. Client complains of headache, chills, malaise, or lethargy. Bleeding from gums or bruising.

---

# Miscellaneous Antiinfectives

## CLINDAMYCIN PHOSPHATE

*Trade Name:* Cleocin
*Canadian Availability:* Dalacin C Phosphate
*Pregnancy Risk:* Category Unknown
*pH:* 6–6.3
*Storage/Stability:* Store below 40° C. Protect from freezing. May be stored at room temperature for up to 24 hours after reconstituting and diluting.

### ASSESSMENT: DRUG CHARACTERISTICS

#### ACTION

An antibacterial agent that inhibits protein synthesis in susceptible organisms preventing replication.

#### INDICATIONS

Used to treat anaerobic infections and infections in penicillin-sensitive clients. ▼

Has been used to treat bone and joint infections, female pelvic infections, pneumonia, intraabdominal infections, bacterial septicemias, and skin and soft tissue infections.

#### CAUTIONS

ADVERSE EFFECTS. Pseudomembranous colitis, allergic reactions, nausea, vomiting, diarrhea, and fungal overgrowth.

CONTRAINDICATIONS. History of gastrointestinal disorders such as ulcerative colitis or history of hypersensitivity to clindamycin.

#### POTENTIAL DRUG/FOOD INTERACTIONS

May interact with hydrocarbon anesthetic agents or neuromuscular blocking agents to increase neuromuscular blockade even to the extent of paralysis. May antagonize the effects of chloramphenicol and erythromycin.

#### INTERVENTIONS: ADMINISTRATION

Each 300-mg/2 mL vial of clindamycin must be diluted in at least 50 mL of diluent before giving to the client. May be diluted in 0.9% NSS or D5W solution.

#### MODE/RATE OF ADMINISTRATION

May be given by intermittent IV infusion over at least 10 min or by continuous infusion.

INTRAVENOUS USE (WITH NORMAL RENAL FUNCTION)

**Adults:** For most infections the usual dosage is 300–600 mg q6–8h or 900 mg q8h. Maximum daily dose should not exceed 2.7 g.

**Children >12 years:** Follow adult dosing schedule.

**Children 1 month–12 years:** The usual dosage is 3.75–10 mg/kg of body weight q6h or 5–13.5 mg/kg of body weight q8h.

**Neonates ≤1 month:** The usual dosage is 3.75–5 mg/kg of body weight q6h or 5–6.7 mg/kg of body weight q8h.

**Geriatrics:** Follow adult dosing schedule.

INTRATHECAL USE OR OTHER INFUSION ROUTES AS INDICATED. Not recommended.

#### POTENTIAL PROBLEMS IN ADMINISTRATION

If allergic reactions occur or seizures occur, the infusion should be discontinued immediately. Severe allergic symptoms should be treated with the usual agents such as antihistamines, adrenocorticoids, or epinephrine. If pseudomembranous colitis occurs, discontinue the drug and support with fluid, electrolyte, and protein replacement.

#### INDEPENDENT NURSING ACTIONS

Monitor vital signs and laboratory values, especially BUN and serum creatinine. Collect specimens as required. Keep skin clean and dry. Change dressings as needed. Use appropriate aseptic techniques and isolation precautions. Teach risk factors for infection.

#### ADMINISTRATION IN ALTERNATE SETTINGS

May be given in acute care settings or in the home by a qualified IV nurse.

**EVALUATION: OUTCOMES OF DRUG THERAPY**

**EXPECTED OUTCOMES**

PHYSICAL ASSESSMENT. Temperature less than 37.5° C. Pulse between 60 and 100 bpm and regular. Skin warm, pink, and dry. No rashes, no flushing, no drainage. Breath sounds clear. Clear yellow urine. Clear CSF. No complaints of headache or abdominal pain, chills, malaise, or lethargy.

LABORATORY. BUN between 10 and 20 mg/dL. Serum creatinine between 0.7 and 1.4 mg/dL. White blood count 5000 to 10,000/mm$^3$. Neutrophils 60% to 70%. Erythrocyte sedimentation rate below 20 mm/h. Negative cultures of urine, blood, or CSF.

**NEGATIVE OUTCOMES**

Temperature more than 37.5° C. Pulse more than 100 bpm and irregular. Client complains of headache, abdominal pain, muscle aches, malaise, or lethargy. Hot, flushed skin. Rashes. Diaphoresis. Client may have neck rigidity or discharge or drainage from wounds.

## METRONIDAZOLE

*Trade Name:* Flagyl IV
*Canadian Availability:* Flagyl IV
*Pregnancy Risk:* Category B
*pH:* 5–7
*Storage/Stability:* Store below 40° C. Protect from light. Protect from freezing. If not available in premixed bags, may store for up to 96 hours after reconstituting if refrigerated below 30° C. Do not refrigerate neutralized solutions. Diluted and neutralized solutions may be stored for up to 24 hours at room temperature.

**ASSESSMENT: DRUG CHARACTERISTICS**

**ACTION**

An antibacterial and antiprotozoal agent with inflammatory bowel disease–suppressing and antihelmintic properties. Acts by inhibiting DNA synthesis in most anaerobic organisms.

**INDICATIONS**

Used to treat brain abscesses; infections of the CNS, abdomen, pelvis, bone and joint, skin and soft tissue; endocarditis, pneumonia, septicemia, and perioperative colorectal infections; and amebiasis and trichomoniasis. Also used to treat *clostridium difficile* infection.

**CAUTIONS**

ADVERSE EFFECTS. Peripheral neuropathy, seizures, CNS toxicity, leukopenia, thrombophlebitis at infusion site, vaginal candidiasis, and gastrointestinal distress.

CONTRAINDICATIONS. Active disease of the CNS, blood dyscrasias, impaired hepatic function, or history of hypersensitivity to metronidazole.

**POTENTIAL DRUG/FOOD INTERACTIONS**

May interact with alcohol to cause a disulfiram-like re-

▼

action. May potentiate the effects of anticoagulants. May interact with disulfiram to cause psychosis or confusion.

#### INTERVENTIONS: ADMINISTRATION

If not provided in premixed bags, add 4.4 mL of sterile water for injection to each 500-mg vial to achieve a concentration of 100 mg/mL. The concentration should be further diluted in 100 mL of 0.9% NSS, D5W, or Ringer's lactate injection. Further, 5 mEq of sodium bicarbonate should be added to each 500 mg of metronidazole to neutralize the solution to a pH of 6–7.

#### MODE/RATE OF ADMINISTRATION

Should be given by intermittent IV infusion over 1 h.

#### INTRAVENOUS USE (WITH NORMAL RENAL FUNCTION)

**Adults:** For bacterial infections the usual dosage is 15 mg/kg of body weight initially, followed by 7.5 mg/kg of body weight up to 1 g q6h for at least 7 d.

For perioperative prophylaxis the usual dosage is 15 mg/kg of body weight started 1 h before surgery and 7.5 mg/kg of body weight 6 and 12 h after surgery.

Maximum daily dose should not exceed 4 g.

**Children >12 years:** Follow adult dosing schedule.

**Infants >7 days and Children ≤12 years:** The usual dosage is an initial dose of 15 mg/kg of body weight followed by 7.5 mg/kg of body weight q6h.

**Newborns ≤7 days:** The usual dosage is an initial 15 mg/kg of body weight followed by 7.5 mg/kg of body weight q12h starting 24 h after the first dose.

**Preterm Infants:** The usual dosage is an initial 15 mg/kg of body weight followed by 7.5 mg/kg of body weight q12h starting 48 h after the first dose.

**Geriatrics:** Elderly clients are more likely to have age-related diminished hepatic function that may require a lesser dose.

#### INTRATHECAL USE OR OTHER INFUSION ROUTES AS INDICATED.

Not recommended.

#### POTENTIAL PROBLEMS IN ADMINISTRATION

Clients with impaired hepatic function should be closely monitored for toxicity. Clients with anuria should have the metabolites of metronidazole removed with dialysis.

#### INDEPENDENT NURSING ACTIONS

Monitor vital signs and laboratory values, especially BUN, serum creatinine, and liver enzymes. Collect specimens as required. Keep skin clean and dry. Change dressings as needed. Use appropriate aseptic techniques and isolation precautions. Teach risk factors for infection and avoidance of alcohol.

#### ADMINISTRATION IN ALTERNATE SETTINGS

May be given in acute care settings or in the home by a qualified IV nurse.

### EVALUATION: OUTCOMES OF DRUG THERAPY

#### EXPECTED OUTCOMES

PHYSICAL ASSESSMENT. Temperature less than 37.5° C. Pulse between 60 and 100 bpm and regular. Skin warm, pink, and dry. No rashes, no flushing, no drainage. Breath sounds clear. Clear yellow urine. Clear CSF. No complaints of headache or abdominal pain, chills, malaise, or lethargy.

LABORATORY. BUN between 10 and 20 mg/dL. Serum creatinine between 0.7 and 1.4 mg/dL. AST between 7 and 40 U/mL. ALT between 10 and 40 U/ml. White blood count 5000 to 10,000/mm$^3$. Neutrophils 60% to 70%. Erythrocyte sedimentation rate below 20 mm/h. No abnormal findings from cultures of urine, blood, or CSF. PT 9.5 to 12 seconds.

#### NEGATIVE OUTCOMES

Temperature more than 37.5° C. Pulse more than 100 bpm and irregular. Client complains of headache, abdominal pain, muscle aches, malaise, or lethargy. Hot, flushed skin. Rashes. Diaphoresis. Client may have neck rigidity or discharge or drainage from wounds.

---

## PENTAMIDINE

*Trade Name:* Pentam 300
*Canadian Availability:* Pentacarinat
*Pregnancy Risk:* Category C
*pH:* Not specified
*Storage/Stability:* Store between 2° and 8° C. Protect both dry powder and reconstituted solution from light. May store reconstituted solutions in concentrations of 1 and 2.5 mg/mL for up to 24 hours at room temperature.

### ASSESSMENT: DRUG CHARACTERISTICS

#### ACTION

An antiprotozoal agent that appears to interfere with RNA and DNA synthesis. The exact mechanism of action is unknown, but pentamidine appears to interfere with the incorporation of nucleotides into RNA and DNA and possibly to interfere with folate metabolism.

#### INDICATIONS

Used to treat *Pneumocystis carinii* pneumonia in immunocompromised clients such as those with AIDS.

#### CAUTIONS

ADVERSE EFFECTS. Diabetes mellitus, hyperglycemia, hypoglycemia, severe hypotension, leukopenia or neutropenia, hepatotoxicity, nephrotoxicity, thrombocytopenia, anemia, cardiac dysrhythmias, hypersensitivity reactions, pancreatitis, phlebitis, unpleasant metallic taste in the month, or gastrointestinal symptoms including nausea, vomiting, anorexia, or diarrhea.

▼

CONTRAINDICATIONS. Should not be given to clients with a known history of hypersensitivity reactions to pentamidine. Should be given with caution to clients with a history of bleeding disorders, bone marrow depression, dysrhythmias, dehydration, impaired hepatic or renal function, diabetes mellitus, or hypotension.

**POTENTIAL DRUG/FOOD INTERACTIONS**

May increase the risk of bone marrow depression if used with other agents or radiation known to cause bone marrow depression. If used with didanosine, may increase the risk of pancreatitis. If used with foscarnet, may precipitate a severe hypocalcemia, hypomagnesemia, and nephrotoxicity. Use with other nephrotoxic drugs increases the incidence of nephrotoxicity.

**INTERVENTIONS: ADMINISTRATION**

Powder should be first diluted with 3–5 mL of sterile water for injection. Resulting solution should be mixed with 50–250 mL of D5W only.

**MODE/RATE OF ADMINISTRATION**

Give by intermittent IV infusion over 1–2 h using an infusion pump.

INTRAVENOUS USE (WITH NORMAL RENAL FUNCTION)

**Adults:** For *Pneumocystis carinii* pneumonia the usual dosage is 4 mg/kg of body weight q.d. for 14–21 d.

**Children >12 years:** Follow adult dosing schedule.

**Infants/Neonates:** Follow adult dosing schedule.

**Geriatrics:** No information available on the effect of age on dosing for pentamidine.

INTRATHECAL USE OR OTHER INFUSION ROUTES AS INDICATED. Not recommended.

**POTENTIAL PROBLEMS IN ADMINISTRATION**

May cause sudden severe hypotension, even on the first dose. Clients should be reclining and blood pressure should be carefully monitored.

**INDEPENDENT NURSING ACTIONS**

Monitor vital signs, especially blood pressure and cardiac rate and rhythm. Monitor laboratory values, especially blood sugar levels, BUN, serum creatinine, ALT, AST, and complete blood counts. Keep skin clean and dry. Use appropriate aseptic techniques and isolation precautions. Teach risk factors for infection.

**ADMINISTRATION IN ALTERNATE SETTINGS**

Initial doses should be administered in acute care settings where the client can be carefully monitored. May be given in other clinical settings or in the home by a qualified IV therapy nurse.

**EVALUATION: OUTCOMES OF DRUG THERAPY**

**EXPECTED OUTCOMES**

PHYSICAL ASSESSMENT. Blood pressure remains within 15% of clients baseline. Heart rate and rhythm remain within 15% of baseline. Temperature less than 37.5° C. Skin warm, pink, and dry. No complaints of headache, chills, malaise, blurred vision, nausea, vomiting, diarrhea, or lethargy.

LABORATORY. Serum potassium between 3.5 and 5 mEq/L. Serum calcium between 9 and 11 mg/dL. BUN between 10 and 20 mg/dL. Serum creatinine between 0.7 and 1.4 mg/dL. Red blood cell count 4.2 to 6.2 million/mm$^3$. White blood cell count returns to baseline.

**NEGATIVE OUTCOMES**

Blood pressure more than 15% less than client's baseline. Heart rate more than 15% more then baseline. Heart rhythm irregular. Temperature more than 37.5° C. Skin hot and dry or cold and clammy. Client complains of headache, chills, malaise, blurred vision, nausea, vomiting, diarrhea, or lethargy.

## TRIMETHOPRIM-SULFAMETHOXAZOLE

*Trade Names:* Bactrim, Septra, Sulfamethoprim
*Canadian Availability:* Bactrim, Septra
*Pregnancy Risk:* Category C
*pH:* 10
*Storage/Stability:* Store below 40° C. Protect from light. Do not refrigerate. Do not use if cloudy or contains a precipitate. After reconstituting, solution should be used within 6 hours.

### ASSESSMENT: DRUG CHARACTERISTICS

**ACTION**

An antibacterial and antiprotozoal agent that combines sulfamethoxazole and trimethoprim. Sulfamethoxazole is a bacteriostatic agent that inhibits folic acid synthesis needed for DNA synthesis in sensitive organisms. Trimethoprim is a bacteriostatic agent that also interferes with folic acid synthesis and acts synergistically with sulfamethoxazole.

**INDICATIONS**

A broad-spectrum agent that is used to treat otitis media, bronchitis, pneumonia, enterocolitis, traveler's diarrhea from *Shigella* and *E. coli,* and urinary tract infections.

**CAUTIONS**

ADVERSE EFFECTS. Allergic reactions, bleeding or bruising, photosensitivity, hepatitis, joint pain or muscle cramping, skin rashes, hematuria nephritis, thyroid dysfunction, or methemoglobinemia.

CONTRAINDICATIONS. Allergies to sulfonamides, furosemide, thiazide diuretics; blood dyscrasias or impaired hepatic or renal function.

**POTENTIAL DRUG/FOOD INTERACTIONS**

May interact with anticoagulants, anticonvulsants, or antidiabetic agents to delay the metabolism of cotrimoxazole and increase toxic effects. May interact with hemolytics and hepatotoxic agents to increase the toxic effects of those agents. Methenamine may cause a precipitate if used concurrently and cause crystalluria. May potentiate the effects of methotrexate, phenylbutazone, or sulfinpyrazone.

**INTERVENTIONS: ADMINISTRATION**

Dilute each 5-mL vial of 80 mg of trimethoprim and 400 mg of sulfamethoxazole in 75–100 mL of D5W solution.

**MODE/RATE OF ADMINISTRATION**

Should be given by intermittent infusion over 60–90 min.

INTRAVENOUS USE (WITH NORMAL RENAL FUNCTION)

**Adults:** For most infections the usual dosage is 2–2.5 mg of trimethoprim and 10–12.5 mg of sulfamethoxazole per kg of body weight q6h, 2.7–3.3 mg of trimethoprim and 13.3–16.7 mg of sulfamethoxazole per kg of body weight q8h, or 4–5 mg of trimethoprim and 20–25 mg of sulfamethoxazole per kg of body weight q12h.

**Children >12 years:** Follow adult dosing schedule.

**Infants/Neonates ≤ 2 months:** Not recommended.

**Infants > 2 months and Children ≤ 12 years:** Follow adult dosing schedule.

**Geriatrics:** Older clients are more at risk for side effects, including bone marrow depression and thrombocytopenia.

INTRATHECAL USE OR OTHER INFUSION ROUTES AS INDICATED. Not recommended.

**POTENTIAL PROBLEMS IN ADMINISTRATION**

Fluid intake should be maintained to at least 1200–1500 mL/d to avoid crystalluria.

**INDEPENDENT NURSING ACTIONS**

Monitor vital signs and laboratory values, especially BUN, serum creatinine, and liver enzymes. Collect specimens as required. Keep skin clean and dry. Change dressings as needed. Use appropriate aseptic techniques and isolation precautions. Teach risk factors for infection.

**ADMINISTRATION IN ALTERNATE SETTINGS**

May be given in acute care settings or in the home by a qualified IV nurse.

**EVALUATION: OUTCOMES OF DRUG THERAPY**

**EXPECTED OUTCOMES**

PHYSICAL ASSESSMENT. Temperature less than 37.5° C. Pulse between 60 and 100 bpm and regular. Skin warm, pink, and dry. No rashes, no flushing, no drainage. Breath sounds clear. Clear yellow urine. Clear CSF. No complaints of headache or abdominal pain, chills, malaise, or lethargy.

LABORATORY. BUN between 10 and 20 mg/dL. Serum creatinine between 0.7 and 1.4 mg/dL. AST between 7 and 40 U/mL. ALT between 10 and 40 U/mL. White blood count 5000 to 10,000/mm³. Neutrophils 60% to 70%. Erythrocyte sedimentation rate below 20 mm/h. No abnormal findings from cultures of urine, blood, or CSF. PT 9.5 to 12 seconds.

**NEGATIVE OUTCOMES**

Temperature more than 37.5° C. Pulse more than 100 bpm and irregular. Client complains of headache, abdominal pain, muscle aches, malaise, or lethargy. Hot, flushed skin. Rashes. Diaphoresis. Client may have neck rigidity or discharge or drainage from wounds.

---

## VANCOMYCIN

*Trade Names:* Lyphocin P, Vancocin
*Canadian Availability:* Vancocin
*Pregnancy Risk:* Category B
*pH:* 2.4–4.5
*Storage/Stability:* Store below 40° C. After reconstitution, may be stored for 24 hours at room temperature or 96 hours if refrigerated.

### ASSESSMENT: DRUG CHARACTERISTICS

**ACTION**

A narrow-spectrum antibacterial that inhibits bacterial cell wall synthesis by binding to sites that are slightly different from the penicillins and cephalosporins. May also alter cytoplasmic membrane permeability and inhibit RNA synthesis.

**INDICATIONS**

Used to treat bone and joint infections, bacterial septicemias, and bacterial endocarditis caused by *Corynebacterium* and methicillin-resistant *Staphylococcus*. May also be used prophylactically to prevent endocarditis in clients with a history of valvular disorders or rheumatic fever. Also used to treat *clostridium difficile* infection.

**CAUTIONS**

ADVERSE EFFECTS. Nephrotoxicity, ototoxicity, or allergic reactions. May also cause dysuria, nausea, vomiting, or anorexia.

CONTRAINDICATIONS. History of hearing loss, hypersensitivity to vancomycin, or renal impairment.

**POTENTIAL DRUG/FOOD INTERACTIONS**

May interact with aminoglycosides, amphotericin B, aspirin, parenteral bacitracin or bumetanide, capreomycin, cyclosporine, cisplatin, ethacrynic acid, furosemide, polymyxins, or streptozocin to increase the risk of nephrotoxicity and ototoxicity.

### INTERVENTIONS: ADMINISTRATION

Add 10 mL of sterile water to each 500-mg vial. Further dilute the 500 mg/mL concentration in 100–200 mL of
▼

D5W or 0.9% NSS for intermittent infusion. Dilute greater quantities in larger volumes of fluid for continuous infusion.

**MODE/RATE OF ADMINISTRATION**

May be given by intermittent IV infusion over 60 min or by continuous infusion.

INTRAVENOUS USE (WITH NORMAL RENAL FUNCTION)

**Adults:** For prophylaxis the usual dose is 1 g starting 1 h before the procedure and 8 h after surgery.

For infections the usual dosage is 7.5 mg/kg of body weight q6h or 15 mg/kg of body weight or 1 g q12h. Maximum daily dose should not exceed 3–4 g.

**Children > 12 years:** Follow adult dosing schedule.

**Infants/Neonates:** For prophylaxis the usual dosage is 20 mg/kg of body weight starting 1 h before surgery and 8 h after surgery.

**Children ≤ 12 years:** For infection the usual dose is 10 mg/kg of body weight q6h or 20 mg/kg of body weight q12h.

**Neonates 1 week–1 month:** For infection the usual dose is 15 mg/kg of body weight initially, then 10 mg/kg of body weight q8h.

**Neonates ≤ 1 week:** For infection the usual dose is 15 mg/kg of body weight initially, then 10 mg/kg of body weight q12h.

**Geriatrics:** Elderly clients are more likely to have age-related diminished renal function that may require a lesser dose. Elderly clients are also more at risk for ototoxicity and nephrotoxicity.

INTRATHECAL USE OR OTHER INFUSION ROUTES AS INDICATED. Not recommended.

**POTENTIAL PROBLEMS IN ADMINISTRATION**

Avoid extravasation. May cause tissue necrosis and severe pain. Should not be given as an IV push. Doing so may precipitate hypotension or cardiac arrest from histamine release.

**INDEPENDENT NURSING ACTIONS**

Monitor vital signs and laboratory values, especially BUN and serum creatinine. Collect specimens as required. Keep skin clean and dry. Change dressings as needed. Use appropriate aseptic techniques and isolation precautions. Teach risk factors for infection.

**ADMINISTRATION IN ALTERNATE SETTINGS**

May be given in acute care settings or in the home by a qualified IV nurse.

**EVALUATION: OUTCOMES OF DRUG THERAPY**

**EXPECTED OUTCOMES**

PHYSICAL ASSESSMENT. Temperature less than 37.5° C. Pulse between 60 and 100 bpm and regular. Skin warm, pink, and dry. No rashes, no flushing, no drainage. Breath sounds clear. Clear yellow urine. Clear CSF. No complaints of headache or abdominal pain, chills, malaise, or lethargy.

LABORATORY. BUN between 10 and 20 mg/dL. Serum creatinine between 0.7 and 1.4 mg/dL. White blood count 5000 to 10,000/$mm^3$. Neutrophils 60% to 70%. Erythrocyte sedimentation rate below 20 mm/h. No abnormal findings from cultures of urine, blood, or CSF.

**NEGATIVE OUTCOMES**

Temperature more than 37.5° C. Pulse more than 100 bpm and irregular. Client complains of headache, abdominal pain, muscle aches, malaise, or lethargy. Hot, flushed skin. Rashes. Diaphoresis. Client may have neck rigidity or discharge or drainage from wounds.

CHAPTER 17

# Antineoplastic Agents

*Elaine Kennedy*



## DEFINITION

Antineoplastic agents are subtances that exert their influence on DNA synthesis or function. Antineoplastic agents are also referred to as cytotoxic drugs or chemotherapeutic agents. Antineoplastic agents affect both normal and cancer cells through alterations in biochemical pathways common to all cells. Rapidly dividing abnormal cells are the targets for chemotherapy. Normal cells that rapidly divide, however, such as hair, skin, and germinal epithelium in gonads, may also be affected. The effects of antineoplastic agents on all cells explain the wide range of toxic/side effects seen in clients during chemotherapy. The goal of antineoplastic therapy is to control or eliminate cancer cells without damaging or destroying normal, healthy cells.

## CLASSIFICATION

Antineoplastic agents may be classified by their effects on various parts of cell cycle activity. The exact mechanism action for all agents has not been determined. Cell cycle activity may be broken into the M phase (actual cell division) and three chemically distinctive postdivision phases: $G_1$ phase (pre-DNA synthesis), S phase (DNA synthesis), and $G_2$ phase (post-DNA synthesis). Antineoplastic agents that affect the cell at specific times in cell activity are called cell cycle specific. Antineoplastic agents whose actions are independent of cell cycle activity are called cell cycle nonspecific.

### CELL CYCLE SPECIFIC ANTINEOPLASTICS

Cell cycle specific antineoplastic agents include antimetabolites, vinca alkaloids, and agents such as cytarabine, hydroxyurea, and bleomycin. The cell cycle specific agents are most effective against neoplasms that have a large number of cells undergoing division at the same time.

- Antimetabolites are analogs of normal metabolites and compete with the normal metabolites in normal metabolic pathways. Some antimetabolites are used in DNA synthesis in place of normal nucleotides.
- Vinca alkaloids appear to affect the mitotic spindle, causing arrest of cell division.

### CELL CYCLE NONSPECIFIC ANTINEOPLASTICS

Cell cycle nonspecific antineoplastic agents include alkylating agents, most antineoplastic antibiotics, and other agents such as cisplatin, fluorouracil, and floxuridine.

- Alkylating agents, in general, cause structural damage to DNA by causing cross-linking and scissoring of DNA strands. Alkylating agents can be subdivided into nitrogen mustards, ethylenimines, alkasulfonates, triazenes, and nitrosoureas.
- Antineoplastic antibiotics bind with DNA or RNA and inhibit DNA synthesis.

## RESISTANCE

Resistance to antineoplastic drugs is a major consideration of therapy. Resistance may be natural or induced. Natural resistance results from cellular discrimination and is passed along cell lines. Induced resistance results from neoplastic cellular adaptation or mutation as an outcome of drug therapy.

## CHEMOTHERAPY PRINCIPLES

- Antineoplastic agents may be the treatment of choice for some cancers or may be used as adjuvant therapy along with surgery or radiation therapy.
- Cancer cells are the most susceptible to the appropriate antineoplastic agent given in high concentrations when the majority of cells are in the affected cycle.
- The fewer the cancer cells, the greater the effect of antineoplastic drugs. Therefore, the earlier treatment is begun, the greater the chances of remission.

- Antineoplastic drugs are highly toxic and carry the potential for myelosuppression, hemorrhage, and infection. Physicians skilled in the management of cancer treatment should oversee any therapy using antineoplastic drugs. Toxicity is greatest in clients who have had previous therapy with antineoplastic agents or radiation therapy.
- No single antineoplastic agent is useful for all cancers or in all clients. Careful consideration must be given to the type of cancer cell; the age, general condition, and sex of the client; the characteristics of the antineoplastic agent; and any previous or adjuvant therapy.
- Antineoplastic agents are frequently given in combinations, with the sequencing of doses of the various agents carefully timed to maximize the impact on cell cycle activity. Antineoplastic agents can usually be given over longer periods with less toxicity if the therapy is given in cycles and sequenced. The combination agents should not have the same general effects on cell cycle activity.

## ANTINEOPLASTIC DRUG DANGERS

Antineoplastic agents pose special hazards to health care workers who are directly exposed to these agents. Exposure may be from inhaled dust, from ingested food exposed to agent dust, or from direct agent-skin contact when the agent is handled.

Several variables may determine the extent of risk to health care workers:

1. The antineoplastic agent's chemical properties
2. The individual health care worker's susceptibility to the given agent
3. The individual health care worker's risk factors such as smoking, age, gender, etc.
4. The number and amount of exposure
5. The type of exposure

In theory, perfect technique for preparing and administering antineoplastic agents prevents environmental and personal exposure. In practice, however, the likelihood of perfect technique 100% of the time by all health care workers is unlikely. All personnel handling antineoplastic agents must assume that the likelihood of exposure exists. They must know how to safely handle the agents and must know how to protect themselves and the environment.

The antineoplastic drugs are grouped by subclassifications in Table 17–1.

**TABLE 17–1**
**Parenteral Antineoplastic Drugs Grouped by Subclassifications**

| Cell Cycle Specific | Cell Cycle Nonspecific |
|---|---|
| ***Antimetabolites*** | ***Alkylating Agents*** |
| Asparaginase* | Carmustine |
| Cytarabine | Cisplatin |
| Etoposide | Cyclophosphamide |
| Floxuridine* | Dacarbazine |
| Fluorouracil | Mechlorethamine hydrochloride |
| Methotrexate sodium | Thiotepa |
| Pegasparagase (PEG-L-Asparaginase) | |
| Trimetrexate glucuronate | |
| ***Vinca Alkaloids*** | ***Antibiotics*** |
| Vinblastine sulfate | Bleomycin sulfate |
| Vincristine sulfate | Dactinomycin* |
| | Daunorubicin hydrochloride |
| | Doxorubicin hydrochloride |
| | Mitomycin |
| | Plicamycin |
| | Streptozocin* |

*Not discussed in this chapter.

# CELL CYCLE SPECIFIC ANTINEOPLASTICS

## THERAPEUTIC EFFECTS

Cell cycle specific antineoplastics act at specific times in cell cycle activity. Some agents appear to act in more than one way, and the precise mechanism of some agents has not yet been determined. Antimetabolites are structures that are similar to naturally occurring metabolites and compete for sites on protein compounds needed for DNA synthesis. Vinca alkaloids interfere with rapid cellular division by crystallizing protein in the mitotic spindle.

## PHARMACOKINETICS

**Distribution.** Diffusion following intravenous (IV) infusion is rapid and widespread. Some agents diffuse across the blood-brain barrier more readily than others.

**Metabolism/Elimination.** Plasma half-life is usually ½ to 2 hours in adults with normal kidney and liver function. Some agents may have half-lives as long as 24 hours or even longer. Traces of some agents may be detected in the liver months after administration.

## CAUTIONS

**Side/Adverse Effects.** Cell cycle specific antineoplastics are potent bone marrow suppressants and highly cytotoxic. Clients may be more prone to infection as well as hemorrhagic complications.

**Contraindications.** Cell cycle specific antineoplastics should not be given to clients who have been previously treated with antineoplastic agents and who have a documented history of hepatotoxicity, nephrotoxicity, or allergic reactions or to clients with severe leukopenia or infections. The agents should be used with extreme caution in clients with a history of pancreatitis.

***Pregnancy and Lactation.*** Cell cycle specific antineoplastic agents are teratogenic and mutagenic substances. They should not be given to pregnant women without careful consideration to the potential for fetal damage. Some agents are transmitted via breast milk.

***Pediatrics.*** No age-specific contraindications have been determined.

***Geriatrics.*** No age-specific contraindications have been determined.

## TOXICITY

See Table 17–2 for toxicities of cell cycle specific antineoplastics.

## POTENTIAL DRUG/FOOD INTERACTIONS

Some agents interact with monoamine oxidase (MAO) inhibitors and potentiate the effects of the MAO inhibitor. Agents generally interact with anticoagulants, salicylates, and nonsteroidal antiinflammatory drugs (NSAIDs) to potentiate the anticoagulant properties of those drugs.

# Antimetabolites

## CYTARABINE (ARA-C, CYTOSINE ARABINOSIDE)

*Trade Name:* Cytosar-U
*Canadian Availability:* Cytosar
*Pregnancy Risk:* Category D
*pH:* 5
*Storage/Stability:* Store below 40° C. Reconstituted solutions are stable at room temperature for 48 hours. Discard solutions with a slight haze. Use solutions for intrathecal use immediately. Infusions with up to 500 mcg (0.5 mg) of cytarabine per milliliter are stable at room temperature for up to 7 days.

### ASSESSMENT: DRUG CHARACTERISTICS

#### ACTION

A cell cycle specific antimetabolite that is effective during the S phase (DNA synthesis phase) of cell activity. DNA synthesis is inhibited with little effect on RNA or protein synthesis.

#### INDICATIONS

Used to treat acute lymphocytic and myelogenous leukemias and non-Hodgkin's lymphomas.

▼

**TABLE 17–2**
**Toxicities of Cell Cycle Specific Antineoplastics**

| Body System | Side/Toxic Effects | Physical Assessment Indicators | Laboratory Indicators | Nursing Interventions |
|---|---|---|---|---|
| Neurologic | Neurotoxicity | Numbness, paresthesias, peripheral neuropathy, neuritis, seizures, dizziness, urinary retention | N/A | Initiate safety precautions for sensory and mobility deficits. |
| Respiratory | | Acute shortness of breath, bronchospasm | N/A | Avoid allergens and people with respiratory infections. Stop drug administration immediately if bronchospasm occurs. |
| Renal | Azotemia | | | Monitor lab values, weigh client frequently, increase fluid intake. |
| Gastrointestinal | Hepatomegaly, pancreatitis | Nausea and vomiting, anorexia, diarrhea, pharyngitis, stomatitis, adynamic ileus | | Give antiemetics before and after administering agent. Give meticulous mouth care. Avoid hot, spicy foods, and alcohol. |
| Hematologic | Bone marrow suppression, leukopenia, anemia | Bruising, bleeding, melena, petechiae, epistaxis, hematuria | | Avoid anticoagulants and aspirin. Provide a safe environment to prevent injury. |
| Dermatologic | Dermatitis | Phototoxicity, cellulitis, tissue irritation, phlebitis, necrosis, acute allergic response | N/A | Be prepared to administer epinephrine and corticosteroids for allergic response. |
| Sensory | Corneal ulcer | Lesions on cornea | N/A | Flush eyes with copious amounts of water if direct contact with agent occurs. |
| Other | Bone pain | | N/A | Medicate for pain. Handle client gently. |

**CAUTIONS**

A potent immunosuppressive and bone marrow depressive agent. There is an increased incidence of infection and delayed healing of dental work. Dental work should be done before therapy is started or delayed until blood counts return to normal. Clients should be instructed in proper oral hygiene. Cytarbine is both mutagenic and teratogenic. Clients should be instructed to use appropriate forms of birth control during treatment and for 4 months after treatment.

ADVERSE EFFECTS. Carries the possibility of secondary malignancy as a result of therapy. Risk of malignancy seems to increase with long-term use. Leukopenia, stomatitis, thrombocytopenia are common effects of therapy. Frequent platelet and leukocyte counts should be done after therapy to monitor for thrombocytopenia and leukopenia.

CONTRAINDICATIONS. Should be given cautiously, if at all, to clients with significant immunosuppression, herpes zoster, impaired hepatic functioning, infection, or sensitivity to cytarabine.

**POTENTIAL DRUG/FOOD INTERACTIONS**

May interact with antigout agents such as probenecid or sulfinpyrazone to raise serum uric acid levels significantly. Allopurinol is frequently given to lower serum uric acid levels. Bone marrow suppression may be potentiated if cytarabine is used in conjunction with radiation therapy or with cyclophosphamide. Cytarabine should not be given with live virus vaccine because the viral replication may increase.

**INTERVENTIONS: ADMINISTRATION**

Strict adherence to agency safety procedures for handling antineoplastic agents should be followed when reconstituting and administering cytarabine. Dilute 100 mg with 5 mL (500 mg with 10 mL) sterile water with benzyl alcohol for IV push administration. Dilute further with 50 to 100 mL or more normal saline solution (NSS) or 5% dextrose in water (D5W) and give as infusion.

**MODE/RATE OF ADMINISTRATION**

May be given IV push through the side arm of a free-flowing infusion at the rate of 100 mg over 1–3 min. Intermittent infusions are given over 30 min. The rate and concentration of continuous infusion are ordered individually by the physician. High-dose infusions generally infuse over 1–3 h. Intermittent infusions are generally mixed with D5W or 0.9% NSS.

INTRAVENOUS USE (WITH NORMAL RENAL AND HEPATIC FUNCTION)

**Adults:** Usual adult and adolescent dosage is 3 mg/kg of body weight per day for 5–10 d, repeated q2wk.

**Children:** Dosage and schedule for children are similar to those for adults and adolescents.

**Infants/Neonates:** Safety for use with infants has not been established.

**Geriatrics:** Follow adult dosing schedule. No specific cautions.

INTRATHECAL USE OR OTHER INFUSION ROUTES AS INDICATED. May be given by intrathecal infusion. The usual dosage is 5–75 mg/m2 of body surface area (BSA) given once a day for 4 d or once q4d. The average dosage is 30 mg/m2 of BSA once q4d until the cerebrospinal fluid (CSF) is clear, plus one additional dose. Maintenance doses of 1 mg/kg of body weight may be given SC once or twice a week.

#### POTENTIAL PROBLEMS IN ADMINISTRATION

Clients seem to tolerate rapid IV injection better than a slow infusion, although they have more severe nausea and vomiting after the injection. Strict adherence to safety procedures should be followed when reconstituting and administering cytarabine. Rarely, clients may experience cytarabine syndrome, which occurs 6–12 hours after administration. With cytarabine syndrome, clients experience bone or muscle pain, occasional chest pain, fever, general malaise, conjunctivitis, and maculopapular rash. Cytarabine syndrome usually responds to corticosteroids. The client must experience some toxicity to yield remission. The physician will restart the drug as soon as signs of bone marrow recovery occur or the effectiveness of the original dosage will be lost.

#### INDEPENDENT NURSING ACTIONS

Monitor hematologic laboratory values carefully. Teach clients to use good oral hygiene with soft bristled toothbrushes and to notify physician if stomatitis interferes with eating. Teach clients to avoid sources of infection when their blood counts are low. Teach clients to monitor themselves for infection, sore throat, or fever greater than or equal to 100.4° F and unusual bleeding such as black, tarry stools or bruising that occurs without injury. Unless contraindicated, encourage fluids to at least 2 L/d to reduce symptoms of gout.

#### ADMINISTRATION IN ALTERNATE SETTINGS

Should be administered in settings where the client can be closely monitored during the administration.

#### EVALUATION: OUTCOMES OF DRUG THERAPY

#### EXPECTED OUTCOMES

PHYSICAL ASSESSMENT. Loss of hair,· nausea, vomiting, and stomatitis. Leukocyte count drops.

LABORATORY. Leukocyte levels typically start to fall in the first 24 hours after administration, hit the first nadir in 7 to 9 days, rebound slightly, and fall to a lower nadir between days 15 and 24. Leukocyte counts start to rise

▼

quickly after day 24. Thrombocytes start to fall about day 5, hit nadir at 12 to 15 days, and recover over the next 10 days. Clients should have a hematocrit (Hct), hemoglobin (Hgb), platelet count, and leukocyte count prior to the start of therapy.

#### NEGATIVE OUTCOMES

Acute pancreatitis, infection, central nervous system (CNS) toxicity, elevated serum uric acid levels, hepatotoxicity, gastrointestinal (GI) tract bleeding, pulmonary edema, or urinary retention.

## ETOPOSIDE (VP-16-213)

*Trade Name:* VePesid
*Canadian Availability:* VePesid
*Pregnancy Risk:* Category D
*pH:* 3–4
*Storage/Stability:* Store below 40° C. Protect from freezing. When diluted to 0.4 mg and 0.2 mg/mL, solutions are stable for 48 to 96 hours, respectively, at 25° C in glass or plastic containers.

### ASSESSMENT: DRUG CHARACTERISTICS

#### ACTION

A cell cycle specific antineoplastic agent that appears to act during the pre-DNA synthesis S stage of cell division.

#### INDICATIONS

Used primarily as first-line treatment of small cell carcinomas of the lung and testicular cancer in combination with other agents and surgery.

#### CAUTIONS

A potent immunosuppressive and bone marrow depressive agent. There is an increased incidence of infection and delayed healing of dental work. Dental work should be done before therapy is started or delayed until blood counts return to normal. Clients should be instructed in proper oral hygiene. Etoposide is both mutagenic and teratogenic. Clients should be instructed to use appropriate forms of birth control during treatment and for 4 months after treatment.

ADVERSE EFFECTS. Carries the possibility of secondary malignancy as a result of therapy. Risk of malignancy seems to increase with long-term use. Acute leukemias have been noted when etoposide has been used with other antineoplastic agents. Leukopenia, stomatitis, thrombocytopenia, and neurotoxicity are common effects of therapy. Frequent platelet and leukocyte counts should be done after therapy to monitor the leukopenia and thrombocytopenia.

CONTRAINDICATIONS. Should be given cautiously, if at all, to clients with bone marrow depression, herpes zoster, impaired hepatic functioning, infection, or sensitivity to etoposide.

**POTENTIAL DRUG/FOOD INTERACTIONS**

Bone marrow suppression may be potentiated if etoposide is used in conjunction with radiation therapy or with cyclophosphamide. Etoposide should not be given with live virus vaccine because the viral replication may increase.

**INTERVENTIONS: ADMINISTRATION**

Strict adherence to agency safety procedures for handling antineoplastic agents should be followed when reconstituting and administering etoposide. Usually diluted in solutions of either D5W or 0.9% NSS to produce a solution containing 200–400 mcg (0.2–0.4 mg)/mL.

**MODE/RATE OF ADMINISTRATION**

Given as a diluted solution by slow infusion over 30–60 min. Should not be given by rapid IV injection or by any other route.

INTRAVENOUS USE (WITH NORMAL RENAL AND HEPATIC FUNCTION)

**Adults:** For testicular carcinoma, IV infusions of 50–100 mg/m$^2$ of BSA are given on days 1 through 5. Dosing schedules of up to 100 mg/m$^2$ of BSA are given on days 1, 3, and 5 each week for 3- to 4-week cycles. For small cell carcinoma of the lung, IV infusions of 35 mg/m$^2$ of BSA are given for 4 d. Dosing schedules may include up to 50 mg/m$^2$ of BSA per day for 5 d on a q3–4 wk schedule.

**Children:** Dosage not established.

**Infants/Neonates:** Dosage not established.

**Geriatrics:** Follow adult dosing schedules. No specific cautions.

INTRATHECAL USE OR OTHER INFUSION ROUTES AS INDICATED. Not recommended.

**POTENTIAL PROBLEMS IN ADMINISTRATION**

An etoposide infusion administered too rapidly may cause hypotension. Treat by stopping infusion, giving fluids, repositioning the client, and resuming the infusion at a slower rate. The elderly are likely to have this side effect.

**INDEPENDENT NURSING ACTIONS**

Monitor hematologic laboratory values carefully. Teach clients to use proper oral hygiene and to avoid sources of infection when their blood counts are low. Teach clients to monitor themselves for infection and unusual bleeding such as black, tarry stools or bruising that occurs without injury.

**ADMINISTRATION IN ALTERNATE SETTINGS**

Should be administered in settings where the client can be closely monitored during the administration.

**EVALUATION: OUTCOMES OF DRUG THERAPY**

**EXPECTED OUTCOMES**

PHYSICAL ASSESSMENT. Loss of hair, nausea, vomiting, and stomatitis. Tumor mass diminishes in size. If given for small cell carcinoma of the lung, shortness of breath and dyspnea improve.

▼

LABORATORY. Leukocyte levels typically start to fall in the first 24 hours after administration and hit nadir in 7 to 14 days. Leukocyte counts should recover by day 20. Thrombocyte levels start to fall about day 5, hit nadir at 9 to 16 days, and recover by day 20. Clients should have an Hct, Hgb, platelet count, and leukocyte count with differential prior to the start of therapy.

#### NEGATIVE OUTCOMES

Infection, CNS toxicity, severe oral ulcers, hepatotoxicity, and GI tract bleeding. Tumor mass does not diminish in size.

---

## FLUOROURACIL (5-FLUOROURACIL, 5-FU)

*Trade Name:* Adrucil
*Canadian Availability:* Adrucil
*Pregnancy Risk:* Category D
*pH:* 9.2
*Storage/Stability:* Store below 40° C. Protect from light and freezing. Undiluted vials are stable for up to 1 month. If diluted, the injection solution should be discarded within 24 hours. Do not refrigerate solution.

### ASSESSMENT: DRUG CHARACTERISTICS

#### ACTION

A cell cycle specific antimetabolite that appears to act during the S phase (DNA synthesis phase) of cell division and inhibits both DNA and RNA synthesis.

#### INDICATIONS

Used to treat colorectal, breast, gastric, and pancreatic carcinomas.

#### CAUTIONS

A potent immunosuppressive and bone marrow depressive agent. There is an increased incidence of infection and delayed healing of dental work. Dental work should be done before therapy is started or delayed until blood counts return to normal. Clients should be instructed in proper oral hygiene. Fluorouracil is both mutagenic and teratogenic. Clients should be instructed to use appropriate forms of birth control during treatment and for 4 months after treatment.

ADVERSE EFFECTS. Carries the possibility of secondary malignancy as a result of therapy. Risk of malignancy seems to increase with long-term use. Leukopenia, stomatitis, thrombocytopenia, diarrhea, and esophagitis are common effects of therapy. Frequent platelet and leukocyte counts should be done after therapy to monitor the leukopenia and thrombocytopenia. Clients may develop acute cerebellar syndrome (difficulty with balance), myocardial ischemia, palmar-plantar erythrodysesthesia syndrome (tingling of hands and feet, with subsequent swelling, redness, and pain). Pretreatment with leucovorin may prevent some of the toxic effects. All symptoms usually clear in 5 to 7 days after stopping fluorouracil. The syndrome may be treated with oral pyridoxine, 100 to 150 mg/d.

CONTRAINDICATIONS. Should be given cautiously, if at all, to clients with significant immunosuppression, herpes zoster, impaired hepatic functioning, infection, impaired renal function, tumor cell infiltration of the bone marrow, or sensitivity to fluorouracil.

**POTENTIAL DRUG/FOOD INTERACTIONS**

Bone marrow depression may be potentiated if fluorouracil is used with radiation therapy or leucovorin. Fluorouracil should not be given with live virus vaccine because the viral replication may increase.

**INTERVENTIONS: ADMINISTRATION**

Strict adherence to agency safety procedures for handling antineoplastic agents should be followed when reconstituting and administering fluorouracil.

**MODE/RATE OF ADMINISTRATIONX**

Given as a diluted solution over 2–24 h. D5W or 0.9% NSS may be used. May also be given by rapid IV injection, which may be more effective but increases risk of toxicity.

INTRAVENOUS USE (WITH NORMAL RENAL AND HEPATIC FUNCTION)

**Adults:** Dependent on protocol, initial IV dosage is 7–12 mg/kg of body weight q24h for 4 d with a 3-d pause. If no toxic symptoms are evident, dosage is 7–10 mg/kg of body weight q3–4d for 2 wk. Clients who are poor risks have slightly lower dosing schedules. The maintenance dosing schedule is 7–12 mg/kg of body weight q7–10d. Maximum daily dose should not exceed 800 mg/24 h.

**Children:** Dosage not determined for children under 12 years. Adolescents follow adult dosing schedules.

**Infants/Neonates:** Dosage not determined.

**Geriatrics:** Follow adult dosing schedule. No specific cautions.

INTRATHECAL USE OR OTHER INFUSION ROUTES AS INDICATED. Intrathecal use not recommended because of neurotoxicity. May be given intra-arterially.

**POTENTIAL PROBLEMS IN ADMINISTRATION**

Appropriate dosage must be based on lean body weight. Estimates must be done if the client has evidence of edema or is obese. Some clients experience a darkening along the vein used for infusion.

**INDEPENDENT NURSING ACTIONS**

Monitor hematologic laboratory values carefully. Teach clients to use good oral hygiene and to avoid sources of infection when

▼

their blood counts are low. Teach clients to monitor themselves for infection and unusual bleeding such as black, tarry stools or bruising that occurs without injury. Apply pressure to venipuncture sites for at least 10 min.

**ADMINISTRATION IN ALTERNATE SETTINGS**

The first course of fluorouracil should be done as an inpatient in a hospital; subsequent IV administration of fluorouracil can be done in a setting where the client can be monitored and personnel are skilled in administering antineoplastic agents.

**EVALUATION: OUTCOMES OF DRUG THERAPY**

**EXPECTED OUTCOMES**

PHYSICAL ASSESSMENT. Loss of hair, nausea, vomiting, and stomatitis. Tumor mass diminishes in size.

LABORATORY. Leukocyte levels typically start to fall in the first 24 hours after administration, hit the first nadir in 7 to 9 days, rebound slightly days 10 to 14, and fall to a lower nadir between days 15 and 24. Recovers in 30 days. Thrombocyte levels start to fall about day 5, hit nadir at 12 to 15 days, and recover over the next 10 days. Clients should have an Hct, Hgb, platelet count, and leukocyte count prior to the start of therapy.

**NEGATIVE OUTCOMES**

Acute pancreatitis, infection, CNS toxicity, elevated serum uric acid levels, hepatotoxicity, GI tract bleeding, pulmonary edema, or urinary retention. Tumor mass does not decrease in size.

## METHOTREXATE SODIUM

*Trade Names:* Folex PFS, Mexate-AQ
*Canadian Availability:* Metho-trexate
*Pregnancy Risk:* Category X
*pH:* 7.5–9
*Storage/Stability:* Store below 40° C. Protect from freezing. Immediately prior to use, mix solutions that contain no preservatives. Stability of preservative-containing solutions depends on the concentration of the drug, the specific diluents used, the resulting pH, and the temperature.

**ASSESSMENT: DRUG CHARACTERISTICS**

**ACTION**

A cell cycle specific antimetabolite that appears active during the pre-DNA synthesis S stage of cell division. Inhibits both DNA and RNA synthesis. Growth of rapidly dividing tissues is more affected than growth of normally dividing tissues such as skin.

**INDICATIONS**

Used primarily to treat carcinomas of the breast,

head, neck, and lung; acute lymphocytic leukemias; mycosis fungoides; and osteosarcomas. Used for the symptomatic control of recalcitrant, disabling psoriasis in carefully selected clients. Used in small doses to manage the active stage of severe classic or definite rheumatoid arthritis.

**CAUTIONS**

A potent immunosuppressive and bone marrow depressive agent. There is an increased incidence of infection and delayed healing of dental work. Dental work should be done before therapy is started or delayed until blood counts return to normal. Clients should be instructed in proper oral hygiene. Methotrexate is both mutagenic and teratogenic and is known to cause abortions if used during the first trimester of pregnancy. Clients should be instructed to use appropriate forms of birth control during treatment and for 4 months following treatment. Ulcerations of the oral mucosa are usually the earliest signs of toxicity.

ADVERSE EFFECTS. Carries the possibility of secondary malignancy as a result of therapy. Risk of malignancy seems to increase with long-term use. Acute leukemias have been noted when methotrexate has been used with other antineoplastic agents. Leukopenia, stomatitis, thrombocytopenia, and neurotoxicity are common effects of therapy. Frequent platelet and leukocyte counts should be done after therapy to monitor the leukopenia and thrombocytopenia. Renal failure from hyperuricemia may result from high-dose therapy.

CONTRAINDICATIONS. Immunodeficiency, ascites, pleural or peritoneal effusions, impaired renal function, bone marrow depression, herpes zoster, impaired hepatic functions, infection, oral mucositis, peptic ulcer, or ulcerative colitis.

**POTENTIAL DRUG/FOOD INTERACTIONS**

When used with acyclovir, there is increased risk of neurotoxicity. When used with alcohol or other hepatotoxic drugs, there is increased risk of hepatotoxicity. Use with NSAIDs may increase bone marrow depression. May inhibit action of asparaginase and may potentiate bone marrow supression when used with radiation therapy or cytarabine. Probenecid and aspirin may delay excretion of methotrexate, thus increasing the risk of toxicity. Aspirin therapy should be discontinued for 24 to 48 hours prior to infusion therapy with methotrexate.

**INTERVENTIONS: ADMINISTRATION**

Strict adherence to agency safety procedures for handling antineoplastic agents should be followed when reconstituting and administering methotrexate. Usually diluted in solutions of D5W or

▼

0.9% NSS to produce a solution containing 200–400 mcg (0.2–0.4 mg)/mL.

**MODE/RATE OF ADMINISTRATION**

May be given as a rapid IV, slow IV, intrathecal, intraarterial, or intraventricular infusion. Caution must be excercised to assure that the drug preparation and diluent are appropriate for the route of administration.

INTRAVENOUS USE (WITH NORMAL RENAL AND HEPATIC FUNCTION)

**Adults:** For osteosarcoma, dosing is 12 g/m$^2$ of BSA infused in 4 h, followed by a leucovorin rescue of usually 15 mg orally q6h for 10 doses starting 24 h after the methotrexate infusion. Therapy is given over many weeks and may be used in conjunction with doxorubicin, cisplatin, bleomycin, cyclophosphamide, and dactinomycin.

**Children:** Dosage not established.

**Infants/Neonates:** Dosage not established.

**Geriatrics:** Follow adult dosing schedules. No specific recommendations.

INTRATHECAL USE OR OTHER INFUSION ROUTES AS INDICATED. Preservative-free preparations only may be given by intrathecal infusion. Dosing schedules are different from rapid IV infusion schedules. Prior to intrathecal administration of methotrexate, a volume of CSF approximately equivalent to the volume of methotrexate solution to be injected (e.g., 5–15 mL) is usually removed. If the lumbar puncture is traumatic, methotrexate should not be administered intrathecally. Allow 2 d before again attempting the injection.

Because the volume of CSF is related to age and not BSA, dosage regimens based on BSA may result in inadequate CSF concentrations in children and high, potentially neurotoxic CSF concentrations in adults. For this reason, some clinicians recommend that intrathecal dosage be based on the patient's age.

**Adults:** 12 mg/m$^2$ BSA intrathecally.

**Children ≥3 years:** Same as adults.

**Children 2 years:** 10 mg/m$^2$ BSA intrathecally.

**Children 1 year:** 8 mg/m$^2$ BSA intrathecally.

**Infants < 1 year:** 6 mg/m$^2$ BSA intrathecally.

**Geriatrics:** Elderly clients may require lower doses because of reduced CSF turnover and decreasing brain volume. Intraarterial administration into the hepatic artery for the treatment of metastatic colon cancer has been effective.

**POTENTIAL PROBLEMS IN ADMINISTRATION**

Leucovorin, an antidote to folic acid antagonists such as methotrexate, is used to counter the GI and hematologic effects of methotrexate. Rapid infusion therapy should not be started unless leucovorin is physically on hand and ready to be administered. Leucovorin should be administered after methotrexate so that leucovorin does not interfere with methotrexate's antineoplastic activity.

**INDEPENDENT NURSING ACTIONS**

Monitor hematologic laboratory values carefully. Teach clients to use proper oral hygiene and to avoid sources of infection when their blood counts are low. Teach clients to monitor themselves for infection and unusual bleeding such as black, tarry stools or bruising that occurs without injury. Do not administer methotrexate if the client's serum uric acid and creatinine clearance values are elevated.

**ADMINISTRATION IN ALTERNATE SETTINGS**

Should be administered in settings where the client can be closely monitored during the administration.

**EVALUATION: OUTCOMES OF DRUG THERAPY**

**EXPECTED OUTCOMES**

PHYSICAL ASSESSMENT. Loss of hair, nausea, vomiting, and stomatitis. Tumor mass diminishes in size. If given for small cell carcinoma of the lung, shortness of breath and dyspnea improve.

LABORATORY. Leukocyte levels typically start to fall in the first 24 hours after administration and hit nadir in 7 to 14 days. Leukocyte counts should recover by day 20. Thrombocyte levels start to fall about day 5, hit nadir at 9 to 16 days, and recover by day 20. Clients should have an Hct, Hgb, platelet count, and leukocyte count with differential prior to the start of therapy. Blood urea nitrogen (BUN) may be elevated.

**NEGATIVE OUTCOMES**

Renal failure, azotemia, hyperuricemia, severe neuropathy, hepatotoxicity, pneumonia, and increased intracranial pressure. Failure of cell counts to reach normal levels in CSF if given by intrathecal infusion or no change in tumor mass.

## PACLITAXEL

*Trade Name:* Taxol
*Canadian Availability:* Not specified
*Pregnancy Risk:* Category D
*pH:* Not specified
*Storage/Stability:* Store between 2° and 8° C. Dilute solution before using. Diluted solutions may be kept at room temperature and light for up to 27 hours. Diluted solutions may be hazy.

**ASSESSMENT: DRUG CHARACTERISTICS**

**ACTION**

A cell cycle specific agent that interferes with interphase and mitotic cellular functions by preventing the reorganization of the microtubule network.

▼

**INDICATIONS**

Used to treat ovarian cancer. Usually used after first-line agents have proved ineffective.

**CAUTIONS**

A potent immunosuppressive and bone marrow depressive agent. There is an increased incidence of infection and delayed healing of dental work. Dental work should be done before therapy is started or delayed until blood counts return to normal. Clients should be instructed in proper oral hygiene. Paclitaxel is both mutagenic and teratogenic in animal studies. Clients should be instructed to use appropriate forms of birth control.

ADVERSE EFFECTS. Carries the possibility of secondary malignancy as a result of therapy. Risk of malignancy seems to increase with long-term use. Leukopenia, stomatitis, and thrombocytopenia are common effects of therapy. Frequent platelet and leukocyte counts should be done after therapy to monitor the leukopenia and thrombocytopenia.

CONTRAINDICATIONS. Should be given cautiously to clients with known cardiac problems such as conduction disorders, congestive heart failure, and acute myocardial infarctions within 6 months of the onset of therapy or to clients who have used other antineoplastic agents. Should not be given to clients who have known sensitivity to paclitaxel.

**POTENTIAL DRUG/FOOD INTERACTIONS**

Bone marrow suppression may be potentiated if paclitaxel is used in conjunction with radiation therapy. Paclitaxel should not be given with live virus vaccine because the viral replication may increase.

**INTERVENTIONS: ADMINISTRATION**

Strict adherence to agency safety procedures for handling antineoplastic agents should be followed when reconstituting paclitaxel. Must be diluted before administration. Dilute with D5W, 0.9% NSS, or D5W and Ringer's lactate solutions to a strength of 0.3–1.2 mg/mL. Avoid using polyvinyl chloride containers. Use an in-line microporous filter with micropores not greater than 0.22 $\mu$m. The filter should be changed every 12 h.

**MODE/RATE OF ADMINISTRATION**

Dose given by slow continuous infusion over 24 h.

INTRAVENOUS USE (WITH NORMAL RENAL FUNCTION)

**Adults:** For ovarian cancer the usual dosage is 135 mg/m$^2$ of BSA every 21 d.

**Children:** Dosage not established.

**Infants/Neonates:** Dosage not established.

**Geriatrics:** Follow adult dosing schedule.

INTRATHECAL USE OR OTHER INFUSION ROUTES AS INDICATED. Not recommended.

#### POTENTIAL PROBLEMS IN ADMINISTRATION

To prevent a hypersensitivity reaction, corticosteroids such as dexamethasone are usually given to clients 12 and 6 h prior to starting therapy with paclitaxel. Antinausea agents are also given prior to the start of the infusion to diminish the adverse effects of the therapy.

#### INDEPENDENT NURSING ACTIONS

Monitor hematologic laboratory values carefully. Teach clients to use proper oral hygiene and to avoid sources of infection when their blood counts are low. Teach clients to monitor themselves for infection and unusual bleeding such as black, tarry stools or bruising that occurs without injury.

#### ADMINISTRATION IN ALTERNATE SETTINGS

Should be administered in settings where the client can be closely monitored during the administration.

### EVALUATION: OUTCOMES OF DRUG THERAPY

#### EXPECTED OUTCOMES

PHYSICAL ASSESSMENT. Loss of hair, nausea, vomiting, and stomatitis. Tumor mass diminishes in size.

LABORATORY. Leukocyte levels typically start to fall in the first 24 hours after administration and hit nadir in 11 days. Leukocyte counts should recover by days 15 to 21. Thrombocyte level starts to fall about day 5, hits nadir at 8 to 9 days, and recovers by day 20. Clients should have an Hct, Hgb, platelet count, and leukocyte count with differential prior to the start of therapy.

#### NEGATIVE OUTCOMES

Infection, cardiovascular system toxicity, severe oral ulcers, hepatotoxicity, and GI tract bleeding. Tumor mass does not diminish in size.

---

## PEGASPARAGASE (PEG-L-ASPARAGINASE)

*Trade Name:* Oncaspar
*Canadian Availability:* Not specified
*Pregnancy Risk:* Category C
*pH:* Not specified
*Storage/Stability:* Avoid excessive agitation. Do not shake. Store at 2° to 8° C. Do not use if solution is not clear or if a precipitate is present. Do not use if stored at room temperature for greater than 48 hours. Do not freeze. Freezing destroys the action of the drug. Discard unused portions.

### ASSESSMENT: DRUG CHARACTERISTICS

#### ACTION

A cell cycle specific antimetabolic agent that is a modified version of the enzyme L-asparaginase. The agent catalyzes the conversion of asparagine, an amino acid, to aspartic acid and ammonia. Some cells, espe-

▼

cially acute lymphoblastic leukemic cells (ALL), are unable to synthesize asparagine, which is needed by the cell to synthesize DNA.

**INDICATIONS**

Used to treat ALL in clients sensitive to *Escherichia coli*–derived L-asparaginase.

**CAUTIONS**

ADVERSE EFFECTS. May deplete serum proteins and increase toxicity of drugs that are protein bound. May cause imbalances in the clotting mechanism and predispose the client to hemorrhage. May cause allergic reactions, including skin rashes, urticaria, hypotension, and anaphylactic shock. May have some impact on hepatic function, including elevating serum aspartate aminotransferase (AST), alamine aminotransferase (ALT), and serum bilirubin. May cause azotemia or prerenal shutdown, fatal renal insufficiency, increased BUN, or increased serum creatinine. May cause pancreatitis, hyperosmolar nonketotic hyperglycemia, or hyponatremia. May cause CNS depression or hyperexcitability to include seizures, irritability, depression, coma, hallucinations, or mental status changes. Nausea and vomiting, anorexia, and weight loss are common. Clients may experience night sweats.

CONTRAINDICATIONS. Pancreatitis, known hypersensitivity to pegasparagase, or a history of hemorrhage with l-asparaginase therapy.

**POTENTIAL DRUG/FOOD INTERACTIONS**

May interfere with the action of methotrexate. May potentiate wafarin, heparin, dipyridamole, aspirin, or NSAIDs.

**INTERVENTIONS: ADMINISTRATION**

Solution is available in containers of 750 IU/mL. Dilute with 5 mL of 0.9% NSS. Mix in 100 mL of 0.9% NSS or D5W solutions.

**MODE/RATE OF ADMINISTRATION**

Given through a free-flowing IV infusion, using an infusion pump.

INTRAVENOUS USE (WITH NORMAL RENAL FUNCTION)

**Adults:** Usual dosage is 2500 IU/kg q14d.

**Children 0.6 $m^2$ BSA:** Dosage is 2500 IU/$m^2$ q14d.

**Children 0.6 $m^2$ BSA:** Dosage is 82.5 IU/$m^2$ q14d.

**Infants/Neonates:** Dosage not established for children 1 year.

**Geriatrics:** Elderly clients are more likely to have preexisting conditions that increase the likelihood of renal and liver complications. Follow adult dosing schedule and monitor carefully.

INTRATHECAL USE OR OTHER INFUSION ROUTES AS INDICATED. Not recommended.

**POTENTIAL PROBLEMS IN ADMINISTRATION**

May cause anaphylactic shock. Hypersensitivity reactions are more common in clients receiving the drug every day compared to those receiving the drug weekly.

**INDEPENDENT NURSING ACTIONS**

Monitor all vital signs carefully. Monitor laboratory reports carefully, especially those reflecting renal and liver function. Observe for any allergic reactions.

**ADMINISTRATION IN ALTERNATE SETTINGS**

Should be administered in clinical settings where emergency equipment is immediately available and the client can be continuously monitored.

**EVALUATION: OUTCOMES OF DRUG THERAPY**

**EXPECTED OUTCOMES**

PHYSICAL ASSESSMENT. Heart rate, rhythm, blood pressure, and weight remain within 15% of client's baseline. Breath sounds are clear. Skin color pink. Client does not have any unusual bleeding, abdominal pain, wheezing, urticaria, anorexia, nausea, vomiting, or night sweats. Client remains alert and oriented.

LABORATORY. Hct is 37 to 54 mg/dL. Serum sodium is 136 to 145 mEq/L. Total serum protein is 6 to 8 g/dL. Fasting blood glucose is 70 to 115 mg/dL. AST is 10 to 30 U/L. ALT is 5 to 30 U/L. Serum bilirubin is 0.3 to 1.1 mg/dL. BUN is 11 to 23 mg/dL. Total serum creatinine is 15 to 25 mg/kg body weight per 24 h.

**NEGATIVE OUTCOMES**

Heart rate, blood pressure, and weight are more than 15% higher or lower than client's baseline. Lungs have wheezes or crackles on auscultation. Client has unusual bleeding, urticaria, vomiting, or night sweats. Client complains of anorexia, nausea, or abdominal pain. Client demonstrates mental status changes such as irritability, somnolence, convulsions, or coma.

## TRIMETREXATE GLUCURONATE

*Trade name:* Neutrexin
*Canadian Availability:* Not specified
*Pregnancy Risk:* Category X
*pH:* Not specified
*Storage/Stability:* Store below 40° C. Must be reconstituted before use.

**ASSESSMENT: DRUG CHARACTERISTICS**

**ACTION**

A cell cycle specific antimetabolite that is an analog of methotrexate. The agent appears active during the pre-DNA synthesis S stage of cell division. Inhibits both DNA and RNA synthesis. Growth of rapidly dividing tissues is more affected than growth of normally dividing tissues such as skin.

**INDICATIONS**

Used primarily to treat colorectal carcinomas, metastatic carcinomas of the head and neck, advanced non-small cell carcinoma of the lungs, pancreatic adenocarcinomas, and *Pneumocystis carinii* pneumonia (PCP) in clients with acquired immunodeficiency syndrome (AIDS).

**CAUTIONS**

A potent immunosuppressive and bone marrow depressive agent. There is an increased incidence of infection and delayed healing of dental work. Dental work should be done before therapy is started or delayed until blood counts return to normal. Clients should be instructed in proper oral hygiene. Trimetrexate is both mutagenic and teratogenic. It is known to cause abortions if used during the first trimester of pregnancy. Clients should be instructed to use appropriate forms of birth control.

ADVERSE EFFECTS. Carries the possibility of secondary malignancy as a result of therapy. Risk of malignancy seems to increase with long-term use. Adverse reactions are generally less frequent with trimetrexate than with methotrexate. Hematologic toxicity is the most evident effect. Frequent platelet and leukocyte counts should be done after therapy to monitor the leukopenia and thrombocytopenia. Abnormal liver function, nausea, vomiting and diarrhea, skin rashes, and fever are common.

CONTRAINDICATIONS. Should be given cautiously to clients with immunodeficiency, ascites, bone marrow depression, herpes zoster, impaired hepatic functions, infection, oral mucositis, peptic ulcer, or ulcerative colitis.

**POTENTIAL DRUG/FOOD INTERACTIONS**

When used with alcohol or other hepatotoxic drugs, there is increased risk of hepatotoxicity. NSAIDs may increase bone marrow depression. Trimetrexate may inhibit action of asparaginase. If used without leucovorin in clients with cancer, the incidence of hematologic toxicities increases.

**INTERVENTIONS: ADMINISTRATION**

Strict aherence to agency safety procedures for handling antineoplastic agents should be followed during reconstitution and administration of trimetrexate. Reconstitute 25-mg vials with 2 mL of sterile water for injection to a concentration of 12.5 mg/mL. Further dilute in D5W solution to a concentration of 0.25–2 mg/mL. Use an in-line micropore filter with pores not larger than 22 $\mu$m.

**MODE/RATE OF ADMINISTRATION**

Give IV as a diluted solution by slow infusion over 60–90 min.

INTRAVENOUS USE (WITH NORMAL RENAL FUNCTION)

**Adults:** For cancer the usual dosage range is 8–12 mg/m$^2$ of BSA daily for 5 d to 125–150 mg/m$^2$ of BSA q14d. Each dose is usually followed by leucovorin; however, regimens vary. Do not mix trimetrexate and leucovorin together. An insoluble precipitate forms instantly.

For PCP the usual dosage is 30 mg/m$^2$ of BSA daily for 21 d followed by leucovorin 20 mg/m$^2$ of BSA q6h for the duration of therapy.

**Children:** Dosage not established.

**Infants/Neonates:** Dosage not established.

**Geriatrics:** Follow adult dosing schedules. No specific recommendations.

INTRATHECAL USE OR OTHER INFUSION ROUTES AS INDICATED. Not recommended.

**POTENTIAL PROBLEMS IN ADMINISTRATION**

Leucovorin, an antidote to folic acid antagonists such as trimetrexate, is used to counter the GI and hematologic effects of trimetrexate. Leucovorin should be administered after trimetrexate so that leucovorin does not interfere with trimetrexate's antineoplastic activity.

**INDEPENDENT NURSING ACTIONS**

Monitor hematologic laboratory values carefully. Teach clients to use proper oral hygiene and to avoid sources of infection when their blood counts are low. Teach clients to monitor themselves for infection and unusual bleeding such as black, tarry stools or bruising that occurs without injury. Do not administer trimetrexate if the client's serum uric acid and creatinine clearance values are elevated.

**ADMINISTRATION IN ALTERNATE SETTINGS**

Should be administered in settings where the client can be closely monitored during administration.

**EVALUATION: OUTCOMES OF DRUG THERAPY**

**EXPECTED OUTCOMES**

PHYSICAL ASSESSMENT. Loss of hair, nausea, vomiting, and stomatitis. Tumor mass diminishes in size. If given for small cell carcinoma of the lung or PCP, shortness of breath and dyspnea improve.

LABORATORY. Clients should have an Hct, Hgb, platelet count, and leukocyte count with differential prior to the start of therapy. BUN may be elevated. Leukocyte count hits nadir in 7 to 10 days with recovery 7 days later.

**NEGATIVE OUTCOMES**

Renal failure, azotemia, hyperuricemia, severe neuropathy, hepatotoxicity, pneumonia, and increased intracranial pressure.

## Vinca Alkaloids

### VINBLASTINE SULFATE

*Trade Names:* Alkaban-AQ, Velban, Velsar

*Canadian Availability:* Velbe

*Pregnancy Risk:* Category D

*pH:* 3.5–5.0

*Storage/Stability:* Store vials between 2° and 8° C. Vials ▼

are reconstituted using 10 mL of 0.9% NSS injection. Reconstituted vials may be kept for up to 30 days at temperatures between 2° and 8° C.

## ASSESSMENT: DRUG CHARACTERISTICS

### ACTION

A cell cycle specific vinca alkaloid that is effective during the M phase of cell cycle activity and prevents mitosis and cell division.

### INDICATIONS

Used to treat carcinomas of the breast or testicles, both Hodgkin's and non-Hodgkin's lymphomas, and Kaposi's sarcoma.

### CAUTIONS

A potent immunosuppressive and bone marrow depressive agent. There is an increased incidence of infection and delayed healing of dental work. Dental work should be done before therapy is started or delayed until blood counts return to normal. Clients should be instructed in good oral hygiene. Vinblastine is both mutagenic and teratogenic.

ADVERSE EFFECTS. Carries the possibility of secondary malignancy as a result of therapy. Risk of malignancy seems to increase with long-term use. Leukopenia, stomatitis, and thrombocytopenia are common effects of therapy. Frequent platelet and leukocyte counts should be done after therapy to monitor the leukopenia and thrombocytopenia.

CONTRAINDICATIONS. Should be given cautiously, if at all, to clients with significant immunosuppression, herpes zoster, impaired hepatic functioning, infection, or sensitivty to vinblastine.

### POTENTIAL DRUG/FOOD INTERACTIONS

May interact with antigout agents such as probenecid or sulfinpyrazone to raise serum uric acid levels significantly. Bone marrow suppression may be potentiated if vinblastine is used in conjunction with radiation therapy. Vinblastine should not be given with live virus vaccine because the viral replication may increase.

## INTERVENTIONS: ADMINISTRATION

Prepare and handle vinblastine according to the policies and procedures established for handling chemotherapeutic (cytotoxic) drugs within the agency.

### MODE/RATE OF ADMINISTRATION

Given IV push through free-flowing IV infusion.

INTRAVENOUS USE (WITH NORMAL RENAL FUNCTION)

**Adults:** Usual initial IV dose is 100 mcg (0.1 mg)/kg of body weight per week. Successive doses increase by 50 mcg (0.05 mg)/kg of body weight until the leukocyte count falls to 3000/mm$^3$, the tumor shrinks, or a maximum dose of 500 mcg (0.5 mg)/kg of body weight is achieved. An IV maintenance dose one increment lower than the last progressive dose may be given q7–14d. Each such following dose should be delayed until the leukocyte count reaches 4000/mm³. The doses are reduced by 50% if the serum bilirubin concentrations are above 3 mg/dL.

**Children:** Usual initial IV dosage is 2.5 mg/m² of BSA per week. Successive doses increase by 1.25 mg/m² of BSA until the leukocyte count falls to 3000/mm³, the tumor shrinks, or a maximum dose of 7.5 mg/m² of BSA is achieved. An IV maintenance dose one increment lower than the last progressive dose may be given q7–14d. Each such following dose should be delayed until the leukocyte count reaches 4000/mm³. The doses are reduced by 50% if the serum bilirubin concentrations are above 3 mg/dL.

#### POTENTIAL PROBLEMS IN ADMINISTRATION

Avoid extravasation. Stop infusion immediately if extravasation does occur. Site may be injected with hyaluronidase, the limb elevated, and moist heat applied as warranted. Inject the remainder of the dose in another site.

#### INDEPENDENT NURSING ACTIONS

Monitor hematologic laboratory values carefully. Teach clients to use good oral hygiene and to avoid sources of infection when their blood counts are low. Teach clients to monitor themselves for infection and unusual bleeding such as black, tarry stools or bruising that occurs without injury.

#### ADMINISTRATION IN ALTERNATE SETTINGS

May be administered in the home if done by a qualified IV nurse.

#### EVALUATION: OUTCOMES OF DRUG THERAPY

#### EXPECTED OUTCOMES

PHYSICAL ASSESSMENT. Tumor mass shrinks. Loss of hair, nausea, vomiting, stomatitis. Leukocyte count drops to near normal levels.

LABORATORY. Leukocyte levels typically fall in the first 24 hours after administration and hit nadir 5 to 10 days after the last dose is given. Leukocyte counts usually recover in 7 to 14 days. Clients should have an Hct, Hgb, platelet count, and leukocyte count prior to the start of therapy. Clients should have serum bilirubin and leukocyte counts done prior to receiving the next scheduled dose.

#### NEGATIVE OUTCOMES

Tumor mass remains unchanged in size, infection, CNS toxicity, elevated serum uric acid levels, hepatotoxicity, GI tract bleeding, pulmonary edema, or urinary retention.

## Vincristine Sulfate

*Trade Names:* Oncovin, Vincasar PFS, Vincrex
*Canadian Availability:* Oncovin
*Pregnancy Risk:* Category D
*pH:* 3.5–4.5
*Storage/Stability:* Store between 2° and 8° C. Reconstituted vincristine is stable for 14 days if refrigerated. Do not add vincristine to solution that will raise or lower the pH outside the range of 3.5 to 5.5.

### ASSESSMENT: DRUG CHARACTERISTICS

#### ACTION

A cell cycle specific vinca alkaloid that is effective during the M phase of cell cycle activity.

#### INDICATIONS

Used to treat acute lymphocytic leukemias, neuroblastomas, Wilms' tumor, both Hodgkin's and non-Hodgkin's lymphomas, rhabdomyosarcoma, and Ewing's sarcoma.

#### CAUTIONS

Potent cytotoxic. Dental work should be done before therapy is started or delayed until blood counts return to normal. Clients should be instructed in proper oral hygiene. Vincristine is both mutagenic and teratogenic. Clients should be instructed to use appropriate forms of birth control.

ADVERSE EFFECTS. Carries the possibility of secondary malignancy as a result of therapy. Risk of malignancy seems to increase with long-term use. Leukopenia, stomatitis, and thrombocytopenia are common effects of therapy. Frequent platelet and leukocyte counts should be done after therapy to monitor the leukopenia and thrombocytopenia.

CONTRAINDICATIONS. Should be given cautiously, if at all, to clients with significant immunosuppression, herpes zoster, impaired hepatic functioning, infection, or sensitivity to vincristine.

#### POTENTIAL DRUG/FOOD INTERACTIONS

May interact with antigout agents such as probenecid or sulfinpyrazone to raise serum uric acid levels significantly. Allopurinol is frequently given to lower serum uric acid levels. Bone marrow suppression may be potentiated if vincristine is used in conjunction with radiation therapy or with doxorubicin. Vincristine given before bleomycin may make cells more susceptible to bleomycin; vincristine may increase neurotoxicity if given with asparaginase. Vincristine should not be given with live virus vaccine because the viral replication may increase.

### INTERVENTIONS: ADMINISTRATION

Strict adherence to agency safety procedures for handling antineoplastic agents should be followed when reconstituting and administering vincristine. Vials are reconstituted by adding 5 mL of sterile water for injection to the vial. Vincristine should not be mixed in solutions other than D5W or 0.9% NSS.

**MODE/RATE OF ADMINISTRATION**

Given by rapid IV injection through a free-flowing IV infusion over 1 min. May also be added to D5W or 0.9% NSS and infused over 15 min.

INTRAVENOUS USE (WITH NORMAL RENAL FUNCTION)

**Adults:** Usual adult IV dosage is 1.4 mg/m$^2$ of BSA each week as a single dose. Dose is reduced by 50% if serum bilirubin concentrations are above 3 mg/dL.

**Children:** Usual IV dosage is 1.5–2 mg/m$^2$ of BSA each week as a single dose. Dose is reduced by 50% if serum bilirubin concentrations are above 3 mg/dL.

**Infants/Neonates:** For children 10 kg and under, usual IV dosage is 50 mcg (0.05 mg)/kg of body weight once a week. Dose is reduced by 50% if serum bilirubin concentrations are above 3 mg/dL.

**Geriatrics:** Follow adult dosing schedule. The elderly may be more likely to exhibit neurotoxic effects.

INTRATHECAL USE OR OTHER INFUSION ROUTES AS INDICATED. Contraindicated. Vincristine is fatal if given by intrathecal infusion.

**POTENTIAL PROBLEMS IN ADMINISTRATION**

Avoid extravasation. Stop infusion immediately if extravasation does occur. Inject hyaluronidase locally, elevate the extremity, and apply moist heat. Infuse the remaining solution in another location.

**INDEPENDENT NURSING ACTIONS**

Monitor hematologic laboratory values carefully. Teach clients to use proper oral hygiene and to avoid sources of infection when their blood counts are low. Teach clients to monitor themselves for infection and unusual bleeding such as black, tarry stools or bruising that occurs without injury.

**ADMINISTRATION IN ALTERNATE SETTINGS**

Should be administered in settings where the client can be closely monitored during the administration.

**EVALUATION: OUTCOMES OF DRUG THERAPY**

**EXPECTED OUTCOMES**

PHYSICAL ASSESSMENT: Tumor mass shrinks or leukocyte count drops to near normal levels. Loss of hair, nausea and vomiting, diarrhea, stomatitis, and weight loss are common.

LABORATORY. Clients should have an Hct, Hgb, platelet count, and leukocyte count prior to the start of therapy. Leukopenia hits nadir at 5 to 10 days after last administration and should recover 7 to 14 days after nadir.

▼

**NEGATIVE OUTCOMES**

Hepatotoxicity, infection, autonomic toxicity, CNS toxicity, and GI tract bleeding. Tumor masses fail to diminish in size, or leukocyte counts remain elevated.

---

## CELL CYCLE NONSPECIFIC ANTINEOPLASTICS

### THERAPEUTIC EFFECTS

Cell cycle nonspecific antineoplastics act independent of cell cycle activity. Alkylating agents work by substituting an alkyl group for hydrogen ions in several organic compounds. The compounds then intefere with DNA synthesis, causing splitting and cross-linking of the DNA strands. Antineoplastic antibiotics bind with DNA and inhibit DNA or RNA synthesis.

### PHARMACOKINETICS

**Distribution.** Diffusion following IV infusion is rapid and widespread. Some agents cross the blood-brain barrier readily; most do not. Tissue uptake is variable, depending on the antineoplastic agent selected.

**Metabolism/Elimination.** Plasma half-life is usually 15 minutes to 7 hours in adults with normal kidney and liver function. Some agents may have half-lives as long as 36 hours or even longer. Traces of some agents may be detected in the liver months after administration.

### CAUTIONS

**Side/Adverse Effects.** Cell cycle nonspecific antineoplastics are potent bone marrow suppressants and highly cytotoxic. Clients may be more prone to infection and hemorrhagic complications.

**Contraindications.** Cell cycle nonspecific antineoplastics should not be given to clients who have been previously treated with antineoplastic agents or radiation therapy; clients who have a documented history of hepatotoxicity, nephrotoxicity, or allergic reactions; and clients with severe leukopenia, thrombocytopenia, or infections.

***Pregnancy and Lactation.*** Cell cycle nonspecific antineoplastic agents are teratogenic and mutagenic substances. They should not be given to pregnant women without careful consideration to the potential for fetal damage. Some agents are transmitted via breast milk.

***Pediatrics.*** No age specific contraindications have been determined.

***Geriatrics.*** No age specific contraindications have been determined.

### TOXICITY

See Table 17–3 for toxicities of cell cycle nonspecific antineoplastics.

**TABLE 17–3**
**Toxicities of Cell Cycle Nonspecific Antineoplastics**

| Body System | Side/Toxic Effects | Physical Assessment Indicators | Laboratory Indicators | Nursing Interventions |
|---|---|---|---|---|
| Neurologic | Neurotoxicity | Peripheral neuropathies, drowsiness, headaches, seizures, vertigo | N/A | Initiate safety precautions for sensory and mobility deficits, dizziness, urinary retention. |
| Cardiac | Cardiotoxicity, pericarditis, CHF, cardiomyopathy | Peripheral edema, shortness of breath, crackles, $S_3$ and $S_4$ heart sounds, decreased urinary output, sudden weight gain | Elevated serum electrolytes, BUN, serum creatinine | Monitor laboratory values. Report early symptoms. |
| Respiratory | Pulmonary toxicity, interstitial pneumonitis | Acute shortness of breath, dyspnea on exertion, elevated temperature, increased respirations | Elevated WBCs | Avoid allergens and people with respiratory infections. |
| Renal | Nephrotoxicity | Decreased urinary output | Creatinine clearance, BUN, serum calcium, phosphorus in urine | Monitor laboratory values, weigh client frequently, increase fluid intake. |
| Gastrointestinal | Hepatomegaly, esophagitis, pharyngitis | Nausea and vomiting, anorexia, diarrhea, stomatitis, oral ulcers, dysphagia, weight loss | Increased blood glucose, bilirubin, ammonium, AST, ALT, alkaline phosphatase, decreased fibrinogin, albumin | Give antiemetics before administering agent. Give meticulous mouth care. Avoid hot, spicy foods and alcohol. |
| Hematologic | Bone marrow suppression, leukopenia, pancytopenia, thrombocytopenia | Bruising, bleeding melena, petechiae, epistaxis, hematuria | Decreased RBCs, WBCs, Hct, Hgb, platelets | Use anticoagulants and aspirin with extreme caution. Provide a safe environment. |

*Continued on following page.*

**TABLE 17–3**
**Toxicities of Cell Cycle Nonspecific Antineoplastics *Continued***

| Body System | Side/Toxic Effects | Physical Assessment Indicators | Laboratory Indicators | Nursing Interventions |
|---|---|---|---|---|
| Dermatologic | Mucocutaneous pain | Erythema, swelling, tissue irritation, oral ulceration, hyperpigmentation, alopecia | N/A | Be prepared to administer epinephrine and corticosteroids for allergic response. Give meticulous skin care with mild products. Avoid gastrointestinal irritants. |
| Sensory | Ototoxicity, optic neuritis | Loss of hearing acuity, tinnitus, vision loss, eye pain | N/A | Monitor for evidence of hearing or vision loss. |
| Other | Anaphylactoid reactions | Acute shortness of breath, urticaria, tachycardia, tachypnea | N/A | Stop therapy immediately. Give epinephrine and corticosteroids. |

ALT = alanine aminotransferase, AST = aspartate aminotransferase, BUN = blood urea nitrogen, CHF = congestive heart failure, Hct = hematocrit, Hgb = hemoglobin, RBCs = red blood cell counts, WBCs = white blood cell counts.

## POTENTIAL DRUG/FOOD INTERACTIONS

Alkylating agents may interact with cimetidine, ototoxic drugs, nephrotoxic drugs, cardiotoxic drugs, hepatotoxic drugs, succinylcholine, aminoglycosides, and antifungals to potentiate the effects of those drugs. Antineoplastic antibiotics may interact with other antineoplastic agents to potentiate them. Antineoplasitc antibiotics may also interfere with the action of phenytoin.

# Alkylating Agents

## CARMUSTINE

*Trade Name:* BiCNU
*Canadian Availability:* BiCNU
*Pregnancy Risk:* Category D
*pH:* 5.6–6
*Storage/Stability:* Store between 2° and 8° C. If exposed to temperatures above 30.5° C, drug may decompose and liquefy. Vial then must be discarded. Reconstituted solutions are stable for 8 hours at 25° C or 24 hours at 4° C.

### ASSESSMENT: DRUG CHARACTERISTICS

#### ACTION

A cell cycle nonspecific alkylating agent of the nitrosourea type. Interferes with DNA and RNA functioning and may cause cross-linking of DNA to inhibit synthesis.

#### INDICATIONS

Used primarily to treat brain tumors, Hodgkin's and non-Hodgkin's lymphomas, and multiple myelomas.

#### CAUTIONS

A potent bone marrow depressive agent. There is an increased incidence of infection and delayed healing of dental work. Dental work should be done before therapy is started or delayed until blood counts return to normal. Clients should be instructed in proper oral hygiene. Carmustine is both mutagenic and teratogenic. Clients should be instructed to use appropriate forms of birth control.

ADVERSE EFFECTS. Carries the possibility of secondary malignancy as a result of therapy. Risk of malignancy seems to increase with long-term use. Leukopenia, stomatitis, pneumonitis, pulmonary fibrosis, and thrombocytopenia are common effects of therapy. Frequent platelet and leukocyte counts should be done after therapy to monitor the leukopenia and thrombocytopenia.

CONTRAINDICATIONS. Should be given cautiously, if at all, to clients with significant immunosuppression, herpes zoster, impaired hepatic functioning, infection, or sensitivity to carmustine.

▼

**POTENTIAL DRUG/FOOD INTERACTIONS**

May interact with antigout agents such as probenecid or sulfinpyrazone to raise serum uric acid levels significantly. Allopurinol is frequently given to lower serum uric acid levels. Bone marrow suppression may be potentiated if carmustine is used in conjunction with radiation therapy or with cyclophosphamide. Carmustine should not be given with live virus vaccine because the viral replication may increase.

**INTERVENTIONS: ADMINISTRATION**

Strict adherence to agency safety procedures for handling antineoplastic agents should be followed when reconstituting and administering carmustine. Carmustine for injection is reconstituted with 3 mL of sterile diluent supplied by the manufacturer and then adding 27 ml of sterile water, making a 3.3 mg/mL solution. May be further diluted with 0.9% NSS or D5W.

**MODE/RATE OF ADMINISTRATION**

Give intravenously over 1 to 2 hours. Flush line before and after administration with 5–10 mL 0.9% NSS.

INTRAVENOUS USE (WITH NORMAL RENAL FUNCTION)

**Adults:** Usual dosage is 150–200 mg/m² of BSA as a single dose q6–8wk. Alternate dosage schedule is 75–100 mg/m² of BSA on 2 consecutive days q6wk or 40 mg/m² of BSA for 5 d q6wk. Successive dosage ranges are dependent on leukocyte and platelet counts.

**Children:** Adolescents follow adult dosage schedule. Dosage for children under 12 not established.

**Infants/Neonates:** Dosage not established.

**Geriatrics:** Follow adult dosage schedule. Dosage may need to be lowered if renal or hepatic function is diminished.

INTRATHECAL USE OR OTHER INFUSION ROUTES AS INDICATED. Has been administered by intraarterial infusion for investigational therapy for hepatic tumors. Dosing schedule is 200 mg/m2 of BSA given over 20 to 60 min.

**POTENTIAL PROBLEMS IN ADMINISTRATION**

Rapid infusion of carmustine may cause intense pain and burning at the infusion device insertion site and along the vessel.

**INDEPENDENT NURSING ACTIONS**

Monitor hematologic laboratory values carefully. Teach clients to use good oral hygiene and to avoid sources of infections when their blood counts are low. Teach clients to monitor themselves for infection and unusual bleeding such as black, tarry stools or bruising that occurs without injury.

**ADMINISTRATION IN ALTERNATE SETTINGS**

Should be administered in settings where the client can be closely monitored during the administration.

**EVALUATION: OUTCOMES OF DRUG THERAPY**

**EXPECTED OUTCOMES**

PHYSICAL ASSESSMENT. Loss of hair, nausea and vomiting, diarrhea, anorexia, skin rash, dysphagia, and weight loss. Tumor mass should diminish in size.

LABORATORY.

Leukocyte levels typically hit nadir in 5 to 6 weeks and recover in 10 to 12 weeks. Thrombocyte levels hit nadir in 4 to 5 weeks and recover in 6 to 7 weeks. Clients should have an Hct, Hgb, platelet count, and leukocyte count prior to the start of therapy. Pulmonary function studies should be done prior to beginning carmustine therapy and repeated at frequent intervals. Pneumonitis or pulmonary fibrosis are common adverse responses to carmustine therapy.

**NEGATIVE OUTCOMES**

Severe leukopenia, pneumonitis, anemia, hepatotoxicity, renal failure, and failure of the tumor mass to diminish.

## CISPLATIN

*Trade Names:* Platinol, Platinol-AQ
*Canadian Availability:* Abiplatin, Platinol-AQ
*Pregnancy Risk:* Category D
*pH:* 3.7–6
*Storage/Stability:* Store between 15° and 25° C. Protect from light. If unreconstituted, may be stored for up to 17 months. If reconstituted, solutions are stable for 20 hours at 27° C. Do not refrigerate reconstituted solutions because a precipitate forms.

**ASSESSMENT: DRUG CHARACTERISTICS**

**ACTION**

A cell cycle nonspecific alkylating agent that interferes with DNA and RNA functioning and may cause cross-linking of the DNA strands.

**INDICATIONS**

Used primarily to treat carcinoma of the bladder, ovaries, and testes.

**CAUTIONS**

There is an increased incidence of infection and delayed healing of dental work. Dental work should be done before therapy is started or delayed until blood counts return to normal. Clients should be instructed in proper oral hygiene. Cisplatin is both mutagenic and teratogenic. Clients should be instructed to use appropriate forms of birth control.

ADVERSE EFFECTS. Carries the possibility of secondary malignancy as a result of therapy. Risk of malignancy seems to increase with long-term use. Leukopenia, stomatitis, ototoxicity, and thrombocytopenia are common effects of therapy. Frequent platelet and leukocyte counts should be done after therapy to monitor the leukopenia and thrombocytopenia.

▼

**CONTRAINDICATIONS.** Should be given cautiously, if at all, to clients with significant immunosuppression, herpes zoster, impaired hepatic functioning, infection, hearing impairment, or sensitivity to cisplatin.

**POTENTIAL DRUG/FOOD INTERACTIONS**

May interact with probenecid or sulfinpyrazone to elevate serum uric acid. Allopurinol may be given to lower serum uric acid levels. Cisplatin may potentiate the effects of bone marrow depressants, radiation therapy, and nephrotoxic and ototoxic drugs. Cisplatin should not be given with live virus vaccine because the viral replication may increase.

**INTERVENTIONS: ADMINISTRATION**

Prepare and handle cisplatin according to the policies and procedures established for handling chemotherapeutic (cytotoxic) drugs within the agency. Cisplatin is reconstituted by adding 10–50 mL of sterile water for injection to 10 to 50-mg vials, respectively, to achieve a 1-mg/mL solution. May be further mixed with D5W or 0.3% to 0.45% NSS for injection if required.

**MODE/RATE OF ADMINISTRATION**

Infusions are given over 24 h–5 d to reduce nausea. Slow infusion does not appear to reduce nephrotoxicity or ototoxicity.

INTRAVENOUS USE (WITH NORMAL RENAL FUNCTION)

**Adults:** Dosage is generally 20–70 mg/m² of BSA a day for 5 d, repeated q3wk for three courses. Cisplatin may be given in conjunction with bleomycin and vinblastine to treat testicular tumors or doxorubicin to treat ovarian tumors. Dosage schedules are adjusted to include the additional antineoplastic agents.

**Children:** Dosage schedule for children follows adult schedule.

**Infants/Neonates:** Dosage not established.

**Geriatrics:** Dosage schedule follows adult schedule. Adjustments may need to be made if renal function is diminished.

INTRATHECAL USE OR OTHER INFUSION ROUTES AS INDICATED. Not recommended.

**POTENTIAL PROBLEMS IN ADMINISTRATION**

Clients should be well hydrated with 1–2 L of fluid 8–12 h before treatment is started. Mannitol may be added to the cisplatin infusion or furosemide given following the infusion to maintain urinary output for 24 h. Do not use aluminum needles or IV sets or any equipment containing aluminum, since cisplatin is incompatible with aluminum and forms a black platinum precipitate.

**INDEPENDENT NURSING ACTIONS**

Perform audiometric testing, neurologic function testing, and serum creatinine levels prior to starting cisplatin therapy. Evaluate neurologic function and serum creatinine levels frequently during cisplatin therapy. Monitor hematologic laboratory values carefully. Teach clients to use good oral hygiene and to avoid sources of infection when their blood counts are low. Teach clients to monitor themselves for infection and unusual bleeding such as black, tarry stools or bruising that occurs without injury.

**ADMINISTRATION IN ALTERNATE SETTINGS**

Should be administered in settings where the client can be closely monitored during the administration.

**EVALUATION: OUTCOMES OF DRUG THERAPY**

**EXPECTED OUTCOMES**

PHYSICAL ASSESSMENT. Loss of hair, nausea, vomiting, diarrhea, anorexia, and skin rash. Tumor mass diminishes in size.

LABORATORY. Leukocyte levels typically hit nadir in 18 to 23 days and recover in 39 days. Clients should have an Hct, Hgb, platelet count, and leukocyte count prior to the start of therapy and frequently during the course of therapy.

**NEGATIVE OUTCOMES**

Severe leukopenia, thrombocytopenia, nephrotoxicity, hyperuricemia, and ototoxicity. Tumor mass fails to diminish in size.

## CYCLOPHOSPHAMIDE

*Trade Name:* Cytoxan, Neosar
*Canadian Availability:* Cytoxan, Procytox
*Pregnancy Risk:* Category D
*pH:* 3–7.5
*Storage/Stability:* Store below 25° C. Reconstituted solutions are stable at room temperature for 24 hours, or for 6 days refrigerated, if mixed with bacteriostatic water for injection.

**ASSESSMENT: DRUG CHARACTERISTICS**

**ACTION**

A cell cycle nonspecific alkylating agent of the nitrogen mustard type. Causes cross-linking of DNA strands and inhibits protein synthesis.

**INDICATIONS**

Used to treat acute and chronic lymphocytic and myelogenous leukemias and chronic monocytic leukemia. Also used to treat breast and ovarian carcinomas, Hodgkin's and non-Hodgkin's lymphomas, multiple myeloma, and mycosis fungoides.

**CAUTIONS**

A potent immunosuppressive and bone marrow depressive agent. There is an increased incidence of infection and delayed healing of dental work. Dental work should be done before therapy is started or delayed until blood counts return to normal. Clients should be instructed in proper oral hygiene. Cyclophosphamide is both mutagenic and teratogenic. Clients should be instructed to use appropriate forms of birth control.

ADVERSE EFFECTS. Carries the possibility of secondary malignancy as a result of therapy. Risk of malignancy seems to increase with long-term use. Leukopenia, stomatitis, gonadal suppression, and thrombocytopenia are common effects of therapy. Frequent platelet and leukocyte counts should be done after therapy to monitor the leukopenia and thrombocytopenia.

CONTRAINDICATIONS. Should be given cautiously, if at all, to clients with significant immunosuppression, herpes zoster, impaired hepatic functioning, infection, or sensitivity to cyclophosphamide.

**POTENTIAL DRUG/FOOD INTERACTIONS**

May interact with antigout agents such as probenecid or sulfinpyrazone to raise serum uric acid levels significantly. Allopurinol is frequently given to lower serum uric acid levels. Bone marrow suppression may be potentiated if cyclophosphamide is used in conjunction with radiation therapy or with other bone marrow depressants. Cyclophsophamide should not be given with live virus vaccine because the viral replication may increase. May inhibit anticoagulant effect of oral anticoagulants. May potentiate the cardiotoxic effects of doxorubicin. May prolong the metabolism of cocaine.

**INTERVENTIONS: ADMINISTRATION**

Strict adherence to agency safety procedures for handling antineoplastic agents should be followed when reconstituting and administering cyclophosphamide. Add sterile water for injection to vial to obtain a solution of 20 mg/mL. The solution can then be added to D5W, 0.9% NSS, D5W and Ringer's lactate, or lactated Ringer's, 0.45% sodium NSS, or sodium lactate injection for IV administration.

**MODE/RATE OF ADMINISTRATION**

May be given by rapid IV infusion, intraperitoneally, or intrapleurally.

INTRAVENOUS USE (WITH NORMAL RENAL FUNCTION)

**Adults:** Usual dosage is 40–50 mg/kg of body weight given in divided doses over 2–5 d, 10–15 mg/kg of body weight q7–10d, 3–5 mg/kg of body weight twice a week, or 1.5–3 mg/kg of body weight daily. Maximum doses may vary substantially.

**Children:** Usual dosage is 2–8 mg/kg of body weight or 60 mg/m$^2$ of BSA in divided doses over 6 d or more. Maintenance dosages are 10–15 mg/kg of body weight q7–10d or 30 mg/kg of body weight q3–4wk or when bone marrow recovers.

**Infants/Neonates:** Follow dosing schedule for children.

**Geriatrics:** Follow adult dosing schedules. Clients with diminished renal function may require adjusted doses.

INTRATHECAL USE OR OTHER INFUSION ROUTES AS INDICATED. Not recommended.

**POTENTIAL PROBLEMS IN ADMINISTRATION**

Clients need adequate hydration for at least 72 h prior to treatment to reduce the incidence of hemorrhagic cystitis.

**INDEPENDENT NURSING ACTIONS**

Monitor hematologic laboratory values carefully. Teach clients to use proper oral hygiene and to avoid sources of infection when their blood counts are low. Teach clients to monitor themselves for infection and unusual bleeding such as black, tarry stools or bruising that occurs without injury.

**ADMINISTRATION IN ALTERNATE SETTINGS**

Should be administered in settings where the client can be closely monitored during the administration.

**EVALUATION: OUTCOMES OF DRUG THERAPY**

**EXPECTED OUTCOMES**

PHYSICAL ASSESSMENT. Loss of hair, nausea, vomiting, stomatitis. Leukocyte count drops to near normal levels. Skin may darken.

LABORATORY. Leukocyte levels typically start to fall in the first 24 hours after administration and hit nadir in 7 to 12 days. Leukocyte counts should recover after 17 to 21 days. Clients should have an Hct, Hgb, platelet count, and leukocyte count prior to the start of therapy and frequently during therapy.

**NEGATIVE OUTCOMES**

Cardiotoxicity, hemorrhagic cystitis, hyperuricemia, and nephrotoxicity. Leukocyte counts remain elevated and unresponsive to cyclophosphamide.

---

## DACARBAZINE (DTIC)

*Trade Name:* DTIC-Dome
*Canadian Availability:* DTIC
*Pregnancy Risk:* Category C
*pH:* 3–4
*Storage/Stability:* Store below 40° C. Protect from light. Reconstituted solutions are stable for 8 hours at room temperature or up to 72 hours at 4° C. Solutions further diluted for IV infusion use are stable for 8 hours at room temperature or 72 hours at 4° C.

**ASSESSMENT: DRUG CHARACTERISTICS**

**ACTION**

A cell cycle nonspecific alkylating agent. Inhibits synthesis of DNA and RNA.

**INDICATIONS**

Used to treat malignant melanomas and Hodgkin's lymphomas.

**CAUTIONS**

A bone marrow depressive agent. There is an increased incidence of infection and delayed healing of dental work. Dental work should be done before therapy is started or delayed until blood counts return to normal. Clients should be instructed in proper oral hygiene. Dacarbazine is both mutagenic and teratogenic. Clients should be instructed to use appropriate forms of birth control.

ADVERSE EFFECTS. Carries the possibility of secondary malignancy as a result of therapy. Risk of malignancy seems to increase with long-term use. Leukopenia, stomatitis, and thrombocytopenia are common effects of therapy; frequent platelet and leukocyte counts should be done after therapy to monitor the leukopenia and thrombocytopenia.

CONTRAINDICATIONS. Should be given cautiously, if at all, to clients with significant immunosuppression, bone marrow depression, herpes zoster, impaired hepatic functioning, infection, or sensitivity to dacarbazine.

**POTENTIAL DRUG/FOOD INTERACTIONS**

May interact with antigout agents such as probenecid or sulfinpyrazone to raise serum uric acid levels significantly. Allopurinol is frequently given to lower serum uric acid levels. Bone marrow suppression may be potentiated if dacarbazine is used in conjunction with radiation therapy or with cyclophosphamide. Dacarbazine should not be given with live virus vaccine because the viral replication may increase.

**INTERVENTIONS: ADMINISTRATION**

Prepare and handle dacarbazine according to the policies and procedures established for handling chemotherapeutic (cytotoxic) drugs within the agency. Reconstitute with sterile water for injection to make 10 mg of dacarbazine per milliliter. Reconstituted solutions of dacarbazine may be added to D5W or 0.9% NSS.

**MODE/RATE OF ADMINISTRATION**

May be given over 1–2 min through a free-flowing IV solution or over 15–30 min as an IV infusion. The slower infusion may prevent pain along the vein.

INTRAVENOUS USE (WITH NORMAL RENAL FUNCTION)

**Adults:** Usual IV dosage for treatment of malignant melanoma is 2–4.5 mg/kg of body weight a day for 10 d. May be repeated q28d. For Hodgkin's lymphoma the usual dosage is 150 mg/m$^2$ of BSA for 5 d. May be repeated q28d.

**Children:** Dosage not determined.

**Infants/Neonates:** Dosage not determined.

**Geriatrics:** Follow adult dosing schedules. Clients with diminished renal function may need dose adjustment.

INTRATHECAL USE OR OTHER INFUSION ROUTES AS INDICATED. Not recommended.

#### POTENTIAL PROBLEMS IN ADMINISTRATION

If the IV infusion extravasates, the infusion should be stopped immediately and restarted in another vein. Extravasation is determined by local burning and stinging at the infusion site.

#### INDEPENDENT NURSING ACTIONS

Monitor hematologic laboratory values carefully. Teach clients to use good oral hygiene and to avoid sources of infection when their blood counts are low. Teach clients to monitor themselves for infection and unusual bleeding such as black, tarry stools or bruising that occurs without injury.

#### ADMINISTRATION IN ALTERNATE SETTINGS

Should be administered in settings where the client can be closely monitored during the administration.

### EVALUATION: OUTCOMES OF DRUG THERAPY

#### EXPECTED OUTCOMES

PHYSICAL ASSESSMENT. Loss of hair, nausea, vomiting, stomatitis. Leukocyte count drops to near normal levels. Tumor masses diminish in size.

LABORATORY. Leukocyte counts hit nadir in 21 to 25 days. Leukocyte counts usually recover in 28 to 30 days. Thrombocytopenia usually hits nadir at 16 days. Recovery occurs at 19 to 21 days. Clients should have an Hct, Hgb, platelet count, and leukocyte count prior to the start of therapy.

#### NEGATIVE OUTCOMES

Infection, CNS toxicity, elevated serum uric acid levels, hepatotoxicity, GI tract bleeding, pulmonary edema, hypersensitivity response or anaphylaxis, or urinary retention. Tumor masses fail to diminish in size.

## MECHLORETHAMINE HYDROCHLORIDE

*Trade Name:* Mustargen
*Canadian Availability:* Mustargen
*Pregnancy Risk:* Category D
*pH:* 3–5
*Storage/Stability:* Store below 40° C. Reconstituted solutions should be used within 15 minutes.

### ASSESSMENT: DRUG CHARACTERISTICS

#### ACTION

A cell cycle nonspecific alkylating agent. Causes cross-linking of DNA and RNA strands. Inhibits synthesis of protein.

▼

**INDICATIONS**

Used primarily to treat carcinoma of the lung, chronic lymphocytic and myelocytic leukemias, Hodgkin's and non-Hodgkin's lymphomas, and malignant effusions of the pericardium, peritoneum, and pleura.

**CAUTIONS**

A potent bone marrow depressive agent and a weak immunosuppressant. There is an increased incidence of infection and delayed healing of dental work. Dental work should be done before therapy is started or delayed until blood counts return to normal. Clients should be instructed in proper oral hygiene. Mechlorethamine is both mutagenic and teratogenic. Clients should be instructed to use appropriate forms of birth control.

ADVERSE EFFECTS.

Carries the possibility of secondary malignancy as a result of therapy. Risk of malignancy seems to increase with long-term use. Leukopenia, stomatitis, hepatotoxicity, and thrombocytopenia are common effects of therapy. Frequent platelet and leukocyte counts should be done after therapy to monitor the leukopenia and thrombocytopenia.

CONTRAINDICATIONS. Should be given cautiously, if at all, to clients with significant immunosuppression, herpes zoster, impaired hepatic functioning, infection, or sensitivity to mechlorethamine.

**POTENTIAL DRUG/FOOD INTERACTIONS**

May interact with antigout agents such as probenecid or sulfinpyrazone to raise serum uric acid levels significantly. Allopurinol is frequently given to lower serum uric acid levels. Bone marrow suppression may be potentiated if mechlorethamine is used in conjunction with radiation therapy. Mechlorethamine should not be given with live virus vaccine because the viral replication may increase.

**INTERVENTIONS: ADMINISTRATION**

Strict adherence to agency safety procedures for handling antineoplastic agents should be followed when reconstituting and administering mechlorethamine. Any equipment used to administer mechlorethamine should be neutralized immediately after use by soaking in a solution containing equal parts of 5% sodium thiosulfate and 5% sodium bicarbonate for 45 min and rinsing well with water. Mechlorethamine is reconstituted using sterile water for injection to a strength of 1 mg/mL for IV use.

**MODE/RATE OF ADMINISTRATION**

May be given by rapid IV infusion, preferably through a free-flowing infusion. The injection should be completed in minutes. Slow infusion may cause solution to deactivate mechlorethamine.

INTRAVENOUS USE (WITH NORMAL RENAL FUNCTION)

**Adults:** Usual dosage is 400 mcg (0.4 mg)/kg of body weight as a single dose. Dose may be halved or quartered and given in consecutive daily doses. Maximum dose is usually 400 mcg (0.4 mg).

**Children:** Follow adult dosage schedule.

**Infants/Neonates:** Dosage not established.

**Geriatrics:** Follow adult dosage schedule.

INTRATHECAL USE OR OTHER INFUSION ROUTES AS INDICATED. May be used as an intracavitary or intrapericardial infusion. Usual infusion strength is 5–10 mg/mL. Usual dose is 400 mcg (0.4 mg)/kg of body weight intracavitary or 200 mcg (0.2 mg)/kg of body weight intrapericardial.

**POTENTIAL PROBLEMS IN ADMINISTRATION**

Hyperuricemia may be prevented in clients with lymphomas or leukemias by adequate hydration and administration of allopurinol. If extravasation occurs, the area should be immediately infiltrated with sterile isotonic thiosulfate or 1% lidocaine. Ice compresses should be applied for 6 to 12 hours.

**INDEPENDENT NURSING ACTIONS**

Monitor hematologic laboratory values carefully. Teach clients to use proper oral hygiene and to avoid sources of infection when their blood counts are low. Teach clients to monitor themselves for infection and unusual bleeding such as black, tarry stools or bruising that occurs without injury. Perform audiometric testing prior to the start of therapy.

**ADMINISTRATION IN ALTERNATE SETTINGS**

Mechlorethamine should be administered in settings where the client can be closely monitored during the administration.

**EVALUATION: OUTCOMES OF DRUG THERAPY**

**EXPECTED OUTCOMES**

PHYSICAL ASSESSMENT. Lymphocyte count falls to near normal levels or the tumor mass diminishes in size.

LABORATORY. Lymphocytopenia with nadir in 6 to 8 days, lasting 10 days to 3 weeks.

**NEGATIVE OUTCOMES**

Hyperuricemia, ototoxicity, thrombophlebitis, hepatotoxicity, peptic ulcer, and gonadal suppression. Tumor mass size does not diminish, WBC remains elevated, or malignant effusion does not diminish in size.

## THIOTEPA

*Trade Name:* Not specified.
*Canadian Availability:* Thiotepa
*Pregnancy Risk:* Category D
*pH:* 7.6
*Storage/Stability:* Store between 2° and 8° C. Protect from light. Reconstituted so-

▼

lutions may be kept for 5 days between 2° and 8° C. Reconstituted solutions should be clear to slightly opaque.

**ASSESSMENT: DRUG CHARACTERISTICS**

**ACTION**

A cell cycle nonspecific alkylating agent. Causes cross-linking of DNA and RNA strands. Inhibits protein syntheses.

**INDICATIONS**

Used to treat carcinomas of the breast, ovaries, and bladder; Hodgkin's and non-Hodgkin's lymphomas; and malignant pericardial, pleural, and peritoneal effusions.

**CAUTIONS**

A potent bone marrow depressive agent. There is an increased incidence of infection and delayed healing of dental work. Dental work should be done before therapy is started or delayed until blood counts return to normal. Patients should be instructed in proper oral hygiene. Thiotepa is both mutagenic and teratogenic. Clients should be instructed to use appropriate forms of birth control.

ADVERSE EFFECTS. Carries the possibility of secondary malignancy as a result of therapy. Risk of malignancy seems to increase with long-term use. Leukopenia, stomatitis, and thrombocytopenia are common effects of therapy. Frequent platelet and leukocyte counts should be done after therapy to monitor the leukopenia and thrombocytopenia.

CONTRAINDICATIONS. Should be given cautiously, if at all, to clients with significant immunosuppression, herpes zoster, impaired hepatic functioning, infection, or sensitivity to thiotepa.

**POTENTIAL DRUG/FOOD INTERACTIONS**

May interact with antigout agents such as probenecid or sulfinpyrazone to raise serum uric acid levels significantly. Allopurinol is frequently given to lower serum uric acid levels. Bone marrow suppression may be potentiated if thiotepa is used in conjunction with radiation therapy. Urokinase may potentiate the effects of thiotepa. Thiotepa may interact with succinylcholine to increase neuromuscular blockade. Respirations should be closely monitored during surgery if succinylcholine is used. Thiotepa should not be given with live virus vaccine because the viral replication may increase.

**INTERVENTIONS: ADMINISTRATION**

Strict adherence to agency safety procedures for handling antineoplastic agents should be followed when reconstituting and administering thiotepa. Thiopeta is reconstituted using sterile water for injection to achieve a strength of 10 mg/ml. Reconstituted solutions may be further diluted with D5W, 0.9% NSS, D5W in 0.9% NSS, or Ringer's lactate solution or lactated Ringer's injection.

**MODE/RATE OF ADMINISTRATION**

May be given by IV, intrapleural, intrapericardial, intraperitoneal, or intratumor routes.

INTRAVENOUS USE (WITH NORMAL RENAL FUNCTION)

**Adults:** Usual dosage for IV treatment of carcinomas, effusions, or lymphomas is 300–400 mcg (0.3–0.4 mg)/kg of body weight q1–4wk. Maintenance dose and schedule are determined by blood counts.

**Children 12 years:** Follow adult dosing schedule.

**Children < 12 years:** Dosage not established.

**Infants/Neonates:** Dosage not established.

**Geriatrics:** Follow adult dosing schedule. Clients with diminished renal function may require adjusted doses.

INTRATHECAL USE OR OTHER INFUSION ROUTES AS INDICATED. If given intracavitary or intratumor, usual dosage is 600–800 mcg (0.6–0.8 mg)/kg of body weight q1–4wk. A maintenance dose of 70–800 mcg (0.07–0.8 mg) may be given.

**POTENTIAL PROBLEMS IN ADMINISTRATION**

Hyperuricemia may be prevented in clients with lymphomas by adequate hydration and administration of allopurinol.

**INDEPENDENT NURSING ACTIONS**

Monitor hematologic laboratory values carefully. Teach clients to use proper oral hygiene and to avoid sources of infection when their blood counts are low. Teach clients to monitor themselves for infection and unusual bleeding such as black, tarry stools or bruising that occurs without injury.

**ADMINISTRATION IN ALTERNATE SETTINGS**

Should be administered in settings where the client can be closely monitored during the administration.

**EVALUATION: OUTCOMES OF DRUG THERAPY**

**EXPECTED OUTCOMES**

PHYSICAL ASSESSMENT. Loss of hair, nausea, vomiting, stomatitis, and weight loss. Tumor masses diminish in size.

LABORATORY. Clients should have an Hct, Hgb, platelet count, and leukocyte count prior to the start of therapy. Leukopenia and thrombocytopenia are common. Therapy is usually stopped if the WBC falls below 4000/mm3 or platelets are below 150,000/mm3.

**NEGATIVE OUTCOMES**

Hyperuricemia, infection, nephrotoxicity, and anaphylaxis. Tumor masses remain unchanged.

# Antibiotics

## BLEOMYCIN SULFATE

*Trade Name:* Blenoxane
*Canadian Availability:* Blenoxane
*Pregnancy Risk:* Category D
*pH:* 4.5–6
*Storage/Stability:* Store between 2° and 8° C. Reconstituted solutions are stable at room temperature for 24 hours or at least 14 days if refrigerated.

### ASSESSMENT: DRUG CHARACTERISTICS

**ACTION**

An antibiotic, but is not used as an antibiotic. Appears to be effective with both cycling and noncycling cells. Has the greatest effect during the $G_2$ phase of cell division and may bind with the DNA to reduce synthesis.

**INDICATIONS**

Used to treat carcinomas of the head, neck, cervix, penis, and testicles, and Hodgkin's and non-Hodgkin's lymphomas.

**CAUTIONS**

Increases incidence of infection and delayed healing of dental work. Dental work should be done before therapy is started or delayed until blood counts return to normal. Patients should be instructed in proper oral hygiene. Bleomycin is both mutagenic and teratogenic. Clients should be instructed to use appropriate forms of birth control.

ADVERSE EFFECTS. Carries risk that therapy will induce a secondary malignancy. This risk seems to increase with long-term use. Stomatitis is a common effect of therapy. Bleomycin is known to impair pulmonary function.

CONTRAINDICATIONS. Should be given cautiously, if at all, to clients who smoke, who have significantly impaired pulmonary, renal, or hepatic function, infection, or sensitivity to the agent, or who have had cytotoxic or radiation therapy, previously.

**POTENTIAL DRUG/FOOD INTERACTIONS**

May interact with general anesthetics to further impair pulmonary function. Bone marrow suppression may be potentiated if bleomycin is used in conjunction with radiation therapy. Bleomycin may potentiate cisplatin's nephrotoxic effects. Vincristine given before bleomycin may make cells more susceptible to bleomycin's cytotoxic activity.

### INTERVENTIONS: ADMINISTRATION

Strict adherence to agency safety procedures for handling antineoplastic agents should be followed when reconstituting and administering bleomycin. Bleomycin is reconstituted with 0.9% NSS or D5W injection.

**MODE/RATE OF ADMINISTRATION**

May be given intravenously or intraarterially over 10 min. May be further diluted with 50 to 100 mL of diluent and infused regionally.

INTRAVENOUS USE (WITH NORMAL RENAL FUNCTION)

**Adults:** Usual adult IV dose for Hodgkin's disease and testicular carcinomas is 0.25 U/kg of body weight for 4–5 d.

**Children:** Dose and schedule for children similar to those for adults and adolescents.

**Infants/Neonates:** Dose has not been established.

**Geriatrics:** Follow adult dosing schedule. Clients over 70 are at greater risk for pulmonary dysfunction. Clients with diminished renal function may need to have dose adjusted.

INTRATHECAL USE OR OTHER INFUSION ROUTES AS INDICATED. The usual adult regional arterial infusion dose for squamous cell carcinoma of the head, neck, or cervix is 30–60 U/d over a period of 1–24 h. The usual intraperitoneal infusion dose is 60–120 U instilled, then removed after 24 h.

**POTENTIAL PROBLEMS IN ADMINISTRATION**

Idiosyncratic reactions to bleomycin may be treated with pressor agents, antihistamines, or corticosteroids. Bleomycin given with vincristine may cause vasospasm.

**INDEPENDENT NURSING ACTIONS**

Monitor hematology laboratory values carefully. Teach clients to use proper oral hygiene and to avoid sources of infection when their blood counts are low. Clients should also be taught to monitor themselves for infection and unusual bleeding such as black, tarry stools or bruising that occurs without injury. A chest x-ray and pulmonary function studies should be made before therapy is started. The client's chest should be auscultated before treatment is started.

**ADMINISTRATION IN ALTERNATE SETTINGS**

Bleomycin should be administered in settings where the client can be closely monitored during the administration.

**EVALUATION: OUTCOMES OF DRUG THERAPY**

**EXPECTED OUTCOMES**

PHYSICAL ASSESSMENT. Fever and chills 3 to 6 hours after administration, loss of hair, nausea, vomiting, stomatitis, and weight loss are common. Tumor masses diminish in size.

LABORATORY. A Hct, Hgb, platelet count, leukocyte count, and creatinine clearance levels should be done before the start of therapy.

**NEGATIVE OUTCOMES**

Idiosyncratic reactions, hepatotoxicity, nephrotoxicity, GI bleeding, pulmonary edema, or urinary retention.

## DAUNORUBICIN HYDROCHLORIDE

*Trade Name:* Cerubidine
*Canadian Availability:* Cerubidine
*Pregnancy Risk:* Category D
*pH:* 4.5–6
*Storage/Stability:* Store below 40° C. Protect from light. Reconstituted solutions are stable at room temperature for 24 hours or for at least 48 hours if stored at temperatures between 2° and 8° C.

### ASSESSMENT: DRUG CHARACTERISTICS

#### ACTION

An anthracycline glycoside; an antibiotic, but is not used as an antibiotic. Has the greatest effect during the S phase of cell division, but is cell cycle nonspecific. Daunorubicin may bind with the DNA to reduce synthesis by scrambling the DNA template.

#### INDICATIONS

Used to treat acute lymphocytic, myelocytic, and monocytic leukemias.

#### CAUTIONS

A potent bone marrow depressant. Increases incidence of infection and delayed healing of dental work. Dental work should be done before therapy is started or delayed until blood counts return to normal. Patients should be instructed in proper oral hygiene. Daunorubicin is both mutagenic and teratogenic. Clients should be instructed to use appropriate forms of birth control.

**ADVERSE EFFECTS.** Carries risk that therapy will induce a secondary malignancy. This risk seems to increase with long-term use. Stomatitis, cardiotoxicity, gastrointestinal ulceration, and hyperuricemia are common effects of therapy.

**CONTRAINDICATIONS.** Should be given cautiously, if at all, to clients with significant immunosuppression, bone marrow depression, herpes zoster, impaired hepatic or renal function, heart disease, infection, tumor cell infiltrate to bone marrow, or sensitivity to the agent.

#### POTENTIAL DRUG/FOOD INTERACTIONS

Bone marrow suppression may be potentiated if daunorubicin is used in conjunction with radiation therapy or with cyclophosphamide. May interact with antigout agents such as probenecid or sulfinpyrazone to raise serum uric acid levels significantly. Allopurinol is frequently given before daunorubicin to lower serum uric acid levels. Daunorubicin may potentiate the cardiotoxic effects of doxorubicin and hepatotoxic effects of other drugs. Should be used cautiously with clients who have had cytotoxic or radiation therapy previously. Daunorubicin should not be given with live virus vaccine because the viral replication may increase.

#### INTERVENTIONS: ADMINISTRATION

Strict adherence to agency safety procedures for handling antineoplastic agents should be followed when reconstituting and administering daunorubicin. Daunorubicin is reconstituted with sterile water for injection to a strength of 5 mg/mL.

#### MODE/RATE OF ADMINISTRATION

Should be given by rapid IV infusion through the side port of a free flowing infusion of D5W or 0.9% NSS infusion over 2–3 min.

#### INTRAVENOUS USE (WITH NORMAL RENAL FUNCTION)

**Adults:** Usual adult IV dose for acute lymphocytic and nonlymphocytic leukemias is 45 mg/m$^2$ of BSA on days 1, 2, and 3 of the first course of a 32-d course. Additional dosing is done with vincristine, asparaginase, and prednisone for acute lymphocytic leukemia and cytarabine for acute nonlymphocytic leukemias. Maximum lifetime dose should not exceed 550 mg/m$^2$ of BSA to avoid cardiotoxicity.

**Children:** Usual dose for acute lymphocytic leukemia is 25 mg/m$^2$ of BSA once a week in combination with vincristine and prednisone. Maximum lifetime dose should not exceed 300 mg/m$^2$ of BSA.

**Infants/Neonates:** Usual dose for children under 2 years or who have a BSA of less than 0.5 m$^2$ for acute lymphocytic leukemia is based on 10 mg/kg of body weight.

**Geriatrics:** Usual dose for clients over 60 years for acute nonlymphocytic leukemia is 30 mg/m$^2$ of BSA on days 1, 2, and 3 of the first course and days 1 and 2 of the second course in combination with cytarabine.

#### INTRATHECAL USE OR OTHER INFUSION ROUTES AS INDICATED.

Not recommended.

#### POTENTIAL PROBLEMS IN ADMINISTRATION

Facial flushing or red streaking along vein indicates that the infusion rate is too rapid. If extravasation occurs, stop the infusion. The remaining medication should be administered in a different vein.

#### INDEPENDENT NURSING ACTIONS

Monitor hematology laboratory values carefully. Teach clients to use proper oral hygiene and to avoid sources of infection when their blood counts are low. Clients should also be taught to monitor themselves for infection and unusual bleeding such as black, tarry stools or bruising that occurs without injury. A chest x-ray, ECG, echocardiogram, and radionuclide angiography determination of ejection fractions should be done before therapy is started.

#### ADMINISTRATION IN ALTERNATE SETTINGS

Daunorubicin should be administered in settings where the client can be closely monitored during the administration.

▼

**EVALUATION: OUTCOMES OF DRUG THERAPY**

**EXPECTED OUTCOMES**

PHYSICAL ASSESSMENT. Loss of hair, nausea, vomiting, stomatitis, and weight loss are common. Leukocyte counts approach normal.

LABORATORY. Leukocyte counts hit nadir in 10 to 14 days. Leukocyte counts usually recover within 21 days. An Hct, Hgb, platelet count, and leukocyte count should be done before the start of therapy.

**NEGATIVE OUTCOMES**

Congestive heart failure, GI bleeding, hyperuricemia, or hypersensitivity reactions are negative outcomes. Leukocyte count remains unchanged.

## DOXORUBICIN HYDROCHLORIDE

*Trade Names:* Adriamycin RDF, Rubex
*Canadian Availability:* Adriamycin RDF
*Pregnancy Risk:* Category D
*pH:* 3.8–6.5
*Storage/Stability:* Store below 40° C. Protect from light. Reconstituted solutions of Adriamycin RDF are stable at room temperature for 7 days or 15 days if stored at temperatures between 2° and 8° C. Reconstituted solutions of generic doxorubicin are stable for 24 hours at room temperature or 48 hours if stored at temperatures between 2° and 8° C.

**ASSESSMENT: DRUG CHARACTERISTICS**

**ACTION**

An anthracycline glycoside; an antibiotic, but is not used as an antibiotic. Has the greatest effect during the S phase of cell division, but is cell cycle nonspecific. May bind with DNA to reduce synthesis by scrambling the DNA template.

**INDICATIONS**

Used to treat acute lymphocytic and myelocytic leukemias; carcinomas of the bladder, breast, ovaries, thyroid, lung, and stomach; Hodgkin's and non-Hodgkin's lymphomas; neuroblastomas; Wilms' tumor; sarcomas; and osteosarcomas.

**CAUTIONS**

A potent bone marrow depressant. There is an increased incidence of infection and delayed healing of dental work. Dental work should be done before therapy is started or delayed until blood counts return to normal. Clients should be instructed in proper oral hygiene. Doxorubicin is both mutagenic and teratogenic. Clients should be instructed to use appropriate forms of birth control.

ADVERSE EFFECTS. Carries the possibility of secondary malignancy as a result of therapy. Risk of malignancy seems to increase with long-term use. Leukopenia, stomatitis, cardiotoxicity, GI tract ulceration, and hyperuricemia are common effects of therapy.

CONTRAINDICATIONS. Should be given cautiously, if at all, to clients with significant immunosuppression, bone marrow depression, herpes zoster, impaired hepatic functioning, heart disease, infection, tumor cell infiltrate to bone marrow, or sensitivity to doxorubicin.

**POTENTIAL DRUG/FOOD INTERACTIONS**

Bone marrow suppression may be potentiated if doxorubicin is used in conjunction with radiation therapy, cyclophosphamide, dactinomycin, or mitomycin. May interact with antigout agents such as probenecid or sulfinpyrazone to raise serum uric acid levels significantly. Allopurinol is frequently given to lower serum uric acid levels. Doxorubicin may potentiate the cardiotoxic effects of daunorubicin and hepatotoxic effects of other drugs. May prolong the effects of streptozocin. Should be used cautiously with clients who have had previous cytotoxic or radiation therapy. Should not be given with live virus vaccine because the viral replication may increase.

**INTERVENTIONS: ADMINISTRATION**

Strict adherence to agency safety procedures for handling antineoplastic agents should be followed when reconstituting and administering doxorubicin. Doxorubicin is reconstituted using 0.9% NSS for injection to a strength of 2 mg/mL. Should not be mixed with heparin, dexamethasone, fluorouracil, hydrocortisone, sodium succinate, aminophylline, or cephalothin because a precipitate forms.

**MODE/RATE OF ADMINISTRATION**

Should be given by rapid IV infusion through the side port of a free-flowing infusion of 0.9% NSS or D5W infusion over not less than 3–5 min.

INTRAVENOUS USE (WITH NORMAL RENAL FUNCTION)

**Adults:** Usual adult IV dosage is 60–75 $mg/m^2$ of BSA repeated q21d. Maximum dose should not exceed 550 $mg/m^2$ of BSA to avoid cardiotoxicity.

**Children:** Usual dosage is 30 $mg/m^2$ of BSA a day for three consecutive days q4wk.

**Infants/Neonates:** Dosage not established.

**Geriatrics:** Clients over 70 years are at greater risk for cardiotoxicity. Dosage may need to be adjusted for age.

INTRATHECAL USE OR OTHER INFUSION ROUTES AS INDICATED. May be given intraarterially or as an instillation.

**POTENTIAL PROBLEMS IN ADMINISTRATION**

If extravasation occurs, stop the infusion. Extravasation is indicated by swelling, burning, and stinging at the IV site. Local antidotes are not recommended. The limb may be elevated and ice compresses applied. The remaining medication should be administered in a different vein.

**INDEPENDENT NURSING ACTIONS**

Monitor hematologic laboratory values carefully. Teach clients to use proper oral hygiene and to avoid sources of infection when their blood counts are low. Teach clients to monitor themselves for infection and unusual bleeding such as black, tarry stools or bruising that occurs without injury. A chest x-ray, ECG, echocardiogram, and radionuclide angiography determination of ejection fractions should be done before therapy is started.

**ADMINISTRATION IN ALTERNATE SETTINGS**

Should be administered in settings where the client can be closely monitored during the administration.

**EVALUATION: OUTCOMES OF DRUG THERAPY**

**EXPECTED OUTCOMES**

PHYSICAL ASSESSMENT. Loss of hair, nausea, vomiting, reddish urine that clears in 48 hours, stomatitis, and weight loss. WBC approach normal.

LABORATORY. Leukocyte counts hit nadir in 10 to 14 days. Leukocyte counts usually recover within 21 days. Clients should have an Hct, Hgb, platelet count, and leukocyte count prior to the start of therapy. BUN and serum creatinine levels should be monitored.

**NEGATIVE OUTCOMES**

Congestive heart failure, GI tract bleeding, hyperuricemia, or hypersensitivity reactions. WBC count remains unchanged. Tumor mass remains unchanged.

## MITOMYCIN

*Trade Name:* Mutamycin
*Canadian Availability:* Mutamycin
*Pregnancy Risk:* Category D
*pH:* 6–8
*Storage/Stability:* Store below 40° C. Protect from light. Reconstituted solutions of mitomycin are stable at room temperature for 7 days or 14 days if stored at temperatures between 2° and 8° C. When further diluted for IV infusion, solutions in D5W are stable for 3 hours, solutions in 0.9% NSS are stable for 12 hours, and solutions in sodium lactate are stable for 24 hours at room temperature.

**ASSESSMENT: DRUG CHARACTERISTICS**

**ACTION**

An antibiotic, but is not used as an antibiotic because of its toxicity. Has the greatest effect during the G and S phases of cell division, but is cell cycle nonspecific.

Causes cross-linking of DNA to inhibit synthesis. RNA and protein synthesis are affected to a lesser degree.

#### INDICATIONS

Used primarily to treat carcinomas of the pancreas and stomach.

#### CAUTIONS

A potent bone marrow depressant. There is an increased incidence of infection and delayed healing of dental work. Dental work should be done before therapy is started or delayed until blood counts return to normal. Clients should be instructed in proper oral hygiene. Mitomycin is both mutagenic and teratogenic. Clients should be instructed to use appropriate forms of birth control.

ADVERSE EFFECTS. Carries the possibility of secondary malignancy as a result of therapy. Risk of malignancy seems to increase with long-term use. Leukopenia, stomatitis, pulmonary toxicity, GI tract ulceration, and hyperuricemia are common effects of therapy.

CONTRAINDICATIONS. Should be given cautiously, if at all, to clients with significant immunosuppression, bone marrow depression, herpes zoster, impaired renal functioning, coagulation disorders, infection, or sensitivity to mitomycin.

#### POTENTIAL DRUG/FOOD INTERACTIONS

Bone marrow suppression may be potentiated if mitomycin is used in conjunction with radiation therapy or doxorubicin. Mitomycin should be used cautiously with clients who have had previous cytotoxic or radiation therapy. Should not be given with live virus vaccine because the viral replication may increase.

#### INTERVENTIONS: ADMINISTRATION

Strict adherence to agency safety procedures for handling antineoplastic agents should be followed when reconstituting and administering mitomycin. Mitomycin is reconstituted using sterile water for injection. May be further diluted with D5W, 0.9% NSS, or sodium lactate.

#### MODE/RATE OF ADMINISTRATION

Should be given by rapid IV infusion through the side port of a free-flowing infusion of 0.9% NSS or D5W over 3–5 min.

INTRAVENOUS USE (WITH NORMAL RENAL FUNCTION)

**Adults:** Usual adult IV dosage is 10–20 mg/m$^2$ of BSA as a single dose, repeated q6–8 wk. Maximum dose should not exceed 20 mg/m$^2$ of BSA. Higher doses increase toxic side effects and are not known to be any more effective.

**Children:** Follow adult dosing schedule.

**Infants/Neonates:** Dosage not established.

**Geriatrics:** Clients over 60 years may have diminished renal function. Dosage may need to be adjusted.

▼

INTRATHECAL USE OR OTHER INFUSION ROUTES AS INDICATED. May be given intraarterially or as an instillation.

**POTENTIAL PROBLEMS IN ADMINISTRATION**

If extravasation occurs, stop the infusion. Extravasation is indicated by swelling, burning, and stinging at the IV site. Local antidotes are not recommended. The limb may be elevated and ice compresses applied. Mitomycin is extremely tissue toxic. Surgery may be needed to excise necrosed tissue. The remaining medication should be administered in a different vein.

**INDEPENDENT NURSING ACTIONS**

Monitor hematologic laboratory values carefully. Teach clients to use proper oral hygiene and to avoid sources of infection when their blood counts are low. Teach clients to monitor themselves for infection and unusual bleeding such as black, tarry stools or bruising that occurs without injury. A chest x-ray, ECG, echocardiogram, and radionuclide angiography determination of ejection fractions, BUN, and serum creatinine should be done before therapy is started.

**ADMINISTRATION IN ALTERNATE SETTINGS**

Should be administered in settings where the client can be closely monitored during the administration.

**EVALUATION: OUTCOMES OF DRUG THERAPY**

**EXPECTED OUTCOMES**

PHYSICAL ASSESSMENT. Loss of hair, nausea, vomiting, reddish urine that clears in 48 hours, stomatitis, and weight loss. Tumor mass diminishes in size.

LABORATORY. Leukocyte and thrombocyte counts hit nadir in 3 to 8 weeks. Leukocyte counts usually recover within 10 weeks. Clients should have an Hct, Hgb, platelet count, and leukocyte count prior to the start of therapy. BUN and serum creatinine levels should be monitored.

**NEGATIVE OUTCOMES**

Pulmonary toxicity (cough, shortness of breath), GI tract bleeding, hyperuricemia, nephrotoxicity (hematuria, oliguria, edema), or hypersensitivity reactions. WBC count remains unchanged. Tumor mass remains unchanged.

## PLICAMYCIN (MITHRAMYCIN)

*Trade Name:* Mithracin
*Canadian Availability:* Not commercially available
*Pregnancy Risk:* Category X
*pH:* 7
*Storage/Stability:* Store between 2° and 8° C. Protect from light. Reconstituted solutions of plicamycin are stable at room temperature 4 to 6 hours. Should be used immediately after being reconstituted.

## ASSESSMENT: DRUG CHARACTERISTICS

### ACTION

A cell cycle nonspecific antineoplastic agent. Mechanism of action is not well understood. Appears to cause cross-linking of DNA and RNA to inhibit synthesis.

### INDICATIONS

Used primarily to treat testicular carcinoma, hypercalcemia, and hypercalciuria associated with neoplasms.

### CAUTIONS

A potent bone marrow depressant. There is an increased incidence of infection and delayed healing of dental work. Dental work should be done before therapy is started or delayed until blood counts return to normal. Clients should be instructed in proper oral hygiene. Plicamycin is both mutagenic and teratogenic. Clients should be instructed to use appropriate forms of birth control.

ADVERSE EFFECTS. Carries the possibility of secondary malignancy as a result of therapy. Risk of malignancy seems to increase with long-term use. Hypocalcemia, leukopenia, stomatitis, and GI tract ulceration are common effects of therapy.

CONTRAINDICATIONS. Should be given cautiously, if at all, to clients with significant immunosuppression, bone marrow depression, herpes zoster, impaired hepatic or renal functioning, coagulation disorders, infection, or sensitivity to plicamycin.

### POTENTIAL DRUG/FOOD INTERACTIONS

Bone marrow suppression may be potentiated if plicamycin is used in conjunction with radiation therapy. Plicamycin should be used cautiously with clients who have had previous cytotoxic or radiation therapy. May potentiate coagulation disorders or GI tract ulceration if client is also receiving heparin, thrombolytic agents, NSAIDs, aspirin, dipyridamole, sulfinpyrazone, or valproic acid. May potentiate the effects of other hepatotoxic or nephrotoxic agents. Vitamin D and calcium-containing preparations may antagonize plicamycin's activity. Plicamycin should not be given with live virus vaccine because the viral replication may increase.

## INTERVENTIONS: ADMINISTRATION

Strict adherence to agency safety procedures for handling antineoplastic agents should be followed when reconstituting and administering plicamycin. Plicamycin is reconstituted using sterile water for injection. May be further diluted with 1000 mL D5W or 0.9% NSS.

### MODE/RATE OF ADMINISTRATION

Should be given by IV infusion over a period of 4–6 h.

INTRAVENOUS USE (WITH NORMAL RENAL FUNCTION)

**Adults:** Usual adult IV dosage for antineoplastic activity is 25–30 mcg (0.025–0.03 mg)/kg of body ▼

weight for 8–10 d unless toxic effects are significant. Further doses may be given at 1-mo intervals. Usual adult dosage for antihypercalcemic or antihypercalciuric activity is 15–25 mcg (0.015–0.025 mg)/kg of body weight for 3–4 d, repeated at 1-wk intervals if necessary.

**Children:** Dosage not established.

**Infants/Neonates:** Dosage not established.

**Geriatrics:** Follow adult dosing schedule. Clients over 60 years may have diminished renal function. Dosage may need to be adjusted.

INTRATHECAL USE OR OTHER INFUSION ROUTES AS INDICATED. Not recommended.

#### POTENTIAL PROBLEMS IN ADMINISTRATION

If extravasation occurs, stop the infusion. Extravasation is indicated by swelling, burning, and stinging at the IV site. Local antidotes are not recommended. The limb may be elevated and ice compresses applied. Plicamycin is extremely tissue toxic. The remaining medication should be administered in a different vein. Too rapid infusion of plicamycin may cause more severe GI tract side effects.

#### INDEPENDENT NURSING ACTIONS

Monitor hematologic laboratory values carefully. Teach clients to use proper oral hygiene and to avoid sources of infection when their blood counts are low. Teach clients to monitor themselves for infection and unusual bleeding such as black, tarry stools or bruising that occurs without injury. Serum calcium, BUN, and serum creatinine levels should be done before therapy is started.

#### ADMINISTRATION IN ALTERNATE SETTINGS

Plicamycin should be administered in settings where the client can be closely monitored during the administration.

#### EVALUATION: OUTCOMES OF DRUG THERAPY

#### EXPECTED OUTCOMES

PHYSICAL ASSESSMENT. Loss of hair, nausea, vomiting, reddish urine that clears in 48 hours, stomatitis, and weight loss. Tumor mass diminishes in size. Serum and urine calcium levels lower.

LABORATORY. BUN, serum creatinine, and urine calcium levels should be monitored.

#### NEGATIVE OUTCOMES

GI tract bleeding, hypocalcemia, hepatotoxicity, leukopenia, or hypersensitivity reactions. Tumor mass remains unchanged. Serum and urine calcium levels remain elevated.

CHAPTER 18

# Autonomic Agents

*Elaine Kennedy*



## DEFINITION

Autonomic drugs are drugs that alter the functioning of the autonomic nervous system. The autonomic nervous system is divided into the parasympathetic nervous system (cholinergic or muscarinic) and the sympathetic nervous system (adrenergic). The predominant function of the parasympathetic nervous system is to control regulatory functions such as cardiac output, blood pressure, and digestive processes. The sympathetic nervous system provides immediate defense in "fight-or-flight" responses. The parasympathetic and the sympathetic nervous systems work in opposition to create a balanced control of body functions. Autonomic drugs may block or enhance the effects of the parasympathetic or the sympathetic nervous system.

## CLASSIFICATION

Autonomic drugs work by one of several means:

1. Enhance or mimic the parasympathetic nervous system (parasympathomimetic or cholinergic)
2. Block the parasympathetic nervous system (anticholinergic)
3. Enhance or mimic the sympathetic nervous system (sympathomimetic or adrenergic)

4. Block the sympathetic nervous system (sympatholytic)

## PARASYMPATHOMIMETIC (CHOLINERGIC) DRUGS

Parasympathomimetic drugs act by mimicking the action of or preventing the breakdown of the neurotransmitter, acetylcholine. Acetylcholine is released by stimulated neurons, diffuses across the nerve synapse, and binds to receptors on the synapse neuron to transmit neural stimulation. Drugs that prevent the breakdown of acetylcholine do so by inhibiting acetylcholinesterase. Parasympathomimetic drugs are commonly used for three purposes:

1. Restore muscle tone, in conditions such as myasthenia gravis
2. Constrict the pupil (useful in some ophthalmic conditions)
3. Stimulate an atonic bladder

## PARASYMPATHOLYTIC (ANTICHOLINERGIC) DRUGS

Parasympatholytic drugs act by blocking the acetylcholine receptor site on the receptor neuron. There are three common receptor sites:

1. The neuromuscular receptors
2. The ganglionic receptors
3. The muscarinic receptors

The neuromuscular receptor blockers, also called skeletal muscle relaxants, cause muscular relaxation or paralysis. The ganglionic receptor blockers block both parasympathetic and sympathetic neuron transmission and have some use in treating hypertension. The muscarinic receptor blockers such as atropine and scopolamine block acetylcholine activity in smooth muscle, the heart, and exocrine glands. In general, the muscarinic receptor blockers decrease secretions, decrease gastrointestinal (GI) tract motility, increase the heart rate, dilate the eye, and relax bronchial smooth muscle.

## SYMPATHOMIMETIC (ADRENERGIC) DRUGS

Sympathomimetic drugs act by mimicking the action of one of the three sympathetic neurotransmitters: epinephrine, norepinephrine, or dopamine. Epinephrine is released from the adrenal medulla, norepinephrine is released at the sympathetic neural synapse, and dopamine is the chemical precursor to norepinephrine. The sympathetic nervous system has a number of different receptors ($\alpha_1$, $\alpha_2$, $\beta_1$, and $\beta_2$) that respond differently to norepinephrine and epinephrine. In general, drugs that stimulate the $\alpha_1$-receptors cause an increase in blood pressure and local vasoconstriction. Drugs that stimulate $\alpha_2$-receptors inhibit the amount of norepinephrine released from the neuron. Drugs that stimulate $\beta_1$-receptors cause an increased heart rate and increased cardiac contractile force. Drugs that stimulate the $\beta_2$-receptors cause vasodilation in heart and skeletal muscle and the brain, bronchodilation, and uterine relaxation.

## SYMPATHOLYTIC DRUGS

Sympatholytic drugs act by blocking a specific $\alpha$- or $\beta$-receptor site at the neural synapse, depleting the store of or inhibiting the release of norepinephrine in peripheral neurons or inhibiting peripheral neural activity through central nervous system (CNS) activity. $\alpha$-Blockers may cause orthostatic hypotension and pinpoint pupils. $\beta$-Blockers are used to manage angina and some arrhythmias. Drugs that deplete norepinephrine in peripheral neurons may be used to treat hypertension. Drugs that inhibit peripheral neural activity through CNS action may be used to treat hypertension. The $\beta$-blockers, norepinephrine depletion agents, and the CNS neural inhibitors are discussed in depth in Chapter 20.

The autonomic drugs are grouped by subclassifications in Table 18–1.

**TABLE 18–1**
**Parenteral Autonomic Agents Grouped by Subclassifications**

**Parasympathomimetics**
Neostigmine*
Physostigmine*
Pyridostigmine bromide

**Parasympatholytics**

***Muscarinics***
Biperiden*
Atropine sulfate
Clidinium*

***Neuromuscular Blocking Agents***
Atracurium besylate
Dantrolene sodium*
Gallamine*
Methocarbamol
Metaxalone*
Metocurine*
Orphenadrine citrate
Pancuronium bromide
Succinylcholine*
Tubocurarine*
Vecuronium bromide

**Sympathomimetics**
Dobutamine hydrochloride
Dopamine hydrochloride
Ephedrine*
Epinephrine hydrochloride
Isoproterenol hydrochloride
Mephentermine*
Metaraminol bitartrate
Methoxamine*
Norepinephrine*
Ritodrine hydrochloride

**Sympatholytics**

***α-Receptor Blockers***
Dihydroergotamine mesylate
Phentolamine*

*Not discussed in this chapter.

# PARASYMPATHOMIMETICS (CHOLINERGICS)

## THERAPEUTIC EFFECTS

Parasympathomimetics cause acetylcholine to accumulate at the cholinergic synapses, thereby prolonging and exaggerating the effects of acetylcholine. The drugs compete with acetylcholine for attachment to acetylcholinesterase, preventing the hydrolysis of acetylcholine. Parasympathomimetic drugs are primarily used to treat myasthenia gravis, reverse the effects of nondepolarizing neuromuscular blocking agents, and prevent or treat postsurgical urinary retention.

## PHARMACOKINETICS

**Distribution.** When administered intravenously, parasympathomimetics are widely distributed throughout the body. Onset varies from 2 to 5 minutes to as long as 20 to 30 minutes. Maximum effects are generally seen in 30 to 60 minutes and last for 2–4 hours. Parasympathomimetics may cross the blood-brain barrier and the placental barrier.

**Excretion.** Parasympathomimetics are excreted in urine in 24 to 72 hours.

## CAUTIONS

**Side/Adverse Effects.** Adverse effects are mainly those of exaggerated response to the parasympathetic nervous system stimulation, including nausea, vomiting, diarrhea, excessive salivation, sweating, increased bronchial secretions, seizures, muscle weakness, and cramps.

**Contraindications.** Parasympathomimetics should not be given to clients with hypersensitivity to cholinergics. The drugs should be used with caution in clients with epilepsy, bronchial asthma, bradycardia, hyperthyroidism, cardiac dysrhythmias, or peptic ulcers.

***Pregnancy and Lactation.*** Parasympathomimetics may cause uterine irritability and induce labor if given to near-term pregnant women. The drugs may cross the placental barrier.

***Pediatrics.*** No age specific effects have been determined.

***Geriatrics.*** No age specific effects have been determined.

## TOXICITY

See Table 18–2 for toxicities associated with parasympathomimetic agents.

## POTENTIAL DRUG/FOOD INTERACTIONS

Parasympathomimetic (cholinergic) drugs may be used to reverse muscle relaxation after surgery because of their antagonistic effect on nondepolarizing neuromuscular blocking agents. However, the cholinergic drugs may potentiate the effects of depolarizing neuromuscular blocking agents. Atropine may be used to reverse adverse effects of choliner-

**TABLE 18–2**
**Toxicities of Parasympathomimetic Agents**

| Body System | Side/ Toxic Effects | Physical Assessment Indicators | Laboratory Indicators | Nursing Interventions |
|---|---|---|---|---|
| Other | Cholinergic crisis | Nausea, vomiting, diarrhea, bradycardia, tachycardia, blurred vision, muscle weakness, cramps, respiratory paralysis | N/A | Monitor respiratory function. Be prepared to administer atropine IV if symptoms are severe. |

gics. Clients who are using cholinergics may have undesirable neuromuscular blocking effects from aminoglycosides, some local and general anesthetics, and some antiarrhythmic drugs.

## Pyridostigmine Bromide

*Trade Names:* Mestinon, Regonol
*Canadian Availability:* Regonol
*Pregnancy Risk:* Category C
*pH:* 5
*Storage/Stability:* Store below 40° C. Protect from light and freezing.

### ASSESSMENT: DRUG CHARACTERISTICS

#### ACTION

Blocks the destruction of acetylcholine by acetylcholinesterase at the myoneural junction, thus facilitating the transmission of nerve impulses. Muscle response to repeated stimulation is improved, as is muscle strength.

#### INDICATIONS

Used as an antidote to nondepolarizing neuromuscular blocking agents such as atracurium and to treat myasthenia gravis.

#### CAUTIONS

ADVERSE EFFECTS. May cause bradycardia, excessive salivation, and GI tract stimulation. May cause allergic reactions, confusion, difficulty in breathing, seizures, blurred vision, irritability, severe diarrhea, shortness of breath, wheezing, stomach cramps, muscle cramps or twitching, weakness, and fatigue.

CONTRAINDICATIONS. Intestinal or urinary tract obstructions, urinary tract infections, asthma, cardiac arrhythmias, or sensitivity to pyridostigmine.

#### POTENTIAL DRUG/FOOD INTERACTIONS

May interact with other antimyasthenic agents to potentiate their effects. May in

▼

teract with guanadrel, guanethidine, mecamylamine, trimethaphan, procainamide, or quinidine to antagonize the antimyasthenic effects of pyridostigmine. The action of neuromuscular blocking agents may be prolonged if used with pyridostigmine. If used with edrophonium, may mask the symptoms of overdose.

**INTERVENTIONS: ADMINISTRATION**

May be given undiluted.

**MODE/RATE OF ADMINISTRATION**

Usually given by rapid intravenous (IV) injection through a free-flowing IV solution.

INTRAVENOUS USE (WITH NORMAL RENAL FUNCTION)

**Adults:** As an antimyasthenic the usual dosage is 2 mg q2–3h. As an antidote to neuromuscular blockers the usual dose is 10–20 mg.

**Children:** Dose not established.

**Infants/Neonates:** IV dose not established.

**Geriatrics:** Action of the drug as an antagonist to neuromuscular blockers is prolonged.

INTRATHECAL USE OR OTHER INFUSION ROUTES AS INDICATED. Not recommended.

**POTENTIAL PROBLEMS IN ADMINISTRATION**

If used to antagonize neuromuscular blockers, atropine sulfate 600 mcg (0.6 mg)–1.2 mg should be given prior to administration of pyridostigmine to counter the respiratory effects of pyridostigmine.

**INDEPENDENT NURSING ACTIONS**

Monitor client for muscle strength and endurance. Monitor vital signs for bradycardia or evidence of respiratory difficulty. Monitor GI tract function for diarrhea or cramping.

**ADMINISTRATION IN ALTERNATE SETTINGS**

May be given in a variety of acute care settings by a qualified IV nurse. Respiratory support equipment should be available.

**EVALUATION: OUTCOMES OF DRUG THERAPY**

**EXPECTED OUTCOMES**

PHYSICAL ASSESSMENT. Client is able to carry out the activities of daily living without assistance. Respirations are free and effortless. Client does not complain of diarrhea, abdominal cramping, or muscle twitching.

LABORATORY. Serum electrolytes remain within client's baseline.

**NEGATIVE OUTCOMES**

Client is unable to carry out activities of daily living without fatigue or assistance; complains of excessive salivation, a tightness in the chest, shortness of breath, or difficulty breathing; has diarrhea, abdominal cramping, or muscle twitching; is confused or complains of visual changes.

## PARASYMPATHOLYTICS (ANTICHOLINERGICS)

### THERAPEUTIC EFFECTS

Parasympatholytics inhibit the action of acetylcholine at cholinergic receptor sites (muscarinic) or at the myoneural end plate (neuromuscular blocking agents). Various muscarinic receptor sites are not equally sensitive to paraysympatholytic (anticholinergic) drug stimulation. There may be marked differences in drug effects. Some muscarinic receptors are very sensitive, such as those controlling the salivary glands, whereas receptors affecting gastric secretion and motility are less sensitive. Thus, an anticholinergic drug given to decrease gastric motility is likely to cause a dry mouth. Neuromuscular blocking agents are given to induce skeletal muscle relaxation, usually as an adjunct to general anesthesia during surgery. They may also be given during electroconvulsive therapy (ECT) to prevent tetanic muscle contractions that may cause vertebral collapse or fractures.

### PHARMACOKINETICS

**Distribution.** Parasympatholytics are widely distributed when given intravenously. They usually cross the blood-brain barrier. Some parasympatholytics cross the placental barrier.

**Excretion.** Parasympatholytics are mainly excreted through the urinary tract.

### CAUTIONS

**Side/Adverse Effects.** Muscarinics may cause heat prostration in clients exposed to high temperatures or fever. Muscarinics may cause blurred vision or drowsiness. Clients should be warned not to operate motor vehicles or engage in activities requiring high mental or visual acuity. Muscarinics should be used with caution in clients with hyperthyroidism, hepatic or renal disease, or hypertension. Clients with tachydysrhythmias, congestive heart failure, or coronary artery disease must be monitored carefully. Clients with chronic pulmonary disease may develop airway problems associated with increased bronchial secretions.

Neuromuscular blocking agents may cause apnea, residual muscle weakness, and allergic reactions.

#### Contraindications

*Muscarinics*

- Clients with known intestinal infections should not be given muscarinic drugs because they may prolong the symptomatology.
- Clients with diarrhea must be evaluated carefully before using muscarinic drugs, since diarrhea is a possible early symptom of obstruction.

- Clients with obstructive urinary tract disorders.
- Clients with myasthenia gravis.

*Neuromuscular Blocking Agents*

- Must be used cautiously in clients with respiratory problems. Personnel experienced and able to intubate and oxygenate the client must be on hand with the necessary supplies when neuromuscular blocking agents are used.
- Used with caution in clients with renal, hepatic, or pulmonary dysfunction.
- Clients with myasthenia gravis.
- Used very carefully in clients with electrolyte imbalance, especially hyperkalemia. Neuronmuscular blocking agents may cause the release of intracellular potassium into the intravascular space.

***Pregnancy and Lactation.*** The effects of muscarinics on the fetus have not been determined. Muscarinics may cause reproductive problems stemming from impotence, may inhibit lactation, and are found in breast milk. Neuromuscular blocking agents should be used in reduced doses in women who receive magnesium sulfate during delivery. Neuromuscular blocking agents cross the placental barrier and may cause respiratory depression in the neonate.

***Pediatrics.*** Muscarinics are used with caution in infants. These drugs may cause respiratory distress, seizures, asphyxia, hypotonia, and coma in infants 6 weeks and younger.

***Geriatrics.*** Muscarinics are used with caution in elderly clients. The elderly may be more susceptible to all effects of muscarinic drugs. Neuromuscular blocking agents should be used cautiously.

## TOXICITY

See Table 18–3 for toxicities of parasympatholytics.

## POTENTIAL DRUG/FOOD INTERACTIONS

Parasympatholytics (anticholinergics) that block acetylcholine at muscarinic receptor sites may be potentiated by phenothiazines, amantadine, anti-Parkinson drugs, glutethimide, meperidine, tricyclic antidepressants, some antiarrhythmics, and some antihistamines. Muscarinics may alter the absorption of drugs given orally because of decreased gastric motility.

Neuromuscular blocking agents may be potentiated by general anesthesia and aminoglycosides. Opiates may intensify respiratory depression if used with neuromuscular blocking agents. Potassium-depleting agents may prolong the neuromuscular blockade induced by these drugs.

**TABLE 18–3**

**Toxicities of Parasympatholytics***

| Body System | Side/Toxic Effects | Physical Assessment Indicators | Laboratory Indicators | Nursing Interventions |
|---|---|---|---|---|
| Neurologic | CNS stimulation, vagal stimulation | Decreased heart rate, restlessness, delirium, irritability, hallucinations | | Monitor level of consciousness. Provide a safe environment. Monitor vital signs. |
| Cardiovascular | Dose dependent, vagal stimulation, flushed face | Tachycardia, atrial and ventricular dysrhythmias<br>Dysrhythmias, hypotension* | ECG: shortened PR, QRS interval | Monitor heart rate, ECG. Report any abnormal rhythms. |
| Respiratory | Bronchodilation<br>Bronchospasm* | Decreased respiratory tract secretions<br>Wheezing, dyspnea* | N/A | Monitor breath sounds, respiratory rate. Give oxygen. Place in semi-Fowler's position. |
| Genitourinary | Decreased tone of ureters, bladder | Decreased urge to void, decreased stream, incomplete emptying of bladder; in males loss of erection | N/A | Monitor urinary output. Palpate bladder |
| Gastrointestinal | Reduced gastrointestinal secretions, decreased gastric motility | Dry oral mucous membranes, decreased bowel sounds | N/A | Monitor bowel sounds. |
| Musculoskeletal | Fasiculations* | Fine tremors* | N/A | Evaluate for muscle pain after operation. |
| Sensory | Mydriasis, cycloplegia | Dilated pupils, inability to accommodate to light changes | N/A | Advise caution with night driving. |
| Dermatologic | Decreased sweating | Dry, flushed skin<br>Flushing, erythema, pruritus, urticaria, wheals* | | Monitor body temperature. |

*Continued on following page.*

**TABLE 18–3**
**Toxicities of Parasympatholytics* *Continued***

| Body System | Side/Toxic Effects | Physical Assessment Indicators | Laboratory Indicators | Nursing Interventions |
|---|---|---|---|---|
| Other | Acute toxicity | Dilated, unreactive pupils; blurred vision; hot, flushed skin; dry mucous membranes; dysphagia; absent bowel sounds; urinary retention; tachycardia; hyperthermia; hypertension; increased respiratory rate; depression; nausea; vomiting; rash over face, neck, and upper trunk; acute psychosis | ECG: widening of QRS, prolonged QT, ST segment | Monitor vital signs carefully. Discontinue immediately with symptoms of acute toxicity. |
| | Malignant hyperthermia* | Rapid, profound elevation in body temperature, extreme muscle rigidity* | | Have dantrolene available to administer intravenously.* Start measures to cool client. Give oxygen. |

*Effects of neuromuscular blocking agents.
CNS = central nervous system, ECG = electrocardiogram.

## Atropine Sulfate

*Trade Name:* None specified.
*Canadian Availability:* Atropine
*Pregnancy Risk:* Category C
*pH:* 3.5–6.5
*Storage/Stability:* Store below 40° C. Protect from freezing.

### ASSESSMENT: DRUG CHARACTERISTICS

#### ACTION

An anticholinergic and belladonna alkaloid that inhibits acetylcholine at the parasympathetic junction. Cardiac muscle, smooth muscle, and gland tissue are most affected. Increases heart rate by blocking vagal stimulation to the sinoatrial node and increasing conduction through the atrioventricular node.

#### INDICATIONS

Used as an anticholinergic to reduce activity of the GI tract, reduce bladder and uterine muscle tone, inhibit salivation and bronchial secretions, dilate the pupil, and increase heart rate. May be used as an antidysmenorrheal, antiarrhythmic, antiemetic, antivertigo, or antidiarrheal agent. May also be used as an antidote to cholinesterase inhibitors and organophosphate pesticide toxicity. May be used with nondepolarizing neuromuscular blockers to diminish secretions. May be used as an adjunct with anesthesia.

#### CAUTIONS

ADVERSE EFFECTS. May cause blurred vision, confusion, dizziness, drowsiness, hallucinations, seizures, slurred speech, restlessness, irritability, dry mouth, dyspnea, tachycardia, fever, muscle weakness, fatigue, flushed skin, constipation, decreased sweating, or redness or irritation at the injection site.

CONTRAINDICATIONS. Cardiac arrhythmias such as tachycardia, reflux esophagitis, GI or urinary tract obstruction, glaucoma, hemorrhage, paralytic ileus, myasthenia gravis, prostatic hypertrophy, or ulcerative colitis.

#### POTENTIAL DRUG/FOOD INTERACTIONS

May interact with antacids to cause delay of excretion. May potentiate the effects of other anticholinergics. May cause ventricular arrhythmias if used with cyclopropane. May cause increased gastric pH if used with ketoconazole. May increase the incidence of lesions if used with potassium chloride.

### INTERVENTIONS: ADMINISTRATION

May be given undiluted. May be diluted with up to 10 mL of sterile water for injection.

#### MODE/RATE OF ADMINISTRATION

Usualy given by rapid IV injection through a freely flowing IV solution.

▼

INTRAVENOUS USE (WITH NORMAL RENAL FUNCTION)

**Adults:** As an anticholinergic, the usual dosage is 400–600 mcg (0.4–0.6 mg) q4–6h. As an antiarrhythmic, the usual dosage is 400 mcg (0.4 mg)–1 mg q1–2h. Maximum dose is 2 mg. As a cholinergic adjunct, the usual dose is 600 mcg (0.6 mg)–1.2 mg a few minutes before giving neostigmine or pyridostigmine. As an antidote to cholinesterase inhibitors, the usual dose is 2–4 mg initially. May be repeated q5–10min until symptoms disappear.

**Children:** As an antiarrhythmic, the usual dose is 10–30 mcg (0.01–0.03 mg)/kg of body weight. As an antidote to cholinesterase inhibitors, the usual dose is 1 mg. Further doses of 0.5–1 mg may be given q5–10 min until symptoms disappear. Fatal dose may be as little as 10 mg.

**Infants/Neonates:** Dosage not established.

**Geriatrics:** Elderly clients are more likely to have dry mouth, constipation, urinary retention, hallucinations, confusion, drowsiness, or memory deficits. Dose may need to be lowered.

INTRATHECAL USE OR OTHER INFUSION ROUTES AS INDICATED. Not recommended.

**POTENTIAL PROBLEMS IN ADMINISTRATION**

In adults, lower doses of atropine (0.5–1 mg) are more likely to cause CNS excitement. Small children are particularly sensitive to the toxic effects of atropine. Children may also show a paradoxical excitement to large doses of atropine.

**INDEPENDENT NURSING ACTIONS**

Monitor for CNS effects. Monitor heart and respiratory rate and rhythm. Monitor temperature. Monitor urinary and bowel elimination. Initiate safety precautions for visual disturbances, muscle weakness, and fatigue. Advise client not to operate hazardous equipment.

**ADMINISTRATION IN ALTERNATE SETTINGS**

Not recommended.

**EVALUATION: OUTCOMES OF DRUG THERAPY**

**EXPECTED OUTCOMES**

PHYSICAL ASSESSMENT. Heart rate between 60 and 100 beats per minute (bpm) and regular. Respiratory rate between 16 and 20/min and regular. Client breathes freely. Temperature within client's baseline. Urine and bowel elimination within client's baseline. Client denies visual changes, weakness, or fatigue.

LABORATORY. May alter test results for gastric acidity and phenolsulfonphthalein (PSP). Client should not have atropine within 24 hours of these tests.

**NEGATIVE OUTCOMES**

Heart rate greater than 100 bpm or irregular. Client complains of difficulty breathing, constipation, visual changes, weakness, or fatigue. Skin flushed, warm, and dry. Client unable to void.

## ATRACURIUM BESYLATE

*Trade Name:* Tracrium
*Canadian Availability:* Tracrium
*Pregnancy Risk:* Category C
*pH:* 3.25–3.65
*Storage/Stability:* Store between 2° and 8° C. Protect from freezing. IV solutions may be stored at room temperature or refrigerated for 24 hours. Unused portions should be discarded.

### ASSESSMENT: DRUG CHARACTERISTICS

#### ACTION

A nondepolarizing neuromuscular blocking agent that produces skeletal muscle paralysis by blocking neural transmission at the myoneural junction. Competes with acetylcholine for the cholinergic receptor at the motor end plate, thus decreasing response to acetylcholine.

#### INDICATIONS

Used to induce skeletal muscle relaxation in clients who are receiving mechanical ventilation or having convulsions. Nondepolarizing agents are less likely to be used during surgery to induce skeletal muscle relaxation.

#### CAUTIONS

ADVERSE EFFECTS. May cause flushing of skin, hypotension or hypertension, tachycardia, respiratory compromise, or histamine reactions.

CONTRAINDICATIONS. History of allergic reaction to atracurium, problems with histamine release, bronchogenic carcinomas, dehydration, electrolyte imbalances, hypotension, hypothermia, myasthenia gravis, or respiratory depression.

#### POTENTIAL DRUG/FOOD INTERACTIONS

May interact with aminoglycosides, parenteral or local anesthetics, capreomycin, citrate-anticoagulated blood, clindamycin, lincomycin, polymixins, procaine, or trimethaphan to enhance the neuromuscular blocking activities of each drug. May interact with analgesics, especially opioids, to increase respiratory depression. May precipitate malignant hypertension and increased neuromuscular blocking if used with hydrocarbon inhalation anesthetic agents. Antimyasthenics antagonize the effects of atracurium. Calcium salts usually reverse the effects of atracurium. Lithium may prolong the activity of altracurium. Procainamide or quinidine may potentiate the neuromuscular blocking activity of atracurium. Atracurium may interact with polarizing neuromuscular blockers and other nondepolarizing blockers to increase the effects of each drug. Potassium-depleting drugs may potentiate the effects of atracurium.

### INTERVENTIONS: ADMINISTRATION

Dilute with 0.9% normal saline solution (NSS), 5%

▼

dextrose in water (D5W), or 5% D5W in 0.9% NSS for injection. Ringer's lactate should not be used for the dilution because atracurium degrades more quickly. Solution strength should be 200 mcg (0.02 mg) or 500 mcg (0.05 mg)/mL.

**MODE/RATE OF ADMINISTRATION**

May be given by rapid IV injection over 30–60 s or by continuous infusion.

INTRAVENOUS USE (WITH NORMAL RENAL FUNCTION)

**Adults:** Usual initial dose is 400–500 mcg (0.4–0.5 mg)/kg of body weight. Dose may be lowered to 300–400 mcg (0.3–0.4 mg)/kg of body weight for clients who may have a problem with histamine release. Further doses of 80–100 mcg (0.08–0.1 mg)/kg of body weight may be given 20 to 45 min after the first dose. Depending on client's condition, doses may be given as often as q15–25min thereafter.

**Children 1 month to 2 years:** For those receiving anesthesia the usual initial dose is 300–400 mcg (0.3–0.4 mg)/kg of body weight. Succeeding doses may be required in shorter times required for adults.

**Children > 2 years:** Follow adult dosing schedule.

**Infants/Neonates:** Dose not established for neonates.

**Geriatrics:** Clients with diminished renal function may require a lower dose.

INTRATHECAL USE OR OTHER INFUSION ROUTES AS INDICATED. Not recommended.

**POTENTIAL PROBLEMS IN ADMINISTRATION**

Hypothermia increases the neuromuscular blockage. Hypokalemia or hypernatremia prolong the action of the drug. Incompatible with alkaline solutions.

**INDEPENDENT NURSING ACTIONS**

Monitor respiratory function. Suction as needed. Must have a manual resuscitator available at bedside. Auscultate breath sounds. Monitor vital signs and electrocardiogram (ECG). Monitor hemodynamic status. Monitor level of muscle relaxation using a peripheral nerve stimulator. Provide emotional support. Evaluate for pain on a regular basis as client condition indicates and medicate when indicated.

**ADMINISTRATION IN ALTERNATE SETTINGS**

IV administration should be done in settings where the client can be closely monitored and where full cardiac technologic support is available.

**EVALUATION: OUTCOMES OF DRUG THERAPY**

**EXPECTED OUTCOMES**

PHYSICAL ASSESSMENT. Breath sounds clear. Bilateral equal expansion of lungs. Pulse between 60 and 100 bpm and regular. Skin intact, warm, and pink. Blood pressure within client's normal range. Body weight remains stable. Joints freely mobile with passive range of motion.

LABORATORY. White blood count (WBC) between 5000 and 10,000/mm3. Hemoglobin (Hgb) and hematocrit (Hct) remain within normal range for client's age and gender. Serum potassium between 3.5 and 5.5 mEq/L. Serum sodium between 135 and 145 mEq/L.

#### NEGATIVE OUTCOMES

Breath sounds have coarse crackles or wheezes. Unequal expansion of lungs. Pulse above 100 bpm or irregular. Elevated temperature. Inadequate muscle relaxation and "fighting" the ventilator. Cyanosis. Hypotension. Weight loss greater than 1 kg (2 lb). Skin breakdown. Joint stiffness with passive range of motion.

## METHOCARBAMOL

*Trade Names:* Carbacot, Robaxin
*Canadian Availability:* Robaxin
*Pregnancy Risk:* Category C
*pH:* 4.0–5.0
*Storage/Stability:* Store below 40° C. Protect from freezing.

### ASSESSMENT: DRUG CHARACTERISTICS

#### ACTION

Skeletal muscle relaxant whose action is not completely understood. Acts on the CNS rather than on skeletal muscle directly. Appears to block activity in the descending reticular formation and the spinal cord.

#### INDICATIONS

Used as an adjunct therapy to treat skeletal muscle spasm.

#### CAUTIONS

ADVERSE EFFECTS. May induce bradycardia, conjunctivitis or nasal stuffiness, dermatitis, fever, blurred or double vision, nystagmus, dizziness, drowsiness, headache, muscle weakness, flushing or redness of face, nausea or vomiting, or pain at the injection site.

CONTRAINDICATIONS. History of allergic reaction to methocarbamol, renal impairment or disease, CNS depression, epilepsy, or impaired hepatic functioning.

#### POTENTIAL DRUG/FOOD INTERACTIONS

May interact with other CNS-depressing agents to increase the CNS depression.

### INTERVENTIONS: ADMINISTRATION

May be given undiluted by rapid IV injection or diluted in D5W or 0.9% NSS.

#### MODE/RATE OF ADMINISTRATION

Usually given by rapid IV injection at a rate not to exceed 300 mg/min. May be given as a continuous IV infusion.

INTRAVENOUS USE (WITH NORMAL RENAL FUNCTION)

**Adults:** Usual dosage is 1–3 g/d for 3 d. After 48 h, another 3-d course may be given if necessary. Maximum

▼

daily dose should not exceed 3 g for more than 3 d.

**Children:** Dosage not established.

**Infants/Neonates:** Dosage not established.

**Geriatrics:** Clients with diminished renal function may require a lower dose.

INTRATHECAL USE OR OTHER INFUSION ROUTES AS INDICATED. Not recommended.

#### POTENTIAL PROBLEMS IN ADMINISTRATION

May cause orthostatic hypotension. Give while the client is in a supine position and wait at least 15 min before assisting client into slowly rising.

#### INDEPENDENT NURSING ACTIONS

Monitor blood count, liver, and renal function tests. Monitor vital signs for hypotension or tachycardia. Monitor for CNS depression or seizures. Institute safety measures to prevent injuries from dizziness, syncope, or visual changes. Provide ice chips, sugarless hard candy, or sugarless gum, unless otherwise contraindicated, to relieve discomfort from dry mouth. Monitor urinary and bowel elimination.

#### ADMINISTRATION IN ALTERNATE SETTINGS

Appropriate for administration in most clinical settings and home care by a qualified IV nurse.

### EVALUATION: OUTCOMES OF DRUG THERAPY

#### EXPECTED OUTCOMES

PHYSICAL ASSESSMENT. Client does not complain of muscle spasm or pain from muscle spasm. Blood pressure and pulse remain at baseline. Urine and bowel elimination follow client's normal pattern.

LABORATORY. Blood count, liver, and renal function tests remain at client's baseline.

#### NEGATIVE OUTCOMES

Client continues to complain of pain from muscle spasm; is unable to urinate or unable to eliminate feces; complains of eye pain, blurred or double vision, or dry mouth. Blood pressure falls more than 20 mm Hg below baseline. Heart rate greater than 100 bpm.

## ORPHENADRINE CITRATE

*Trade Names:* Marflex, Noradex, Norflex, Orflagen
*Canadian Availability:* Norflex
*Pregnancy Risk:* Category C
*pH:* 5.0–6.0
*Storage/Stability:* Store below 40° C. Protect from light and from freezing.

### ASSESSMENT: DRUG CHARACTERISTICS

#### ACTION

Skeletal muscle relaxant whose action is not completely understood. Acts on the CNS rather than on skeletal muscle directly. Appears to block activity in the descending reticular formation and the spinal cord. Seems to have some analgesic properties and a mild anticholinergic action.

**INDICATIONS**

Used as an adjunct therapy to treat skeletal muscle spasm and some forms of Parkinson's disease.

**CAUTIONS**

ADVERSE EFFECTS. May cause difficulty with urination, increased intraocular pressure, tachycardia, orthostatic hypotension, dry mouth, constipation, blurred or double vision, weakness, confusion, dizziness, drowsiness, headache, tremors, irritability, excitement, and nausea or vomiting.

CONTRAINDICATIONS. Bladder neck obstructions, glaucoma, myasthenia gravis, peptic ulcer, prostatic hypertrophy, intestinal obstruction, cardiac arrhythmias such as tachycardia, CNS depression, or impaired hepatic or renal functioning.

**POTENTIAL DRUG/FOOD INTERACTIONS**

May interact with other CNS-depressing agents to increase the CNS depression. May interact with anticholinergics to potentiate their effects.

**INTERVENTIONS: ADMINISTRATION**

May be given undiluted.

**MODE/RATE OF ADMINISTRATION**

Usually given by rapid IV injection over 5 min.

INTRAVENOUS USE (WITH NORMAL RENAL FUNCTION)

**Adults:** Usual dosage is 60 mg q12h.

**Children:** Dosage not established.

**Infants/Neonates:** Dosage not established.

**Geriatrics:** May cause hallucinations and confusion. Clients must be evaluated for prostatic hypertrophy. Clients with diminished renal function may require a lower dose.

INTRATHECAL USE OR OTHER INFUSION ROUTES AS INDICATED. Not recommended.

**POTENTIAL PROBLEMS IN ADMINISTRATION**

May cause orthostatic hypotension. Give while the client is in a supine position and wait at least 5–10 min before assisting client into slowly rising.

**INDEPENDENT NURSING ACTIONS**

Monitor blood count, liver, and renal function tests. Monitor vital signs for hypotension or tachycardia. Institute safety measures to prevent injuries from dizziness, syncope, or visual changes. Provide ice chips, sugarless hard candy, or sugarless gum, unless otherwise contraindicated, to relieve discomfort from dry mouth. Monitor urinary and bowel elimination.

**ADMINISTRATION IN ALTERNATE SETTINGS**

Appropriate for administration in most clinical settings and home care by a qualified IV nurse.

▼

**EVALUATION: OUTCOMES OF DRUG THERAPY**

**EXPECTED OUTCOMES**

PHYSICAL ASSESSMENT. Client does not complain of muscle spasm or pain from muscle spasm. Blood pressure and pulse remain at baseline. Urine and bowel elimination follow client's normal pattern.

LABORATORY. Blood count, liver, and renal function tests remain at client's baseline.

**NEGATIVE OUTCOMES**

Client continues to complain of pain from muscle spasm; is unable to urinate or unable to eliminate feces; complains of eye pain, blurred or double vision, or dry mouth. Blood pressure falls more than 20 mm Hg below baseline. Heart rate greater than 100 bpm.

## Pancuronium Bromide

*Trade Name:* Pavulon
*Canadian Availability:* Pavulon
*Pregnancy Risk:* Category C
*pH:* 4.0–5.0
*Storage/Stability:* Store between 2° and 8° C. Protect from freezing. IV solutions may be stored at room temperature or refrigerated for 24 hours. Unused portions should be discarded.

**ASSESSMENT: DRUG CHARACTERISTICS**

**ACTION**

A nondepolarizing neuromuscular blocking agent that produces skeletal muscle paralysis by blocking neural transmission at the myoneural junction. Competes with acetylcholine for the cholinergic receptor at the motor end plate, thus decreasing response to acetylcholine.

**INDICATIONS**

Used to induce skeletal muscle relaxation in clients who are receiving mechanical ventilation or having convulsions. Nondepolarizing agents are less likely to be used during surgery to induce skeletal muscle relaxation.

**CAUTIONS**

ADVERSE EFFECTS. May cause hypertension, tachycardia, pruritus or skin rash, or excessive salivation.

CONTRAINDICATIONS. History of allergic reaction to pancuronium, bronchogenic carcinomas, problems with histamine release, inability to tolerate tachycardia, dehydration, electrolyte imbalances, impaired hepatic or renal functioning, hypertension, hyperthermia, hypothermia, myasthenia gravis, or respiratory depression.

**POTENTIAL DRUG/FOOD INTERACTIONS**

May interact with aminoglycosides, parenteral or local anesthetics, capreomycin, citrate-anticoagulated blood, clindamycin, lincomycin, polymixins, procaine, or trimethaphan to enhance the neuromuscular blocking activities of each drug. May interact with analgesics, especially opioids, to increase respiratory depression and decrease bradycardia or hypotension. May precipitate malignant hypertension and increased neuromuscular blocking if used with hydrocarbon inhalation anesthetic agents. Antimyasthenics antagonize the effects of pancuronium. Calcium salts usually reverse the effects of pancuronium. Lithium may prolong the activity of pancuronium. $\beta$-Adrenergic blocking agents, procainamide, or quinidine may potentiate the neuromuscular blocking activity of pancuronium. Pancuronium may interact with polarizing neuromuscular blockers and other nondepolarizing blockers to increase the effects of each drug. Potassium-depleting drugs may potentiate the effects of pancuronium. Digitalis glycosides may have greater effect if used with pancuronium, but this is associated with a greater incidence of cardiac arrhythmias.

**INTERVENTIONS: ADMINISTRATION**

Dilute with bacteriostatic water for injection, 0.9% NSS, D5W, or D5W in 0.9% NSS for injection, or Ringer's lactate solution. Solution strength for rapid IV injection should be 10 mg/5–10 mL, using bacteriostatic sterile water for injection. Solution strength for infusion should be 10–20 mg/dL of solution.

**MODE/RATE OF ADMINISTRATION**

Usually given by rapid IV injection over 30–60 s.

INTRAVENOUS USE (WITH NORMAL RENAL FUNCTION)

**Adults:** Usual initial dose is 40–100 mcg (0.04–0.1 mg)/kg of body weight. Additional dosage is 10 mcg (0.01 mg)/kg of body weight q30–60 min.

**Children ≤10 years:** Dose is individualized. Initial dose may be slightly higher than adult schedule and may need to be given more frequently.

**Children >10 years:** Follow adult dosing schedule.

**Infants 7 weeks to 1 year:** Dose is individualized. Initial dose may be slightly higher than adult schedule and may need to be given more frequently.

**Neonates:** Dose not established for neonates.

**Geriatrics:** Clients with diminished renal function may require a lower dose.

INTRATHECAL USE OR OTHER INFUSION ROUTES AS INDICATED. Not recommended.

**POTENTIAL PROBLEMS IN ADMINISTRATION**

Hypothermia increases the neuromuscular blockage. Hypokalemia or hypernatremia prolong the action of the drug.

**INDEPENDENT NURSING ACTIONS**

Monitor respiratory function. Suction as needed. ▼

Must have a manual resuscitator available at bedside. Auscultate breath sounds. Monitor vital signs and ECG. Monitor hemodynamic status. Monitor level of muscle relaxation using a peripheral nerve stimulator. Provide emotional support. Medicate for pain on a regular basis as client condition indicates.

**ADMINISTRATION IN ALTERNATE SETTINGS**

IV administration should be done in settings where the client can be closely monitored and where full cardiac technologic support is available.

**EVALUATION: OUTCOMES OF DRUG THERAPY**

**EXPECTED OUTCOMES**

PHYSICAL ASSESSMENT. Breath sounds clear. Bilateral equal expansion of lungs. Pulse between 60 and 100 bpm and regular. Skin intact, warm, and pink. Blood pressure within client's normal range. Eyes lubricated. Body weight remains stable. Joints freely mobile with passive range of motion.

LABORATORY. WBC between 5000 and 10,000/mm$^3$. Hgb and Hct remain within normal range for client's age and gender. Serum potassium between 3.5 and 5.5 mEq/L. Serum sodium between 135 and 145 mEq/L.

**NEGATIVE OUTCOMES**

Breath sounds have coarse crackles or wheezes. Unequal expansion of lungs. Pulse above 100 bpm or irregular. Elevated temperature. Inadequate muscle relaxation and "fighting" the ventilator. Cyanosis. Hypotension. Corneal abrasions. Weight loss greater than 1 kg/2 lb. Skin breakdown. Joint stiffness with passive range of motion.

## VECURONIUM BROMIDE

*Trade Name:* Norcuron
*Canadian Availability:* Norcuron
*Pregnancy Risk:* Category C
*pH:* 4
*Storage/Stability:* Store between 15° and 30° C. Protect from light. If reconstituted with sterile bacteriostatic water for injection, may be refrigerated or stored at room temperature for 5 days. If reconstituted with any other IV solution, unused portions should be discarded after 24 hours.

**ASSESSMENT: DRUG CHARACTERISTICS**

**ACTION**

A nondepolarizing neuromuscular blocking agent that produces skeletal muscle paralysis by blocking neural transmission at the myoneural junction. Competes with acetylcholine for the cholinergic receptor at the motor end plate, thus decreasing response to acetylcholine.

**INDICATIONS**

Used to induce skeletal muscle relaxation in clients who are receiving mechanical ventilation or having convulsions. Nondepolarizing agents are less likely to be used during surgery to induce skeletal muscle relaxation.

**CAUTIONS**

ADVERSE EFFECTS. May cause some minimal cardiovascular effects. Few adverse reactions.

CONTRAINDICATIONS. History of allergic reaction to vecuronium, bronchogenic carcinomas, problems with histamine release, dehydration, impaired cardiac or hepatic functioning, myasthenia gravis, or respiratory depression.

**POTENTIAL DRUG/FOOD INTERACTIONS**

May interact with aminoglycosides, parenteral or local anesthetics, capreomycin, citrate-anticoagulated blood, clindamycin, lincomycin, polymixins, procaine, or trimethaphan to enhance the neuromuscular blocking activities of each drug. May interact with analgesics, especially opioids, to increase respiratory depression and decrease bradycardia or hypotension. May precipitate malignant hypertension and increased neuromuscular blocking if used with hydrocarbon inhalation anesthetic agents. Antimyasthenics antagonize the effects of vecuronium. Calcium salts usually reverse the effects of vecuronium. Procainamide or quinidine may potentiate the neuromuscular blocking activity of vecuronium. Vecuronium may interact with polarizing neuromuscular blockers and other nondepolarizing blockers to increase the effects of each drug. Potassium-depleting drugs may potentiate the effects of vecuronium.

**INTERVENTIONS: ADMINISTRATION**

Dilute with bacteriostatic water for injection, 0.9% NSS, D5W, or D5W in 0.9% NSS for injection or Ringer's lactate solution. Solution strength for rapid IV injection should be 10 mg/5–10 mL, using bacteriostatic sterile water for injection.

**MODE/RATE OF ADMINISTRATION**

Usually given by rapid IV injection over 30–60 s.

INTRAVENOUS USE (WITH NORMAL RENAL FUNCTION)

**Adults:** Usual initial dose is 80–100 mcg (0.08–0.1 mg)/kg of body weight. Additional dosage is 10–15 mcg (0.01–0.015 mg)/kg of body weight q25–40 min.

**Children ≤ 10 years:** Dose is individualized. Initial dose may be slightly higher than adult schedule and may need to be given more frequently.

**Children > 10 years:** Follow adult dosing schedule.

**Infants 7 weeks to 1 year:** Dose is individualized. Initial dose may be slightly higher than adult schedule and may need to be given more frequently.

▼

**Neonates:** Dose not established.

**Geriatrics:** Clients with diminished renal function may require a lower dose.

INTRATHECAL USE OR OTHER INFUSION ROUTES AS INDICATED. Not recommended.

#### POTENTIAL PROBLEMS IN ADMINISTRATION

Hypothermia increases the neuromuscular blockage. Hypokalemia or hypernatremia prolong the action of the drug.

#### INDEPENDENT NURSING ACTIONS

Monitor respiratory function. Suction as needed. Must have a manual resuscitator available at bedside. Auscultate breath sounds. Monitor vital signs and ECG. Monitor hemodynamic status. Monitor level of muscle relaxation using a peripheral nerve stimulator. Provide emotional support. Medicate for pain on a regular basis as client condition indicates.

#### ADMINISTRATION IN ALTERNATE SETTINGS

IV administration should be done in settings where the client can be closely monitored and where full cardiac technologic support is available.

### EVALUATION: OUTCOMES OF DRUG THERAPY

#### EXPECTED OUTCOMES

PHYSICAL ASSESSMENT. Breath sounds clear. Bilateral equal expansion of lungs. Pulse between 60 and 100 bpm and regular. Skin intact, warm, and pink. Blood pressure within client's normal range. Eyes lubricated. Body weight remains stable. Joints freely mobile with passive range of motion.

LABORATORY. WBC between 5000 and 10,000/mm3. Hgb and Hct remain within normal range for client's age and gender. Serum potassium between 3.5 and 5.5 mEq/L. Serum sodium is between 135 and 145 mEq/L.

#### NEGATIVE OUTCOMES

Breath sounds have coarse crackles or wheezes. Unequal expansion of lungs. Pulse above 100 bpm or irregular. Elevated temperature. Inadequate muscle relaxation and "fighting" the ventilator. Cyanosis. Hypotension. Corneal abrasions. Weight loss greater than 1 kg (2 lb). Skin breakdown. Joint stiffness with passive range of motion.

## SYMPATHOMIMETICS (ADRENERGICS)

### THERAPEUTIC EFFECTS

$\alpha_1$-Receptor stimulators cause the same effects as norepinephrine: contraction of the radial muscles of the iris, vasoconstriction of arterioles and veins, contraction of smooth muscle sphincters in the GI and urinary tract systems, contraction of the uterus and stimulation of ejaculation, decreased pancreatic secretions, and elevation of blood sugar by increased breakdown of glycogen and increased synthesis of glucose. The role of $\alpha_2$-receptor stimulators remains less clear, but they appear to function as a negative feedback mechanism to decrease the amount of norepinephrine released from the neuron. Their therapeutic benefits are still being determined. $\beta_1$-Receptor stimulators cause increased heart rate, increased cardiac muscle contraction, and increased breakdown of stored fat for energy. $\beta_2$-Receptor stimulators appear to cause bronchodilation, relaxation of the uterus, dilation of vessels in skeletal muscle, and increases in blood sugar.

## PHARMACOKINETICS

**Distribution.** Sympathomimetic agents are widely distributed when given intravenously. Onset is rapid (2 to 5 minutes), peak effect usually occurs within 5 to 10 minutes, and the effect time lasts only minutes after an IV dose has been discontinued. These agents may cross the placental barrier but usually do not cross the blood-brain barrier.

**Metabolism/Elimination.** The plasma half-life is about 2 minutes. These agents are metabolized primarily by the liver but also by the kidneys and other tissues. They are excreted in urine.

## CAUTIONS

**Side/Adverse Effects.** Sympathomimetic agents may cause ectopic heart beats, increased heart rate, angina, increased blood pressure, anxiety, tremors, restlessness, and nausea.

**Contraindications.** Sympathomimetic agents should not be used with clients who have had a myocardial infarction or a previous hypersensitivity reaction to the agent. In addition, clients who have pheochromocytoma, ventricular dysrhythmias, glaucoma, hyperthyroidism, or cardiac glycoside intoxication should not receive an adrenergic agent. Some of the contraindications are more strongly associated with the $\alpha$-receptor stimulators, and some with the $\beta$-receptor stimulators.

***Pregnancy and Lactation.*** The drugs' effects on the fetus have not been established. Adrenergic agents may cross the placental barrier. Some agents inhibit uterine contractions and delay the second stage of labor.

***Pediatrics.*** The drugs' usefulness with children has not been determined. Adrenergic agents are contraindicated if a child is hypersensitive to sympathomimetic drugs. They may cause hypoglycemia or hyperglycemia in neonates.

***Geriatrics.*** The elderly may be more susceptible to adrenergic drug effects.

## TOXICITY

See Table 18–4 for toxicities of sympathomimetic agents.

**TABLE 18–4**
**Toxicities of Sympathomimetic Agents**

| Body System | Side/Toxic Effects | Physical Assessment Indicators | Laboratory Indicators | Nursing Interventions |
|---|---|---|---|---|
| Neurologic | | Apprehension, anxiety, restlessness, tremors, weakness, syncope, dizziness, headache | N/A | Monitor level of consciousness. Provide a safe environment. |
| Cardiovascular | Vasoconstriction | Ectopic heart beats, tachycardia, hypertension, dysrhythmias, increased blood pressure | ECG, cardiac output, pulmonary wedge pressure | Monitor central venous pressure. Monitor respiratory status and oxygenation. |
| Respiratory | Bronchodilation | Increased respiratory rate; shortness of breath and dyspnea ameliorated | Arterial blood gases: acidosis | Provide oxygen as necessary. Support ventilation with semi-Fowler's position. |
| Genitourinary | Decreased renal blood flow, decreased uterine contractions | Decreased urine output, delayed second-stage labor | Decreased serum potassium, sodium, and chlorides | Monitor urine output frequently. Monitor serum electrolytes. |
| Gastrointestinal | Relaxation of gastrointestinal smooth muscle | Abdominal distention, diminished bowel sounds, intestinal necrosis | N/A | Monitor bowel sounds. Report complaints of abdominal pain. |
| Dermatologic | Peripheral vasoconstriction | Pallor, cold extremities, tissue necrosis, mottling, hemostasis | N/A | Monitor peripheral circulation. |
| Other | Hyperglycemia | Glycosuria; dry, flushed skin | Elevated blood glucose | |

ECG = electrocardiogram.

## POTENTIAL DRUG/FOOD INTERACTIONS

Sympathomimetic (adrenergic) drugs may react with monamine oxidase (MAO) inhibitors, prolonging and intensifying the action of the adrenergic drug. $\beta$-Receptor blocking agents are antagonistic to adrenergic agents. Cardiac dysrhythmias may develop if these agents are used with general anesthesia. Adrenergic agents may react with phenytoin to cause hypotension and bradycardia. Atropine may block the cardiac effects of adrenergic agents. Most adrenergic agents should be used cautiously, if at all, with other drugs in the same class.

## DOBUTAMINE HYDROCHLORIDE

*Trade Name:* Dobutrex
*Canadian Availability:* Dobutrex
*Pregnancy Risk:* Category C
*pH:* 2.5–5.5
*Storage/Stability:* Store between 15° and 30° C if undiluted. Solution may be used if discolored faintly pink. May store diluted solutions for 48 hours if refrigerated. Discard unused diluted solutions after 24 hours.

### ASSESSMENT: DRUG CHARACTERISTICS

#### ACTION

A sympathomimetic agent. Acts primarily on $\beta_1$-receptors to increase cardiac contractility and stroke volume. Systemic vascular resistance (afterload) is usually lowered. Blood pressure may remain unaffected, since cardiac output is increased. Facilitates atrioventricular conduction and lowers ventricular filling pressure (preload). Has little effect on $\beta_2$-receptors. Usually does not increase heart rate, but does increase renal blood flow and urine output.

#### INDICATIONS

Used as a short-term therapy for cardiogenic shock.

#### CAUTIONS

ADVERSE EFFECTS. May cause a marked increase (50 mm Hg or more) in systolic pressure, an increase (30 bpm or greater) in heart rate, premature ventricular contractions, chest pain, shortness of breath, headache, elevated blood sugar in diabetic clients, or nausea.

CONTRAINDICATIONS. Idiopathic hypertrophic subaortic stenosis, hypovolemia if fluid replacement is not conducted either before or concurrently, or myocardial infarction.

#### POTENTIAL DRUG/FOOD INTERACTIONS

May antagonize $\beta$-adrenergic blocking agents. If nitroprusside is used with dobutamine, cardiac output may increase and pulmonary artery wedge pressure (PAWP) may decrease. Rauwolfia derivatives may prolong the action of dobut-

▼

amine. If used with guanethidine, may cause hypertension and cardiac arrhythmias.

#### INTERVENTIONS: ADMINISTRATION

Each 250-mg ampule must be diluted in at least 10 mL of sterile water. Must be further diluted in at least 50 mL of solution. May be diluted by adding to D5W, 0.9% NSS, D5W and 0.45% NSS, D5W and 0.9% NSS, Ringer's lactate, D5W and Ringer's lactate, D10W, or sodium lactate injection. Standard concentrations are 250, 500, or 1000 mcg (0.25, 0.5, 1 mg)/mL by adding 250 mg to 1 L, 250 mg to 500 mL, or 250 mL to 250 mL of solution, respectively. Concentration should not exceed 5 mg/mL. The formulas for determining dose and rate follow:

1. Baseline concentration ÷ Weight (kg) ÷ Drop factor (60) = Client's mcg/kg/gtts
2. mcg/kg/gtt × Infusion rate (gtts/min) = mcg/kg/min

#### MODE/RATE OF ADMINISTRATION

Given by continuous infusion, using an infusion pump.

INTRAVENOUS USE (WITH NORMAL RENAL FUNCTION)

**Adults:** Usual dose is 2.5–10 mcg (0.005–0.010 mg)/kg of body weight. Dose is gradually increased until the desired blood pressure is achieved.

**Children:** Dose not established.

**Infants/Neonates:** Dose not established.

**Geriatrics:** Follow adult dosing schedule.

INTRATHECAL USE OR OTHER INFUSION ROUTES AS INDICATED. Not recommended.

#### POTENTIAL PROBLEMS IN ADMINISTRATION

May cause a marked increase in systolic blood pressure. Infusion should be slowed or, rarely, stopped until systolic pressure decreases to established limits. Dobutamine is rapidly metabolized. Therapeutic effects are quickly reversed if infusion is stopped abruptly.

#### INDEPENDENT NURSING ACTIONS

Monitor heart rate and ECG for the presence of cardiac arrhythmias, especially premature ventricular contractions, blood pressure, urine flow, and if possible central venous pressure (CVP) or PAWP. Weigh client daily. Monitor intake.

#### ADMINISTRATION IN ALTERNATE SETTINGS

Should be administered in critical care settings for urgent treatment to stabilize cardiogenic shock. The client should be closely monitored, and full cardiac technologic support should be available. After the client is stabilized, dobutamine may be given in the home setting by a qualified IV nurse when constant monitoring of the client can be done.

**EVALUATION: OUTCOMES OF DRUG THERAPY**

**EXPECTED OUTCOMES**

PHYSICAL ASSESSMENT. Heart rate is less than 15% greater than baseline and regular. Blood pressure is sufficient for urine flow to be greater than 30 mL/h and less than 20% greater than baseline. CVP is 4 to 10 mm Hg or mean PAWP is 4.5 to 13 mm Hg.

LABORATORY. Monitor serum glucose, sodium, and potassium levels.

**NEGATIVE OUTCOMES**

Heart rate is more than 15% greater than baseline or irregular from premature ventricular contractions. Blood pressure is greater than 50 mm Hg or 20% above client's baseline. Client complains of chest pain. CVP is greater than 10 mm Hg, or mean PAWP is greater than 13 mm Hg. Client complains of shortness of breath. Crackles heard on auscultation of breath sounds. Urine output not greater than 30 mL/h, and client has marked edema in lower extremities.

---

## DOPAMINE HYDROCHLORIDE

*Trade Name:* Intropin
*Canadian Availability:* Intropin, Revimine
*Pregnancy Risk:* Category C
*pH:* 3.0–4.5
*Storage/Stability:* Store below 40° C. Protect from freezing. Discard if solution is darker than light yellow or discolored. Should be diluted immediately prior to using. Discard unused portion after 24 hours.

**ASSESSMENT: DRUG CHARACTERISTICS**

**ACTION**

Acts directly on the sympathetic nerve terminals and causes the release of norepinephrine, which stimulates $\alpha$-, $\beta$-, and dopaminergic responses. Effects of dopamine are dose dependent. In low doses, there is renal and mesenteric vasodilation with subsequent increase in urine output and sodium excretion. In moderate doses, dopamine has a positive inotropic effect from direct stimulation of $\beta_1$-receptor sites and subsequent increased cardiac contractility, increased cardiac output, and increased myocardial oxygenation. In high doses, dopamine stimulates the $\alpha$-adrenergic receptors, causing increased peripheral vascular constriction and renal vasoconstriction.

**INDICATIONS**

Used to treat hypotension, cardiogenic shock, decreased cardiac output, and congestive heart failure.

**CAUTIONS**

ADVERSE EFFECTS. May cause headache, chest pain, difficulty in breathing, hypotension or hypertension, palpitations, tachycardia or bradycardia, ventricular arrhythmias, severe peripheral vasoconstriction (which may lead to tissue necrosis), nausea, vomiting, or restlessness.

CONTRAINDICATIONS. Should not be given to clients with a pheochromocytoma, or who have ventricular arrhythmias or tachyarrhythmias. Should be given with caution to clients with occlusive peripheral vascular diseases such as Buerger's disease, who are hypoxic, hypercapnic, or acidotic. Should not be given to treat shock unless hypovolemia is treated prior to or concurrently with dopamine administration.

**POTENTIAL DRUG/FOOD INTERACTIONS**

May interact with antidepressants or maprotiline to cause arrhythmias, severe hypertension, or pyrexia. May antagonize the effects of $\beta$-adrenergic blocking agents if used concurrently. May potentiate the cardiovascular effects of cocaine. If used with digoxin, may increase the incidence of cardiac arrhythmias. If used with ergotamine, may increase the vasoconstrictor effect of both agents and increase the risk of severe tissue ischemia or gangrene. If used with MAO inhibitors, may increase both the cardiac and vasoconstrictor effects of dopamine. If used with hydrocarbon anesthetic agents, there may be an increased incidence of ventricular arrhythmias.

**INTERVENTIONS: ADMINISTRATION**

Must be diluted before using. Do not use alkaline solutions, since they inactivate dopamine. May use 0.9% NSS, D5W, D5W and 0.45% NSS, D5W and 0.9% NSS, D5W and Ringer's lactate or sodium lactate solutions. Common concentrations of dopamine are 800 mcg (0.8 mg)/mL or 1.6 mg/mL. Add 200 mg of dopamine to 250 mL for 800 mcg/mL or 400 mg to 250 mL for 1.6 mg/mL.

**MODE/RATE OF ADMINISTRATION**

Usually given by continuous infusion using an infusion pump.

INTRAVENOUS USE (WITH NORMAL RENAL FUNCTION)

**Adults:** Usual initial dosage is 1–5 mcg (0.001–0.005 mg)/kg of body weight per minute. The dosage is increased by 1–4 mcg (0.001–0.004 mg)/kg of body weight per minute q10–30min until the desired response is achieved. For chronic congestive heart failure the usual dosage is 0.5–2 mcg (0.0005–0.002 mg)/kg of body weight per minute with gradual increases until the desired response is achieved. Most clients can be maintained on a dosage of 20 mcg (0.02 mg)/kg of body weight per minute or less.

**Children:** Dosage not established.

**Infants/Neonates:** Dosage not established.

**Geriatrics:** Elderly clients are more likely to have age-related vascular conditions that require a lower dose.

INTRATHECAL USE OR OTHER INFUSION ROUTES AS INDICATED. Not recommended.

### POTENTIAL PROBLEMS IN ADMINISTRATION

The IV infusion site should be a large vein to decrease the possibility of extravasation and subsequent tissue necrosis. If extravasation does occur, the area should be infiltrated with 10–15 mL of 0.9% NSS that contains 5–10 mg of phentolamine. A fine needle should be used. If the area can be treated within 12 h, the area should show the hyperemic effects of the sympathetic blockade. If severe hypertension occurs, the infusion rate should be slowed or, rarely, temporarily discontinued until the blood pressure returns to acceptable levels. When discontinuing the therapy, the dose should be gradually tapered down. Abrupt withdrawal may cause a marked hypotension.

### INDEPENDENT NURSING ACTIONS

Monitor heart rate and ECG for cardiac arrhythmias, especially premature ventricular contractions, BP, urine flow, and if possible CVP or PAWP. Weigh client daily. Monitor intake. BP should be monitored q2min initialy, q5min until stable, and frequently thereafter. Monitor serum sodium and potassium levels. Use of potassium-free solutions may precipitate a marked hypokalemia.

### ADMINISTRATION IN ALTERNATE SETTINGS

Not recommended.

### EVALUATION: OUTCOMES OF DRUG THERAPY

#### EXPECTED OUTCOMES

PHYSICAL ASSESSMENT. Heart rate is within 15 beats of baseline. BP is within 50 mm Hg of baseline. Weight is not more or less than 1 kg (2 lb) from baseline, ECG is regular with no premature ventricular contractions. Urine flow is above 45 mL/h. CVP is between 3 and 8 cm $H_2O$. PAWP is between 4 and 12 cm $H_2O$. Client denies chest pain or shortness of breath.

LABORATORY. Serum sodium is between 136 and 145 mEq/L. Serum potassium is between 3.5 and 5.5 mEq/L.

#### NEGATIVE OUTCOMES

Client's heart rate is more than or less than 15 beats from baseline or irregular from premature ventricular contractions. BP is more than 50 mm Hg from client's baseline. Client complains of chest pain. CVP is higher than 10 cm $H_2O$ or mean PAWP is higher than 13 cm $H_2O$. Client complains of shortness of breath. Crackles heard on auscultation of breath sounds. Urine output not greater than 30 mL/h, and client has marked edema in lower extremities.

## Epinephrine Hydrochloride

*Trade Name:* Adrenalin
*Canadian Availability:* Adrenalin
*Pregnancy Risk:* Category C
*pH:* 2.5–5.0
*Storage/Stability:* Store below 40° C. Protect from light. Protect from freezing. Do not use if discolored pink or brown or if there is visible precipitate. Discard unused portion.

### ASSESSMENT: DRUG CHARACTERISTICS

#### ACTION

A sympathomimetic agent. Stimulates $\beta_2$-receptors to relax bronchial smooth muscle. Inhibits histamine release from allergic responses. Stimulates $\beta_1$-receptors to cause vasoconstriction and a positive inotropic response of the heart muscle. Increases heart rate. Acts on $\alpha$-adrenergic receptors in skin, mucous membranes, and viscera to cause vasoconstriction. Stops bleeding and congestion.

#### INDICATIONS

Used to treat asthma, bronchospasm, emphysema, obstructive pulmonary diseases, allergic reactions, anaphylactic shock, angioedema, laryngeal edema, transfusion reactions, acute hypotension, cardiac arrest, heart block, cardiac arrhythmias, hypovolemic shock, nasal congestion, carotid sinus hypersensitivity, and superficial bleeding.

#### CAUTIONS

ADVERSE EFFECTS. May cause convulsions, dizziness, hallucinations, headache, hypertension, chest pain, tachycardia, bradycardia, arrhythmias, palpitations, chills or fever, nausea or vomiting, shortness of breath, trembling, anxiety, enlarged pupils, pallor, or weakness.

CONTRAINDICATIONS. Organic brain damage; cardiovascular diseases that include rate irregularities, hypertension, congestive heart failure, or ischemic heart conditions; diabetes mellitus; glaucoma; hyperthyroidism; pheochromocytoma; prostatic hypertrophy; shock; or allergy to epinephrine. Should not be used to treat phenothiazine-induced hypotension.

#### POTENTIAL DRUG/FOOD INTERACTIONS

May block the effects of $\alpha$-adrenergic vasodilators, causing severe hypotension. May block the bronchodilating action of $\beta$-adrenergic agents if used concurrently. May increase the risk of ventricular arrhythmias if used with hydrocarbon anesthetic agents. If used with parenteral local anesthetics, may increase the incidence of local ischemia. If used with tricyclic antidepressants, there may be arrhythmias, tachycardia, severe hypertension, or pyrexia. Antagonizes action of insulin and antihypertensive agents. May potentiate CNS stimulants and cause convulsions. May interact with cardiac glycosides to increase incidence of arrhythmias. Potentiates the action of ergotamine to increase risk of peripheral vascular ischemia or postpartum rupture of cerebral vessels. Potentiates the pressor effects of doxapram, mazindol, methylphenidate, MAO inhibitors, rauwolfia, other sympathomimetic drugs, thyroid, and xanthine drugs. May decrease the hypotensive effects of trimethaphan and guanethidine.

#### INTERVENTIONS: ADMINISTRATION

Solutions of 1:1000 must be diluted before using. Do not use alkaline solutions for dilution. May use D5W or 0.9% NSS. For intracardiac injection, dilute 0.5 mg of epinephrine 1:1000 in 10 mL of 0.9% NSS for injection.

#### MODE/RATE OF ADMINISTRATION

May be given by rapid IV injection through a free-flowing IV solution. May be given by continuous infusion using an infusion pump.

INTRAVENOUS USE (WITH NORMAL RENAL FUNCTION)

**Adults:** For bronchodilation the usual dose is 200–500 mcg (0.2–0.5 mg). Dose may be repeated q20min–4h. Maximum dose is 1 mg per dose. For anaphylactic shock the usual dose is 100–250 mcg (0.1–0.25 mg) given slowly. Dose may be repeated q5–15min as needed. May be given as a continuous infusion at 1 mcg (0.001 mg)/min, up to 4 mcg (0.004 mg)/min. For cardiac arrest, 100 mcg (0.1 mg)–1 mg either intracardiac, intratracheal, or IV. May be repeated q5min as needed.

**Children:** For bronchodilation, 10 mcg (0.01 mg)/kg of body weight q5–15min as needed. For cardiac arrest, 5–10 mcg (0.005–0.010 mg)/kg of body weight intracardiac or IV q5min as necessary. May be given as a continuous infusion at 0.11 mcg (0.0001 mg)/kg of body weight per minute, up to 1.5 mcg (0.0015 mg)/kg of body weight per minute.

**Infants/Neonates:** Dosage not established.

**Geriatrics:** Follow adult dosing schedule.

INTRATHECAL USE OR OTHER INFUSION ROUTES AS INDICATED. May be given intracardiac or by intratracheal route. May be given intraspinal to prolong the effects of local anesthesia.

#### POTENTIAL PROBLEMS IN ADMINISTRATION

Should not be given intraarterially, since vasoconstriction may cause gangrene.

#### INDEPENDENT NURSING ACTIONS

Monitor blood pressure q5min. Monitor heart rate and ECG for the presence of cardiac arrhythmias, especially premature ventricular contractions, urine flow, and if possible CVP or PAWP. Contains sulfites. May cause allergic response in sensitive clients.

#### ADMINISTRATION IN ALTERNATE SETTINGS

IV infusion not recommended in home setting. May be used in most short-term care settings as an
▼

emergency treatment for severe drug reactions.

**EVALUATION: OUTCOMES OF DRUG THERAPY**

**EXPECTED OUTCOMES**

PHYSICAL ASSESSMENT. Heart rate is less than 15% greater than baseline and regular. Blood pressure is sufficient for urine flow to be greater than 30 mL/h and less than 20% greater than baseline. Breath sounds clear on auscultation. Client warm, pink, and resting quietly.

LABORATORY. Serum glucose may be elevated. Serum sodium and potassium levels may be decreased.

**NEGATIVE OUTCOMES**

Heart rate is greater than 100 bpm or irregular. Blood pressure is greater than 50 mm Hg above client's baseline. Client complains of chest pain, palpitations, or shortness of breath. Crackles or wheezes heard on auscultation. Urine output not greater than 30 mL/h. Client has pale, cool extremities; tremors; or complains of feeling anxious.

## Isoproterenol Hydrochloride

*Trade Name:* Isuprel
*Canadian Availability:* Isuprel
*Pregnancy Risk:* Category C
*pH:* 3.5–4.5
*Storage/Stability:* Store below 40° C. Protect from light. Protect from freezing. Do not use if discolored pink or brown or if there is visible precipitate. Discard unused portion.

**ASSESSMENT: DRUG CHARACTERISTICS**

**ACTION**

A sympathomimetic agent. Stimulates $\beta_2$-receptors to relax bronchial smooth muscle. Inhibits histamine release from allergic responses. Stimulates $\beta_1$-receptors to cause vasoconstriction and a positive inotropic response of the heart muscle. Increases heart rate. Acts on $\alpha$-adrenergic receptors in skin, mucous membranes, and viscera to cause vasoconstriction. Stops bleeding and congestion.

**INDICATIONS**

Used to treat cardiac arrest, heart block, cardiac arrhythmias, hypovolemic shock, carotid and sinus hypersensitivity, asthma, emphysema, or obstructive pulmonary diseases.

**CAUTIONS**

ADVERSE EFFECTS. May cause dry mouth, nervousness, convulsions, dizziness, hallucinations, headache, hypertension, chest pain, tachycardia, bradycardia, arrhythmias, palpitations, chills or fever, nausea or vomiting, shortness of breath, trembling, anxiety, enlarged pupils, pallor, or weakness.

CONTRAINDICATIONS. Cardiovascular diseases, including tachycardia, hypertension, and ischemic heart conditions; diabetes mellitus; glaucoma; hyperthyroidism; pheochromocytoma; or shock. Should not be used to treat tachycardia caused by digitalis toxicity.

**POTENTIAL DRUG/FOOD INTERACTIONS**

May block the effects of $\alpha$-adrenergic vasodilators, causing severe hypotension. May block the bronchodilating action of $\beta$-adrenergic agents if used concurrently. If used with parenteral local anesthetics, may increase the incidence of local ischemia. If used with tricyclic antidepressants, there may be arrhythmias, tachycardia, severe hypertension, or pyrexia. Antagonizes the action of antihypertensive agents. May potentiate CNS stimulants and cause convulsions. May interact with cardiac glycosides to increase incidence of arrhythmias. Potentiates the pressor effects of other sympathomimetic drugs, thyroid, and xanthine drugs.

**INTERVENTIONS: ADMINISTRATION**

May be given undiluted (0.2 mg of 1:5000). May be diluted in D5W solution. May be further diluted in 250 mL of IV solution.

**MODE/RATE OF ADMINISTRATION**

May be given by rapid IV injection over 1 min through a free-flowing IV solution. May be given by continuous infusion using an infusion pump.

INTRAVENOUS USE (WITH NORMAL RENAL FUNCTION)

**Adults:** For bronchodilation the usual dose is 10–20 mcg (0.2–0.5 mg). Dose may be repeated as needed. For hypovolemic shock the usual dosage is 0.5–1 mcg (0.0005–0.005 mg)/min of 1 mg of Isuprel per 500 mL of D5W solution. Dosage may be adjusted according to client response. For cardiac arrhythmias or cardiac arrest the usual dose is 20 mcg (0.02 mg) intracardiac. For rapid IV injection the usual dose is 20–60 mcg (0.02–0.06 mg) initially. Doses of 10–200 mcg (0.01–0.2 mg) may be repeated as needed. For continuous infusion the usual dose is 5 mcg (0.005 mg) of 2 mg of Isuprel in 500 mL of D5W solution, which is then titrated according to client response.

**Children:** Usual dose is one tenth to one half adult dose, titrated according to client response.

**Infants/Neonates:** Dose not established.

**Geriatrics:** Follow adult dosing schedule.

INTRATHECAL USE OR OTHER INFUSION ROUTES AS INDICATED. May be given intracardiac. Not recommended for intrathecal infusion.

**POTENTIAL PROBLEMS IN ADMINISTRATION**

Contains sulfites. May cause allergic response in sensitive clients.

**INDEPENDENT NURSING ACTIONS**

Monitor blood pressure q5min. Monitor heart rate and ECG for the presence of cardiac arrhythmias, especially premature ventricular contractions, urine flow, and if possible CVP or PAWP.

▼

**ADMINISTRATION IN ALTERNATE SETTINGS**

IV administration not recommended.

**EVALUATION: OUTCOMES OF DRUG THERAPY**

**EXPECTED OUTCOMES**

PHYSICAL ASSESSMENT. Heart rate is less than 15% greater than baseline and regular. Blood pressure is sufficient for urine flow to be greater than 30 mL/h and less than 20% greater than baseline. Breath sounds clear on auscultation. Client warm, pink, and resting quietly.

LABORATORY. Serum glucose may be elevated. Serum sodium and potassium levels may be decreased.

**NEGATIVE OUTCOMES**

Heart rate is greater than 100 bpm or irregular. Blood pressure is greater than 50 mm Hg above client's baseline. Client complains of chest pain, palpitations, or shortness of breath. Crackles or wheezes heard on auscultation. Urine output not greater than 30 mL/h. Client has pale, cool extremities; tremors; or complains of feeling anxious.

---

## METARAMINOL BITARTRATE

*Trade Name:* Aramine
*Canadian Availability:* Not commercially available.
*Pregnancy Risk:* Category C
*pH:* 3.5–4.5
*Storage/Stability:* Store below 40° C. Protect from light and from freezing. Discard unused diluted solutions after 24 hours.

**ASSESSMENT: DRUG CHARACTERISTICS**

**ACTION**

A vasopressor that directly affects $\alpha$-adrenergic receptor sites on vascular smooth muscle. Causes the release of norepinephrine from storage. Acts on $\beta_1$-adrenergic receptor sites in cardiac muscle to increase both systolic and diastolic pressure. May cause bradycardia and pulmonary, cerebral, and renal vasoconstriction.

**INDICATIONS**

Used to treat acute hypotension resulting from hemorrhage, reactions to medication, surgery, and traumatic shock. Treatment for shock must be accompanied by appropriate fluid replacement.

**CAUTIONS**

ADVERSE EFFECTS. May cause ventricular tachycardia, vasoconstriction, abscess formation or ischemia from extravasation, hypotension, cardiac arrhythmias, convulsions, or allergic reactions from sulfites.

CONTRAINDICATIONS. Acidosis, hypercapnia, or hypoxia. Should be used with caution in clients who have obstructive vascular diseases, cirrhosis of the liver, heart disease, hypertension, or hyperthyroidism.

**POTENTIAL DRUG/FOOD INTERACTIONS**

May decrease the effects of α-adrenergic vasodilators, causing severe hypotension. May block the bronchodilating action of β-adrenergic agents if used concurrently. May increase the risk of ventricular arrhythmias if used with hydrocarbon anesthetic agents. If used with tricyclic antidepressants, there may be arrhythmias, tachycardia, severe hypertension, or pyrexia. May interact with cardiac glycosides to increase incidence of arrhythmias. Potentiates the action of ergotamine to increase risk of peripheral vascular ischemia or postpartum rupture of cerebral vessels. Potentiates the pressor effects of doxapram, mazindol, ethylphenidate, MAO inhibitors, rauwolfia, other sympathomimetic drugs, thyroid, and xanthine drugs. May decrease the hypotensive effects of trimethaphan and guanethidine.

**INTERVENTIONS: ADMINISTRATION**

1% Aramine must be diluted prior to use. Preferred solutions are 0.9% NSS or D5W solution. May use Ringer's lactate.

**MODE/RATE OF ADMINISTRATION**

May be given by rapid IV injection through a free-flowing IV line at a rate of 1 mg/min. May be given by continuous infusion using an infusion pump.

INTRAVENOUS USE (WITH NORMAL RENAL FUNCTION)

**Adults:** For severe shock the usual dose is 500 mcg (0.5mg)–5 mg by rapid IV injection followed by a continuous infusion of 15–100 mg of metaraminol in 100 mL of D5W solution titrated to the client's response. For hypotension the usual dose is a continuous infusion of 15–100 mg of metaraminol in 100 mL of D5W solution titrated to the client's response. The maximum concentration should not exceed 500 mg in 500 mL.

**Children:** For severe hypotension the usual dose is 400 mcg (0.04 mg)/kg of body weight in a concentration of 1 mg/25 ml 0.9% NSS or D5W solution. The rate is titrated according to client response.

**Infants/Neonates:** Dose not established.

**Geriatrics:** Clients may have diminished renal function that would require a lower dose.

INTRATHECAL USE OR OTHER INFUSION ROUTES AS INDICATED. Not recommended.

**POTENTIAL PROBLEMS IN ADMINISTRATION**

The IV infusion site should be a large vein to decrease the possibility of extravasation and subsequent tissue necrosis. If extravasation does occur, the area should be infiltrated with 10–15 mL of 0.9% NSS that contains 5–10 mg of phentolamine. A fine needle should be used. If the area can be treated within 12 h, the area

▼

should show the hyperemic effects of the sympathetic blockade. When discontinuing the therapy, the dose should be gradually tapered down. Abrupt withdrawal may cause a marked hypotension. Clients must be monitored carefully after metaraminol is withdrawn to ensure that their blood pressure does not fall abruptly.

**INDEPENDENT NURSING ACTIONS**

Monitor heart rate and ECG for cardiac arrhythmias, especially premature ventricular contractions, BP, urine flow, and if possible CVP or PAWP. Weigh client daily. Monitor intake. BP should be monitored q2min initially, q5min until stable, and frequently thereafter. Monitor serum sodium and potassium levels. Use of potassium-free solutions may precipitate a marked hypokalemia.

**ADMINISTRATION IN ALTERNATE SETTINGS**

Not recommended.

**EVALUATION: OUTCOMES OF DRUG THERAPY**

**EXPECTED OUTCOMES**

PHYSICAL ASSESSMENT. Heart rate is within 15 beats of baseline. BP is within 50 mm Hg of baseline. Weight is not more or less than 1 kg (2 lb) from baseline. ECG is regular with no premature ventricular contractions. Urine flow is above 45 mL/h. CVP is between 3 and 8 cm H2O. PAWP is between 4 and 12 cm H2O. Client denies chest pain or shortness of breath.

LABORATORY. Serum sodium is between 136 and 145 mEq/L. Serum potassium is between 3.5 and 5.5 mEq/L.

**NEGATIVE OUTCOMES**

Client's heart rate is more than or less than 15 beats from baseline or irregular from premature ventricular contractions. BP is more than 50 mm Hg from client's baseline. Client complains of chest pain. CVP is higher than 10 cm $H_2O$ or mean PAWP is higher than 13 cm $H_2O$. Client complains of shortness of breath. Crackles heard on auscultation of breath sounds. Urine output not greater than 30 mL/h, and client has marked edema in lower extremities.

## RITODRINE HYDROCHLORIDE

*Trade Name:* Yutopar
*Canadian Availability:* Yutopar
*Pregnancy Risk:* Category B
*pH:* 4.8–5.5
*Storage/Stability:* Store between 15° and 30° C. Solutions containing 300 mcg (0.3 mg)/mL may be stored for up to 48 hours after preparation. Do not use if solution is discolored or contains precipitate.

**ASSESSMENT: DRUG CHARACTERISTICS**

**ACTION**

A $\beta_2$-adrenergic stimulant that causes uterine muscle

relaxation by inhibiting uterine contractions.

**INDICATIONS**

Used to treat uncomplicated premature labor in pregnancies of 20 weeks' or more gestation. Ritodrine should be given as soon as labor is confirmed.

**CAUTIONS**

ADVERSE EFFECTS. May cause tachycardia or arrhythmias, angina, pulmonary edema, or hepatic impairment.

CONTRAINDICATIONS. Cardiac arrhythmias, hyperthyroidism, hemorrhage, intrauterine fetal death, eclampsia, pulmonary hypertension, diabetes mellitus.

**POTENTIAL DRUG/FOOD INTERACTIONS**

$\beta$-Adrenergic blocking agents may antagonize the effect of ritodrine. If used with corticosteroids, may precipitate maternal pulmonary edema. May potentiate the effects of other sympathomimetics.

**INTERVENTIONS: ADMINISTRATION**

Must be diluted. Ritodrine 150 mg in 500 mL of D5W produces a concentration of 300 mcg (0.03 mg)/mL. If fluid restriction is essential, solution concentration may be higher than 300 mcg/mL.

**MODE/RATE OF ADMINISTRATION**

Given by continuous infusion using an infusion pump.

INTRAVENOUS USE (WITH NORMAL RENAL FUNCTION)

**Adults:** Usual initial dosage is 50–100 mcg (0.05–0.1 mg)/min. May be increased by 50 mcg (0.05 mg) q10min until desired response is achieved. Mainten-ance dosage is 150–350 mcg (0.15–0.35 mg)/min.

**Children:** No approved use.

**Infants/Neonates:** No approved use.

**Geriatrics:** No approved use.

INTRATHECAL USE OR OTHER INFUSION ROUTES AS INDICATED. Not recommended.

**POTENTIAL PROBLEMS IN ADMINISTRATION**

Saline solutions should be avoided because of the incidence of pulmonary edema. IV infusion should be contin-ued for 12–24 h after labor has stopped. Ritodrine may be restarted if preterm labor restarts.

**INDEPENDENT NURSING ACTIONS**

Monitor maternal vital signs, especially heart rate and rhythm. Monitor for uterine contractions, fetal heart rate, and hyperglycemia. Auscultate breath sounds frequently.

**ADMINISTRATION IN ALTERNATE SETTINGS**

Not recommended.

**EVALUATION: OUTCOMES OF DRUG THERAPY**

**EXPECTED OUTCOMES**

PHYSICAL ASSESSMENT. Heart rate less than 100 bpm and regular. Breath sounds clear, and respiratory rate between 16 and 20/min. Fetal heart rate remains at baseline. Uterine contractions stop.

LABORATORY. Serum glucose remains less than 150 mg/dL.

▼

**NEGATIVE OUTCOMES**

Heart rate greater than 100 bpm or irregular. Fetal heart rate deviates from baseline. Uterine contractions continue. Crackles are heard on auscultation of maternal breath sounds. Respiratory rate is above 20/min.

## SYMPATHOLYTICS

### THERAPEUTIC EFFECTS

α-Receptor blockers inhibit responses to sympathomimetic (adrenergic) agents by competing for the α-receptor sites, which are located primarily in smooth muscle and exocrine glands. In general, the response is vasodilation and smooth muscle relaxation. Sympatholytic drugs are useful in the treatment of vascular headaches and hypertension associated with pheochromocytoma and in the prevention of tissue damage if norepinephrine extravasates during infusion therapy.

### PHARMACOKINETICS

**Distribution.** Most α-receptor blockers are incompletely and irregularly absorbed from the GI tract. When given intravenously, about 90% are bound to plasma protein. Onset of action is within minutes. Duration of action is up to 3 to 4 hours.

**Metabolism/Elimination.** Plasma half-life is 1 to 2 hours. These agents are metabolized by the liver, and the metabolites are excreted in the urine within 72 hours.

### CAUTIONS

**Side/Adverse Effects.** Sympatholytics may cause localized itching or edema, bradycardia or tachycardia, hypotension, weakness, and nasal congestion.

**Contraindications.** Clients with peripheral vascular disease, coronary artery disease, uncontrolled hypertension, or impaired hepatic or renal functioning should not be given sympatholytic drugs.

***Pregnancy and Lactation.*** Sympatholytic drugs are contraindicated during pregnancy. They may be passed in breast milk.

***Pediatrics.*** Effects on children have not been determined.

***Geriatrics.*** Elderly clients are more likely to have preexisting conditions, such as coronary artery disease, that contraindicate using sympatholytic drugs.

### TOXICITY

See Table 18–5 for toxicities of sympatholytic agents.

**TABLE 18–5**
**Toxicities of Sympatholytic Agents**

| Body System | Side/Toxic Effects | Physical Assessment Indicators | Laboratory Indicators | Nursing Interventions |
|---|---|---|---|---|
| Neurologic | | Confusion, dizziness, seizures, syncope, nervousness, weakness | N/A | Monitor level of consciousness. Provide a safe environment. |
| Cardiovascular | Myocardial infarction, vasospasm | Chest pain, shortness of breath, tachycardia, hypertension, dysrhythmias, muscle pain, marbling, cyanosis | ECG, cardiac isoenzymes | Discontinue drug and be prepared to give vasodilators such as nitroprusside. |
| Gastrointestinal | | Nausea, vomiting, diarrhea, abdominal distention | Stool for occult blood | Monitor gastrointestinal functioning, palpate abdomen. |
| Dermatologic | | Rare: urticaria, pruritus, erythema | N/A | Provide comfort measures for itching. Report findings if reaction intense. |
| Genitourinary | Priapism | Prolonged painful erection | N/A | Report findings. Provide privacy and psychologic support. |

## POTENTIAL DRUG/FOOD INTERACTIONS

Sympatholytics that are ergot alkaloids may interact with erythromycin or troleandomycin to cause severe vasospasm.

---

# DIHYDROERGOTAMINE MESYLATE

*Trade Name:* D.H.E. 45
*Canadian Availability:* Dihydroergotamine
*Pregnancy Risk:* Category X
*pH:* 3.7–4.1
*Storage/Stability:* Store below 40° C. Protect from light. Protect from freezing. Do not use if solution is discolored.

### ASSESSMENT: DRUG CHARACTERISTICS

#### ACTION

An antimigraine or vascular headache suppressant. Acts on several neurotransmitter receptors, including α-adrenergic, serotoninergic, and dopaminergic sites. Has both agonist and antagonist actions on many of the receptors. Stimulates smooth muscle to cause vasoconstriction of both arteries and veins. In addition to the constriction of cerebral vascular beds, there is a decrease in cerebral vascular pulsation. May act directly on the chemoreceptor trigger zone to cause nausea and vomiting.

#### INDICATIONS

Used to treat migraine headaches or suppress vascular headaches such as cluster headaches. Is the drug of choice for severe, refractory headaches.

#### CAUTIONS

ADVERSE EFFECTS. May cause edema of hands, face, or lower extremities. May cause angina pectoris, tachycardia or bradycardia, hypotension or hypertension, cerebral or peripheral vascular spasm, or ischemia. Ergot toxicity may be determined by CNS symptoms of seizures, confusion, or weakness or by diarrhea, vomiting, abdominal pain, or shortness of breath.

CONTRAINDICATIONS. Hypertension, Angioplasty, vascular sur-gery, trauma, angina pectoris, coronary artery disease, impaired hepatic or renal function, pruritus, sepsis, or sensitivity to dihydroergotamine.

#### POTENTIAL DRUG/FOOD INTERACTIONS

May interact with other ergot alkaloids, other vasoconstrictors, or anesthetic agents to intensify vasoconstriction and the risk of ischemia or gangrene.

### INTERVENTIONS: ADMINISTRATION

Usually given undiluted.

#### MODE/RATE OF ADMINISTRATION

Usually given by rapid IV injection over 1–2 min.

INTRAVENOUS USE (WITH NORMAL RENAL FUNCTION)

**Adults:** For an acute migraine or vascular headache the usual dose is 500 mcg (0.5 mg) at the start of an attack. Should be given with an antiemetic. May be repeated in 1 h if needed. Maximum dose is 2 mg. For chronic intractable headache the usual dose if 500 mcg (0.5 mg) over 1 min. Should be given 3–5 min after an antiemetic has been given. The dose is repeated q8–10h until the headache has stopped. One source recommends that the dosing schedule continue for 2–3 doses after the headache has stopped to prevent recurrence. Maximum dosage is 6 mg/wk.

**Children ≥ 6 years:** Usual dose is 250 mcg (0.25 mg) at the start of the attack. Should be given after an antiemetic.

**Infants/Neonates:** Dose not established.

**Geriatrics:** Clients are more likely to have diminished renal function and age-related vascular changes that put them more at risk for peripheral vasoconstriction and hypothermia. Dose may need to be lowered.

INTRATHECAL USE OR OTHER INFUSION ROUTES AS INDICATED. Not recommended. Intraarterial infusion may cause severe vasospasm and gangrene.

#### POTENTIAL PROBLEMS IN ADMINISTRATION

Clients may experience significant nausea and vomiting. Antiemetics such as metoclopramide, atropine, or phenothiazine are recommended prior to giving dihydroergotamine. After dihydroergotamine is given, the client should be placed in a quiet, dark room for greater comfort.

#### INDEPENDENT NURSING ACTIONS

Monitor vital signs, especially blood pressure and heart rate. ECG should be done for clients receiving therapy for chronic, intractable headaches. Observe extremities and palpate peripheral pulses frequently.

#### ADMINISTRATION IN ALTERNATE SETTINGS

May be administered in outpatient settings by a qualified IV nurse. Not recommended for the home setting.

#### EVALUATION: OUTCOMES OF DRUG THERAPY

#### EXPECTED OUTCOMES

PHYSICAL ASSESSMENT. Client states that headache is relieved. Blood pressure and pulse within client's baseline. Extremities warm, pink, and free of edema.

LABORATORY. Hepatic and renal function studies remain within client's baseline.

#### NEGATIVE OUTCOMES

Client experiences no significant relief from headache and complains of nausea and vomiting. Blood pressure or pulse varies more than 15% above or below baseline. Extremities are pale, cold, or swollen.

CHAPTER 19

# Blood Derivatives, Blood Formers, Anticoagulants, Hemostatics, and Thrombolytics

*Elaine Kennedy*



Blood is a complex fluid made up of cells and plasma. The cells are erythrocytes, leukocytes, and platelets. Plasma is primarily albumin, globulin, water, and electrolytes. Blood supplies the medium for the transport of oxygen and nutrients to all body cells and for the removal of end products of metabolism. Whole blood—all components—may be provided by a healthy donor and given to a recipient. More commonly, a healthy donor provides one pint of whole blood, which is then separated into its various components, such as packed red blood cells (RBCs) and albumin. Further, some clotting factors exist in minute amounts. These factors are removed and mixed with several hundred other donated factors, and the pooled material is used to treat clients with various blood clotting disorders.

## DEFINITIONS

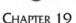

**Blood Derivatives.** Blood derivatives are commercially available plasma expanders. Manufacturers pool albumin and plasma from healthy human donors and package the product for sale to pharmacies.

**Blood Formers.** Hematopoiesis, or blood formation, takes place mainly in the red bone marrow of axial skeletal bones and the proximal heads of the femur and humerus. Within the red marrow are parent cells and other earliest forms of blood cells. The earliest forms of blood cells can be divided into stem cells and progenitor cells. Stem cells can mature and differentiate into all the hematopoietic cells or form new stem cells, and progenitor cells can become mature differentiated cells but cannot form new stem cells.

Drugs that affect blood formation affect the development of stem cells as they mature and differentiate into granulocyte/monocyte, erythrocyte, megakaryocyte, or lymphocyte progenitor cells. Sargramostim appears to stimulate the production of stem cells, as well as granulocyte/monocyte, erythrocyte, and megakaryocyte progenitor cells. These cells mature into monocytes, eosinophils, basophils, erythrocytes, and thrombocytes. Filgrastim appears to stimulate the granulocyte progenitor cells to produce more neutrophils. Erythropoietin stimulates the erythrocyte progenitor cell to increase the production of erythrocytes or RBCs.

**Blood Coagulants.** Drugs may promote or inhibit blood clotting by intervening at specific points in the clotting cascade. As blood clots, it changes from a viscous fluid to a gel. One clotting pathway, called the extrinsic pathway, is triggered by injury. When tissue is damaged, a lipoprotein, called tissue thromboplastin, is released, which activates several enzymes in turn and finally gives rise to fibrin. Fibrin strands are long protein chains that trap and hold cells to form the gelatinous mass that forms a dam to avoid further fluid loss.

A second clotting pathway, called the intrinsic pathway, is within the blood itself. When the endothelial lining of vessels is damaged, blood is exposed to collagen and other elements. That exposure triggers the enzyme known as factor XII or Hageman factor, which activates a series of enzymes that eventually also gives rise to fibrin and a clot. Endothelial injury is common with a number of cardiovascular diseases such as hypertension, atherosclerosis, and arteriosclerosis.

Drugs may facilitate clotting by (1) supplying factors that the body is unable to produce, such as antihemophilic factor (AHF); (2) by inhibiting the activation of enzymes necessary to break down fibrin, such as aminocaproic acid; or (3) by inactivating substances that prevent the formation of fibrin, such as protamine sulfate's action on heparin.

**Thrombolytic Enzymes.** Thrombolytic enzymes are used to remove blood clots that have already formed, in contrast to anticoagulant drugs that act to prevent clot formation.

Thrombolytic enzymes are used in the treatment of the early stages of myocardial infarction. Heart muscle damage is minimized by dissolving the blood clot occluding the coronary artery and reestablishing blood flow to the heart muscle. In addition, thrombolytic enzymes may be used to lyse a clot in an arteriovenous shunt or in other vascular access devices.

Thrombolytic enzymes are tissue activators that cause the conversion of plasminogen to plasmin. Plasmin in turn causes fibrin, fibrinogen, and other clotting factors to deteriorate. As fibrin degrades, the long protein strands soften, weaken, and straighten. With the lysis of the matrix, the clot breaks apart and permits blood flow through the previously obstructed area. Thrombolytic therapy carries the risk of hemorrhage if the client's clotting mechanism is sufficiently impaired.

**Classification.** Blood products and drugs affecting blood formation, coagulation, and thrombolysis are grouped by subclassifications in Table 19–1.

## BLOOD DERIVATIVES

### THERAPEUTIC EFFECTS

Blood derivatives are used to expand plasma volume and to maintain cardiac output in certain types of shock resulting from hemorrhage, surgery, burns, or other conditions where circulating plasma volume is deficient. The products are derived from pooled human blood from healthy human donors.

### PHARMACOKINETICS

**Distribution.** Blood derivatives are given intravenously and distributed throughout the vascular system.

**TABLE 19–1**
**Blood Derivatives and Agents Affecting Blood Formation, Coagulation, and Thrombolysis**

| | |
|---|---|
| **Blood Derivatives** | **Blood Coagulants** |
| Human albumin, 5% and 25% | Aminocaproic acid |
| Plasma protein fraction | Antihemophilic factor (Factor VIII, AHF) |
| **Blood Formers** | Aprotinin |
| Epoetin alfa | Coumarin* |
| Filgrastim (G-CSF) | Factor IX* |
| Iron preparations* | Heparin sodium |
| Iron dextran | Protamine sulfate |
| Sargramostim (GM-CSF) | Warfarin* |
| | **Thrombolytic Enzymes** |
| | Alteplase (tPA) |
| | Streptokinase |
| | Urokinase |

*Not discussed in this chapter.

**Excretion:** Metabolized by the liver and excreted by the kidneys.

## CAUTIONS

**Side/Adverse Effects.** Allergic symptoms, nausea, vomiting, pulmonary edema, hypertension, or tachycardia may result.

**Contraindications**

***Pregnancy and Lactation.*** Effects on the fetus have not been established. Blood derivatives should be used only when the potential maternal benefit outweighs the risk to the fetus.

***Pediatrics.*** Blood derivatives may be used to treat nephrotic syndrome in children. The products should not be given to children with known hypersensitivity to blood derivatives.

***Geriatrics.*** The elderly are more likely to have preexisting conditions that put them at risk for cardiac dysrhythmias, hypertension, and pulmonary edema.

## TOXICITY

See Table 19–2 for toxicities of blood derivatives.

## POTENTIAL DRUG/FOOD INTERACTIONS

Blood products are not known to have any specific drug or food interactions.

# HUMAN ALBUMIN, 5% AND 25%

*Trade Name:* Buminate 5%, and 25%
*Canadian Availability:* Plasbumin
*Pregnancy Risk:* Category C
*pH:* 6.4–7.3
*Storage/Stability:* Store below 37° C. Discard if turbid or contains a precipitate. Discard unused opened containers after 4 hours.

### ASSESSMENT: DRUG CHARACTERISTICS

#### ACTION

A blood derivative that provides albumin, one of the major plasma proteins. Albumin increases colloidal oncotic pressure, which helps draw fluid into the vascular space.

#### INDICATIONS

Used to treat shock, burns, hypoproteinemia from diseases such as nephrotic syndrome or acute cirrhosis, and hyperbilirubinemia from erythroblastosis fetalis.

#### CAUTIONS

ADVERSE EFFECTS. Nausea, vomiting, pulmonary edema, hypertension, tachycardia, or allergic symptoms.

CONTRAINDICATIONS. Severe anemia, cardiac failure, or

**TABLE 19–2**
**Toxicities of Blood Derivatives**

| Body System | Side/Toxic Effects | Physical Assessment Indicators | Laboratory Indicators | Nursing Interventions |
|---|---|---|---|---|
| Cardiovascular | Vascular overload | Moist, noisy respirations; dyspnea; mental status changes; edema | N/A | Monitor respirations; measure intake and output; observe for restlessness, irritability, or confusion. |
| Other | Hypersensitivity reaction | Nausea, vomiting, fever, chills, increased salivation, urticaria, tachycardia, hypertension, tachypnea | N/A | Monitor for signs of hypersensitivity; stop infusion and give antihistamines if ordered. |

N/A = not applicable.

hypersensitvity to human albumin.

#### POTENTIAL DRUG/FOOD INTERACTIONS

No significant interactions reported.

#### INTERVENTIONS: ADMINISTRATION

May be given undiluted. May be diluted in 0.9% normal saline solution (NSS), 5% dextrose in water (D5W), combinations of NSS and dextrose, and Ringer's lactate solutions.

#### MODE/RATE OF ADMINISTRATION

May be given by intravenous (IV) push at a rate not to exceed 1 mL/min.

INTRAVENOUS USE (WITH NORMAL RENAL FUNCTION)

**Adults:** For volume replacement the usual dose is 25 g, which may be repeated in 15–30 min. Further treatment is determined by blood chemistry laboratory values. Maximum dosage should not exceed 125 g/24 h or 250 g/48 h.

For hypoproteinemia the usual dosage is 200–300 mL of 25% albumin given not faster than 100 mL in 30–45 min.

**Children:** In emergencies the usual dose is 25 g. In nonemergency situations the usual dose is 25%–50% the usual adult dose.

**Infants/Neonates:** The usual dose for premature infants is 1 g/kg of a 25% solution given prior to transfusion.

**Geriatrics:** Follow adult dosing schedules.

INTRATHECAL USE OR OTHER INFUSION ROUTES AS INDICATED. Not recommended.

#### POTENTIAL PROBLEMS IN ADMINISTRATION

Too rapid administration of albumin may cause circulatory overload or pulmonary edema.

#### INDEPENDENT NURSING ACTIONS

Monitor vital signs, intake and output, and level of consciousness. Observe for evidence of bleeding or fluid loss.

#### ADMINISTRATION IN ALTERNATE SETTINGS

May be given in a variety of clinical settings by a qualified IV nurse.

#### EVALUATION: OUTCOMES OF DRUG THERAPY

#### EXPECTED OUTCOMES

PHYSICAL ASSESSMENT. Temperature less than 37.5° C, pulse between 60 and 100 beats per minute (bpm) and regular, respirations between 16 and 20/min and regular, and blood pressure within 15% of baseline. Breath sounds clear. Urinary output more than 30 mL/h. Client alert or easily aroused.

LABORATORY. Serum albumin between 3.5 and 5 g/dL.

#### NEGATIVE OUTCOMES

Temperature more than 37.5° C, pulse more than 100 bpm, respirations more than 20/min, and blood pressure more than 15% higher or lower than baseline. Breath sounds demonstrate crackles or wheezes. Urinary output less than 30 mL/h. Client lethargic or stuporous.

## Plasma Protein Fraction

*Trade Name:* Protenate 5%
*Canadian Availability:* Not specified.
*Pregnancy Risk:* Category C
*pH:* 6.7–7.3
*Storage/Stability:* Store below 37° C. Discard if turbid or contains a precipitate. Discard unused opened containers after 4 hours.

### ASSESSMENT: DRUG CHARACTERISTICS

#### ACTION

A blood derivative that provides approximately 83% albumin, one of the major plasma proteins. Albumin increases colloidal oncotic pressure, which helps draw fluid into the vascular space.

#### INDICATIONS

Used to treat shock, burns, and hypoproteinemia from diseases such as nephrotic syndrome or acute cirrhosis. Clinicians may choose to use albumin because it is purer and less likely to cause a reaction.

#### CAUTIONS

ADVERSE EFFECTS. Allergic symptoms, nausea, vomiting, pulmonary edema, hypertension, or tachycardia.

CONTRAINDICATIONS. Severe anemia, cardiac failure, or hypersensitivity to plasma protein fraction.

#### POTENTIAL DRUG/FOOD INTERACTIONS

No significant interactions reported.

### INTERVENTIONS: ADMINISTRATION

Usually given undiluted.

#### MODE/RATE OF ADMINISTRATION

May be given by IV push at a rate not to exceed 10 mL/min.

INTRAVENOUS USE (WITH NORMAL RENAL FUNCTION)

**Adults:** For volume replacement the usual dose is 12.5–25 g initially. Further treatment is determined by blood chemistry laboratory values. Maximum dosage should not exceed 250 g/48 h.

For severe hypoproteinemia the usual dosage is 1000–1500 mL/d. Further treatment is determined by blood chemistry laboratory values.

**Children:** The usual initial dose is 6.6–33 ml/kg of body weight. Further treatment is determined by blood chemistry laboratory values.

**Infants/Neonates:** Follow children's dosing schedule.

**Geriatrics:** Follow adult dosing schedule.

INTRATHECAL USE OR OTHER INFUSION ROUTES AS INDICATED. Not recommended.

#### POTENTIAL PROBLEMS IN ADMINISTRATION

Too rapid administration of albumin may cause circulatory overload or pulmonary edema.

#### INDEPENDENT NURSING ACTIONS

Monitor vital signs, intake and output, and level of consciousness. Observe for evidence of bleeding or fluid loss.

▼

**ADMINISTRATION IN ALTERNATE SETTINGS**

May be given in a variety of clinical settings by a qualified IV nurse.

**EVALUATION: OUTCOMES OF DRUG THERAPY**

**EXPECTED OUTCOMES**

PHYSICAL ASSESSMENT. Temperature less than 37.5° C, pulse between 60 and 100 bpm and regular, respirations between 16 and 20/min and regular, and blood pressure within 15% of baseline. Breath sounds clear. Urinary output more than 30 mL/h. Client alert or easily aroused.

LABORATORY. Serum albumin between 3.5–5 g/dL.

**NEGATIVE OUTCOMES**

Temperature is more than 37.5° C, pulse more than 100 bpm, respirations more than 20/min, and blood pressure more than 15% higher or lower than baseline. Breath sounds demonstrate crackles or wheezes. Urinary output less than 30 mL/h. Client lethargic or stuporous.

---

## BLOOD FORMERS

### THERAPEUTIC EFFECTS

Blood formation agents affect hematopoiesis by (1) stimulating the production and differentiation of blood stem cells and (2) enhancing the functioning of mature blood cells. Blood formation agents, also known as colony-stimulating factors, are used to increase neutrophils after cancer chemotherapy, speed up bone marrow recovery after an autologous bone marrow transplant, or increase RBC production in clients with chronic renal failure.

Iron dextran is used to increase RBC formation in clients with iron deficiency anemia.

### PHARMACOKINETICS

**Distribution.** Blood formation agents are widely distributed throughout the body and are rapidly distributed with IV administration.

**Excretion.** The serum half-life of the colony-stimulating factors is approximately 3.5 hours. Colony-stimulating factors do not appear to be affected by hemodialysis. The serum half-life of iron dextran is approximately 6 hours.

### CAUTIONS

**Side/Adverse Effects.** Many of the adverse effects of colony-stimulating factors are also known to be associated with chronic renal failure. Both colony-stimulating factors and iron dextran may cause severe allergic reactions.

Contraindications

***Pregnancy and Lactation.*** Colony-stimulating factors appear to cross the placental barrier and may be passed in breast milk. Studies have not documented fetal harm or injury to infants, but caution should be used.

***Pediatrics.*** Studies have not documented that children have specific age-related effects with colony-stimulating factors. Iron dextran has been associated with an increase in gram-negative sepsis when given intramuscularly to infants younger than 4 months.

***Geriatrics.*** Studies have not documented that the elderly have specific age-related effects with colony-stimulating factors or with iron dextran.

### TOXICTY

See Table 19–3 for toxicities of blood formers.

### POTENTIAL DRUG/FOOD INTERACTIONS

Clients using epoetin may require higher doses of heparin, iron supplements, or antihypertensives. No evidence of interaction with other drugs or food has been reported with filgrastim or sargramostim. Iron dextran may interact with oxytetracycline or sulfadiazine and should not be added to blood for transfusion.

---

## EPOETIN ALFA

*Trade Names:* Epogen, Procrit
*Canadian Availability:* Eprex
*Pregnancy Risk:* Category C
*pH:* 6.6–7.2
*Storage/Stability:* Store between 2° and 8° C. Protect from freezing. Do not shake the vial because it may damage the glycoprotein and inactivate the drug.

### ASSESSMENT: DRUG CHARACTERISTICS

#### ACTION

A product of recombinant DNA technology that resembles human erythropoietin, a hormone that stimulates production of RBCs in the bone marrow. Human erythropoietin is manufactured by the kidney, and in chronic renal failure, anemia is associated with inadequate production of this hormone. Epoetin may also correct bleeding tendencies associated with chronic renal failure.

#### INDICATIONS

Used to treat anemia associated with chronic renal failure or with acquired immunodeficiency syndrome (AIDS).

#### CAUTIONS

**ADVERSE EFFECTS.** Many of the adverse effects of epoetin are also known to be associated with chronic renal failure. Clients should be care-

▼

**TABLE 19–3**
**Toxicities of Blood Formers**

| Body System | Side/Toxic Effects | Physical Assessment Indicators | Laboratory Indicators | Nursing Interventions |
|---|---|---|---|---|
| Neurologic | Central nervous system effects | Headache, dizziness* | N/A | Monitor for client complaints. |
| | Peripheral nervous system effects* | Numbness or tingling of extremities | | |
| Cardiovascular | Cardiotoxic effects | Hypertension, tachycardia*, chest pain, edema, arrhythmias, pericarditis, weakness. | Bleeding time > 9.5 min | Monitor vital signs and report abnormal results; be prepared to give cardiotonics or diuretics. |
| | Capillary leak syndrome | Peripheral edema | | |
| | Vascular effects | Thrombophlebitis, thromboses | | |
| Respiratory | | Pleural effusion, shortness of breath | N/A | |
| Renal | Chronic renal failure | Fluid retention | Hematocrit > 52%, hemoglobin > 16 g/100 | Measure and record intake and output; report significant weight gain. |
| | Hematopoietic | Polycythemia | | |
| Gastrointestinal | Hepatic effects | Splenomegaly | N/A | Observe for and report any client distress. |
| | Gastrointestinal disturbance* | Nausea or vomiting | | |
| Other | Anaphylactic reaction | Rash, wheezing, urticaria, hypotension | N/A | Monitor vital signs; discontinue intravenous administration if severe symptoms are present; be prepared to give oxygen, epinephrine, or other medications as ordered. |
| | Sweet's syndrome | Fever, sores on skin, or other skin rashes | | |

*Iron dextran effects.
N/A = not applicable.

fully evaluated. May cause hypertension, tachycardia, headache, chest pain, edema, or polycythemia.

CONTRAINDICATIONS. Hypersensitivity to human albumin or uncontrolled hypertension.

**POTENTIAL DRUG/FOOD INTERACTIONS**

Clients using epoetin may require higher doses of heparin, iron supplements, or antihypertensives.

**INTERVENTIONS: ADMINISTRATION**

May be given undiluted.

**MODE/RATE OF ADMINISTRATION**

Usually given by rapid IV injection over at least 1 min.

INTRAVENOUS USE (WITH NORMAL RENAL FUNCTION)

**Adults:** Usual dosage is 50–100 U/kg of body weight three times a week. After 8 weeks, if hematocrit (Hct) has not improved by 5–6 points, the dosage may be increased. Dosage increases are usually by 25 U/kg of body weight until a dose is achieved that will maintain the Hct at 30%–33%. The maximum recommended dose is 300 U/kg of body weight three times a week.

**Children ≤12 years:** Dose not established.

**Children >12 years:** Follow adult dosing schedule.

**Infants/Neonates:** Dose not established.

**Geriatrics:** Follow adult dosing schedule.

INTRATHECAL USE OR OTHER INFUSION ROUTES AS INDICATED. Not recommended.

**POTENTIAL PROBLEMS IN ADMINISTRATION**

Dose should be decreased if the Hct increases by more than 4–6 points in a 2-week period. Doses should be omitted if the Hct is above 36%.

**INDEPENDENT NURSING ACTIONS**

Monitor vital signs. Determine client complaints of numbness, tingling, depression, fatigue, weakness, malaise, sensitivity to cold, headache, dizziness, syncope, chest pain, sore mouth, anorexia, nausea, or weight loss. Observe for diaphoresis, conjunctival pallor, pale mucous membranes, oral ulcerations, shortness of breath, or dyspnea on exertion.

**ADMINISTRATION IN ALTERNATE SETTINGS**

May be given in a variety of clinical settings by a qualified IV nurse.

**EVALUATION: OUTCOMES OF DRUG THERAPY**

**EXPECTED OUTCOMES**

PHYSICAL ASSESSMENT. Pulse between 60 and 100 bpm and regular. Blood pressure less than 160 mm Hg systolic. Respiratory rate between 16 and 20/min. Client able to carry out activities of daily living (ADLs) without complaints of fatigue, malaise, or dizziness.

LABORATORY. Complete blood count shows RBCs between 4.4 and 5.5 106/mm$^3$, reticulocyte count between 25,000 and 75,000/mm$^3$, platelets between 150,000 and 450,000/mm$^3$, hemoglobin (Hgb) more than 11 g/dL,

Hct between 30% and 33%, and no erythrocyte abnormalities.

**NEGATIVE OUTCOMES**

Pulse more than 100 bpm and irregular. Blood pressure more than 160 mm Hg systolic. Respiratory rate more than 24/min. Client complains of headache, fatigue, shortness of breath, or chest pain. Client unable to carry out ADLs without complaints of fatigue, dyspnea on exertion, or dizziness.

## FILGRASTIM (G-CSF)

*Trade Name:* Neupogen
*Canadian Availability:* Neupogen
*Pregnancy Risk:* Category C
*pH:* 4
*Storage/Stability:* Store between 2° and 8° C. Protect from freezing. Do not shake. May be left at room temperature for a maximum of 6 hours after completely thawing.

### ASSESSMENT: DRUG CHARACTERISTICS

**ACTION**

A granulocyte colony stimulating factor (G-CSF) that acts on hematopoietic cells to stimulate production and some end-cell functional activation. As a lineage specific agent, acts to increase production of neutrophils only. Acts later in the development cycle in the bone marrow after differentiation is determined. May decrease serum cholesterol.

**INDICATIONS**

Used to treat chemotherapy-induced neutropenia in nonmyeloid leukemias. Has been used investigationally to accelerate myeloid recovery in clients undergoing autologous bone marrow transplantation and to treat AIDS-related granulocytopenia from zidovudine administration.

**CAUTIONS**

ADVERSE EFFECTS. Allergic response or anaphylactic reaction, arrhythmias, splenomegaly, Sweet's syndrome (fever, sores on skin), or other skin rashes.

CONTRAINDICATIONS. Excessive leukemic myeloid blasts in the bone marrow or sensitivity to filgrastim or *Escherichia coli*–derived proteins.

**POTENTIAL DRUG/FOOD INTERACTIONS**

No evidence of interaction with other drugs or food has been reported.

### INTERVENTIONS: ADMINISTRATION

Should be diluted in D5W solution to achieve a concentration of 15 mcg (0.015 mg) of filgrastim per milliliter or more. If the concentration is less than 15 mcg/mL, human albumin should be added to the solution to prevent the filgrastim from being adsorbed to the IV components. The concentration of human albumin should be 0.2%, achieved by adding 2 mL of 5% human albumin to 50 mL of D5W.

▼

**MODE/RATE OF ADMINISTRATION**

May be given as an intermittent IV infusion over 30 min or as a continuous IV infusion.

INTRAVENOUS USE (WITH NORMAL RENAL FUNCTION)

**Adults:** For neutropenia the usual dosage is 5 mcg (0.005 mg)/kg of body weight once a day, beginning at least 24 h after the last dose of chemotherapy. The daily schedule is maintained until the absolute neutrophil count (ANC) is at least 10,000/mm$^3$ following the nadir. The dose may be increased by 5 mcg (0.005 mg)/kg of body weight for succeeding courses of chemotherapy if necessary. The dose should be rounded off to the nearest full vial to reduce wastage. Maximum dose not established.

**Children:** Dose not established.

**Infants/Neonates:** Dose not established.

**Geriatrics:** Little information about effects of colony-stimulating factors on the elderly. Follow adult dosing schedule.

INTRATHECAL USE OR OTHER INFUSION ROUTES AS INDICATED. Not recommended.

**POTENTIAL PROBLEMS IN ADMINISTRATION**

Should not be given within 24 h before or after chemotherapy because the stimulation of cells may cause them to be more susceptible to the effects of radiation or chemotherapy.

**INDEPENDENT NURSING ACTIONS**

Monitor vital signs, especially pulse rate and regularity and respiratory rate and regularity. Determine client complaints of bone pain, fatigue, weakness, malaise, headache, dizziness, syncope, or chest pain. Observe for shortness of breath or dyspnea on exertion.

**ADMINISTRATION IN ALTERNATE SETTINGS**

Not recommended for administration in the home setting. May be given in a wide variety of clinical settings by a qualified IV nurse.

**EVALUATION: OUTCOMES OF DRUG THERAPY**

**EXPECTED OUTCOMES**

PHYSICAL ASSESSMENT. Pulse between 60 and 100 bpm and regular. Temperature less than 37.5° C. Respiratory rate between 16 and 20/min. Breath sounds clear. Client able to carry out ADLs without complaints of fatigue or malaise.

LABORATORY. White blood cell count (WBC) shows neutrophils at 10,000/mm$^3$.

**NEGATIVE OUTCOMES**

Pulse more than 100 bpm and irregular. Temperature more than 37.5° C. Respiratory rate more than 24/min. Breath sounds demonstrate crackles and wheezes. Client complains of headache, fatigue, shortness of breath, or chest pain. Client unable to carry out ADLs without complaints of fatigue or dyspnea on exertion.

# Iron Dextran

*Trade Names:* InFeD, Imferon
*Canadian Availability:* Imferon
*Pregnancy Risk:* Category C
*pH:* 5.2–6.5
*Storage/Stability:* Store below 40° C. Protect from freezing.

## ASSESSMENT: DRUG CHARACTERISTICS

### ACTION

Iron is absorbed from stomach mucosa and transported to bone marrow for incorporation into RBCs as Hgb. Iron is also an important component of myoglobin and several essential enzymes.

### INDICATIONS

Used to restore Hgb and iron supplies in iron deficiency anemias.

### CAUTIONS

ADVERSE EFFECTS. Acute allergic response, backache or muscle pain, headache, nausea or vomiting, numbness or tingling of extremities, chest pain, dizziness, or tachycardia.

CONTRAINDICATIONS. Hemochromatosis, hemosiderosis, or other anemias if not accompanied by iron deficiency.

### POTENTIAL DRUG/FOOD INTERACTIONS

May interact with oxytetracycline and sulfadiazine. Should not be added to blood for transfusion.

## INTERVENTIONS: ADMINISTRATION

May be given undiluted or mixed in 0.9% NSS for injection.

### MODE/RATE OF ADMINISTRATION

May be given by IV push at not more than 1 mL/min or by continuous infusion over 4–5 h.

INTRAVENOUS USE (WITH NORMAL RENAL FUNCTION)

**Adults:** If no allergic symptoms develop from the test dose, the usual dosage is 100 mg/d until the total calculated therapeutic dose is achieved. The dose calculation follows:

$$\text{Iron Dextran (mL)} = 0.0476 \times \text{Body Weight (kg)} \times \text{Hemoglobin} + \text{Iron Stores (1 mL/5 kg Body Weight)}$$

The amount of iron dextran for replacing iron stores should not exceed 14 mL.

**Children:** If no allergic symptoms develop from the test dose, the usual dosage for children weighing less than 10 kg is 50 mg/d until the total calculated therapeutic dose is achieved. The dose calculation follows:

$$\text{Iron Dextran (mL)} = 0.0476 \times \text{Body Weight (kg)} \times (12 - \text{Hemoglobin}) + \text{Iron Stores (1 mL/5 kg Body Weight)}$$

The amount of iron dextran for replacing iron stores should not exceed 14 mL.

▼

**Infants/Neonates:** If no allergic symptoms develop from the test dose, the usual dosage for infants weighing up to 5 kg is 50 mg/d until the total calculated therapeutic dose is achieved.

**Geriatrics:** Follow adult dosing schedule.

INTRATHECAL USE OR OTHER INFUSION ROUTES AS INDICATED. Not recommended.

#### POTENTIAL PROBLEMS IN ADMINISTRATION

Clients may be allergic to iron dextran. A test dose of 25 mg of iron dextran should be given to all clients before their first therapeutic dose. At least 1 h should elapse between the test dose and the first therapeutic dose to assure that any allergic symptoms can be noted.

#### INDEPENDENT NURSING ACTIONS

Monitor vital signs. Determine client complaints of numbness, tingling, depression, fatigue, weakness, malaise, headache, dizziness, syncope, chest pain, anorexia, or nausea. Observe for diaphoresis, conjunctival pallor, pale mucous membranes, oral ulcerations, beefy red tongue, shortness of breath, dyspnea on exertion, tarry stools, constipation, diarrhea, or hematemesis.

#### ADMINISTRATION IN ALTERNATE SETTINGS

Not usually given intravenously in the home setting. May be given in a wide variety of clinical settings by a qualified IV nurse.

#### EVALUATION: OUTCOMES OF DRUG THERAPY

#### EXPECTED OUTCOMES

PHYSICAL ASSESSMENT. Pulse between 60 and 100 bpm and regular. Respiratory rate between 16 and 20/min. Client able to carry out ADLs without complaints of fatigue or malaise.

LABORATORY. Complete blood count shows RBCs between 4.4 and 5.5 × 106/mm$^3$, reticulocyte count between 25,000 and 75,000/mm$^3$, platelets between 150,000 and 450,000/mm$^3$, Hgb between 13.0 and 16.5 g/dL, Hct between 40% and 50%, and no erythrocyte abnormalities.

#### NEGATIVE OUTCOMES

Pulse more than 100 bpm and irregular. Respiratory rate more than 24/min. Client complains of headache, fatigue, shortness of breath, or chest pain. Client unable to carry out ADLs without complaints of fatigue or dyspnea on exertion.

---

## SARGRAMOSTIM (GM-CSF)

*Trade Names:* Leukine, Prokine
*Canadian Availability:* Not commercially available
*Pregnancy Risk:* Category C

*pH:* 4
*Storage/Stability:* Store between 2° and 8° C. Protect from freezing. Do not shake. May store at room tempera-

ture for 6 hours after reconstituting.

## ASSESSMENT: DRUG CHARACTERISTICS

### ACTION

A granulocyte macrophage colony stimulating factor (GM-CSF) that acts on hematopoietic cells to stimulate production, differentiation, and some end-cell functional activation. As a lineage nonspecific agent, acts to increase production of granulocytes (neutrophils and eosinophils) and macrophages. Is active during the early development of cells in the bone marrow. Has been reported to increase the replication of human immunodeficiency virus and to reduce low-density lipoprotein (LDL).

### INDICATIONS

Used to treat chemotherapy-induced neutropenia in nonmyeloid leukemias. Has been used investigationally to accelerate myeloid recovery in clients undergoing autologous bone marrow transplantation and to treat AIDS-related granulocytopenia from zidovudine administration.

### CAUTIONS

ADVERSE EFFECTS. Capillary leak syndrome, pleural or pericardial effusion, peripheral edema, fluid retention, fever, shortness of breath, pericarditis, thrombophlebitis, thromboses, first-dose reaction, and weakness.

CONTRAINDICATIONS. Excessive leukemic myeloid blasts in the bone marrow, sensitivity to sargramostim or to yeast-derived proteins, congestive heart failure, or impaired renal or hepatic functioning.

### POTENTIAL DRUG/FOOD INTERACTIONS

No evidence of interaction with other drugs or food has been reported.

## INTERVENTIONS: ADMINISTRATION

Reconstitute with 1 mL of sterile water to a vial containing 250–500 mcg (0.25–0.5 mg). Do not shake. Add reconstituted sargramostim to 0.9% NSS. If the concentration of sargramostim is less than 10 mcg (0.01 mg)/mL, human albumin should be added to the solution to prevent the sargramostim from being adsorbed to the IV components. The concentration of human albumin should be 0.1%, achieved by adding 1 mL of 5% human albumin to 50 mL of 0.9% NSS for injection.

### MODE/RATE OF ADMINISTRATION

Given as an intermittent infusion over 2 h via a central venous line.

INTRAVENOUS USE (WITH NORMAL RENAL FUNCTION)

**Adults:** For myeloid engraftment the usual dosage is 250 mcg (0.025 mg)/m$^2$ of body surface area (BSA) per day for 21 d beginning 2–4 h after autologous bone marrow transplantation. Should not be given less than 24 h before or after chemotherapy. The dose should be rounded off, within reason, to the nearest full vial to reduce wastage. Maximum dose not established.

▼

**Children:** Dose not established.

**Infants/Neonates:** Dose not established.

**Geriatrics:** Little information about effects of colony-stimulating factors on the elderly. Follow adult dosing schedule.

INTRATHECAL USE OR OTHER INFUSION ROUTES AS INDICATED. Not recommended.

#### POTENTIAL PROBLEMS IN ADMINISTRATION

If shortness of breath occurs during administration, the IV rate should be slowed to one half the rate. If dyspnea persists, the IV infusion should be discontinued. Should not be given within 24 h before or after chemotherapy because the stimulation of cells may cause them to be more susceptible to the effects of radiation or chemotherapy.

#### INDEPENDENT NURSING ACTIONS

Monitor vital signs, especially pulse rate and regularity and respiratory rate and regularity. Determine client complaints of bone pain, fatigue, weakness, malaise, headache, dizziness, syncope, or chest pain. Observe for shortness of breath or dyspnea on exertion.

#### ADMINISTRATION IN ALTERNATE SETTINGS

Not recommended for administration in the home setting. May be given in a wide variety of clinical settings by a qualified IV nurse.

#### EVALUATION: OUTCOMES OF DRUG THERAPY

#### EXPECTED OUTCOMES

PHYSICAL ASSESSMENT. Pulse between 60 and 100 bpm and regular. Temperature less than 37.5° C. Respiratory rate between 16 and 20/min. Breath sounds clear. Client able to carry out ADLs without complaints of fatigue or malaise.

LABORATORY. WBC shows neutrophils at 10,000/mm$^3$.

#### NEGATIVE OUTCOMES

Pulse more than 100 bpm and irregular. Temperature more than 37.5° C. Respiratory rate more than 24/min. Breath sounds demonstrate crackles and wheezes. Client complains of headache, fatigue, shortness of breath, or chest pain. Client unable to carry out ADLs without complaints of fatigue or dyspnea on exertion.

## ANTICOAGULANTS AND HEMOSTATICS

### THERAPEUTIC EFFECTS

Anticoagulants have antifibrinolytic and antihemorrhagic activities that inhibit the activation of plasminogen. Plasminogen converts to plasmin (fibrinolysin), which breaks down fibrin and fibrinogen in clots. These agents are used to treat venous thrombosis, pulmonary embolism, disseminated intravascular coagulation (DIC), and peripheral arterial embolism. In addition, anticoagulants are used to prevent coagulation during procedures such as hemodialysis and cardiac surgery when blood is circulated outside the body or in various indwelling venipuncture devices.

Hemostatic agents may inhibit the anticoagulant activity of heparin, counter hyperactivity of fibrinolysis, or provide an essential component needed to convert prothrombin to thrombin for blood clotting. These agents are used to treat hemorrhage caused by hyperfibrinolysis or surgery, to treat uncontrolled severe bleeding that results from heparin overdose, or prevent or treat bleeding in clients who have hemophilia A, or factor VIII deficiency.

## PHARMACOKINETICS

**Distribution.** Heparin is widely distributed when given intravenously. Hemostatic agents are quickly and widely distributed when given intravenously.

**Metabolism/Elimination.** Heparin appears to be metabolized partially within the walls of blood vessels and partially by the kidneys and excreted as metabolites. The half-life of heparin is 1 to 2 hours, with the half-life increasing as the dosage is increased. Heparin is not removed by hemodialysis.

Hemostatic agents are excreted by the kidneys. The half-life varies according to the agent but is usually between 4 and 24 hours. Hemodialysis removes aminocaproic acid.

## CAUTIONS

**Side/Adverse Effects.** Heparin may cause excessive bleeding. Hemostatic agents may cause blood clotting.

### Contraindications

***Pregnancy and Lactation.*** Heparin should be used with caution during the third trimester because of the risk of postpartum hemorrhage. Heparin does not appear to cross the placental barrier or to be passed in breast milk.

Hemostatic agents have not been documented to cause maternal or fetal harm; however, extensive studies have not been conducted. It is not known if these agents are passed in breast milk.

***Pediatrics.*** Heparin should be used cautiously in neonates. A preservative-free solution should be used to avoid neurotoxicity. Doses must be carefully monitored to prevent intraventricular hemorrhage.

Hemostatic agents have not been documented to cause harm; however, extensive studies have not been conducted.

***Geriatrics.*** The elderly may be more susceptible to hemorrhage from heparin. Hemostatic agents have not been documented to cause harm; however, extensive studies have not been conducted.

## TOXICITY

See Table 19–4 for toxicities of blood coagulants.

## POTENTIAL DRUG/FOOD INTERACTIONS

Heparin may interact with platelet aggregation inhibitors, cefamandole, cefoperazone, cefotetan, moxalactam, plicamycin, valproic acid, methimazole, propylthiouracil, probenecid, or other thrombolytic enzymes. Heparin is incompatible with solutions that contain a phosphate buffer, sodium bicarbonate, or sodium oxalate. Since heparin is very acidic, it may be incompatible with a number of medications and should be administered through a separate line unless compatibility is completely assured.

Hemostatic agents such as protamine sulfate (heparin's antidote) and AHF have no significant reported interactions. Aminocaproic acid may interact with antiinhibitor coagulatnt complex, factor IX, contraceptives such as estrogen, or thrombolytic enzymes such as alteplase, streptokinase, and urokinase.

Protamine sulfate is incompatible with several of the cephalosporins and penicillins.

---

# Aminocaproic Acid

*Trade Name:* Amicar
*Canadian Availability:* Amicar
*Pregnancy Risk:* Category C
*pH:* 6.8
*Storage/Stability:* Store below 40° C. Protect from freezing.

### ASSESSMENT: DRUG CHARACTERISTICS

#### ACTION

An antifibrinolytic and antihemorrhagic agent that inhibits the activation of plasminogen. Plasminogen converts to plasmin (fibrinolysin), which breaks down fibrin and fibrinogen in clots. Reduced plasminogen increases blood clot activity.

#### INDICATIONS

Used to treat hemorrhage caused by hyperfibrinolysis or surgery.

#### CAUTIONS

ADVERSE EFFECTS. Hypotension, bladder obstruction caused by clot formation, headache, dizziness, myopathy, renal failure, tinnitus, skin rash, arrhythmias, stomach cramps, or thromboembolism.

CONTRAINDICATIONS. DIC, cardiac disease, hematuria, impaired hepatic or renal function, a history of thrombus, or hypersensitivity to aminocaproic acid.

#### POTENTIAL DRUG/FOOD INTERACTIONS

May interact with antiinhibitor coagulant complex, factor IX, or contraceptives such as estrogen to increase the risk of thrombus formation. Mutually antagonistic to thrombolytic agents such

▼

**TABLE 19–4**
**Toxicities of Anticoagulants and Hemostatics**

| Body System | Side/Toxic Effects | Physical Assessment Indicators | Laboratory Indicators | Nursing Interventions |
|---|---|---|---|---|
| Neurologic | Peripheral neuropathy | Itching, burning pain in extremities, paresthesias* | N/A | Check circulation of extremities; monitor client complaints of pain; report abnormal findings. |
| | Intracranial bleeding | Headache, dizziness, somnolence, changes in level of consciousness* | | Monitor level of consciousness and neurologic indicators such as pupil size. |
| Cardiovascular | Bleeding | Bleeding from gums, bloody urine or stool | Bleeding time >9.5 min, PT >2 s deviation from control, PTT >38 s, TT > control +5 s | Observe for evidence of bleeding; monitor vital signs; using heparin, be prepared to give protamine as antidote. |
| | Arrhythmias* | Chest pain, bradycardia, tachycardia, arrhythmias, sudden hypotension, shock | | |
| | Thromboembolism* | Pain, cyanosis, cold extremities | | |
| Respiratory | | Dyspnea, pulmonary edema | ABG $Po_2$ <80 mm Hg | Report promptly; be prepared to give oxygen, epinephrine, or other medications as ordered. |
| Renal | Bladder obstruction* | Difficulty with urination | RBCs in urine Sp. Gr. < 1.003, BUN > 50 mg/dL, creatinine > 1.5 mg/dL | Measure and record intake and output; observe color for evidence of bleeding; report promptly. |
| | Renal failure* | Decreased urine output | | |
| Gastrointestinal | Gastrointestinal disturbance* | Stomach cramps, nausea, vomiting | N/A | Monitor client complaints; observe stool for evidence of bleeding. |
| Special senses | Eyes*, ears | Visual changes, tinnitus | N/A | Monitor client complaints; report promptly. |
| Dermatologic | Skin lesions | Skin necrosis | N/A | Observe client. |
| Other | Allergic reactions | Fever, chills, urticaria, or flushing | N/A | Discontinue agent immediately; be prepared to give epinephrine or other medications as ordered. |

*Hemostatic agents.

as alteplase, streptokinase, and urokinase.

**INTERVENTIONS: ADMINISTRATION**

Should not be given undiluted. Dilute with 0.9% NSS, D5W, or Ringer's lactate.

**MODE/RATE OF ADMINISTRATION**

May be given by intermittent or continuous infusion.

INTRAVENOUS USE (WITH NORMAL RENAL FUNCTION)

**Adults:** For acute bleeding the usual initial dosage is 4–5 g over 1 h. Further treatment with 1 g/h for 8 h by continuous infusion or until bleeding is stopped. Postsurgical bleeding may be treated with 6 g or less in 24 h. Maximum dose is 30 g in 24 h.

**Children:** The usual initial dose is 100 mg/kg of body weight over 1 h, then 33.3 mg/kg/h by continuous infusion. Maximum dose is 18 g/m$^2$ in 24 h.

**Infants/Neonates:** Follow children's dosing schedule.

**Geriatrics:** Elderly clients may have age-related diminished renal function, which may require a lower dose.

INTRATHECAL USE OR OTHER INFUSION ROUTES AS INDICATED. Not recommended.

**POTENTIAL PROBLEMS IN ADMINISTRATION**

Rapid IV administration may cause hypertension or bradycardia. Care should be taken to stabilize the IV needle to avoid increased incidence of clot formation.

**INDEPENDENT NURSING ACTIONS**

Monitor heart rate and rhythm, electrocardiograph (ECG) reports, and hemodynamic status (if available) frequently. Monitor fluid intake and output, coagulation profile (fibrinogen, fibrin degradation products, prothrombin time/partial thromboplastin time [PT/PTT]), and blood urea nitrogen (BUN).

**ADMINISTRATION IN ALTERNATE SETTINGS**

IV administration should be done in settings where the client can be closely monitored and where full cardiac technologic support is available.

**EVALUATION: OUTCOMES OF DRUG THERAPY**

**EXPECTED OUTCOMES**

PHYSICAL ASSESSMENT. No evidence of bleeding. Systolic blood pressure remains above 75 mm Hg and below 160 mm Hg. Heart rate between 60 and 100 bpm and regular. No complaints of weakness, fatigue, or headache. Extremities warm, pink, and free of edema. Urinary output more than 30 mL/h.

LABORATORY. Fibrinogen level between 200 and 400 mg/dL, fibrin degradation products less than 10 mg/L, PT 9.5 to 12 seconds, PTT 20 to 45 seconds, and BUN 10 to 20 mg/dL.

**NEGATIVE OUTCOMES**

Evidence of active bleeding. Marked hypotension and a weak, irregular heart rate less than 60 bpm. Client complains of weakness, fatigue, or headache. Urine output less than 30 mL/h. Extremities pale and cool. Client confused or lethargic.

## Antihemophilic Factor (Factor VIII, AHF)

*Trade Name:* Hemofil M
*Canadian Availability:* Koate-HP specified.
*Pregnancy Risk:* Category C
*pH:* Not specified.
*Storage/Stability:* Store between 2° and 8° C. Protect from freezing. Some preparations may be stored up to 3 to 6 months at room temperature. Check label. Reconstituted solutions are stable for 24 hours at room temperature, but should be used within 3 hours. Some preparations should be given within 1 hour. Discard if discolored or contains precipitate.

### ASSESSMENT: DRUG CHARACTERISTICS

#### ACTION

A hemostatic substance essential for the conversion of prothrombin to thrombin for blood clotting.

#### INDICATIONS

Used to prevent or treat bleeding in clients who have hemophilia A, or factor VIII deficiency.

#### CAUTIONS

ADVERSE EFFECTS. Tachycardia, hypotension, headache, paresthesias, visual changes, somnolence, changes in level of consciousness, back pain, nausea, vomiting, or symptoms of allergic reaction such as fever, chills, urticaria, or flushing.

CONTRAINDICATIONS. Sensitivity to mouse or bovine protein.

#### POTENTIAL DRUG/FOOD INTERACTIONS

No significant interactions reported.

### INTERVENTIONS: ADMINISTRATION

Must be reconstituted. Warm vial and diluent to room temperature, but not more than 37° C. Do not shake vial to mix. Gently rotate. May take up to 10 min to completely reconstitute. Do not refrigerate the reconstituted solution. Solution should not fall below room temperature during administration because a precipitate may form.

#### MODE/RATE OF ADMINISTRATION

May be given by slow IV push at a rate of 2 mL but not more than 4 mL/min or by continuous infusion.

INTRAVENOUS USE (WITH NORMAL RENAL FUNCTION)

**Adults:** Dosage is individualized based on the severity of factor VIII deficiency, severity of hemorrhage, weight, and coagulation studies completed prior to beginning treatment. The expected increase in AHF can be estimated from the following formula:

1. Expected Factor VIII Increase (% Normal) = Units Given/Body Weight in kg × 2–2.5
2. Units Required = Body Weight (kg) × 0.4–0.5 × Desired Factor VIII Increase

For joint hemorrhages the usual dosage is 8 U/kg q8–12h for 1–2 d.

▼

For minor hemorrhage in muscles or extremities the usual dosage is 8 U/kg q24h for 2–3 d.

For severe hemorrhage in nonvital areas the usual dosage is 8 U/kg q12h for 2 d, then q.d. for 2 d.

For severe hemorrhage in or near vital organs the usual initial dose is 15 U/kg, followed by 8 U/kg q8h for 48 h, then 4 U/kg q8h for another 48 h.

For overt bleeding the usual dose is 15 U/kg, followed by 8 U/kg q8–12h for 3–4 d.

For prophylactic treatment of severe factor VIII deficiency, an individualized dose is given q1–2 d to maintain the AHF level at not more than 15% below normal.

**Children:** Follow adult dosing schedule.

**Infants/Neonates:** Follow adult dosing schedule.

**Geriatrics:** Follow adult dosing schedule.

INTRATHECAL USE OR OTHER INFUSION ROUTES AS INDICATED. Not recommended.

#### POTENTIAL PROBLEMS IN ADMINISTRATION

May cause tachycardia if given too rapidly. Pulse should be taken prior to beginning therapy and monitored during therapy. The infusion rate should be slowed if a rapid increase in pulse rate is detected. Should be administered with a plastic syringe only because the AHF may cling to glass.

#### INDEPENDENT NURSING ACTIONS

Observe for evidence of bleeding. Monitor heart rate and rhythm frequently. Monitor fluid intake and output and AHF levels.

#### ADMINISTRATION IN ALTERNATE SETTINGS

May be given in a variety of clinical settings by a qualified IV nurse. May be given in the home setting.

#### EVALUATION: OUTCOMES OF DRUG THERAPY

#### EXPECTED OUTCOMES

PHYSICAL ASSESSMENT. No evidence of bleeding. Systolic blood pressure remains above 75 mm Hg and below 160 mm Hg. Heart rate between 60 and 100 bpm and regular. No complaints of weakness, fatigue, or headache. Extremities warm, pink, and free of edema. Urinary output more than 30 mL/h.

LABORATORY. AHF levels within 30% to 60% of normal.

#### NEGATIVE OUTCOMES

Evidence of active bleeding. Marked hypotension and a weak, irregular heart rate less than 60 bpm; client complains of weakness, fatigue, or headache; is confused or lethargic. Urine output less than 30 mL,/h. Extremities pale and cool.

# APROTINININ

*Trade Name:* Trasylol
*Canadian Availability:* Not specified
*Pregnancy Risk:* Category C
*pH:* Unspecified
*Storage/Stability:* Not specified

## ASSESSMENT: DRUG CHARACTERISTICS

### ACTION

A bovine proteinase inhibitor that acts as an antifibrinolytic.

### INDICATIONS

Used to reduce blood loss from surgery such as coronary artery bypass grafting (CABG), thus reducing the need for homologous blood transfusions. Also used to reduce hemorrhage for hyperfibrinolysis and pancreatitis.

### CAUTIONS

ADVERSE EFFECTS. Has been associated with atrial fibrillation, myocardial infarction, and congestive heart failure with open heart surgery. May also cause renal dysfunction or anaphylactic shock.

CONTRAINDICATIONS. Should not be given to clients with a known hypersensitivity reaction to the drug.

### POTENTIAL DRUG/FOOD INTERACTIONS

May inhibit the action of fibrinolytic agents. May block the action of captopril. May prolong clotting times if given with heparin.

## INTERVENTIONS: ADMINISTRATION

Premixed containers have 10,000 KIU/1 mL.

### MODE/RATE OF ADMINISTRATION

The loading dose should be given over at least 4 min through a free-flowing IV line of 0.9% NSS or a D5W solution.

INTRAVENOUS USE (WITH NORMAL RENAL FUNCTION)

**Adults:** For surgery the usual dose is 2,000,000 KIU (200 mL) as a loading dose 20–30 min after anesthesia is begun but before the chest is opened, and 500,000 KIU (50 mL)/h by slow infusion for the duration of the surgery.

For hyperfibrinolysis-induced hemorrhage the usual dose is 200,000–500,000 KIU (20–50 mL) with 200,000 KIU (20 mL) given in the first 4 min and the rest by slow infusion.

For pancreatitis the usual dose is 100,000–200,000 KIU (10–20 mL) by slow infusion, and 100,000 KIU (10 mL) q6h for 4–5 d.

**Children:** Dose not established.

**Infants/Neonates:** Dose not established.

**Geriatrics:** More likely to have preexisting conditions that increase the likelihood of renal dysfunction. Follow adult dosing schedule and monitor.

INTRATHECAL USED OR OTHER INFUSION ROUTES AS INDICATED. Not recommended.

### POTENTIAL PROBLEMS IN ADMINISTRATION

A test dose of 10,000 KIU (1mL) is given 10 min before ▼

the loading dose. If the client does not demonstrate any adverse reactions, the loading dose is given after the induction of anesthesia, A dose of 2,000,000 KIU (200 mL) is also added to the priming fluid in the surgical equipment before surgery begins. Clients with previous exposure to the drug are more likely to demonstrate severe hypersensitivity reactions.

**INDEPENDENT NURSING ACTIONS**

Be sure the client's medical record has a location to record whether the client has previously received the drug. Place an allergic sticker on the client's chart to indicate that he has had the drug to alert others to the risk of anaphylactic shock. Suggest that the surgeon note the use of the drug in his surgical summary and postoperative orders. Before the client's discharge, be sure the client and family are aware of the risks involved with further use of the drug. Encourage the use of a medical-alert bracelet to indicate previous exposure to the drug.

**ADMINISTRATION IN ALTERNATE SETTINGS**

IV administration should be done in settings where the client can be closely monitored and where full cardiac and respiratory technologic support is available.

**EVALUATION: OUTCOMES OF DRUG THERAPY**

**EXPECTED OUTCOMES**

PHYSICAL ASSESSMENT. Heart rate, blood pressure, and pulse remain within 15% of client's baseline. Lung sounds clear. No lower extremity edema. Skin clear. Client remains alert and responsive.

LABORATORY. BUN and serum creatinine remain within 15% of client's baseline.

NEGATIVE OUTCOMES. Artrial fibrillation. Blood pressure more than 15% lower than baseline. Wheezes and crackles heard on lung auscultation. Respirations labored. Urine scant and concentrated. Lower extremity edema. Skin has rashes or urticaria. Client complains of difficulty breathing and severe itching. Client appears restless, confused, or anxious.

---

## HEPARIN SODIUM

*Trade Name:* Liquaemin
*Canadian Availability:* Hepalean, Heparin Leo
*Pregnancy Risk:* Category C
*pH:* 5.0–7.5
*Storage/Stability:* Store below 40° C. Protect from freezing. Do not use if solution is discolored or has a precipitate. Should be used within 24 hours if mixed with D5W for injection. Should not be mixed with other medications in a solution.

**ASSESSMENT: DRUG CHARACTERISTICS**

**ACTION**

An anticoagulant that indirectly acts at many sites in the intrinsic and extrinsic clotting pathways. Heparin, with several cofactors, prevents the conversion of prothrombin to thrombin and fibrinogen to fibrin. In addition, appears to decrease the stickiness of platelets.

**INDICATIONS**

Used to treat cerebral thrombosis, deep vein thrombosis, arterial and systemic thromboembolism, DIC, and prophylactically to prevent blood clotting during renal dialysis, open heart surgery, and indwelling intermittent IV device use.

**CAUTIONS**

ADVERSE EFFECTS. Allergic reactions; active bleeding; chest pain; skin necrosis; peripheral neuropathy; or pain, cyanosis, and cold extremities.

CONTRAINDICATIONS. Aneurysm; active bleeding; recent cerebrovascular accident; surgery, trauma, or recent childbirth; or severe hypertension.

**POTENTIAL DRUG/FOOD INTERACTIONS**

May interact with platelet aggregation inhibitors such as aspirin to cause uncontrolled bleeding. May increase the hypoprothrombinemia associated with cefamandole, cefoperazone, cefotetan, moxalactam, plicamycin, or valproic acid, methimazole, or propylthiouracil. Probenecid may increase and prolong the effects of heparin. Use with thrombolytic agents such as alteplase, streptokinase, and urokinase may increase the risk of bleeding but may decrease the incidence of reocclusion.

**INTERVENTIONS: ADMINISTRATION**

May be given undiluted or mixed in D5W, 0.9% NSS, or Ringer's injection.

**MODE/RATE OF ADMINISTRATION**

May be given by rapid IV injection and by intermittent and continuous IV infusion, using an infusion pump.

INTRAVENOUS USE (WITH NORMAL RENAL FUNCTION)

**Adults:** For a full-dose intermittent regimen the usual dosing schedule is 10,000 U initially, then 5000–10,000 U q4–6 h or 100 U/kg of body weight q4h, depending on the results of blood coagulation studies.

For a full-dose continuous regimen the usual dosing schedule is 35–70 U/kg of body weight or 5000 U initially, then 20,000–40,000 U in 1000 mL of 0.9% NSS at a rate of 1000 U/h, depending on the results of blood coagulation studies.

For cardiac and vascular surgery the usual dose is less than 150 U/kg of body weight, depending on the expected length of surgery.

For disseminated intravascular coagulation the usual dosage is 50–100 U/kg of body weight q4h by rapid IV injection or continuous infusion.

▼

**Children:** For a full-dose intermittent regimen the usual dosing schedule is 50 U/kg of body weight initially, then 50–100 U/kg of body weight q4–6h, depending on the results of blood coagulation studies.

For a full-dose continuous regimen the usual dosing schedule is 50 U/kg of body weight initially, then at a rate of 100 U/kg of body weight q4h, depending on the results of blood coagulation studies.

For cardiac and vascular surgery the usual dose is less than 150 U/kg of body weight, depending on the expected length of surgery.

For disseminated intravascular coagulation the usual dosage is 25–50 U/kg of body weight q4h by rapid IV injection or continuous infusion.

**Infants/Neonates:** Dose not established.

**Geriatrics:** Elderly clients may be more prone to active bleeding from therapy. May be more likely to have age-related changes in renal function that may prolong the effects of therapy or require a lower dose.

INTRATHECAL USE OR OTHER INFUSION ROUTES AS INDICATED. Not recommended.

#### POTENTIAL PROBLEMS IN ADMINISTRATION

Clients who require heparin after surgery, who have an infection, or who have active thromboembolic disorders such as pulmonary embolism may require a higher dose because of resistance to heparin. Clients may be allergic to heparin and whenever possible should have an IV test dose before starting full-dose therapy.

#### INDEPENDENT NURSING ACTIONS

Monitor vital signs for hypotension or tachycardia. Apply direct pressure to surface bleeding. Initiate and maintain bleeding precautions, e.g., avoid intramuscular injections, straight razors, or vigorous toothbrushing. Monitor neurologic status q4h for 24 h. Monitor gums, urine, and stools for evidence of bleeding.

#### ADMINISTRATION IN ALTERNATE SETTINGS

Full-dose therapy is not recommended in settings where blood coagulation studies cannot be performed to aid in decisions about dose adjustment.

#### EVALUATION: OUTCOMES OF DRUG THERAPY

#### EXPECTED OUTCOMES

PHYSICAL ASSESSMENT. Pulse remains regular and between 60 and 100 bpm. Blood pressure remains within 15% of client's established baseline. Client remains alert and responsive.

LABORATORY. Blood coagulation studies remain within therapeutic range. The activated clotting time (ACT) is two to three times the control value; the PTT is 1½ to two times control; and the activated partial thromboplastin time (APTT) is 1½ to 2½ times control. Hct 40% to 50%. Platelet count between 150,000 and 450,000/mm$^3$.

#### NEGATIVE OUTCOMES

Pulse more than 100 bpm. Blood pressure more than 15% below baseline. Blood in stool or urine. Client complains of fatigue and weakness.

---

## PROTAMINE SULFATE

*Trade Name:* Not specified.
*Canadian Availability:* Protamine
*Pregnancy Risk:* Category C
*pH:* 3
*Storage/Stability:* Store between 2° and 8° C. Protect from freezing. Does not contain preservatives. Unused portion should be discarded after opening.

#### ASSESSMENT: DRUG CHARACTERISTICS

#### ACTION

A heparin antidote/anticoagulant that binds with heparin and appears to reduce the heparin-antithrombin III complex that inhibits the anticoagulant activity of heparin. Has some anticoagulant activity of its own, but is rarely used for that purpose.

#### INDICATIONS

Used to treat the uncontrolled severe bleeding that results from heparin overdose. May also be used following cardiac or vascular surgery or renal dialysis to counter the effects of heparin used during these procedures.

#### CAUTIONS

ADVERSE EFFECTS. Bradycardia, shock, sudden hypotension, dyspnea, bleeding, hypertension, allergic reactions, pulmonary edema, nausea, vomiting, flushed face, or rash.

CONTRAINDICATIONS. History of allergic reactions to protamine or exposure to other protamine-containing substances such as protamine insulin.

#### POTENTIAL DRUG/FOOD INTERACTIONS

No significant interactions.

#### INTERVENTIONS: ADMINISTRATION

May be given undiluted or added to D5W or 0.9% NSS for injection.

#### MODE/RATE OF ADMINISTRATION

May be given by IV push over 1–3 min or by continuous infusion over 2–3 h, using an infusion pump.

INTRAVENOUS USE (WITH NORMAL RENAL FUNCTION)

**Adults:** Usual dosage is 1 mg for each 100 U of heparin to be neutralized over 1–2 min, but not to exceed 50 mg in any 10-min period. Maximum dosage of protamine should not exceed 100 mg in a 2-h period. Additional doses should be determined by blood coagulation results.

**Children:** Follow adult dosing schedule.

▼

**Infants/Neonates:** Dose not established.

**Geriatrics:** Follow adult dosing schedule.

INTRATHECAL USE OR OTHER INFUSION ROUTES AS INDICATED. Not recommended.

#### POTENTIAL PROBLEMS IN ADMINISTRATION

As time elapsed from overdose of heparin increases, the amount of protamine to neutralize the remaining heparin decreases. Since protamine is also an anticoagulant, dose determination must be based on blood coagulation studies.

#### INDEPENDENT NURSING ACTIONS

Monitor vital signs for hypotension or tachycardia. Apply direct pressure to surface bleeding. Initiate and maintain bleeding precautions, e.g., avoid intramuscular injections, straight razors, or vigorous toothbrushing. Monitor neurologic status q4h.

#### ADMINISTRATION IN ALTERNATE SETTINGS

Therapy not recommended in settings where blood coagulation studies cannot be performed. Equipment to manage anaphylactic shock should be immediately available.

#### EVALUATION: OUTCOMES OF DRUG THERAPY

#### EXPECTED OUTCOMES

PHYSICAL ASSESSMENT. Pulse remains regular and between 60 and 100 bpm. Blood pressure remains within 15% of client's established baseline. Client remains alert amd responsive.

LABORATORY. Blood coagulation studies remain within therapeutic range. The ACT is two to three times the control value; the PTT is 1½ to two times control; and the APTT is 1½ to 2½ times control. Hct 40% to 50%. Platelet count between 150,000 and 450,000/mm³.

#### NEGATIVE OUTCOMES

Pulse more than 100 bpm. Blood pressure decreases more than 15% below baseline. Blood in stool, urine, or other evidence of uncontrolled severe bleeding. Client complains of fatigue and weakness.

## THROMBOLYTIC ENZYMES

### THERAPEUTIC EFFECTS

Thrombolytic enzymes are used to save heart muscle by limiting the size of infarction. Thrombolytic enzymes act directly or indirectly to convert plasminogen to plasmin, which digests the fibrin network for thrombolysis. The enzymes are used to treat acute coronary artery or other arterial thrombi, deep vein thrombosis, and pulmonary embolism or to clear an occluded arteriovenous cannula.

## PHARMACOKINETICS

**Distribution.** Thrombolytic enzymes are quickly distributed in plasma following IV administration.

**Metabolism/Elimination.** Thrombolytic enzymes are metabolized by the liver and excreted through the kidneys. The plasma half-life for thrombolytic enzymes is approximately 12 to 18 minutes.

## CAUTIONS

**Side/Adverse Effects.** Administration of thrombolytic enzymes may cause bleeding from cuts, wounds, gums, or allergic reactions.

**Contraindications.** Thrombolytic enzymes should not be given to clients with an aneurysm, endocarditis, mitral stenosis, active bleeding, a recent cerebrovascular accident or neurosurgical procedures within the past 2 months, surgery, trauma or childbirth within the past 10 days, or severe hypertension.

***Pregnancy and Lactation.*** Studies have not documented fetal harm if thrombolytic enzymes are administered in the first two trimesters of pregnancy. However, the uterine attachment of the placenta during the first 18 weeks of pregnancy is primarily fibrin, and thrombolytic enzymes may cause premature detachment of the placenta. Thrombolytics are passed in breast milk, although studies have not documented harm to infants.

***Pediatrics.*** Studies have not documented specific pediatric problems.

***Geriatrics.*** Elderly clients are more likely to have conditions that increase the probability of hemorrhagic complications such as intracranial bleeding. In addition, elderly clients have a poorer prognosis for survival following a myocardial infarction.

## TOXICITY

See Table 19–5 for toxicities of thrombolytic enzymes.

## POTENTIAL DRUG/FOOD INTERACTIONS

Thrombolytic enzymes may interact with other anticoagulants, heparin, or antifibrinolytic agents to produce severe uncontrolled bleeding. The enzymes may interact with nonsteroidal antiinflammatory drugs (NSAIDs) or other platelet aggregate inhibitors such as sulfinpyrazone to increase risk of bleeding. The enzymes may also interact with cefamandole, cefoperazone, cefotetan, moxalactam, plicamycin, or valproic acid to cause hypoprothrombinemia. They are incompatible with any other medication. No other medication should be administered through the same IV line used to administer a thrombolytic enzyme.

**TABLE 19–5**
**Toxicities of Thrombolytic Enzymes**

| Body System | Side/Toxic Effects | Physical Assessment Indicators | Laboratory Indicators | Nursing Interventions |
|---|---|---|---|---|
| Neurologic | Intracranial hemorrhage | Dizziness, headaches | RBCs in cerebrospinal fluid | Monitor for complaints of headache or symptoms of neurologic deficits. |
| Vascular | Bleeding | Unusual bruising, bloody urine, bloody gums, hemoptysis, nosebleeds | Bleeding time > 2–8 min; RBCs in urine, sputum | Observe for bruising or other unusual bleeding. |
| Gastrointestinal | Bleeding | Abdominal pain, tarry stools, hematemesis | RBCs in stool or vomitus | Monitor bowel sounds; observe for evidence of bleeding; report immediately. |
| Other | Anaphylactic shock | Skin rash, skin flush, wheals, urticaria, wheezing, shortness of breath, sudden sharp drop of blood pressure | N/A | Monitor vital signs; report any evidence of respiratory difficulty; be prepared to administer oxygen, epinephrine or other emergency medications. |
| | Febrile reaction | Temperature elevation of 37° C or more | N/A | |

N/A = not applicable, RBC = red blood cell.

## ALTEPLASE (tPA)

*Trade Name:* Activase
*Canadian Availability:* Activase rt-PA
*Pregnancy Risk:* Category C
*pH:* 7.3
*Storage/Stability:* Store between 2° and 30° C. Protect from light. Should be stable for up to 8 hours after being reconstituted if stored between 2° and 30° C.

### ASSESSMENT: DRUG CHARACTERISTICS

#### ACTION

A thrombolytic enzyme that acts directly to convert plasminogen to plasmin—a tissue plasminogen activator (tPA). Has a strong affinity for fibrin and may be the most clot selective of the thrombolytic enzymes.

#### INDICATIONS

Used to treat acute coronary artery thrombosis and acute pulmonary thromboembolism.

#### CAUTIONS

ADVERSE EFFECTS. Bleeding from cuts, wounds, gums, or allergic reactions.

CONTRAINDICATIONS. Aneurysm, active bleeding, recent cerebrovascular accident, surgery, trauma, or severe hypertension.

#### POTENTIAL DRUG/FOOD INTERACTIONS

May interact with other anticoagulants, heparin, or antifibrinolytic agents to produce severe uncontrolled bleeding. May interact with NSAIDs or other platelet aggregate inhibitors such as sulfinpyrazone to increase risk of bleeding. May interact with cefamandole, cefoperazone, cefotetan, moxalactam, plicamycin, or valproic acid to cause hypoprothrombinemia.

### INTERVENTIONS: ADMINISTRATION

Reconstitute using sterile water for injection. Do not use bacteriostatic water for injection. Use an 18-gauge needle and direct diluent directly into the powder. The concentration of the pale yellow alteplase should be 1 mg/mL. This concentration may be used without further dilution or may be diluted to 0.5 mg/mL, using 0.9% NSS or D5W injections. Do not use other solutions or solutions containing preservatives.

#### MODE/RATE OF ADMINISTRATION

May be given by rapid IV injection over 1–2 min and by continuous infusion without a filter and using an infusion pump.

#### INTRAVENOUS USE (WITH NORMAL RENAL FUNCTION)

**Adults:** For clients weighing over 65 kg the usual dose for acute coronary arterial thrombosis is 100 mg total. The first 10 mg is given as a rapid direct IV injection over 1–2 min. The remaining 90 mg is given by continuous infusion, with 50 mg administered the first hour and 20 mg each hour thereafter.

▼

For clients weighing less than 65 kg the usual dose for acute coronary arterial thrombosis is 1.25 mg/kg of body weight. Ten percent is given by rapid direct IV infusion over 1–2 min. The remaining 90% is given by continuous infusion, with 50% being given in the first hour and 20% each hour thereafter.

For acute pulmonary thromboembolism the usual dose is 100 mg, given over a 2-h period.

**Children:** Dose not established.

**Infants/Neonates:** Dose not established.

**Geriatrics:** Elderly clients are more likely to have preexisting conditions that increase the likelihood of complications such as intracranial bleeding. Follow adult dosing schedule and monitor.

INTRATHECAL USE OR OTHER INFUSION ROUTES AS INDICATED. Not recommended.

#### POTENTIAL PROBLEMS IN ADMINISTRATION

To minimize the chances of bleeding, clients should have strict bedrest. Therapy should be discontinued immediately if bleeding at any site cannot be controlled by direct pressure. Reperfusion arrhythmias, bradycardia, and sudden hypotension are common.

#### INDEPENDENT NURSING ACTIONS

Monitor vital signs for hypotension or irregular pulse. Monitor ECG for dysrhythmias. Apply direct pressure to surface bleeding. Initiate and maintain bleeding precautions for 24–48h, e.g., avoid intramuscular injections, straight razors, or vigorous toothbrushing. Monitor neurologic status q4h for 24 h.

#### ADMINISTRATION IN ALTERNATE SETTINGS

IV administration should be done in settings where the client can be closely monitored and where full cardiac technologic support is available.

#### EVALUATION: OUTCOMES OF DRUG THERAPY

#### EXPECTED OUTCOMES

PHYSICAL ASSESSMENT. Pulse remains regular. Blood pressure remains within 15% of client's established baseline. Client remains alert and responsive.

LABORATORY. PTT, fibrinogen, and fibrin split products remain within therapeutic range. Cardiac enzymes show progressive resolution toward normal values. No evidence of bleeding in stool or urine.

#### NEGATIVE OUTCOMES

Pulse more than 100 bpm and irregular. Blood pressure decreases more than 15% below baseline. ECG shows dysrhythmias. Cardiac enzymes continue to rise. Blood in stool or urine.

## Streptokinase

*Trade Names:* Kabikinase, Streptase
*Canadian Availability:* Streptase
*Pregnancy Risk:* Category C
*pH:* 6–8
*Storage/Stability:* Store between 15° and 30° C. Reconstituted drug may be stored at room temperature for 2 hours or up to 8 hours if refrigerated.

### ASSESSMENT: DRUG CHARACTERISTICS

#### ACTION

A thrombolytic enzyme that acts indirectly to promote the conversion of plasminogen to plasmin for thrombolysis. More antigenic than alteplase or urokinase.

#### INDICATIONS

Used to treat acute coronary artery or other arterial thrombi, deep vein thrombosis, and pulmonary embolism or to clear an occluded arteriovenous cannula.

#### CAUTIONS

ADVERSE EFFECTS. Severe allergic reactions or bleeding from cuts, wounds, or gums.

CONTRAINDICATIONS. Aneurysm, active bleeding, recent cerebrovascular accident, surgery, trauma, or severe hypertension.

#### POTENTIAL DRUG/FOOD INTERACTIONS

May interact with other anticoagulants, heparin, or antifibrinolytic agents to produce severe uncontrolled bleeding. May interact with NSAIDs or other platelet aggregate inhibitors such as sulfinpyrazone to increase risk of bleeding. May interact with cefamandole, cefoperazone, cefotetan, moxalactam, plicamycin, or valproic acid to cause hypoprothrombinemia.

### INTERVENTIONS: ADMINISTRATION

Reconstitute two 750,000-U vials with 10 mL of D5W from a 50-mL bag. Inject 5 mL into each vial. Do not shake; swirl gently. Add contents of both vials to the 50-mL bag.

#### MODE/RATE OF ADMINISTRATION

May be given by rapid IV injection over 5–10 min, intermittent infusion, and continuous infusion using an infusion pump.

INTRAVENOUS USE (WITH NORMAL RENAL FUNCTION)

**Adults:** For arterial and deep vein thrombosis or pulmonary embolism, the usual dosage is 250,000 IU over 30 min as a loading dose, then 100,000 IU/h as a continuous infusion.

For acute coronary artery thrombosis the usual dose is 1,500,000 IU given within 1 h.

**Children:** Dose not established.

**Infants/Neonates:** Dose not established.

**Geriatrics:** Elderly clients are more likely to have preexisting conditions that increase the likelihood of complications such as intracranial bleeding. Follow adult dosing schedule and monitor.

INTRATHECAL USE OR OTHER INFUSION ROUTES AS INDICATED. May be infused intraarterially via a coronary artery catheter. Not recommended for other routes.

**POTENTIAL PROBLEMS IN ADMINISTRATION**

Equipment to manage anaphylactic shock should be immediately available. To minimize the chances of bleeding, clients should have strict bedrest. Therapy should be discontinued immediately if bleeding at any site cannot be controlled by direct pressure. Reperfusion arrhythmias, bradycardia, and sudden hypotensions are common. Resistance to streptokinase may be evident if the client has had a recent streptococcal infection or recent therapy with streptokinase.

**INDEPENDENT NURSING ACTIONS**

Monitor vital signs for hypotension or irregular pulse. Monitor ECG for dysrhythmias. Apply direct pressure to surface bleeding. Initiate and maintain bleeding precautions for 24–48 h, e.g., avoid intramuscular injections, straight razors, or vigorous toothbrushing. Monitor neurologic status q4h for 24 h.

**ADMINISTRATION IN ALTERNATE SETTINGS**

IV administration should be done in settings where the client can be closely monitored and where full cardiac technologic support is available.

**EVALUATION: OUTCOMES OF DRUG THERAPY**

**EXPECTED OUTCOMES**

PHYSICAL ASSESSMENT. Pulse remains regular. Blood pressure remains within 15% of client's established baseline. Client remains alert and responsive.

LABORATORY. PTT, fibrinogen, and fibrin split products remain within therapeutic range. Cardiac enzymes show progressive resolution toward normal values. No evidence of bleeding in stool or urine.

**NEGATIVE OUTCOMES**

Pulse more than 100 bpm and irregular. Blood pressure decreases more than 15% below baseline. ECG shows dysrhythmias. Cardiac enzymes continue to rise. Blood in stool or urine.

## UROKINASE

*Trade Names:* Abbokinase, Abbokinase Open-Cath
*Canadian Availability:* Not specified.
*Pregnancy Risk:* Category B
*pH:* 6.0–7.5
*Storage/Stability:* Store between 2° and 8° C. Should be used immediately if reconstituted.

**ASSESSMENT: DRUG CHARACTERISTICS**

**ACTION**

A thrombolytic enzyme that acts directly to promote the conversion of plasminogen to plasmin for thrombolysis.

**INDICATIONS**

Used to treat acute coronary artery or other arterial thrombi, deep vein thrombosis, and pulmonary embolism or to clear an occluded arteriovenous cannula.

**CAUTIONS**

ADVERSE EFFECTS. Severe allergic reactions or bleeding from cuts, wounds, or gums.

CONTRAINDICATIONS. Aneurysm, active bleeding, recent cerebrovascular accident, surgery, trauma, or severe hypertension.

**POTENTIAL DRUG/FOOD INTERACTIONS**

May interact with other anticoagulants, heparin, or antifibrinolytic agents to produce severe uncontrolled bleeding. May interact with NSAIDs or other platelet aggregate inhibitors such as sulfinpyrazone to increase risk of bleeding. May interact with cefamandole, cefoperazone, cefotetan, moxalactam, plicamycin, or valproic acid to cause hypoprothrombinemia.

**INTERVENTIONS: ADMINISTRATION**

Reconstitute three 250,000-U vials with 5-mL of sterile water for injection. Inject 5 mL into each vial. Do not shake; swirl gently. Add contents of both vials to a 500-mL bag D5W for injection for a concentration of 1500 IU/mL.

**MODE/RATE OF ADMINISTRATION**

May be given by rapid direct IV injection over 10 min and by continuous IV infusion with an infusion pump.

INTRAVENOUS USE (WITH NORMAL RENAL FUNCTION)

**Adults:** For pulmonary embolism the usual dosage is 4400 IU/kg of body weight over 10 min, then 4400 IU/kg.

For acute coronary artery thrombosis the usual dosage via intrarterial catheter is 6000 IU (4 mL of 1500 IU/mL)/min until the artery is open. The medication is usually run over 2 h. The average maximum total dose is 500,000 IU.

For IV catheter clearance, disconnect the IV line, fill the IV catheter with 5000 IU/mL of urokinase.

**Children:** Dose not established.

**Infants/Neonates:** Dose not established.

**Geriatrics:** Elderly clients are more likely to have preexisting conditions that increase the likelihood of complications such as intracranial bleeding. Follow adult dosing schedule and monitor.

INTRATHECAL USE OR OTHER INFUSION ROUTES AS INDICATED. May be infused intraarterially via a coronary artery catheter. Not recommended for other routes.

▼

**POTENTIAL PROBLEMS IN ADMINISTRATION**

To minimize the chances of bleeding, clients should have strict bedrest. Therapy should be discontinued immediately if bleeding at any site cannot be controlled by direct pressure. Allergic reactions, reperfusion arrhythmias, bradycardia, and sudden hypotension are common.

**INDEPENDENT NURSING ACTIONS**

Monitor vital signs for hypotension or irregular pulse. Monitor ECG for dysrhythmias. Apply direct pressure to surface bleeding. Initiate and maintain bleeding precautions for 24–48 h, e.g., avoid intramuscular injections, straight razors, or vigorous toothbrushing. Monitor neurologic status q4h for 24 h.

**ADMINISTRATION IN ALTERNATE SETTINGS**

IV administration should be done in settings where the client can be closely monitored and where full cardiac technologic support is available.

**EVALUATION: OUTCOMES OF DRUG THERAPY**

**EXPECTED OUTCOMES**

PHYSICAL ASSESSMENT. Pulse remains regular. Blood pressure remains within 15% of client's established baseline. Client remains alert and responsive.

LABORATORY. PTT, fibrinogen, and fibrin split products remain within therapeutic range. Cardiac enzymes show progressive resolution toward normal values. No evidence of bleeding in stool or urine.

**NEGATIVE OUTCOMES**

Pulse more than 100 bpm and irregular. Blood pressure decreases more than 15% below baseline. ECG shows dysrhythmias. Cardiac enzymes continue to rise. Blood in stool or urine.

CHAPTER 20

# Cardiovascular Agents

*Elaine Kennedy*



## DEFINITION

Cardiovascular agents exert their therapeutic effects on the heart muscle or on blood vessels and are used to (1) improve cardiac muscle contractility, (2) control heart rate, (3) lower blood pressure, or (4) improve coronary circulation by vasodilation.

## CLASSIFICATION

Cardiovascular agents can be classified by their dominant therapeutic effect. Cardiac agents may have a positive effect on cardiac contractility, also known as a positive inotropic effect. They also may control cardiac rate by blocking β-adrenergic stimulation, by altering cell membrane sensitivity, or by slowing the cell membrane's return to resting potential by slowing the return of calcium into cardiac muscle cells. Hypotensive drugs lower blood pressure. Vasodilating agents improve circulation and are used primarily to increase blood supply to the heart muscle for the relief of angina or heart pain. The cardiovascular agents that may be given parenterally are grouped by subclassification in Table 20–1.

**Cardiac Agents.** Cardiac agents improve both the force and velocity of ventricular contraction by direct action on the heart muscle. The result of improved ventricular action is increased cardiac output, more complete emptying of the left ventricle, and decreased diastolic heart size. One outcome of the im-

**TABLE 20–1**
**Parenteral Cardiovascular Agents Grouped by Subclassifications**

| Cardiac Agents | Hypotensive Agents |
|---|---|
| Acebutolol* | Diazoxide |
| Amiodarone* | Hydralazine hydrochloride |
| Amrinone lactate* | Labetalol hydrochloride |
| Atenolol* | Methyldopate hydrochloride |
| Bretylium tosylate | Nitroprusside sodium |
| Deslanoside* | Trimethaphan camsylate |
| Digoxin Immune Fab (Ovine) | Verapamil hydrochloride |
| Enalapril maleate | **Vasodilating Agents** |
| Encainide hydrochloride* | Nimodipine* |
| Esmolol hydrochloride* | Nitroglycerine |
| Flecainide acetate* | Papaverine hydrochloride* |
| Lidocaine hydrochloride | Tolazoline hydrochloride* |
| Metoprolol tartrate | |
| Procainamide hydrochloride | |
| Propranolol hydrochloride | |
| Quinidine* | |

*Not discussed in this Chapter.

proved ventricular action is a decrease in sympathetic nervous stimulation with a consequent drop in heart rate. A second outcome is a decrease in pulmonary venous pressure, since the ventricular end-diastolic pressure is reduced. More efficient ventricular contractions with a slower heart rate and improved pulmonary venous flow may actually increase myocardial oxygen supply. Alternatively, there may be greater cardiac output with no increase in myocardial oxygen consumption.

**Hypotensive Agents.** Hypotensive agents decrease peripheral vascular resistance or block some combination of $\alpha$- or $\beta$-adrenergic stimulation from the autonomic nervous system. Some agents that lower peripheral vascular resistance may act directly on arterial smooth muscle. Others act on both arterial and venous smooth muscle by relaxing the smooth muscle, that is, by vasodilation. Other agents lower intracellular calcium levels in the vessels, thus decreasing muscle tone.

Agents that block autonomic nervous system stimulation have many effects (see Chapter 18). Among the effects are reduction in renin release from the kidney, reduction in cardiac output, parasympathetic blockade at the postsynaptic membrane, and direct peripheral vasodilation caused by the release of histamine

**Vasodilating Agents.** The mechanisms by which vasodilating agents act are not fully understood. Smooth muscle in vessels is affected, causing generalized vasodilation. Peripheral smooth muscle relaxes, and blood flow to the heart diminishes. The effect on arteries is not so great, but the combination of less blood returning to the heart (preload) and somewhat less resistance to blood leaving the heart (afterload) causes a net decrease in myocardial oxygen consumption. Additionally, blood flow throughout the myocardium may be improved even if there is not actual increase in coronary artery blood flow.

## CARDIAC AGENTS

### THERAPEUTIC EFFECTS

Cardiac agents are used to treat congestive heart failure, to control ventricular rate in clients with atrial fibrillation or flutter, and to lower blood pressure. They may be used to treat recurrent atrial tachycardia. They may also be used in conjunction with a $\beta$-adrenergic blocking agent to treat angina pectoris or heart pain.

### PHARMACOKINETICS

**Distribution.** Cardiac agents are widely distributed throughout the body. The greatest concentrations are found in the heart, kidneys, and liver.

**Metabolism/Elimination.** In clients with normal kidney function the plasma half-life of the most common cardiac agents varies from approximately less than 2 hours to more than 33 hours. With impaired renal function the half-life extends. Most cardiac agents are metabolized by the liver and excreted primarily in the urine. Hemodialysis or peritoneal dialysis may or may not remove the drug.

### CAUTIONS

Most cardiac agents should be given initially in the hospital setting where the client can be closely monitored for electrocardiogram (ECG) and hemodynamic changes. Resuscitation equipment must be readily available.

**Side/Adverse Effects.** Postural hypotension, vertigo, dizziness, headache, fatigue, rash, disorientation, confusion, blurred or double vision, psychosis, gastric disturbances, and hypersensitivity to cardiac agents are possible effects.

**Contraindications.** Cardiac agents must be used with caution for clients with known renal impairment, known hypersensitivity, to cardiac agents, bronchospastic disease, marked atrioventricular (AV) conduction disturbances, and Raynaud's disease.

***Pregnancy and Lactation.*** Cardiac agents may be distributed in breast milk and may cross the placental barrier.

***Children.*** Safety has been established for many of the cardiac drugs. Digoxin, propranolol, and verapamil have dosing schedules for children.

***Infants/Neonates.*** Safety has not been established. Digoxin and verapamil have dosing information for infants younger than the age of 12 months.

## TOXICITY

See Table 20–2 for toxicities of cardiac agents.

## POTENTIAL DRUG/FOOD INTERACTIONS

Cardiac agents may potentiate or antagonize the effect of other cardiac drugs such as phenytoin if used together. Cardiac agents may potentiate the effects of hypotensive agents, phenothiazines, carbamazepine, potassium-sparing drugs, lithium, antidiabetic agents, skeletal muscle relaxants, or vasodilating drugs. Cardiac agents may inhibit nonsteroidal antiinflammatory drugs (NSAIDs) and rifampin.

---

## BRETYLIUM TOSYLATE

*Trade Name:* Bretylol
*Canadian Availability:* Bretylate
*Pregnancy Risk:* Category C
*pH:* 4.5–7
*Storage/Stability:* Store between 15° and 30° C. Protect from freezing. Stable for 24 hours at room temperature.

### ASSESSMENT: DRUG CHARACTERISTICS

#### ACTION

An antiarrhythmic whose action is not fully understood. Appears to have a direct action on cardiac muscle and blocks the release of norepinephrine in response to sympathetic nervous system stimulation. Exerts a positive inotropic effect.

#### INDICATIONS

Used to treat ventricular fibrillation and ventricular arrhythmias that are not responding to lidocaine and cardioversion.

#### CAUTIONS

ADVERSE EFFECTS. Hypotension, bradycardia, hyperthermia, or impaired renal function.

CONTRAINDICATIONS. Should be given with caution to clients with severe hypotension because decreased peripheral vascular resistance may significantly lower cardiac output. Should not be given to clients with impaired renal function or who are sensitive to bretylium.

#### POTENTIAL DRUG/FOOD INTERACTIONS

May potentiate toxicity if used with digoxin. Procainamide and quinidine may counteract the inotropic effects of bretylium.

### INTERVENTIONS: ADMINISTRATION

Dilute each 500 mg of bretylium in at least 50 mL of 5% dextrose in water (D5W) or 0.9% normal saline solution (NSS) injection.

#### MODE/RATE OF ADMINISTRATION

May be given by intravenous (IV) push over 1 min in the presence of ventricular fibrillation. May be given as an intermittent IV infusion over at least 8 min, usually 10–30 min. May be given as a continuous IV infusion, using an infusion pump.

▼

**TABLE 20–2**
**Toxicities of Cardiac Agents**

| Body System | Side/Toxic Effects | Physical Assessment Indicators | Laboratory Indicators | Nursing Interventions |
|---|---|---|---|---|
| Neurologic | CNS depression or excitation | Seizures, headache, fatigue, malaise, drowsiness, dizziness, irritability, restlessness, agitation, psychosis, hallucinations | N/A | Monitor LOC; provide a safe environment. |
| Cardiovascular | Conduction disturbances | Heart block, premature ventricular contractions, tachycardia, bradycardia, orthostatic hypotension | ECG changes | Monitor pulse and blood pressure; report ECG changes. |
| Respiratory | Respiratory depression | Shortness of breath | ABG changes | Monitor respirations. |
| Genitourinary | Decreased renal function | Oliguria | Elevated BUN, serum creatinine, glycosuria, proteinuria | Monitor lab values; report any elevations; monitor urinary output; provide small, bland meals. |
| Gastrointestinal | Diarrhea, nausea, vomiting, abdominal pain, dysphagia, constipation, heartbur, bitter taste | Loss of appetite | N/A | Provide small, bland meals. |
| Sensory | Visual disturbances | Blurred vision, double vision, conjunctivitis | N/A | Caution client not to operate hazardous equipment. |
| Dermatologic | Rash, dry skin | Facial flushing, pruritus | N/A | Keep skin clean and dry. |
| Hermatopoietic | Leukopenia, neutropenia, agranulocytosis, thrombocytopenia | Fever, chills | Decreased WBC, decreased neutrophil count, decreased platelet count, decreased hemoglobin and hematocrit | Monitor temperature; report changes in laboratory values or evidence of infection. |
| Other | Hypersensitivity reaction | Tachycardia, dyspnea, urticaria, wheezing | N/A | Stop drug immediately. |

INTRAVENOUS USE (WITH NORMAL RENAL FUNCTION)

**Adults:** Usual dose for ventricular fibrillation is 5 mg/kg of body weight, undiluted. Follow with 10 mg/kg of body weight q15–30 min if necessary. Maximum dose should not exceed 30 mg/kg/d. Usual dose for other ventricular arrhythmias is 5–10 mg/kg of body weight in a diluted solution over a 10 to 30-min period, repeated q1–2h as necessary. Maintenance doses of bretylium in diluted solution at 1–2 mg/min may be given by continuous infusion.

**Children:** Dose not established.

**Infants/Neonates:** Dose not established.

**Geriatrics:** Clients with diminished renal function may require an adjusted dose.

INTRATHECAL USE OR OTHER INFUSION ROUTES AS INDICATED. Not recommended.

**POTENTIAL PROBLEMS IN ADMINISTRATION**

There may be an initial increase in arrhythmias and a transient hypertension within the first few minutes to an hour after therapy has begun because bretylium causes an initial release of norepinephrine before the blockade. Clients usually adjust to the drug-induced hypotension. Systolic pressure should remain above 75 mm Hg. If the systolic pressure drops below that level, treatment with dobutamine, dopamine, or norepinephrine may be required.

**INDEPENDENT NURSING ACTIONS**

Monitor hemodynamics, blood pressure, and ECG.

**ADMINISTRATION IN ALTERNATE SETTINGS**

Should be administered in settings where intensive continuous monitoring can be conducted. A full range of cardiac technologic support should be available.

**EVALUATION: OUTCOMES OF DRUG THERAPY**

**EXPECTED OUTCOMES**

PHYSICAL ASSESSMENT. Heart rate regular and between 60 and 100 beats per minute (bpm). Blood pressure more than 75 mm Hg systolic. Client alert and responsive. Skin pink and warm. Extremities pink, warm, and free of edema.

LABORATORY. None specific.

**NEGATIVE OUTCOMES**

Heart rate less than 60 bpm or more than 100 bpm and irregular. Client lethargic. Skin cool, pale, clammy. Extremities pale. Blood pressure less than 75 mm Hg systolic.

## DIGOXIN

*Trade Name:* Lanoxin
*Canadian Availability:* Lanoxin
*Pregnancy Risk:* Category C
*pH:* 6.6–7.4

*Storage/Stability:* Store below 40° C. Protect from freezing. Diluted solutions of digoxin should be used immediately.

## ASSESSMENT: DRUG CHARACTERISTICS

### ACTION

A cardiac glycoside that (1) exerts a positive inotropic effect on myocardial muscle, increasing the force and velocity of contraction, and (2) slows the heart rate by decreasing the conduction rate and increasing the refractory period.

### INDICATIONS

Used to treat congestive failure and cardiac arrhythmias such as atrial fibrillation, atrial flutter, and paroxysmal atrial tachycardia.

### CAUTIONS

Caution should be exercised when administering digoxin to clients with AV block, glomerulonephritis, impaired hepatic function, hypercalcemia and hypocalcemia, hyperkalemic and hypokalemia, hypomagnesemia, hypothyroidism, ischemic heart disease, myxedema, pulmonary disease, premature ventricular contractions, ventricular tachycardia, sick sinus syndrome, and Wolff-Parkinson-White syndrome. Clients with renal impairment may have an increased incidence of digoxin toxicity.

ADVERSE EFFECTS. Nausea, vomiting, and arrhythmias are early evidence of toxicity.

CONTRAINDICATIONS. Contraindicated for clients who demonstrate toxic effects of digoxin from prior treatment or who have ventricular fibrillation.

### POTENTIAL DRUG/FOOD INTERACTIONS

The use of digoxin with adrenocorticoids, glucocorticoids, mineralocorticoids, amphotericin B, carbonic anhydrase inhibitors, corticotropin (ACTH), or potassium-depleting diuretics (which cause hypokalemia) may increase the potential for toxicity. Amiodarone and quinidine may increase serum digoxin levels. Antiarrhythmics, calcium salts, cocaine, pancuronium, succinycholine, sympathomimetics, or captopril may increase the incidence of arrhythmias. Antidiarrheal adsorbents, cholestyramine, neomycin, or sulfasalazine may decrease the absorption of digoxin from the gastrointestinal tract. Digoxin taken with calcium channel blockers may result in marked bradycardia.

## INTERVENTIONS: ADMINISTRATION

May be given undiluted or mixed at least 4:1 with sterile water for injection, D5W, or 0.9% NSS for injection.

### MODE/RATE OF ADMINISTRATION

Given by IV push over at least 5 min through a free-flowing IV set.

### INTRAVENOUS USE (WITH NORMAL RENAL FUNCTION)

**Adults:** Initial digitalizing dose is 400–600 mcg (0.4–0.6 mg) followed by 100–300 mcg (0.1–0.3 mg) q4–8h until desired therapeutic effect is achieved. Maintenance IV dosage is 125–500 mcg (0.125–0.5 mg) daily.

▼

**Children 2–5 years:** Digitalizing dosage is 25–35 mcg (0.025–0.035 mg)/kg of body weight per day in three doses, with half the total dose given as one dose and the remaining half in two doses.

**Children 5–10 years:** Digitalizing dosage is 15–30 mcg (0.15–0.03 mg)/kg of body weight per day in three doses, with half the total dose given as one dose and the remaining half in two doses.

**Children ≥ 10 years:** Digitalizing dosage is 8–12 mcg (0.008–0.012 mg)/kg of body weight per day in three doses, with half the total dose given as one dose and the remaining half in two doses. Maintenance dosage is 25%–35% of digitalizing dose q.d.

**Premature Infants:** Digitalizing dosage is 15–25 mcg (0.015–0.025 mg)/kg of body weight per day in three doses, with half the total dose given as one dose and the remaining half in two doses. Maintenance dosage is 20%–30% of digitalizing dose divided and given in two to three equal portions per day.

**Full-term infants:** Digitalizing dosage is 20–30 mcg (0.02–0.03 mg)/kg of body weight per day in three doses, with half the total dose given as one dose and the remaining half in two doses.

**Infants 1 month–2 years:** Digitalizing dosage is 30–50 mcg (0.03–0.05 mg)/kg of body weight per day in three doses, with half the total dose given as one dose and the remaining half in two doses.

**Geriatrics:** Clients with diminished renal function, who are debilitated or who have electronic cardiac pacemakers, may require smaller doses to avoid toxicity.

INTRATHECAL USE OR OTHER INFUSION ROUTES AS INDICATED. Not recommended.

#### POTENTIAL PROBLEMS IN ADMINISTRATION

If an overdose is given, IV administration of digoxin immune fab (ovine) will bind serum digoxin. Administration and dosing information is available with digoxin immune fab (ovine).

#### INDEPENDENT NURSING ACTIONS

Frequently monitor heart rate and rhythm, using apical pulse. ECG should be done routinely. Monitor laboratory values for renal and hepatic functioning and serum electrolytes, especially potassium, calcium, magnesium, and serum digoxin levels. Teach clients to monitor their own pulse rates and to report changes in heart rate or rhythm to their physician.

#### ADMINISTRATION IN ALTERNATE SETTINGS

IV digoxin should be administered in settings where the client can be closely monitored and where cardiac technologic support is readily available.

### EVALUATION: OUTCOMES OF DRUG THERAPY

#### EXPECTED OUTCOMES

PHYSICAL ASSESSMENT. Heart rate between 60 and 100 bpm and regular. Urine output more than 30 mL/h. Skin pink and warm. No edema in extremities. Breath sounds clear. No shortness of breath or dyspnea.

LABORATORY. Serum digoxin levels remain in therapeutic range. Serum potassium, calcium, and magnesium levels remain in range.

**NEGATIVE OUTCOMES**

Heart rate less than 50 bpm or more than 100 bpm and irregular. Urine output less than 30 mL/h. Skin cool and clammy. Marked edema of extremities. Crackles and wheezes heard over the lung fields. Client complains of anorexia and shortness of breath on exertion.

## DIGOXIN IMMUNE FAB (OVINE)

*Trade Name:* Digibind
*Pregnancy Risk:* Category C
*pH:* 6–8
*Storage/Stability:* Store between 2° and 8° C. Reconstituted solutions should be used immediately, but may be stored for up to 4 hours between 2° and 8° C.

**ASSESSMENT: DRUG CHARACTERISTICS**

**ACTION**

Binds to serum digoxin molecules, and the complex is then eliminated through the kidneys. As serum digoxin is removed, tissues give up digoxin, which is then bound and removed.

**INDICATIONS**

Used to treat digoxin toxicity.

**CAUTIONS**

Give with caution to clients with a history of allergies.

ADVERSE EFFECTS. Clients may experience fever or hypersensitivity reactions to digoxin immune fab (ovine). Other effects may be the result of withdrawal of digoxin's therapeutic effects.

CONTRAINDICATIONS. Known sensitivity to digoxin immune fab (ovine) or severe renal impairment.

**POTENTIAL DRUG/FOOD INTERACTIONS**

Catecholamine may potentiate digitalis arrhythmias.

**INTERVENTIONS: ADMINISTRATION**

Reconstituted using sterile water for injection. May be further diluted using 0.9% NSS.

**MODE/RATE OF ADMINISTRATION**

Given over 30 min by IV infusion, using a 0.22 $\mu$m filter.

INTRAVENOUS USE (WITH NORMAL RENAL FUNCTION)

**Adults:** A dose of 40 mg of digoxin immune fab (ovine) binds approximately 0.6 mg of digoxin. If tablets were ingested, the following formula can be used to determine the appropriate dose:

$$\text{Dose (mg)} = \frac{\text{Dose Ingested (mg)} \times 0.8}{0.6} \times 40$$

▼

If digoxin was administered intravenously, the following formula can be used to determine the appropriate dose:

$$\text{Dose (mg)} = \frac{\text{Dose Ingested (mg)}}{0.6} \times 40$$

If the amount of digoxin ingested is unknown, 800 mg of digoxin immune fab (ovine) may be administered.

**Children:** Use adult dosing schedule.

**Infants/Neonates:** Use adult dosing schedule.

**Geriatrics:** Clients with diminished renal functioning may require more careful monitoring.

INTRATHECAL USE OR OTHER INFUSION ROUTES AS INDICATED. Not recommended.

#### POTENTIAL PROBLEMS IN ADMINISTRATION

Tuberculin syringes should be used when administering digoxin immune fab (ovine) to infants or neonates. Children must be carefully monitored for fluid volume overload.

#### INDEPENDENT NURSING ACTIONS

Monitor fluid intake, heart rate and rhythm, and ECG reports. Clients should be tested for sensitivity to digoxin immune fab (ovine) before the drug is given intravenously.

#### ADMINISTRATION IN ALTERNATE SETTINGS

Should be administered in settings where the client can be closely monitored and where cardiac technologic support is readily available.

### EVALUATION: OUTCOMES OF DRUG THERAPY

#### EXPECTED OUTCOMES

PHYSICAL ASSESSMENT. Adult heart rate between 60 and 100 bpm and regular.

LABORATORY. Serum digitalis levels return to therapeutic range. Serum potassium level within normal range.

#### NEGATIVE OUTCOMES

Adult heart rate less than 60 bpm and irregular. Serum potassium level elevated.

## ENALAPRIL MALEATE

*Trade Name:* Vasotec IV
*Canadian Availability:* Not commercially available.
*Pregnancy Risk:* Category D
*pH:* 6.5–7.5
*Storage/Stability:* Store below 40° C. Protect from light. Reconstituted infusions are stable for 24 hours at room temperature.

### ASSESSMENT: DRUG CHARACTERISTICS

#### ACTION

An angiotensin converting enzyme inhibitor that acts by causing systemic vasodilation. Prevents angiotensin I from converting to angiotensin II, resulting in decreased peripheral vascular resistance and lowered blood pressure.

#### INDICATIONS

Used to treat hypertension, especially in clients whose pretreatment plasma renin levels are elevated. May also be used to treat congestive heart failure that has not responded to digitalis and diuretics.

#### CAUTIONS

ADVERSE EFFECTS. Headache, paresthesias, angina, dyspnea, anorexia, diarrhea, or hyperkalemia.

CONTRAINDICATIONS. Should be used with caution with clients who are undergoing anesthesia for surgery, are being treated with other hypotensive agents, or have coronary or cerebrovascular insufficiency or aortic stenosis. Potassium-sparing diuretics may increase the possibility of hyperkalemia. Should not be given to clients with renal failure or sensitivity to enalapril.

#### POTENTIAL DRUG/FOOD INTERACTIONS

May interact with halogen anesthetic agents to produce cardiac dysrhythmias. Monamine oxidase inhibitors (MAO) or oxytocic drugs may precipitate a marked hypertension with the possibility of intracranial hemorrhage. Allopurinol may increase the risk of a hypersensitivity reaction. Tricyclic antidepressants may inhibit the action of enalapril, requiring a higher dose for therapeutic effect.

#### INTERVENTIONS: ADMINISTRATION

#### MODE/RATE OF ADMINISTRATION

May be given undiluted through a free-flowing IV infusion over at least 5 min. If diluted, use D5W, 0.9% NSS, or Ringer's lactate solution. May be administered by intermittent IV infusion.

INTRAVENOUS USE (WITH NORMAL RENAL FUNCTION)

**Adults:** Usual dose is 1.25 mg. May be repeated q6h. Dose may be lowered to 0.625 mg for clients with renal impairment or who are receiving diuretic therapy.

**Children:** Dose not established.

**Infants/Neonates:** Dose not established.

**Geriatrics:** Clients with diminished renal function may require dose adjustment.

INTRATHECAL USE OR OTHER INFUSION ROUTES AS INDICATED. Not recommended.

#### POTENTIAL PROBLEMS IN ADMINISTRATION

First dose may cause a marked drop in blood pressure. Clients are more at risk if they are not well hydrated. May cause oliguria or azotemia in clients who have compromised renal function.

#### INDEPENDENT NURSING ACTIONS

Monitor laboratory values for potassium, blood urea nitrogen (BUN), and serum creatinine levels. Monitor blood pressure, heart rate, and hemodynamic status frequently. Maintain accurate intake and output records.

▼

**ADMINISTRATION IN ALTERNATE SETTINGS**

IV administration should be done in settings where the client can be closely monitored and where full cardiac technologic support is available.

**EVALUATION: OUTCOMES OF DRUG THERAPY**

**EXPECTED OUTCOMES**

PHYSICAL ASSESSMENT. Systolic blood pressure remains above 75 mm Hg and below 160 mm Hg. Heart rate between 60 and 100 bpm and regular. Extremities warm, pink, and free of edema. Urinary output more than 30 mL/h.

LABORATORY. BUN, serum creatinine, and potassium levels remain within client's normal range.

**NEGATIVE OUTCOMES**

Marked hypotension and a weak, irregular heart rate. Client complains of angina. Urine output less than 30 mL/h. Extremities pale and cool. Client confused or lethargic.

## LIDOCAINE HYDROCHLORIDE

*Trade Names:* Xylocaine
*Canadian Availability:* Xylocard
*Pregnancy Risk:* Category B
*pH:* 5–7
*Storage/Stability:* Store below 40° C. Diluted solutions of lidocaine are stable for 24 hours at room temperature.

**ASSESSMENT: DRUG CHARACTERISTICS**

**ACTION**

An antiarrhythmic that decreases the depolarization, automaticity, and excitability of the ventricles during diastole. Usual therapeutic doses of lidocaine do not alter contractility, AV conduction velocity, or systolic blood pressure.

**INDICATIONS**

Used to treat ventricular arrhythmias, especially those ventricular arrhythmias that develop after myocardial infarction, cardiac surgery, digitalis toxicity, or cardiac catheterization.

**CAUTIONS**

Should be used with caution with clients who have congestive heart failure, impaired hepatic or renal functioning, hypovolemia, sinus bradycardia, and Wolff-Parkinson-White syndrome.

ADVERSE EFFECTS. Hypotension, arrhythmias, heart block, respiratory arrest, or cardiac arrest.

CONTRAINDICATIONS. Severe heart block, Adams-Stokes syndrome, or sensitivity to lidocaine.

**POTENTIAL DRUG/FOOD INTERACTIONS**

Other antiarrhythmics or neuromuscular blocking agents may potentiate the action of lidocaine. $\beta$-Adrenergic blocking agents and cimetidine may increase the risk of lidocaine toxicity from reduced hepatic blood flow or delayed elimination. Anticonvulsants such as hydantoin may potentiate the cardiac depressant effect of lidocaine.

**INTERVENTIONS: ADMINISTRATION**

IV infusions are prepared by adding 1 or 2 g of lidocaine to 1000 mL of D5W solution. The resulting solution has 1–2 mg/mL of lidocaine. Solutions used to dilute lidocaine should not contain preservatives such as epinephrine.

**MODE/RATE OF ADMINISTRATION**

A loading dose may be given by IV push. Given by continuous infusion, using an infusion pump and a microdrip infusion set.

INTRAVENOUS USE (WITH NORMAL RENAL FUNCTION)

**Adults:** Loading dose is 1–1.5 mg/kg of body weight. Doses of 0.5–1.5 mg/kg may be repeated q5min up to a maximum of 200–300 mg in 1 h.

Maintenance dosage is 20–50 mcg (0.02–0.05 mg)/kg of body weight per minute or 1–4 mg/min. Maximum dose is 300 mg in 1 h.

**Children:** Loading dose is 0.5–1 mg/kg of body weight.

Maintenance dosage is 20–50 mcg (0.02–0.05 mg)/kg of body weight per minute. Maximum dose is 5 mg/kg of body weight.

**Infants/Neonates:** Use dosing schedule for children.

**Geriatrics:** Elderly clients may be more sensitive to the effects of lidocaine. Dose may need to be decreased.

INTRATHECAL USE OR OTHER INFUSION ROUTES AS INDICATED. May be given by intrathecal infusion.

**POTENTIAL PROBLEMS IN ADMINISTRATION**

Lidocaine may cause seizure activity if given too rapidly. Rapid IV injection should be done over at least 1 min.

**INDEPENDENT NURSING ACTIONS**

Monitor heart rate and rhythm frequently. Monitor ECG reports. Monitor laboratory values for potassium, calcium, magnesium, and serum digitalis levels. Teach clients the side effects of lidocaine and to report any arrhythmias.

**ADMINISTRATION IN ALTERNATE SETTINGS**

Should be administered in settings where the client can be closely monitored and where cardiac technologic support equipment is readily available.

**EVALUATION: OUTCOMES OF DRUG THERAPY**

**EXPECTED OUTCOMES**

PHYSICAL ASSESSMENT. Heart rate between 60 and 100 bpm and regular. Blood pressure less than 160 mm Hg and more than 75 mm Hg systolic. Skin warm, pink, and dry. Client has no complaints of palpitations.

LABORATORY. Creatinine kinase (CK) may be elevated

▼

when lidocaine is used. Without testing isoenzymes levels, the CK is an unreliable indicator of myocardial infarction.

**NEGATIVE OUTCOMES**

Heart rate irregular. ECG shows ventricular arrhythmia. Client complains of palpitations. Skin pale, cool, clammy. Urine output less than 30 mL/h.

---

## METOPROLOL TARTRATE

*Trade Name:* Lopressor
*Canadian Availability:* Lopressor, Betaloc
*Pregnancy Risk:* Category B
*pKa:* 9.68
*Storage/Stability:* Store below 40° C. Protect from freezing and from light.

### ASSESSMENT: DRUG CHARACTERISTICS

**ACTION**

A cardioselective, $\beta_1$-adrenergic blocking agent. The mechanism of action is not fully understood. Competes with sympathetic neurotransmitters for $\beta_1$-receptor binding sites in cardiac tissue.

**INDICATIONS**

Used to decrease the size of a myocardial infarction and the incidence of fatal arrhythmias in clients who are hemodynamically stable following a myocardial infarction.

**CAUTIONS**

ADVERSE EFFECTS. Bradycardia, bronchospasm, congestive heart failure, heart block, respiratory distress, or hypotension.

CONTRAINDICATIONS. Concurrent use of verapamil (because there may be myocardial depression and AV conduction disturbance), second- or third-degree heart block, moderate or severe congestive heart failure, or bradycardia of 45 bpm or less.

**POTENTIAL DRUG/FOOD INTERACTIONS**

May antagonize the effects of antihistamines, NSAIDs, and ritodrine. May potentiate oral hypoglycemics, insulin, lidocaine, narcotics, muscle relaxants, or theophylline. May be potentiated by anesthetics, cimetidine, furosemide, phenytoin, and phenothiazines.

### INTERVENTIONS: ADMINISTRATION

Given undiluted.

**MODE/RATE OF ADMINISTRATION**

Given by IV push.

INTRAVENOUS USE (WITH NORMAL RENAL FUNCTION)

**Adults:** Usual dosage is 5 mg q2min for three doses.

**Children:** Dose not established.

**Infants/Neonates:** Dose not established.

**Geriatrics:** Elderly clients may be more or less sensitive to the effects of metoprolol. Dose may require adjustment.

INTRATHECAL USE OR OTHER INFUSION ROUTES AS INDICATED. Not recommended.

**POTENTIAL PROBLEMS IN ADMINISTRATION**

May cause bradycardia, heart block, or hypotension. Atropine may reverse the bradycardia. Hypotension should be managed with fluids and vasopressors, but great caution should be used. Congestive heart failure should be managed with cardiac glycosides, diuretics, and dobutamine or isoproterenol as warranted.

**INDEPENDENT NURSING ACTIONS**

Monitor heart rate and rhythm and ECG reports frequently. Auscultate lungs. Monitor fluid intake and output, blood glucose levels, and BUN.

**ADMINISTRATION IN ALTERNATE SETTINGS**

IV administration should be done in settings where the client can be closely monitored and where full cardiac technologic support is available.

**EVALUATION: OUTCOMES OF DRUG THERAPY**

**EXPECTED OUTCOMES**

PHYSICAL ASSESSMENT. Systolic blood pressure remains above 75 mm Hg and below 160 mm Hg. Heart rate between 60 and 100 bpm and regular. Extremities warm, pink, and free of edema. Urinary output more than 30 mL/h.

LABORATORY. BUN, serum creatinine, and blood glucose levels remain within client's normal range.

**NEGATIVE OUTCOMES**

Marked hypotension and a weak, irregular heart rate less than 60 bpm. Crackles and wheezes heard on chest auscultation. Urine output less than 30 mL/h. Extremities pale and cool. Client confused or lethargic.

## PROCAINAMIDE HYDROCHLORIDE

*Trade Name:* Pronestyl
*Canadian Availability:* Pronestyl
*Pregnancy Risk:* Category C
*pH:* 4–6
*Storage/Stability:* Store between 15° and 20° C. Protect from freezing and from light. Should not be used if darker than light amber.

**ASSESSMENT: DRUG CHARACTERISTICS**

**ACTION**

An antiarrhythmic that acts directly on cardiac tissue to decrease the depolarization, automaticity, and excitability of the ventricles during diastole. Usual therapeutic doses do not alter contractility, AV conduction velocity, or systolic blood pressure.

**INDICATIONS**

Used to treat atrial fibrillation, paroxysmal atrial tachycardia, ventricular tachycardia, and premature ventricular contractions.

▼

**CAUTIONS**

ADVERSE EFFECTS. Tachycardia, hypotension, ventricular fibrillation, ventricular asystole, hallucinations, confusion, leukopenia, hemolytic anemia, thrombocytopenia, oliguria, nausea, vomiting, diarrhea, or anorexia.

CONTRAINDICATIONS. Contraindicated for use with clients with AV block. Clients with hepatic or renal impairment are at higher risk for toxicity. Clients with lupus erythematosus or myasthenia gravis may have escalated symptoms.

**POTENTIAL DRUG/FOOD INTERACTIONS**

Cardiac effects of other antiarrhythmics may be potentiated. Anticholinergic activity of atropine, antihistamines, or antidyskinetics may be potentiated. Procainamide may inhibit the cholinergic activity of bethanechol. Bretylium or antihypertensive agents may enhance the hypotensive effect of procainamide. Pimozide used with procainamide may precipitate cardiac arrhythmias.

**INTERVENTIONS: ADMINISTRATION**

For IV infusion, dilute 200 mg to 1 g of procainamide in D5W solution to achieve a 2–4 mg/mL concentration.

**MODE/RATE OF ADMINISTRATION**

May be given by IV push at a rate not to exceed 50 mg/min. May be given by continuous IV infusion, using a microdrip administration set, filter, and infusion pump.

INTRAVENOUS USE (WITH NORMAL RENAL FUNCTION)

**Adults:** Initial dose is 100 mg by IV push over at least 2 min. Dose may be repeated q5min or until 1 g has been given. Maintenance continuous infusion dosage is 2–6 mg/min to maintain regular cardiac rhythm.

**Children:** Initial dosage is 2–5 mg/kg of body weight not to exceed 100 mg, given by IV injection over at least 2 min. Dose may be repeated q10– 30min. Maximum dosage should not exceed 30 mg/kg in 24 h. Maintenance continuous infusion dosage 0.020–0.08 mg/kg of body weight per minute to maintain regular cardiac rhythm.

**Infants/Neonates:** Dose not established.

**Geriatrics:** Clients may be more prone to hypotensive effect. Clients with diminished renal function may require a decreased dose.

INTRATHECAL USE OR OTHER INFUSION ROUTES AS INDICATED. Not recommended.

**POTENTIAL PROBLEMS IN ADMINISTRATION**

IV administration of procainamide may cause a temporary but profound hypotension. Too rapid administration may precipitate ventricular arrhythmias.

**INDEPENDENT NURSING ACTIONS**

Frequently monitor heart rate and rhythm. Monitor ECG reports. Monitor laboratory values for possible decreases in leukocyte or platelet counts or elevations in alanine aminotransferase (ALT), aspartate aminotransferase (AST), serum bilirubin, or lactate dehydrogenase (LDH).

**ADMINISTRATION IN ALTERNATE SETTINGS**

Should be administered in settings where the client can be closely monitored and where cardiac support equipment is readily available.

**EVALUATION: OUTCOMES OF DRUG THERAPY**

**EXPECTED OUTCOMES**

PHYSICAL ASSESSMENT. Heart rate between 60 and 100 bpm and regular. Blood pressure less than 160 mm Hg and more than 75 mm Hg systolic. Skin warm, pink, and dry. Client has no complaints of palpitations.

LABORATORY. Complete blood count remains within client's normal range. No elevations of ALT, AST, LDH, or serum bilirubin.

**NEGATIVE OUTCOMES**

Heart rate irregular. ECG shows ventricular arrhythmias. Client complains of palpitations. Skin pale, cool, clammy. Urine output less than 30mL/h.

## PROPRANOLOL HYDROCHLORIDE

*Trade Name:* Inderal
*Canadian Availability:* Inderal
*Pregnancy Risk:* Category C
*pH:* 2.8–3.5
*Storage/Stability:* Store below 40° C. Protect from freezing and from light.

**ASSESSMENT: DRUG CHARACTERISTICS**

**ACTION**

A nonselective $\beta_1$- and $\beta_2$-adrenergic blocking agent. The mechanism of action is not fully understood. Competes with sympathetic neurotransmitters for $\beta_1$-receptor binding sites in cardiac tissue and $\beta_2$-receptor sites in other tissues, including pulmonary and vascular.

**INDICATIONS**

Used intravenously to treat supraventricular and ventricular arrhythmias, to control hypertension during surgery, and to control the incidence of fatal arrhythmias in clients who are hemodynamically stable following a myocardial infarction.

**CAUTIONS**

ADVERSE EFFECTS. Allergic reactions, arrhythmias, back or joint pain, bradycardia, bronchospasm, angina, confusion, congestive heart failure, hepatotoxicity, heart block, respiratory distress, hypotension, leukopenia, mental depression, thrombocytopenia, decreased peripheral circulation, or rashes.

CONTRAINDICATIONS. Second- or third-degree heart block, cardiac failure, cardiogenic ▼

shock, moderate or severe congestive heart failure, or sinus bradycardia of 45 bpm or less. Should be given with caution to clients with a history of allergy, bronchial asthma, emphysema, diabetes mellitus, or hyperthyroidism.

**POTENTIAL DRUG/FOOD INTERACTIONS**

May potentiate oral hypoglycemics, insulin, or lidocaine. Anesthetics may increase myocardial depression and hypotension. Fentanyl used during surgery may prevent hypertension or diminish the severity of hypertension. Calcium channel blockers, clonidine, diazoxide, neuromuscular blocking agents, or reserpine may be potentiated. NSAIDs, estrogens, and cocaine may reduce the therapeutic effects of propranolol. Cimetidine, phenytoin, and phenothiazines may potentiate the effects of propranolol. Sympathomimetics and xanthines used with propranolol may cause a mutual inhibition of effects.

**INTERVENTIONS: ADMINISTRATION**

Dilute 1 mg in 10 mL of 0.9% NSS for injection. Diluted solution can be further diluted in 0.9% NSS.

**MODE/RATE OF ADMINISTRATION**

Given by IV push through a free-flowing IV infusion. May be given by slow IV infusion over 10–15 min.

INTRAVENOUS USE (WITH NORMAL RENAL FUNCTION)

**Adults:** Usual IV dosage is 1–3 mg, given at a rate not to exceed 1 mg/min. Dosage may be repeated after 2 min and again after 4 h if necessary.

**Children:** Usual IV dose is 10–100 mcg (0.01–0.1 mg)/kg of body weight by slow IV infusion. Dose may be repeated q6–8h. Maximum dose is 1 mg per infusion.

**Infants/Neonates:** Use children's dosing schedule.

**Geriatrics:** Elderly clients may be less sensitive to the effects, especially to the antihypertensive effects. Diminished hepatic and renal function and decreased peripheral vascular circulation may require that doses be decreased.

INTRATHECAL USE OR OTHER INFUSION ROUTS AS INDICATED. Not recommended.

**POTENTIAL PROBLEMS IN ADMINISTRATION**

May cause bradycardia, heart block, or hypotension. Atropine may reverse the bradycardia. Hypotension should be managed with fluids and vasopressors, but great caution should be used. Congestive heart failure should be managed with cardiac glycosides, diuretics, and dobutamine or isoproterenol as warranted.

**INDEPENDENT NURSING ACTIONS**

Monitor heart rate and rhythm, ECG reports, and hemodynamic status (if available) frequently. Auscultate lungs. Monitor fluid intake and output, blood glucose levels, and BUN.

**ADMINISTRATION IN ALTERNATE SETTINGS**

IV administration should be done in settings where

the client can be closely monitored and where full cardiac technologic support is available.

**EVALUATION: OUTCOMES OF DRUG THERAPY**

**EXPECTED OUTCOMES**

PHYSICAL ASSESSMENT. Systolic blood pressure remains above 75 mm Hg and below 160 mm Hg. Heart rate between 60 and 100 bpm and regular. Breath sounds clear. Extremities warm, pink, and free of edema. Urinary output more than 30 mL/h.

LABORATORY. BUN, serum creatinine, and blood glucose levels remain within client's normal range.

**NEGATIVE OUTCOMES**

Marked hypotension and a weak, irregular heart rate less than 60 bpm. Wheezes and crackles heard on lung auscultation. Urine output less than 30 mL/h. Extremities pale and cool. Client confused or lethargic.

## HYPOTENSIVE AGENTS

### THERAPEUTIC EFFECTS

Hypotensive agents are used to treat hypertension, severe hypertension, and hypertensive emergencies. Some of the agents may be used as in adjunct to anesthesia to control bleeding through hypotension.

### PHARMACOKINETICS

**Distribution.** Hypotensive agents are widely distributed throughout the body. The highest concentrations are found in the kidney, plasma, and liver. Most agents cross the blood-brain and placental barriers and are passed in breast milk.

**Metabolism/Elimination.** Hypotensive agents are metabolized mainly by the gastrointestinal tract and liver and excreted in urine. In the adult with normal kidneys the average half-life is between 8 hours and 3 days. With renal impairment the half-life is extended. Many of the drugs are removed by hemodialysis and peritoneal dialysis.

### CAUTIONS

**Side/Adverse Effects.** The most common adverse effects are hypotension, nausea, vomiting, dizziness, weakness, headache, palpitation, tachycardia, drowsiness, and urinary retention.

**Contraindications.** Hypotensive agents should not be used with clients who have hypersensitivity to the agents, hypertension associated with aortic coarctation or AV shunt, impaired renal function, bronchial asthma, impaired hepatic function, heart block, cardiogenic shock, inadequate cerebral circulation, anemia, hypothermia, or shock.

***Pregnancy and Lactation.*** Hypotensive agents are not known to be mutagenic. There is evidence that hydralazine is teratogenic. Clients should be instructed in proper birth control measures and not to breastfeed if the hypotensive drug is being used for longterm management of hypertension.

*Children.* Hypotensive agents are not recommended for use with children.

*Infants/Neonates.* Hypotensive agents are not recommended for use with infants.

*Geriatrics.* Hypotensive drug effects may last longer and accumulate faster if hepatic and renal function is diminished.

## TOXICITY

See Table 20–3 for toxicities of hypotensive agents.

## POTENTIAL DRUG/FOOD INTERACTIONS

Use of diuretics with hypotensive agents may potentiate the hyperglycemic, hyperuricemic, or hypotensive effects of hypotensive agents. Mild elevations in blood sugars are generally not treated. Allopurinol is commonly prescribed to lower serum uric acid levels. Hypotensive agents may inhibit the effectiveness of phenytoin and warfarin. Methyldopa, phenothiazines, and tricyclic antidepressants may diminish the hypotensive effects of hypotensive agents.

---

## DIAZOXIDE

*Trade Name:* Hyperstat IV
*Canadian Availability:* Hyperstat IV
*Pregnancy Risk:* Category C
*pH:* 11.6
*Storage/Stability:* Store below 40° C. Protect from light and from freezing.

### ASSESSMENT: DRUG CHARACTERISTICS

#### ACTION

An antihypertensive agent whose mechanism of action is not fully understood. Causes arteriolar dilation and a marked decrease in peripheral vascular resistance.

#### INDICATIONS

Used for emergency treatment of the severe hypertension found in malignant hypertension or hypertensive crisis.

#### CAUTIONS

ADVERSE EFFECTS. Sodium and water retention, hypotension, tachycardia, hyperglycemia, allergic reaction, thrombocytopenia, cerebral ischemia, angina, myocardial infarction, back pain, tinnitus, thrombophlebitis, and vasodilation.

CONTRAINDICATIONS. Dissecting aortic aneurysm, aortic coarctation, myocardial or cerebral ischemia, diabetes mellitus, uncompensated congestive heart failure, or sensitivity to diazoxide.

#### POTENTIAL DRUG/FOOD INTERACTIONS

May potentiate the action of other hypotensive drugs or vasodilators. β-adrenergic blocking agents may de-
▼

**TABLE 20–3**
**Toxicities of Hypotensive Agents**

| Body System | Side/Toxic Effects | Physical Assessment Indicators | Laboratory Indicators | Nursing Interventions |
|---|---|---|---|---|
| Neurologic | Extrapyramidal symptoms, mental depression | Drowsiness, oculogyric crisis, trismus, rigidity, tremor, paresthesias, membranes, tingling, fatigue, dizziness, nightmares, somnolence, memory lapses | N/A | Monitor LOC; provide a safe, quiet environment; caution client not to operate hazardous equipment; report extrapyramidal symptoms. |
| Cardiovascular | Congestive heart failure | Orthostatic hypertension, angina, ventricular arrhythmias, pulse rate changes, edema, weight gain | ECG changes | Monitor blood pressure, pulse rate; weigh client frequently; assess complaints of chest pain. |
| Genitourinary | Impotence, urinary retention | Painful urinations, ejaculatory failure, palpable bladder, priapism, decreased libido | Monitor output | Report evidence of urine retention; report client concerns about changes in sexuality. |
| Gastrointestinal | Ileus | Nausea, vomiting, abdominal pain, anorexia, altered taste, diarrhea, constipation, dry mouth, flatulence | N/A | Monitor bowel sounds and fecal elimination. |
| Musculoskeletal | Arthralgia, myalgia | Muscle cramps, weakness | N/A | Provide comfort measures. |
| Sensory | Visual disturbances | Blurred vision | N/A | Instruct clients to exercise caution when engaging in activities requiring visual acuity. |
| Dermatologic | Urticaria | | | |

ECG = electrocardiogram, LOC = level of consciousness, N/A = not applicable.

crease the risk of diazoxide-induced tachycardia but may potentiate the hypotensive effect. Loop diuretics, thiazide diuretics, and indapamide may potentiate the hypotensive, hyperglycemic, and hyperuricemic effects of diazoxide. Diazoxide may potentiate the effects of anticoagulants. Antigout medication may be needed to lower serum uric acid levels caused by diazoxide.

**INTERVENTIONS: ADMINISTRATION**

Should be given undiluted.

**MODE/RATE OF ADMINISTRATION**

Given by IV push for a period not longer than 10–30 s through a free-flowing infusion.

INTRAVENOUS USE (WITH NORMAL RENAL FUNCTION)

**Adults:** Usual dose is 1–3 mg/kg of body weight, up to 150 mg. Dose may be repeated q5–15min if necessary to obtain the desired blood pressure. Additional doses may be given q4–14h to maintain the desired blood pressure.

**Children:** Usual dose is 1–3 mg/kg of body weight or 30–90 mg/m$^2$ of body surface area (BSA). Dose may be repeated in 5–10 min if necessary to obtain the desired blood pressure. Additional doses may be given q4–24h to maintain the desired blood pressure.

**Infants/Neonates:** Follow children's dosing schedule.

**Geriatrics:** Clients with diminished renal function may require reduced doses.

INTRATHECAL USE OR OTHER INFUSION ROUTES AS INDICATED. Not recommended. Severe pain may result.

**POTENTIAL PROBLEMS IN ADMINISTRATION**

Should be administered through a peripheral vein to decrease the risk of cardiac arrhythmias. Client should remain supine for 15–30 min after administration.

**INDEPENDENT NURSING ACTIONS**

Monitor heart rate and rhythm, ECG reports, and hemodynamic status (if available) frequently. Monitor fluid intake and output, blood glucose levels, BUN, and serum potassium levels.

**ADMINISTRATION IN ALTERNATE SETTINGS**

IV administration should be done in settings where the client can be closely monitored and where full cardiac technologic support is available.

**EVALUATION: OUTCOMES OF DRUG THERAPY**

**EXPECTED OUTCOMES**

PHYSICAL ASSESSMENT. Systolic blood pressure remains above 75 mm Hg and below 160 mm Hg. Heart rate between 60 and 100 bpm and regular. Extremities warm, pink, and free of edema. Urinary output more than 30 mL/h. Client has no complaints of chest pain or confusion.

LABORATORY. Serum potassium, BUN, serum creatinine, and blood glucose levels remain within client's normal range.

#### NEGATIVE OUTCOMES

Marked hypotension and a weak, irregular heart rate less than 60 bpm or more than 100 bpm. Urine output less than 30 mL/h. Extremities pale and cool. Client confused or lethargic.

## HYDRALAZINE HYDROCHLORIDE

*Trade Name:* Apresoline
*Canadian Availability:* Apresoline
*Pregnancy Risk:* Category C
*pH:* 3–4
*Storage/Stability:* Store below 40° C. Protect from freezing. Should be used immediately. Should not be added to infusion solutions.

#### ASSESSMENT: DRUG CHARACTERISTICS

#### ACTION

An antihypertensive agent whose mechanism of action is not fully understood. Causes vasodilation of arterioles while having little effect on veins. The resulting decrease in peripheral resistance causes an increase in stroke volume and cardiac output.

#### INDICATIONS

Used to treat severe hypertension and hypertensive crisis.

#### CAUTIONS

ADVERSE EFFECTS. Allergic reactions, angina, swelling of lymph glands, sodium and water retention, peripheral neuritis, systemic lupus erythematosus syndrome, diarrhea, palpitations, headache, anorexia, and nausea and vomiting.

CONTRAINDICATIONS. Coronary artery disease or rheumatic heart disease. Should be given with caution to clients with an aortic aneurysm, cerebral vascular disease, congestive heart failure, impaired renal function, or sensitivity to hydralazine.

#### POTENTIAL DRUG/FOOD INTERACTIONS

May interact with diazoxide or other antihypertensive agents to cause a profound hypotension. When used with NSAIDs, may cause increased sodium and water retention. Sympathomimetics may inhibit the action of hydralazine.

#### INTERVENTIONS: ADMINISTRATION

Should be given undiluted.

#### MODE/RATE OF ADMINISTRATION

Given by IV push through a free-flowing infusion over 1 min. Should not be given faster than 5 mg/min.

INTRAVENOUS USE (WITH NORMAL RENAL FUNCTION)

**Adults:** Usual dose is 10–40 mg. May be repeated as necessary. Maximum total dosage is 300–400 mg in 24 h.

**Children:** Usual dose is 1.7–3.5 mg/kg of body weight or 50–100 mg/m$^2$ of BSA in 4–6 doses.

**Infants/Neonates:** Follow children's dosing schedule.

▼

**Geriatrics:** Elderly clients may be more sensitive to the hypotensive effects or have diminished renal function that may require decreased doses.

INTRATHECAL USE OR OTHER INFUSION ROUTES AS INDICATED. Not recommended.

**POTENTIAL PROBLEMS IN ADMINISTRATION**

Clients may develop tolerance to the hypotensive effects of hydralazine. Adverse side effects may be diminished if the dosage of the drug is slowly increased or if $\beta$-adrenergic blocking agents are also used.

**INDEPENDENT NURSING ACTIONS**

Monitor heart rate and rhythm, ECG reports, and hemodynamic status (if available) frequently. Monitor fluid intake and output, BUN, serum sodium, and other indicators of renal function.

**ADMINISTRATION IN ALTERNATE SETTINGS**

IV administration should be done in settings where the client can be closely monitored and where full cardiac technologic support is available.

**EVALUATION: OUTCOMES OF DRUG THERAPY**

**EXPECTED OUTCOMES**

PHYSICAL ASSESSMENT. Systolic blood pressure remains above 75 mm Hg and below 160 mm Hg. Heart rate between 60 and 100 bpm and regular. No complaints of chest pain or headache. Extremities warm, pink, and free of edema. Urinary output more than 30 mL/h.

LABORATORY. Serum sodium, BUN, and serum creatinine remain within client's normal range.

**NEGATIVE OUTCOMES**

Marked hypotension and a weak, irregular heart rate less than 60 bpm. Client complains of chest pain or headache. Urine output less than 30 mL/h. Extremities pale and cool. Client confused or lethargic.

## LABETALOL HYDROCHLORIDE

*Trade Names:* Normodyne, Trandate
*Canadian Availability:* Trandate
*Pregnancy Risk:* Category C
*pH:* 3–4
*Storage/Stability:* Store between 2° and 30° C. Protect from light and from freezing. Dilutions in sodium chloride are stable for 24 hours at room temperature or up to 72 hours if refrigerated.

**ASSESSMENT: DRUG CHARACTERISTICS**

**ACTION**

An $\alpha_1$- and nonselective $\beta_1$- and $\beta_2$-adrenergic blocking agent. The mechanism of action is not fully understood. Competes with sympathetic neurotransmitters for $\beta_1$-receptor binding sites in cardiac tissue and $\beta_2$-receptor sites in other tissues, including pulmonary and vascular.

**INDICATIONS**

Used intravenously to treat severe hypertension.

**CAUTIONS**

ADVERSE EFFECTS. Bradycardia, bronchospasm, angina, confusion, congestive heart failure, hepatotoxicity, and hypoglycemia with an increased risk of orthostatic hypotension.

CONTRAINDICATIONS. Second- or third-degree heart block, cardiac failure, cardiogenic shock, moderate or severe congestive heart failure, or sinus bradycardia of 45 bpm or less. Should be given with caution to clients with a history of allergy, bronchial asthma, emphysema, diabetes mellitus, or hyperthyroidism.

**POTENTIAL DRUG/FOOD INTERACTIONS**

May potentiate oral hypoglycemics, insulin, or lidocaine. Anesthetics may increase myocardial depression and hypotension. Fentanyl used during surgery may prevent hypertension or diminish the severity of hypertension. Calcium channel blockers, clonidine, diazoxide, neuromuscular blocking agents, or reserpine may be potentiated. NSAIDs, estrogens, and cocaine may reduce the therapeutic effects of labetalol. Cimetidine, phenytoin, and phenothiazines may potentiate the effects of labetalol. Sympathomimetics and xanthines used with labetalol may cause a mutual inhibition of effects.

**INTERVENTIONS: ADMINISTRATION**

Add 200 mg of labetalol to 160 mg of D5W, 0.9% NSS, Ringer's lactate, D5W and NSS (0.2%, 0.33%, or 0.9%), or 2.5% dextrose and 0.45% NSS IV solutions. Resulting concentration is 1 mg labetalol per 1 mL. An alternative concentration results from mixing 200 mg labetalol in 250 mL of solution for a concentration of 2 mg/3 mL.

**MODE/RATE OF ADMINISTRATION**

May be given by IV push over 2 min through a free-flowing infusion. May be given as a continuous IV infusion using a microdrip administration set and an infusion pump.

INTRAVENOUS USE (WITH NORMAL RENAL FUNCTION)

**Adults:** Usual dosage is 20 mg (0.25 mg/kg of body weight for an 80 kg client), given over 2 min. Additional doses of 40–80 mg may be given at 10-min intervals. Maximum total dose is 300 mg.

**Children:** Dose not established.

**Infants/Neonates:** Dose not established.

**Geriatrics:** Elderly clients may be more or less sensitive to the effects, especially to the antihypertensive effects. Diminished hepatic function may require that doses be decreased.

INTRATHECAL USE OR OTHER INFUSION ROUTES AS INDICATED. Not recommended.

▼

**POTENTIAL PROBLEMS IN ADMINISTRATION**

Hypotension is most pronounced while client is in the standing position. Clients should remain supine for at least 3 h after receiving labetalol intravenously. Clients should be carefully observed for evidence of orthostatic hypotension.

**INDEPENDENT NURSING ACTIONS**

Monitor heart rate and rhythm, ECG reports, and hemodynamic status (if available) frequently. Auscultate lungs. Monitor fluid intake and output, blood glucose levels, BUN, and serum bilirubin or other indicators of hepatic function.

**ADMINISTRATION IN ALTERNATE SETTINGS**

IV administration should be done in settings where the client can be closely monitored and where full cardiac technologic support is available.

**EVALUATION: OUTCOMES OF DRUG THERAPY**

**EXPECTED OUTCOMES**

PHYSICAL ASSESSMENT. Systolic blood pressure remains above 75 mm Hg and below 160 mm Hg. Heart rate between 60 and 100 bpm and regular. Breath sounds clear. Extremities warm, pink, and free of edema. Urinary output more than 30 mL/h.

LABORATORY. Serum bilirubin, BUN, serum creatinine, and blood glucose levels remain within client's normal range.

**NEGATIVE OUTCOMES**

Marked hypotension and a weak, irregular heart rate less than 60 bpm. Wheezes and crackles heard on lung auscultation. Urine output less than 30 mL/h. Extremities pale and cool. Client confused or lethargic.

## METHYLDOPATE HYDROCHLORIDE

*Trade Name:* Aldomet
*Canadian Availability:* Aldomet
*Pregnancy Risk:* Category B
*pH:* 3–4.2
*Storage/Stability:* Store below 40° C. Protect from freezing. Stable for 24 hours at room temperature.

**ASSESSMENT: DRUG CHARACTERISTICS**

**ACTION**

An antihypertensive agent whose exact mechanism of action is not known. Appears to stimulate central $\alpha$-adrenergic receptors and decrease sympathetic nervous system stimulation to the heart, kidneys, and peripheral vessels. The decreased sympathetic stimulation causes a decreased peripheral resistance.

**INDICATIONS**

Used to treat severe hypertension, including hypertension resulting from renal disease.

**CAUTIONS**

ADVERSE EFFECTS. Peripheral edema, mental status changes, hemolytic anemia, hepatic toxicity, pancreatitis, myocarditis, systemic lupus erythematosus syndrome, headache, dry mouth.

CONTRAINDICATIONS. Hemolytic anemia, impaired hepatic or renal function, pheochromocytoma, or sensitivity to methyldopate.

**POTENTIAL DRUG/FOOD INTERACTIONS**

May interact with MAO inhibitors to cause a hyperexcitable state. May interact with sympathomimetics such as cocaine and norepinephrine to increase the pressor effects of those drugs and decrease the hypotensive effects of methyldopate. NSAIDs may inhibit the hypotensive effects of methyldopate. Hypotensive effects may be potentiated with concurrent use of other hypotensive agents. Use of haloperidol may increase disorientation or slow cognitive processing. Use with levodopa may potentiate the central nervous system (CNS) effects and cause psychosis. Use with lithium may increase the incidence of lithium toxicity.

**INTERVENTIONS: ADMINISTRATION**

Dilute 250–500 mg in 100 mL of D5W solution.

**MODE/RATE OF ADMINISTRATION**

Given by intermittent IV infusion over 30–60 min.

INTRAVENOUS USE (WITH NORMAL RENAL FUNCTION)

**Adults:** For antihypertensive effect the usual dosage is 250– 500 mg q6h if needed. Maximum dosage is 1 g q6–12 h.

**Children:** For antihypertensive effect the usual dosage is 5–10 mg/kg of body weight q6h if needed. Maximum total daily dose is 65 mg/kg of body weight or 3 g.

**Infants/Neonates:** Use children's dosing schedule.

**Geriatrics:** Elderly clients may be more sensitive to the hypotensive effects. Clients with reduced hepatic or renal function may require a reduced dose.

INTRATHECAL USE OR OTHER INFUSION ROUTES AS INDICATED. Not recommended.

**POTENTIAL PROBLEMS IN ADMINISTRATION**

May have potential to cause sedation. If given with a thiazide diuretic, the dose of the thiazide diuretic should be adjusted.

**INDEPENDENT NURSING ACTIONS**

Monitor heart rate and rhythm, ECG reports, and hemodynamic status (if available) frequently. Monitor fluid intake and output, serum bilirubin levels, BUN, and serum potassium levels.

**ADMINISTRATION IN ALTERNATE SETTINGS**

IV administration should be done in settings where the client can be closely monitored and where full cardiac technologic support is available.

▼

**EVALUATION: OUTCOMES OF DRUG THERAPY**

**EXPECTED OUTCOMES**

PHYSICAL ASSESSMENT. Systolic blood pressure remains above 75 mm Hg and below 160 mm Hg. Heart rate between 60 and 100 bpm and regular. Extremities warm, pink, and free of edema. Urinary output more than 30 mL/h. Client has no complaints of chest pain or confusion.

LABORATORY. Serum potassium, BUN, serum creatinine, serum bilirubin levels, and complete blood counts remain within client's normal range.

**NEGATIVE OUTCOMES**

Marked hypotension and a weak, irregular heart rate less than 60 bpm or more than 100 bpm. Urine output less than 30 mL/h. Extremities pale and cool. Client confused or lethargic and experiences difficulty with cognitive functions.

## NITROPRUSSIDE SODIUM

*Trade Names:* Nitropress, Nipride
*Canadian Availability:* Nipride
*Pregnancy Risk:* Category C
*pH:* 3.5–6
*Storage/Stability:* Store below 40° C. Protect from light. Freshly prepared solutions have a slight brownish tint. Solutions that are dark brown, orange, or blue should be discarded. No other drug should be added to the solution containing nitroprusside. Solutions that change color after administration has begun are showing evidence of degradation and should be discarded. Solution is stable at room temperature for 24 hours when protected from light.

**ASSESSMENT: DRUG CHARACTERISTICS**

**ACTION**

A potent hypotensive agent. Acts directly on arterial and venous smooth muscle to cause vasodilation. Appears to have more effect on veins than on arteries. The resultant decreased peripheral vascular resistance has a variable effect on cardiac output.

**INDICATIONS**

Used to treat congestive heart failure and hypertension. May be used during surgery to produce hypotension.

**CAUTIONS**

ADVERSE EFFECTS. Thiocyanate toxicity or cyanide toxicity, headache, excessive sweating, anxiety, restlessness, tachycardia, abdominal pain, shortness of breath, metabolic acidosis, shallow breathing, or pink color.

CONTRAINDICATIONS. Cerebral or myocardial ischemia, increased intracranial pressure, impaired hepatic or renal function, or vitamin B12 deficiency. Should not be used to treat compensatory hypertension associated with an AV shunt or coarctation of the aorta.

**POTENTIAL DRUG/FOOD INTERACTIONS**

May interact with other antihypertensive agents to increase the degree of hypotension. If used with dobutamine, may increase cardiac output. Sympathomimetics or estrogens may inhibit the hypotensive effects of nitroprusside.

**INTERVENTIONS: ADMINISTRATION**

Dilute 50 mg in 2.3 mL of D5W for injection. Dissolve completely. Solution must be further diluted in 250–1000 mL of D5W solution. The container must be wrapped in an opaque sleeve, aluminum foil, or other opaque material to protect the solution from light. The tubing does not need to be protected.

**MODE/RATE OF ADMINISTRATION**

Given as a continuous infusion using a microdrip infusion set and an infusion pump.

INTRAVENOUS USE (WITH NORMAL RENAL FUNCTION)

**Adults:** For antihypertensive effect the usual dosage is 0.3 mcg (0.0003)/kg of body weight per minute initially, adjusted in several minutes according to blood pressure. Maintenance dosage is 3 mcg (0.003 mg)/kg of body weight per minute. Maximum dose is 10 mcg (0.01 mg)/kg of body weight per minute or not more than 3.5 mg/kg of body weight for a maximum of 10 min. For long-term continuous infusions the maximum dosage should not exceed 3 mcg (0.003 mg)/kg of body weight per minute or 1 mcg (0.001 mg)/kg of body weight for anuric clients.

**Children:** Use adult dosing schedule.

**Infants/Neonates:** Dose not established.

**Geriatrics:** Clients with diminished renal function may require a lower dose. Elderly clients may be more sensitive to the hypotensive effects.

INTRATHECAL USE OR OTHER INFUSION ROUTES AS INDICATED. Not recommended.

**POTENTIAL PROBLEMS IN ADMINISTRATION**

Care should be taken to avoid extravasation, which causes significant pain. Consideration should be given to discontinue a nitroprusside infusion if a dose of 10 mcg (0.01 mg)/kg of body weight has been given for 10 min without desired therapeutic effect. Concurrent administration of sodium thiosulfate may decrease the risk of cyanide toxicity but may potentiate nitroprusside's hypotensive effect. Large doses of sodium thiosulfate increase the risk of thiocyanate toxicity.

**INDEPENDENT NURSING ACTIONS**

Monitor heart rate and rhythm, ECG reports, and hemodynamic status (if available) frequently. Moni-

▼

tor fluid intake and output. Monitor serum cyanide and thiocyanate levels and arterial blood gases for metabolic acidosis.

**ADMINISTRATION IN ALTERNATE SETTINGS**

IV administration should be done in settings where the client can be closely monitored and where full cardiac technologic support is available.

**EVALUATION: OUTCOMES OF DRUG THERAPY**

**EXPECTED OUTCOMES**

PHYSICAL ASSESSMENT. Systolic blood pressure remains above 75 mm Hg and below 160 mm Hg. Heart rate between 60 and 100 bpm and regular. Extremities warm, pink, and free of edema. Urinary output more than 30 mL/h. Client has no complaints of chest pain or confusion.

LABORATORY. Serum cyanide and thiocyanate levels below toxic levels. Arterial blood gases within normal range for client.

**NEGATIVE OUTCOMES**

Marked hypotension and a weak, irregular heart rate less than 60 bpm or more than 100 bpm. Urine output less than 30 mL/h. Extremities pale and cool or pink and cool. Client confused or lethargic and complains of headache or shortness of breath.

## TRIMETHAPHAN CAMSYLATE

*Trade Name:* Arfonad
*Canadian Availability:* Arfonad
*Pregnancy Risk:* Category D
*pH:* 4.9–5.6
*Storage/Stability:* Store between 2° and 8° C. Protect from freezing. IV solutions are stable for 24 hours at room temperature.

**ASSESSMENT: DRUG CHARACTERISTICS**

**ACTION**

An antihypertensive agent that competes with acetylcholine for postsynaptic receptors. The result is peripheral vasodilation and may include histamine release. The decreased peripheral vascular resistance may increase cardiac output in clients with congestive heart failure.

**INDICATIONS**

Used to rapidly reduce blood pressure during hypertensive crises, especially with dissecting aortic aneurysms or with pulmonary edema associated with cardiac failure. May also be used as a hypotensive agent during surgery.

**CAUTIONS**

ADVERSE EFFECTS. Anorexia, nausea, vomiting, orthostatic hypotension, cycloplegia, impotence, paralytic ileus, angina, tachycardia, and urinary retention.

CONTRAINDICATIONS. Should be used with caution with clients with Addison's disease, anemia, hypovolemic shock, cerebral or myocardial ischemia, degenerative diseases of the CNS, glaucoma, impaired hepatic or renal function, respiratory insufficiency, or sensitivity to trimethaphan.

**POTENTIAL DRUG/FOOD INTERACTIONS**

May interact with ambenonium, neostigmine, or pyridostigmine to inhibit the antimyasthenic effects of those drugs. NSAIDs may reduce the antihypertensive effects of trimethaphan. Other antihypertensive agents may potentiate trimethaphan's hypotensive effects. The action of neuromuscular blocking agents may be prolonged. The pressor effects of sympathomimetics may be potentiated.

**INTERVENTIONS: ADMINISTRATION**

Dilute before using, 500 mg in 500 mL of D5W solution.

**MODE/RATE OF ADMINISTRATION**

Given as a continuous infusion, using a microdrip administration set and an infusion pump.

INTRAVENOUS USE (WITH NORMAL RENAL FUNCTION)

**Adults:** For hypertensive emergencies the usual dosage is 500 mcg (0.5 mg) to 1 mg/min, adjusted according to the blood pressure. Maintenance dose is 1–5 mg/min.

**Children:** Usual dosage is 50–150 mcg (0.05–0.15 mg)/kg/min, adjusted according to the blood pressure.

**Infants/Neonates:** Use children's dosing schedule.

**Geriatrics:** Elderly clients may be more sensitive to the hypotensive effects. Dose may need to be decreased.

INTRATHECAL USE OR OTHER INFUSION ROUTES AS INDICATED. Not recommended.

**POTENTIAL PROBLEMS IN ADMINISTRATION**

Hypotensive effects may be enhanced if client is placed in semi-Fowler's position. Caution should be exercised not to cause cerebral ischemia.

**INDEPENDENT NURSING ACTIONS**

Monitor heart rate and rhythm, ECG reports, and hemodynamic status (if available) frequently. Monitor fluid intake and output, blood glucose levels, BUN, and serum potassium levels.

**ADMINISTRATION IN ALTERNATE SETTINGS**

IV administration should be done in settings where the client can be closely monitored and where full cardiac technologic support is available.

**EVALUATION: OUTCOMES OF DRUG THERAPY**

**EXPECTED OUTCOMES**

PHYSICAL ASSESSMENT. Systolic blood pressure remains above 75 mm Hg and below 160 mm Hg. Heart rate between 60 and 100 bpm and regular. Extremities warm, pink, and free of edema. Urinary output more than 30 mL/h. Client has no complaints of chest pain or confusion.

LABORATORY. Serum potassium, BUN, serum creatinine, and serum bilirubin

▼

levels remain within client's normal range.

**NEGATIVE OUTCOMES**

Marked hypotension and a weak, irregular heart rate less than 60 bpm or more than 100 bpm. Urine output less than 30 mL/h. Extremities pale and cool. Client confused or lethargic.

---

## VERAPAMIL HYDROCHLORIDE

*Trade Name:* Isoptin
*Canadian Availability:* Isoptin
*Pregnancy Risk:* Category C
*pH:* 4.1–6
*Storage/Stability:* Store between 15° and 30° C. Protect from light and from freezing. Precipitation occurs in any solution with a pH greater than 6. Diluted solutions are stable for 24 hours at room temperature.

**ASSESSMENT: DRUG CHARACTERISTICS**

**ACTION**

A calcium channel blocker. Mechanism of action is not fully understood. Thought to inhibit flow of calcium and possibly sodium through "slow" channels across certain voltage-sensitive cell membranes, especially in cardiac and vascular tissue. The result is dilation of coronary arteries, peripheral arteries, and arterioles. In addition, heart rate is reduced, myocardial contractility is reduced, and AV conduction is slowed.

**INDICATIONS**

Used to treat angina pectoris, supraventricular tachycardias, and hypertension.

**CAUTIONS**

Should be used with caution in clients with aortic stenosis, bradycardia, cardiogenic shock, congestive heart failure, hypokalemia, myocardial infarction, neuromuscular transmitter deficiency states, renal impairment, ventricular tachycardia, or sensitivity to the agent.

**ADVERSE EFFECTS.** Allergic reactions, bradycardia, congestive heart failure or pulmonary edema, constipation, dizziness, headache, hypotension, nausea, peripheral edema, or weakness.

**CONTRAINDICATIONS.** Second- or third-degree heart block, severe hypotension, sick sinus syndrome. Wolff-Parkinson-White syndrome, or Lown-Ganong-Levine syndrome.

**POTENTIAL DRUG/FOOD INTERACTIONS**

May interact with $\beta$-adrenergic blocking agents to cause marked hypotension from prolonged sinoatrial and AV conduction time. May increase the risk of toxicity for carbamazepine, cyclosporine, quinidine, or theophylline because it slows metabolism of these drugs. Digoxin levels may rise with concurrent use of verapamil. Disopyramide or flecainide used with verapamil may cause death from compounding the negative inotropic properties of both drugs. May interact with potassium-depleting drugs to increase the incidence of arrhythmias. May interact with procainamide, quinidine, or other drugs that prolong the QT interval to compound the negative inotropic effect.

**INTERVENTIONS: ADMINISTRATION**

May be given undiluted.

**MODE/RATE OF ADMINISTRATION**

May be given by IV push through a free-flowing IV solution of D5W or 0.9% NSS. Not recommended for continuous infusion.

INTRAVENOUS USE (WITH NORMAL RENAL FUNCTION)

**Adults:** Initial dose is 5–10 mg or 75–150 mcg (0.075–0.150 mg)/kg of body weight over 2 min. An additional dose of 10 mg or 150 mcg (0.150 mg)/kg of body weight may be given in 30 min if client response indicates.

**Children 1–15 years:** Initial dose is 100–300 mcg (0.1–0.3 mg)/kg of body weight over 2 min. Maximum dose is 5 mg. An additional dose not to exceed 5 mg may be given in 30 min if necessary.

**Infants $<$ 1 year:** Initial dose is 100–200 mcg (0.1–0.2 mg)/kg of body weight over 2 min.

**Geriatrics:** Dose should be administered over 3-min period to avoid undesired effects.

INTRATHECAL USE OR OTHER INFUSION ROUTES AS INDICATED. Not recommended.

**POTENTIAL PROBLEMS IN ADMINISTRATION**

May cause respiratory distress in clients with neuromuscular transmitter deficiencies such as muscular dystrophy.

**INDEPENDENT NURSING ACTIONS**

Monitor heart rate and rhythm, ECG reports, and hemodynamic status (if available) frequently. Auscultate lungs. Monitor fluid intake and output, BUN, and serum potassium levels.

**ADMINISTRATION IN ALTERNATE SETTINGS**

IV administration should be done in settings where the client can be closely monitored and where full cardiac technologic support is available.

**EVALUATION: OUTCOMES OF DRUG THERAPY**

**EXPECTED OUTCOMES**

PHYSICAL ASSESSMENT. Systolic blood pressure remains above 75 mm Hg and below 160 mm Hg. Heart rate between 60 and 100 bpm and regular. Extremities warm, pink, and free of edema. Urinary output more than 30 mL/h.

LABORATORY. BUN, serum creatinine, and serum potassium levels remain within client's normal range.

**NEGATIVE OUTCOMES**

Marked hypotension and a weak, irregular heart rate less than 60 bpm or more than 100 bpm. Urine output less than 30 mL/h. Extremities pale and cool. Client confused or lethargic.

# VASODILATING AGENTS

## THERAPEUTIC EFFECTS

Vasodilating agents are used primarily for the treatment of acute angina and for long-term prophylactic management of angina. Vasodilators may be used to treat clients with congenital intracranial aneurysms that have hemorrhaged to forestall recurrent bleeding. Other uses include relief of peripheral ischemia from arterial spasm and treatment of persistent pulmonary vasoconstriction in newborns.

## PHARMACOKINETICS

**Distribution.** Vasodilating agents are widely distributed throughout the body but are found primarily in the liver and kidneys. Vasodilators may cross the placental barrier and be passed in breast milk.

**Metabolism/Elimination.** In adults with normal renal function, vasodilators are metabolized by the liver and excreted in urine. Plasma half-life varies from minutes to as much as 3 days. Onset of action is rapid, with maximum vasodilation occuring in minutes.

## CAUTIONS

**Side/Adverse Effects.** The most common adverse effects are headache, transient flushing, dizziness, hypotension, vertigo, and piloerection or goose flesh.

**Contraindications.** Vasodilators should be used with caution, if at all, with clients who have glaucoma, impaired hepatic function, marked hypotension, and heart block or other conduction defects.

***Pregnancy and Lactation.*** Vasodilating agents are not known to be mutagenic or teratogenic. Women should be advised not to breastfeed while taking these drugs.

***Children.*** Vasodilating agents are generally not recommended for use in children younger than 18 years of age.

***Infants/Neonates.*** Tolazoline is used specifically with newborns to treat persistent fetal circulation. Other drugs in this group are not recommended for use with infants or neonates.

***Geriatrics.*** No specific recommendations are made.

## TOXICITY

See Table 20–4 for toxicities of vasodilators.

## POTENTIAL DRUG/FOOD INTERACTIONS

Diltiazem and alcohol may potentiate the effects of some vasodilators. Some vasodilators potentiate the effects of hypotensive drugs if used at the same time. Antineoplastic agents may be potentiated by vasodilators. Some vasodilators may antagonize the action of heparin.

**TABLE 20–4**
**Toxicities of Vasodilators**

| Body System | Side/Toxic Effects | Physical Assessment Indicators | Laboratory Indicators | Nursing Interventions |
|---|---|---|---|---|
| Neurologic | Antianxiety properties | Calm depression, dizziness, vertigo, headache, drowsiness, sedation | N/A | Monitor LOC; provide a safe, quiet environment. |
| Cardiovascular | Changes in blood pressure | Flushed face, orthostatic hypotension | N/A | Monitor pulse and blood pressure; change positions slowly. |
| Genitourinary | Priapism | Continued erection | N/A | Observe penis and notify physician if circulation appears compromised. |
| Gastrointestinal | Abdominal distress | Constipation, nausea, diarrhea, anorexia | N/A | Provide symptomatic treatment. |
| Hepatic | Hepatotoxicity | Jaundice | Elevated AST, ALT, total bilirubin | Report changes in laboratory values. |

ALT = alanine aminotransferase, AST = aspartate aminotransferase, LOC = level of consciousness, N/A = not applicable.

## NITROGLYCERIN

*Trade Names:* Nitro-Bid IV, Nitroject
*Canadian Availability:* Nitro-Bid IV, Nitroject
*Pregnancy Risk:* Category C
*pH:*
*Storage/Stability:* Store between 15° and 30° C. Protect from light and from freezing. Diluted solutions should not be kept or used longer than 24 hours.

### ASSESSMENT: DRUG CHARACTERISTICS

#### ACTION

A potent antianginal agent. Reduces blood return to the heart by venous vasodilation (preload) and increases ventricular emptying by reducing arterial resistance (afterload). Reduces myocardial oxygen consumption.

#### INDICATIONS

Used to treat congestive heart failure associated with or not associated with myocardial infarction and to control blood pressure during surgery.

#### CAUTIONS

Doses are based on special non–polyvinyl chloride (PVC) IV infusion sets. Use of standard administration sets may cause as much as 40% to 80% of the diluted nitroglycerin to be absorbed into the infusion set.

ADVERSE EFFECTS. Severe hypotension. Cyanosis, dizziness, shortness of breath, weak rapid pulse, and convulsions may indicate overdose.

CONTRAINDICATIONS. Cerebral hemorrhage, recent head trauma, pericardial tamponade, constrictive pericarditis, or hypovolemia.

#### POTENTIAL DRUG/FOOD INTERACTIONS

May interact with alcohol, antihypertensives, other hypotension-producing agents such as narcotics, or other vasodilators in increase orthostatic hypotension. May decrease the anticoagulant effects of heparin. Sympathomimetics may decrease the antianginal effects of nitroglycerin.

### INTERVENTIONS: ADMINISTRATION

#### MODE/RATE OF ADMINISTRATION

May be given by buccal, lingual, oral, sublingual, topical, and IV routes. Injectable nitroglycerin must be diluted before it is administered intravenously as a continuous infusion.

INTRAVENOUS USE (WITH NORMAL RENAL FUNCTION)

**Adults:** Initial adult dosage is 5 mcg (0.005 mg)/min. The dosage is increased by 5 mcg/min at 3- to 5-min intervals until an effect is achieved or a maximum dose of 20 mcg (0.03 mg) is reached. If no results have been achieved and the dose is 20 mcg/min, the dosage may be increased at 10 mcg (0.01 mg)/q3–5min until an effect has been achieved.

**Children:** No dosage has been determined.

**Infants/Neonates:** No dosage has been determined.

**Geriatrics:** Follow adult dosing suggestions. Be aware that elderly clients may be more sensitive to the hypotensive effects.

INTRATHECAL USE OR OTHER INFUSION ROUTES AS INDICATED. Not recommended.

**POTENTIAL PROBLEMS IN ADMINISTRATION**

Dose titration may be difficult if standard PVC infusion sets are used. With non-PVC sets, infusion pumps may not completely stop the flow if turned off, may not accurately deliver the infusion solution at low flow rates, or may require the addition of standard PVC pieces that negate the advantage of the non-PVC infusion set.

**INDEPENDENT NURSING ACTIONS**

Monitor blood pressure, pulse, hemodynamic values, and urine output. Auscultate heart and breath sounds. Encourage the client to remain as quiet as possible.

**ADMINISTRATION IN ALTERNATE SETTINGS**

Close hemodynamic monitoring of clients is required. Not recommended for administration in settings where such monitoring cannot be done.

**EVALUATION: OUTCOMES OF DRUG THERAPY**

**EXPECTED OUTCOMES**

PHYSICAL ASSESSMENT. Skin pink. Breath sounds clear. Client does not complain of heart pain. Heart rate between 60 and 100 bpm and regular. Urine output between 45 and 60 mL/h.

LABORATORY. BUN, serum creatinine, ALT, and AST within normal range for the client.

**NEGATIVE OUTCOMES**

Client complains of severe angina at rest and during activities of daily living. Adventitious breath sounds heard on auscultation. Peripheral edema noted in lower extremities. Client restless, irritable, or confused.

# CHAPTER 21

# Central Nervous System Agents

*Elaine Kennedy*

**Classification**

**Analgesics**

- Buprenorphine Hydrochloride
- Butorphanol Tartrate
- Fentanyl Citrate
- Hydromorphone Hydrochloride
- Merperidine Hydrochloride
- Morphine Sulfate
- Naloxone Hydrochloride (opioid antagonist)
- Pentazocine

**Anticonvulsants**

- Magnesium Sulfate
- Phenobarbital Sodium
- Phenytoin Sodium

**Anxiolytics, Sedatives, and Hypnotics**

- Diazepam
- Lorazepam
- Midazolam Hydrochloride
- Promethazine Hydrochloride

**Tranquilizers**

- Chlorpromazine Hydrochloride
- Droperidol
- Perphenazine
- Prochlorperazine Edisylate
- Promazine Hydrochloride

Central nervous system (CNS) drugs act primarily on the brain and spinal cord. Following are the common medical uses for CNS drugs:

1. To control pain
2. To prevent or control seizure activity
3. To diminish anxiety or produce sleep
4. To control psychotic behavior
5. To treat a number of unpleasant symptoms such as nausea and vomiting that originate from CNS stimulation

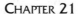

The exact mechanism of action for most CNS drugs has not been determined, but several features of CNS drugs are noteworthy. First, the therapeutic effect of some drugs may increase over time. In particular, the maximum therapeutic effect of antipsychotic and antidepressant drugs may not be achieved for several weeks. Second, unwanted side effects tend to diminish over time. Phenobarbital, for example, usually causes drowsiness when clients first start taking the drug to control seizure activity. The drowsiness diminishes over time. Finally, clients develop a tolerance to and physical dependence on some CNS drugs. For example, clients who have taken morphine for pain for a period of time may require a dose that would cause severe respiratory depression in a client just starting to take morphine.

## CLASSIFICATION

### ANALGESICS

Opioid analgesics alter perceptions and emotional responses to pain. They are usually classified as agonist, partial agonist, or agonist-antagonist based on their action at opioid receptor sites in the CNS and elsewhere. Agonists produce activity at mu, kappa, and delta sites. Partial agonists produce moderate activity at a receptor site but block the action of a full agonist if both agents are used at the same time. Agonist-antagonists produce pain relief if used alone but antagonize the action of agonists if both agents are used at the same time. The agonist-antagonist drugs primarily act to block mu-receptor site activity.

Opioid agonist analgesics, such as hydromorphone, meperidine, and morphine, bind primarily to mu-receptor sites widely found in the CNS and especially in the limbic system, thalamus, striatum, hypothalamus, and the midbrain. Some opioid partial agonist analgesics, such as buprenorphine, partially bind to mu-receptor and kappa sites and produce little activity at the sigma sites. These agents may compete with mu-receptor agonists to displace them, thus increasing the possibility of withdrawal symptoms in clients who are physically dependent on opioid substances. Opioid agonist-antagonist analgesics such as butorphanol and pentazocine bind to kappa- and sigma-receptor sites and fail to bind to mu receptors. These agents have a lower incidence of physical dependence than other opioid substances.

Naloxone is an opioid antagonist that appears to displace opioid analgesics from various opioid receptor sites in the brain and to competitively inhibit receptor uptake of opioid substances.

### ANTICONVULSANTS

Anticonvulsants are used primarily to prevent or diminish the incidence or severity of seizures. The primary drugs used to manage seizures are derivatives of barbiturates such as phenobarbital, benzodiazepines such as diazepam, and hydantoins such as phenytoin. In addition, magnesium sulfate, a CNS depressant, is also used as an antiseizure drug.

Barbiturates are thought to act by depressing the excitability of the nerve cell and by increasing the threshold of electric stimulation of the motor cortex. Benzodiazepines appear to work by damping the spread of electric stimulation from a focal discharge area. Hydantoins appear to work by preventing the nerve synapse from responding to tetanic stimulation.

### ANXIOLYTICS, SEDATIVES, AND HYPNOTICS

Anxiolytic agents decrease anxiety and may also have antiemetic, antivertigo, amnestic, anticonvulsant, antipanic, and skeletal muscle relaxant effects, or sedative-hypnotic action. Barbiturates produce sedation and anticonvulsive activity and induce sleep by general depression of the CNS. In opposition to the benzodiazepines, barbiturates have some effect on the reticular activating system (RAS). By depressing the RAS, sleep can be induced. The benzodiazepines depress the CNS by facilitating the inhibitory neurotransmitter $\gamma$-aminobutyric acid (GABA). Promethazine acts as an antihistaminic by competing for $H_1$-receptor sites, thus blocking histamine effects rather than blocking histamine release.

### TRANQUILIZERS

Tranquilizers may act as antipsychotics, antiemetics, or antidyskinetics. The phenothiazines are classified as low-, medium-, or high-potency antipsychotic agents. Potency is based on the dose of the drug needed to produce the therapeutic effect. Thus, a low-potency phenothiazine requires a higher dose to produce the desired effect. The higher dose may carry a burden of undesirable side effects. Phenothiazines act by blocking postsynaptic dopaminergic receptors in the brain.

Tranquilizers may also have an $\alpha$-adrenergic blocking effect and may decrease hormone release from the hypothalamus and hypophysis. Antiemetic action is created by blocking dopamine receptors in the chemoreceptor trigger zone (CTZ) in the medulla and by blocking vagus stimulation in the gastrointestinal (GI) tract.

CNS infusion agents are grouped by subclassifications in Table 21–1.

## ANALGESICS

### THERAPEUTIC EFFECTS

*Opioid agonist* analgesics bind to specific receptor sites in the CNS and alter perceptions and emotional responses to pain. Some agents such as buprenorphine appear to partially bind to mu-receptor and kappa sites and produce little activity at the sigma sites. These agents may compete with mu-receptor agonists to displace them, thus increasing the possibility of withdrawal symptoms in clients who are physically dependent on opioid substances.

Other opioid agonist analgesics such as hydromorphone, merperidine, and morphine bind primarily to mu-receptor sites widely found in the CNS and especially in the limbic system, thalamus, striatum, hypothalamus, and the midbrain.

**TABLE 21–1**
**Central Nervous System Infusion Agents Grouped by Subclassifications**

**Analgesics**
Buprenorphine hydrochloride
Butorphanol tartrate
Codeine sulfate*
Codeine phosphate*
Fentanyl citrate
Hydromorphone hydrochloride
Levorphanol tartrate*
Meperidine hydrochloride
Methadone hydrochloride*
Morphine sulfate
Nalbuphine hydrochloride*
Naloxone hydrochloride (opioid antagonist)
Oxymorphone hydrochloride*
Pentazocine
Sodium thiosalicylate*
Sufentanil citrate*

**Anticonvulsants**
Clonazepam*
Magnesium sulfate
Phenobarbital sodium
Phenytoin sodium

**Anxiolytics, Sedatives, and Hypnotics**
Amobarbital sodium*
Chlordiazepoxide hydrochloride*
Diazepam
Lorazepam
Methohexital sodium*
Midazolam hydrochloride
Paraldehyde*
Pentobarbital sodium*
Phenobarbital sodium (see under Anticonvulsants this chapter)
Promethazine hydrochloride
Propiomazine hydrochloride*
Secobarbital*

**Tranquilizers**
Chlorpromazine hydrochloride
Droperidol
Perphenazine
Prochlorperazine edisylate
Promazine hydrochloride
Triflupromazine hydrochloride*

*Not discussed in this Chapter.

*Opioid agonist-antagonist* analgesics such as butorphanol and pentazocine bind to kappa- and sigma-receptor sites and fail to bind to mu receptors widely found in the CNS. The failure to bind to mu-receptor sites may diminish withdrawal symptoms in clients with physical dependence on opioid substances. Pentazocine may antagonize mu-receptor agonists, thus precipitating withdrawal symptoms in clients with physical dependence on opioid substances. These agents have a lower incidence of physical dependence than other opioid substances.

Naloxone is an *opioid antagonist* that appears to displace opioid analgesics from various opioid receptor sites in the brain and to competitively inhibit receptor uptake of opioid substances.

## PHARMACOKINETICS

**Distribution.** Analgesics are widely distributed through the body when administered intravenously.

**Metabolism/Elimination.** Opioid agonists and agonist-antagonists are metabolized by the liver and excreted through the urine.

## CAUTIONS

**Side-Adverse Effects.** Administration of analgesics may cause histamine release, hypotension, mild respiratory depression, and withdrawal symptoms such as trembling, nausea, and abdominal cramping.

**Contraindications**

***Pregnancy and Lactation.*** Regular use of analgesics has been determined safe for pregnant women but may lead to withdrawal symptoms in newborns. Analgesics may be passed in the breast milk and should be used carefully with mothers who are breast-feeding.

***Pediatrics.*** Infants younger than 2 years may have increased incidence of respiratory depression. Children may also have paradoxical excitement.

***Geriatrics.*** Elderly clients are more prone to the incidence of respiratory depression. Elderly men are more likely to have prostatic enlargement that makes them more susceptible to urinary retention. Older clients are also more likely to experience GI symptoms such as constipation.

### TOXICITY

See Table 21–2.

### POTENTIAL DRUG/FOOD INTERACTIONS

Analgesics may interact with alcohol, amphetamines, antihypertensives, monoamine oxidase (MAO) inhibitors, anticholinergics, antidiarrheals, buprenorphine, metoclopramide, other CNS depressants, neuromuscular blocking agents, other opioid agonist and opioid agonist-antagonist analgesics, warfarin, and zidovudine. Naloxone reverses the respiratory depression caused by morphine. Naloxone may also interact with opioid analgesics to cause withdrawal symptoms in physically dependent clients.

## BUPRENORPHINE HYDROCHLORIDE

*Trade Name:* Buprenex
*Canadian Availability:* Not specified.
*Pregnancy Risk:* Category C
*pH:* 3.5–5.5
*Storage/Stability:* Store below 40° C. Protect from freezing and from light.

### ASSESSMENT: DRUG CHARACTERISTICS

#### ACTION

An opioid agonist-antagonist analgesic that binds to specific receptor sites in the CNS and alters perceptions and emotional responses to pain. Appears to partially bind to mu-receptor and kappa sites, and produces little activity at the sigma sites. May compete with mu-receptor agonists to displace them, thus increasing the possibility of withdrawal symptoms in clients who are physically dependent on opioid substances. Is 30 times as potent as morphine in analgesic effect. Pain relief begins in 2 to 3 minutes and lasts up to 6 hours.

▼

**TABLE 21–2**
**Analgesic Toxicities**

| Body System | Side/Toxic Effects | Physical Assessment Indicators | Laboratory Indicators | Nursing Interventions |
|---|---|---|---|---|
| Neurologic | Central nervous system depression | Confusion, dizziness, lightheadedness, drowsiness, headache, nightmares, restlessness, euphoria<br>Convulsions* | N/A | Monitor client's level of consciousness; report changes promptly, provide for client safety. |
| Cardiovascular | Cardiac dysrhythmias | Hypotension, hypertension, tachycardia or bradycardia or palpitations<br>Ventricular tachycardia, ventricular fibrillation* | N/A | Monitor client's vital signs, especially pulse rate and rhythm and blood pressure frequently; report significant changes. |
| Respiratory | Mild respiratory depression | Breaths not as deep as previously | N/A | Auscultate breath sounds frequently; have client change position, cough, and deep breath frequently. |
| Renal/urologic | Bladder muscle dysfunction | Urinary retention, painful urination<br>Antidiuretic effect | Serum sodium >145 mEq/L | Measure and record intake and output; report output less than 30 mL/h. |
| Gastrointestinal | Gastrointestinal disturbance | Nausea, vomiting, stomach cramps, constipation, dry mouth, biliary spasm | Serum sodium and potassium chloride more than or less than client's baseline | Monitor client for evidence of vomiting or constipation; assess client for abdominal cramps or dry mouth; provide comfort measures such as frequent mouth care. |
| Sensory | Vision | Conjunctivitis, blurred vision | N/A | Provide for client safety. |

**INDICATIONS**

Used to treat moderate to severe pain. Used also in the treatment of acute myocardial infarctions.

**CAUTIONS**

ADVERSE EFFECTS. Generally incites fewer adverse reactions than other opioid substances do, but sedation can be excessive. May cause hypotension, mild respiratory depression, confusion, conjunctivitis, histamine release, hypertension, urinary retention. May also cause withdrawal symptoms of confusion, dizziness, lightheadedness, drowsiness, nausea, vomiting, abdominal cramps, malaise, anorexia, headache, restlessness, or fatigue.

CONTRAINDICATIONS. Diarrhea associated with use of cephalosporins, lincomycins, penicillins, or other poisoning until all toxic material has been eliminated from the GI tract; concomitant diazepam or lorazepam therapy; respiratory depression, asthma, chronic respiratory diseases, or inflammatory bowel diseases. Reduced dose required for clients with liver dysfunction.

**POTENTIAL DRUG/FOOD INTERACTIONS**

May interact with alcohol or other CNS depressants to increase CNS depression. May potentiate the effects of MAO inhibitors if given at the same time. May antagonize the effects of other opioid substances. Naloxone reverses the respiratory depression caused by buprenorphine but is not as effective as with other opioids.

**INTERVENTIONS: ADMINISTRATION**

Does not require dilution if given by intravenous (IV) push.

**MODE/RATE OF ADMINISTRATION**

Given IV push over 3–5 min.

INTRAVENOUS USE (WITH NORMAL RENAL AND HEPATIC FUNCTION)

**Adults:** For pain the usual dosage is 300 mcg (0.3 mg) q6h or as needed. It may be necessary to give an additional dose of 300 mcg (0.3 mg) ½ to 1h after the initial dose to achieve desired pain control.

**Children:** Dose not established.

**Infants/Neonates:** Dose not established.

**Geriatrics:** Elderly clients are more likely to experience respiratory depression and urinary retention and to have age-related decreases in hepatic and renal functioning that decrease the rate of drug metabolism. Older clients may require dose adjustment and lower doses, usually one half the dose in high-risk clients.

INTRATHECAL USE OR OTHER INFUSION ROUTES AS INDICATED. Not recommended.

**POTENTIAL PROBLEMS IN ADMINISTRATION**

Clients should be lying down when buprenorphine is administered because of its potential for causing dizziness and hypotension. Bolus injection of buprenorphine may elicit severe allergic reactions, hypotension, or cardiac arrest. Buprenorphine should be administered slowly over several minutes.

**INDEPENDENT NURSING ACTIONS**

Assess client frequently for acute or chronic pain. Monitor vital signs. Monitor for changes in level of consciousness, irritability, or restlessness. Observe physical appearance for acute pain behaviors such as crying, moaning, or grimacing. Observe for chronic pain behaviors such as irritability or depression.

**ADMINISTRATION IN ALTERNATE SETTINGS**

May be given in a variety of clinical settings and in the home by a qualified IV nurse.

**EVALUATION: OUTCOMES OF DRUG THERAPY**

**EXPECTED OUTCOMES**

PHYSICAL ASSESSMENT. Vital signs are within client's baseline with no tachycardia, hypertension, or tachypnea. Clients with acute pain verbalize less discomfort and are able to move without complaints of severe discomfort. Clients with chronic pain are able to carry out desired activities without complaints of severe pain or mental cloudiness. No nausea, vomiting, or diarrhea. Skin warm, pink, and dry. Client shows no writhing, grimacing, or unnatural stillness.

LABORATORY. No significant laboratory studies.

**NEGATIVE OUTCOMES**

Vital signs are more than 15% higher or lower than client's baseline. Clients may have tachycardia, hypertension, tachypnea, or gasping. Clients with acute pain verbalize severe discomfort and are unable to move without complaints of severe discomfort. Clients with chronic pain are unable to carry out desired activities without complaints of severe pain or mental cloudiness. Clients may complain of nausea, vomiting, or diarrhea. Skin pale and diaphoretic. Client shows writhing, grimacing, or unnatural stillness.

## BUTORPHANOL TARTRATE

*Trade Name:* Stadol
*Canadian Availability:* Stadol
*Pregnancy Risk:* Category unknown (drug is secreted in breast milk and crosses the placental barrier)
*pH:* 4.5
*Storage/Stability:* Store between 15° and 30° C. Protect from freezing and from light.

**ASSESSMENT: DRUG CHARACTERISTICS**

**ACTION**

An opioid agonist-antagonist analgesic that binds to specific receptor sites in the CNS and alters perceptions and emotional responses to pain. Appears to bind to kappa- and sigma-receptor sites and fails to bind to mu

▼

receptors widely found in the CNS. The failure to bind to mu-receptor sites may diminish withdrawal symptoms in clients who are physically dependent on opioid substances. Has lower incidence of physical dependence than other opioid substances. Pain relief begins immediately, peaks at 30 minutes, and lasts up to 3 hours.

**INDICATIONS**

Used to treat moderate to severe pain. Used also as an adjunct to anesthesia.

**CAUTIONS**

ADVERSE EFFECTS. Histamine release, antidiuretic effect, dizziness, light-headedness, drowsiness, malaise, headache, hypotension, anorexia, mild respiratory depression nausea, vomiting, fatigue, or painful urination.

CONTRAINDICATIONS. Diarrhea associated with use of cephalosporins, lincomycins, penicillins, or other poisoning until all toxic material has been eliminated from the GI tract; respiratory depression, asthma, chronic respiratory disease, inflammatory bowel diseases, biliary disease, or hypertension. Should be used with caution in clients with myocardial infarction, since butorphanol may increase cardiac workload.

**POTENTIAL DRUG/FOOD INTERACTIONS**

May interact with alcohol or other CNS depressants such as phenothiazines and droperidol to increase CNS depression. May potentiate the constipating effects of anticholinergics and antidiarrheals if given at the same time. May inhibit the GI effects of metoclopramide if given at the same time. May potentiate the effects of antihypertensives and MAO inhibitors if given at the same time. Neuromuscular blocking agents and other opioid agonist analgesics may potentiate the respiratory depression caused by butorphanol. Naloxone reverses the respiratory depression caused by butorphanol.

**INTERVENTIONS: ADMINISTRATION**

Does not require dilution if given by IV push.

**MODE/RATE OF ADMINISTRATION**

Usually given IV push over 3–5 min for each 2 mg, or less.

INTRAVENOUS USE (WITH NORMAL RENAL AND HEPATIC FUNCTION)

**Adults:** For pain the usual dosage is 500 mcg (0.5 mg)–2 mg q3–4h as needed.

As an anesthesia adjunct the usual preoperative dose is 2 mg 1–1½h before surgery. Doses up to 4 mg may be given during surgery as supplemental doses.

**Children 18 years:** Doses not established.

**Infants/Neonates:** Doses not established.

**Geriatrics:** Elderly clients are more likely to experience respiratory depression and urinary retention and to have age-related decreases in hepatic and renal functioning that decrease the rate drug metabolism. Older clients may require dose adjustment and lower doses.

INTRATHECAL USE OR OTHER INFUSION ROUTES AS INDICATED. Not recommended.

**POTENTIAL PROBLEMS IN ADMINISTRATION**

Clients should be lying down when butorphanol is administered because of its potential for causing dizziness and hypotension. Butorphanol should be administered slowly over several minutes.

**INDEPENDENT NURSING ACTIONS**

Assess client frequently for acute or chronic pain. Monitor vital signs. Monitor for changes in level of consciousness, irritability, or restlessness. Observe physical appearance for acute pain behaviors such as crying, moaning, or grimacing. Observe for chronic pain behaviors such as irritability or depression.

**ADMINISTRATION IN ALTERNATE SETTINGS**

May be given in a variety of clinical settings and in the home by a qualified infusion therapy nurse.

**EVALUATION: OUTCOMES OF DRUG THERAPY**

**EXPECTED OUTCOMES**

PHYSICAL ASSESSMENT. Vital signs are within client's baseline with no tachycardia, hypertension, or tachypnea. Clients with acute pain verbalize less discomfort and are able to move without complaints of severe discomfort. Clients with chronic pain are able to carry out desired activities without complaints of severe pain or mental cloudiness. No nausea, vomiting, or diarrhea. Skin warm, pink, and dry. Client shows no writhing, grimacing, or unnatural stillness.

LABORATORY. No sigificant laboratory studies.

**NEGATIVE OUTCOMES**

Vital signs are more than 15% higher or lower than client's baseline. Clients may have tachycardia, hypertension, tachypnea, or gasping. Clients with acute pain verbailize severe discomfort and are unable to move without complaints of severe discomfort. Clients with chronic pain are unable to carry out desired activities without complaints of severe pain or mental cloudiness. Clients may complain of nausea, vomiting, or diarrhea. Skin pale and diaphoretic. Client shows writhing, grimacing, or sedation.

## FENTANYL CITRATE

*Trade Names:* Sublimaze, Innovar (with droperidol)
*Canadian Availability:* Sublimaze
*Pregnancy Risk:* Category C
*pH:* 4–7.5
*Storage/Stability:* Store below 40° C. Protect from freezing and from light.

▼

## ASSESSMENT: DRUG CHARACTERISTICS

### ACTION

An opiate agonist similar to morphine and meperidine. Respiratory effects are shorter in duration with fentanyl than with morphine or meperidine. Binds to specific receptor sites in the CNS and alters perceptions and emotional responses to pain.

### INDICATIONS

Used parenterally in the perioperative period, especially for its strong analgesic effects. Also used for its anxiolytic and sedative effects and is particularly useful for diagnostic procedures where the client must be lightly anesthetized (IV conscious sedation).

### CAUTIONS

ADVERSE EFFECTS. Constipation, dizziness, light-headedness, drowsiness, hypotension, or fatigue; allergic response with difficulty breathing, skeletal or thoracic rigidity, confusion, tachycardia or bradycardia or palpitations, tremors, antidiuretic effect, biliary spasm, blurred vision, dry mouth, euphoria, stomach cramps, malaise, anorexia, headache, restlessness, or painful urination. Nausea and vomiting are less likely to occur than with other opiate agonists. If used with droperidol, the effects of droperidol must be considered.

CONTRAINDICATIONS. Diarrhea associated with use of cephalosporins, lincomycins, penicillins, or other poisoning until all toxic material has been eliminated from the GI tract; respiratory depression, asthma, chronic respiratory diseases, or inflammatory bowel diseases.

### POTENTIAL DRUG/FOOD INTERACTIONS

May interact with alcohol or other CNS depressants to increase CNS depression. May potentiate the constipating effects of anticholinergics and antidiarrheals if given at the same time. May potentiate the effects of antihypertensives and MAO inhibitors if given at the same time. Buprenorphine may inhibit the analgesic action of fentanyl. Neuromuscular blocking agents and other opioid agonist analgesics may potentiate the respiratory depression caused by fentanyl.

## INTERVENTIONS: ADMINISTRATION

Usually given undiluted. Ampules of 50 mcg/mL are available in 2-, 5-, 10-, 20-, and 50-mL volumes.

### MODE/RATE OF ADMINISTRATION

Given IV push over 1–2 min.

INTRAVENOUS USE (WITH NORMAL RENAL FUNCTION)

**Adults:** For low-dose regimen the usual dose is 2 mcg/kg of body weight.

For moderate-dose regimen the usual dose is 2–20 mcg/kg initially; then 25–100 mcg/kg as necessary.

For high-dose regimen the usual dose is 20–50 mcg/kg initially, then 25 mcg/kg to one half the initial dose as necessary.

**Children 12 years:** Follow the adult dosing schedule.

**Children 2–12 years:** The usual perioperative dose is 1.7–3.3 mcg/kg.

**Infants/Neonates:** Not recommended for infants younger than 2 years.

**Geriatrics:** Elderly clients are more likely to experience respiratory depression and to have age-related decreases in hepatic and renal functioning that decrease the rate of drug metabolism. Older clients may require dose adjustment and lower doses.

INTRATHECAL USE OR OTHER INFUSION ROUTES AS INDICATED. May be given epidurally by a specially trained and qualified individual.

**POTENTIAL PROBLEMS IN ADMINISTRATION**

Clients should be lying down when fentanyl is administered because of its potential for causing dizziness and hypotension.

**INDEPENDENT NURSING ACTIONS**

Assess client frequently for acute or chronic pain. Monitor vital signs. Monitor for changes in level of consciousness, irritability, or restlessness. Observe physical appearance for acute pain behaviors such as crying, moaning, or grimacing.

**ADMINISTRATION IN ALTERNATE SETTINGS**

May be given intravenously in a variety of clinical settings and in the home by a qualified IV nurse.

**EVALUATION: OUTCOMES OF DRUG THERAPY**

**EXPECTED OUTCOMES**

PHYSICAL ASSESSMENT. Vital signs are within 15% of client's baseline with no tachycardia, hypertension, tachypnea, or gasping. Clients with acute pain verbalize less discomfort and are able to move without complaints of severe discomfort. No nausea, vomiting, or diarrhea. Skin warm, pink, and dry. Client shows no writhing, grimacing, or unnatural stillness.

LABORATORY.

No significant laboratory studies.

**NEGATIVE OUTCOMES**

Vital signs are more than 15% higher or lower than client's baseline. Clients may have tachycardia, hypertension, tachypnea, or gasping. Clients with acute pain verbalize severe discomfort and are unable to move without complaints of severe discomfort. Clients may complain of nausea, vomiting, or diarrhea. Skin pale and diaphoretic. Client shows writhing, grimacing, or sedation.

## HYDROMORPHONE HYDROCHLORIDE

*Trade Name:* Dilaudid
*Canadian Availability:* Dilaudid
*Pregnancy Risk:* Category C
*pH:* 4–5.5
*Storage/Stability:* Store below 40° C. Protect from freezing and from light.

▼

## ASSESSMENT: DRUG CHARACTERISTICS

### ACTION

An opioid agonist analgesic and antitussive that binds to specific receptor sites in the CNS and alters perceptions and emotional responses to pain. Appears to bind mu-receptor sites widely found in the CNS and especially in the limbic system, thalamus, striatum, hypothalamus, and the midbrain. Is five times more potent than morphine. Pain relief begins immediately and lasts 3 to 4 hours.

### INDICATIONS

Used to relieve moderate to severe, acute or chronic pain. Commonly used in high doses for critically ill clients with cancer.

### CAUTIONS

ADVERSE EFFECTS. Dizziness, light-headedness, drowsiness, hypotension, mild respiratory depression, or fatigue; allergic response with difficulty breathing, confusion, tremors, antidiuretic effect, biliary spasm, blurred vision, constipation, dry mouth, euphoria, abdominal cramps, malaise, headache, nausea, vomiting, restlessness, or painful urination.

CONTRAINDICATIONS. Diarrhea associated with use of cephalosporins, lincomycins, penicillins, or other poisoning until all toxic material has been eliminated from the GI tract; respiratory depression, asthma, chronic respiratory diseases, or inflammatory bowel diseases.

### POTENTIAL DRUG/FOOD INTERACTIONS

May interact with other CNS depressants to increase CNS depression. May potentiate the constipating effects of anticholinergics and antidiarrheals if given at the same time. May inhibit the GI effects of metoclopramide if given at the same time. May potentiate the effects of antihypertensives and MAO inhibitors if given at the same time. Buprenorphine may inhibit the analgesic action of hydromorphone. Neuromuscular blocking agents and other opioid agonist analgesics may potentiate the respiratory depression caused by hydromorphone. Naloxone reverses the respiratory depression caused by hydromorphone.

## INTERVENTIONS: ADMINISTRATION

Dilute with 5 mL of sterile water or saline for IV push. For continuous infusion, each 0.1 mg is diluted in 1 mL of normal saline.

### MODE/RATE OF ADMINISTRATION

Usually given IV push over 4–5 min for 2 mg. May be added to 0.9% normal saline solution (NSS) or 5% dextrose in water (D5W) solutions for continuous infusion with infusion pump.

INTRAVENOUS USE (WITH NORMAL RENAL AND HEPATIC FUNCTION)

**Adults:** For moderate pain the usual IV push dosage is 500 mcg (0.5 mg)–1 mg q3h as needed. For more severe pain, 2–4 mg is given q4–6 h. Continuous infusion doses are titrated by physician order on an individual basis, often as high as 2–9 mg/h.

**Children 12 years:** Follow adult dosing schedule.

**Infants/Neonates:** Dose not established.

**Geriatrics:** Elderly clients are more likely to experience respiratory depression and urinary retention and to have age-related decreases in hepatic and renal functioning that decrease the rate of drug metabolism. Older clients may require dose adjustment and lower doses.

INTRATHECAL USE OR OTHER INFUSION ROUTES AS INDICATED. Not recommended.

#### POTENTIAL PROBLEMS IN ADMINISTRATION

Clients should be lying down when hydromorphone is administered because of its potential for causing dizziness and hypotension.

#### INDEPENDENT NURSING ACTIONS

Assess client frequently for acute or chronic pain. Monitor vital signs. Monitor for changes in level of consciousness, irritability, or restlessness. Observe physical appearance for acute pain behaviors such as crying, moaning, or grimacing. Observe for chronic pain behaviors such as irritability or depression.

#### ADMINISTRATION IN ALTERNATE SETTINGS

May be given in a variety of clinical settings and in the home by a qualified infusion nurse. Clients receiving continuous infusions should not be in bed more than 50% of the day unless there is a full-time caregiver in the home.

### EVALUATION: OUTCOMES OF DRUG THERAPY

#### EXPECTED OUTCOMES

PHYSICAL ASSESSMENT. Vital signs are within client's baseline with no tachycardia, hypertension, or tachypnea. Clients with acute pain verbalize less discomfort and are able to move without complaints of severe discomfort. Clients with chronic pain are able to carry out desired activities without complaints of severe pain or mental cloudiness. No nausea, vomiting, or diarrhea. Skin warm, pink, and dry. Client shows no writhing, grimacing, or unnatural stillness.

LABORATORY. No significant laboratory studies.

#### NEGATIVE OUTCOMES

Vital signs are more than 15% higher or lower than client's baseline. Clients may have tachycardia, hypertension, tachypnea, or gasping. Clients with acute pain verbalize severe discomfort and are unable to move without complaints of severe discomfort. Clients with chronic pain are unable to carry out desired activities without complaints of severe pain or mental cloudiness. Clients may complain of nausea, vomiting, or diarrhea. Skin pale and diaphoretic. Client shows writhing, grimacing, or sedation.

## Meperidine Hydrochloride

*Trade Name:* Demerol
*Canadian Availability:* Demerol
*Pregnancy Risk:* Category B
*pH:* 3.5–6
*Storage/Stability:* Store below 40° C. Protect from freezing and from light.

### ASSESSMENT: DRUG CHARACTERISTICS

#### ACTION

An opioid agonist analgesic that binds to specific receptor sites in the CNS and alters perceptions and emotional responses to pain. Appears to bind to mu-receptor sites widely found in the CNS and especially in the limbic system, thalamus, striatum, hypothalamus, and the midbrain. Is readily absorbed but has an extended half-life (15 to 30 hours) that can lead to cumulative effects. Is slightly less potent than morphine. Pain relief begins in 5 mintues and lasts about 2 hours.

#### INDICATIONS

Used on a short-term basis to relieve moderate to severe pain. Used also as an adjunct to anesthesia.

#### CAUTIONS

ADVERSE EFFECTS. Histamine release, constipation, dizziness, light-headedness, drowsiness, hypotension, mild respiratory depression, nausea, vomiting, or fatigue; allergic response with difficulty breathing, confusion, convulsions, tachycardia or bradycardia or palpitations, tremors, antidiuretic effect, biliary spasm, blurred vision, dry mouth, euphoria, abdominal cramps, malaise, anorexia, headache, restlessness, nightmares, or painful urination.

CONTRAINDICATIONS. Diarrhea associated with use of cephalosporins, lincomycins, penicillins, or other poisoning until all toxic material has been eliminated from the GI tract; respiratory depression, asthma, chronic respiratory diseases, or inflammatory bowel diseases. Must be used with caution in clients with glaucoma and head injuries.

#### POTENTIAL DRUG/FOOD INTERACTIONS

May interact with alcohol or other CNS depressants such as tricyclic antidepressants to increase CNS depression. May potentiate the constipating effects of anticholinergics and antidiarrheals if given at the same time. May potentiate the effects of warfarin. May inhibit the GI effects of metoclopramide if given at the same time. May potentiate the effects of antihypertensives and MAO inhibitors if given at the same time. Buprenorphine may inhibit the analgesic action of meperidine. Neuromuscular blocking agents and other opioid agonist analgesics may potentiate the respiratory depression caused by meperidine. Amphetamines may potentiate the analgesic effects of meperidine. Naloxone reverses the respiratory depression caused by meperidine. The rate of hepatic clearance may be slowed if meperidine is given at the same time as zidovudine, thus increasing the risk of toxicity of both drugs. Action inhibited by hydantoins (e.g., phenytoin). Incompatible with aminophylline, furosemide, heparin, hydrocortisone, methylprednisolone, and methicillin.

**INTERVENTIONS: ADMINISTRATION**

Dilute to 10 mg/mL for IV push; use at least 5 mL of sterile water or NSS. For continuous infusion, meperidine is available as 10, 25, 50, 75, or 100 mg/mL. Each 10 mg is diluted in at least 1 mL of NSS or D5W.

**MODE/RATE OF ADMINISTRATION**

May be given IV push. May be given by continuous IV infusion, using an infusion pump or a patient-controlled analgesia (PCA) device.

INTRAVENOUS USE (WITH NORMAL RENAL AND HEPATIC FUNCTION)

**Adults:** For pain the usual dosage is 15–35 mg/h by infusion pump. For anesthesia adjunct the usual dose is small doses of 10 mg/mL during anesthesia or continuous infusion of 1 mg/mL.

**Children 12 years:** Follow adult dosing schedule.

**Infants/Neonates:** Not established for IV injection.

**Geriatrics:** Elderly clients are more likely to experience respiratory depression and urinary retention and to have age-related decreases in hepatic and renal functioning that decrease the rate of drug metabolism. Older clients may require dose adjustment and lower doses, especially in debilitated clients or those with hepatic or renal disease.

INTRATHECAL USE OR OTHER INFUSION ROUTES AS INDICATED. Not recommended.

**POTENTIAL PROBLEMS IN ADMINISTRATION**

Clients should be lying down when meperidine is administered because of its potential for causing dizziness and hypotension. Meperidine should be administered slowly over several minutes.

**INDEPENDENT NURSING ACTIONS**

Assess client frequently for acute or chronic pain. Monitor vital signs. Monitor for changes in level of consciousness, irritability, or restlessness. Observe physical appearance for acute pain behaviors such as crying, moaning, or grimacing. Observe for chronic pain behaviors such as irritability or depression. Observe for hypotension and dizziness.

**ADMINISTRATION IN ALTERNATE SETTINGS**

May be given in a variety of clinical settings and in the home by a qualified infusion nurse. Clients receiving continuous infusions should not be in bed more than 50% of the day unless there is a full-time caregiver in the home.

**EVALUATION: OUTCOMES OF DRUG THERAPY**

**EXPECTED OUTCOMES**

PHYSICAL ASSESSMENT. Vital signs are within client's base-

▼

line with no tachycardia, hypertension, or tachypnea. Clients with acute pain verbalize less discomfort and are able to move without complaints of severe discomfort. Clients with chronic pain are able to carry out desired activities without complaints of severe pain or mental cloudiness. No nausea, vomiting, or diarrhea. Skin warm, pink, and dry. Client shows no writhing, grimacing, or unnatural stillness.

LABORATORY. No significant laboratory studies.

**NEGATIVE OUTCOMES**

Vital signs are more than 15% higher or lower than client's baseline. Clients may have tachycardia, hypertension, tachypnea, or gasping. Clients with acute pain verbalize severe discomfort and are unable to move without complaints of severe discomfort. Clients with chronic pain are unable to carry out desired activities without complaints of severe pain or mental cloudiness. Clients may complain of nausea, vomiting, or diarrhea. Skin pale and diaphoretic. Client shows writhing, grimacing, or sedation.

## MORPHINE SULFATE

*Trade Names:* Astramorph PF, Duramorph, Infumorph (not for IV use)
*Canadian Availability:* Epimorph
*Pregnancy Risk:* Category C
*pH:* 3–6
*Storage/Stability:* Store below 40° C. Protect from freezing and from light.

### ASSESSMENT: DRUG CHARACTERISTICS

**ACTION**

An opioid agonist analgesic that binds to specific receptor sites in the CNS and alters perceptions and emotional responses to pain. Appears to bind to mu-receptor sites widely found in the CNS and especially in the limbic system, thalamus, striatum, hypothalamus, and the midbrain. Pain relief begins almost immediately and lasts about 2 hours.

**INDICATIONS**

Used to relieve severe to excruciating pain. Used also in the treatment of acute myocardial infarctions and acute pulmonary edema by lowering myocardial oxygen requirements, reducing anxiety, and relieving pulmonary congestion. Restores uterine tone and contractions in a uterus made hyperactive by oxytocic drugs.

**CAUTIONS**

ADVERSE EFFECTS. Histamine release, constipation, dizziness, light-headedness, drowsiness, hypotension, mild respiratory depression, nausea, vomiting, or fatigue; allergic response with difficulty breathing, confusion, tachycardia or bradycardia or palpitations, tremors, antidiuretic effect, biliary spasm, blurred vision, dry mouth, euphoria, abdominal cramps, malaise, anorexia, headache, restlessness, or painful urination. Overdose can cause coma, anaphylaxis, severe hypotension, inverted T wave on electrocardiogram (ECG), myocardial depression, or death.

CONTRAINDICATIONS. Diarrhea associated with use of cephalosporins, lincomycins, penicillins, or other poisoning until all toxic material has been eliminated from the GI tract; acute alcoholism, respiratory depression, asthma, chronic respiratory diseases, or inflammatory bowel diseases; benign prostatic hypertrophy, biliary tract surgery, or surgical anastomosis. Used with caution in clients with head injury, hepatic or renal dysfunction, or supraventricular tachycardia.

**POTENTIAL DRUG/FOOD INTERACTIONS**

May interact with alcohol or other CNS depressants such as phenothiazines to increase CNS depression. May potentiate the constipating effects of anticholinergics and antidiarrheals if given at the same time. May inhibit the GI effects of metoclopramide if given at the same time. May potentiate the effects of antihypertensives and MAO inhibitors if given at the same time. Buprenorphine may inhibit the analgesic action of morphine. Neuromuscular blocking agents and other opioid agonist analgesics may potentiate the respiratory depression caused by morphine. Naloxone reverses the respiratory depression caused by morphine. The rate of hepatic clearance may be slowed if morphine is given at the same time as zidovudine, thus increasing the risk of toxicity of both drugs. Incompatible with aminophylline, heparin, chlorothiazide, meperidine, methicillin, phenytoin, and phenobarbital.

**INTERVENTIONS: ADMINISTRATION**

Dilute in 4–5 mL of sterile water to administer by IV push. May require further dilution if administered by other routes.

**MODE/RATE OF ADMINISTRATION**

May be given by IV push. May be given by continuous IV or subcutaneous infusion, using an infusion pump or a PCA device. May also be given by epidural or intrathecal injection.

INTRAVENOUS USE (WITH NORMAL RENAL AND HEPATIC FUNCTION)

**Adults:** For pain the usual IV dose of 4–15 mg in 4–5 mL of sterile water over several minutes and may be repeated every 2–4h as needed. Clients with severe chronic pain from cancer often require up to 150 mg/h.

The usual epidural dose is 5 mg. If no relief, doses of 1–2 mg may be given after 1h up to 10 mg/24 h.

The usual intrathecal dose is 200 mcg (0.2 mg) to 1 mg for one dose.

▼

**Children 12 years:** Follow adult dosing schedule.

**Infants/Neonates:** For pain the usual dose is 50–100 mcg (0.05–0.1 mg)/kg of body weight over several minutes. For severe pain associated with cancer or sickle cell crisis, 0.25–2.5 mg/kg/h may be given. For postoperative analgesia, 0.01–0.04 mg/kg/h is given, reduced to 0.015–0.02 mg/kg/h for neonates.

**Geriatrics:** Elderly clients are more likely to experience respiratory depression and urinary retention and to have age- related decreases in hepatic and renal functioning that decrease the rate of drug metabolism. Older clients may require dose adjustment and lower doses.

INTRATHECAL USE OR OTHER INFUSION ROUTES AS INDICATED. May be given as an epidural or intrathecal infusion. See dosing schedule above.

#### POTENTIAL PROBLEMS IN ADMINISTRATION

Clients should be lying down when morphine is administered because of its potential for causing dizziness and hypotension. Morphine should be administered slowly over several minutes.

#### INDEPENDENT NURSING ACTIONS

Assess client frequently for acute or chronic pain. Monitor vital signs. Monitor for changes in level of consciousness, irritability, or restlessness. Observe physical appearance for acute pain behaviors such as crying, moaning, or grimacing. Observe for chronic pain behaviors such as irritability or depression.

#### ADMINISTRATION IN ALTERNATE SETTINGS

May be given in a variety of clinical settings and in the home by a qualified infusion nurse. Clients receiving continuous infusions should not be in bed more than 50% of the day unless there is a full-time caregiver in the home.

#### EVALUATION: OUTCOMES OF DRUG THERAPY

#### EXPECTED OUTCOMES

PHYSICAL ASSESSMENT. Vital signs are within client's baseline with no tachycardia, hypertension, tachypnea, or gasping. Clients with acute pain verbalize less discomfort and are able to move without complaints of severe discomfort. Clients with chronic pain are able to carry out desired activities without complaints of severe pain or mental cloudiness. No nausea, vomiting, or diarrhea. Skin warm, pink, and dry. Client shows no writhing, grimacing, or unnatural stillness.

LABORATORY. No significant laboratory studies.

#### NEGATIVE OUTCOMES

Vital signs are more than 15% higher or lower than client's baseline. Clients may have tachycardia, hypertension, tachypnea, or gasping. Clients with acute pain verbalize severe discomfort and are unable to move wihout complaints of severe discomfort. Clients with chronic pain are unable to carry out desired activities without complaints of severe pain or mental cloudiness. Clients may complain of nausea, vomiting, or diarrhea. Skin pale and diaphoretic. Client shows writhing, grimacing, or unnatural stillness.

## NALOXONE HYDROCHLORIDE

*Trade Name:* Narcan
*Canadian Availability:* Narcan
*Pregnancy Risk:* Category B
*pH:* 3–4.5
*Storage/Stability:* Store below 40° C. Protect from freezing and light. Use within 24 hours after diluting for IV infusion.

### ASSESSMENT: DRUG CHARACTERISTICS

#### ACTION

An opioid antagonist whose exact action is not fully understood. Appears to displace opioid analgesics from various opioid receptor sites in the brain and to competitively inhibit receptor uptake of opioid substances. Action is immediate and lasts 1 to 4 hours.

#### INDICATIONS

Used to relieve respiratory depression and toxicity resulting from opioid analgesic therapy. Is not effective in reversing respiratory depression caused by anesthetics or nonopioid analgesics.

#### CAUTIONS

ADVERSE EFFECTS. Convulsions, ventricular tachycardia, ventricular fibrillation, or symptoms of withdrawal such as diaphoresis, runny nose, body aches, nausea, vomiting, abdominal cramps, irritability, trembling, restlessness, or excitement in clients with physical dependence on opioids. Overdose can cause excitement, hypertension or hypotension, and pulmonary edema.

CONTRAINDICATIONS. History of allergic reaction to naloxone, known physical dependency on opioids, or cardiac irritability.

#### POTENTIAL DRUG/FOOD INTERACTIONS

May interaect with butorphanol, nalbuphine, pentazocine, or opioid analgesics to cause withdrawal symptoms in physically dependent clients.

### INTERVENTIONS: ADMINISTRATION

Add 2 mL of 1 mg/mL of naloxone to 500 mL of D5W or 0.9% NSS to achieve a concentration of 4 mcg (0.004 mg)/mL. May also be given undiluted.

#### MODE/RATE OF ADMINISTRATION

May be given IV push (0.4 mg or less) over 15 s or by continuous IV infusion.

▼

#### INTRAVENOUS USE (WITH NORMAL RENAL FUNCTION)

**Adults:** The usual emergency IV dose is 400 mcg (0.4 mg) to 2 mg. The dose may be repeated at 2- to 3-min intervals. However, if symptoms of CNS depression have not substantially improved after 10 mg of naloxone has been administered, the cause of symptoms is unlikely to be from opioid substances.

For postoperative opioid depression the usual dosage is 100–200 mcg (0.1–0.2 mg) q2–3 min until adequate ventilation and mental alertness are achieved without severe pain.

**Children 12 years:** Follow adult dosing schedule.

**Infants and Children 12 years:** The usual emergency dose is 10 mcg (0.01 mg)/kg of body weight. The dose may be repeated q2–3 min up to two additional doses.

The usual postoperative opioid depression dosage is 5–10 mcg (0.005–0.010 mg) q2–3 min until adequate ventilation and mental alertness are achieved without severe pain.

**Neonates:** The usual emergency dosage is 10 mcg (0.1 mg)/kg of body weight q2–3 min until the desired response is achieved.

**Geriatrics:** Follow adult dosing schedule.

INTRATHECAL USE OR OTHER INFUSION ROUTES AS INDICATED. Not recommended.

#### POTENTIAL PROBLEMS IN ADMINISTRATION

Close titration is required to achieve reversal of opioid CNS depression without plunging clients into severe pain. Pain returns if drug is effective. For this reason in clients who are terminally ill, some clinicians prefer discontinuation of the opioid until the CNS depression is resolved rather than subjecting these clients to the return of excruciating pain.

#### INDEPENDENT NURSING ACTIONS

Monitor vital signs, especially respiratory rate and depth. Monitor for changes in level of consciousness, irritability, or restlessness. Assess client frequently for acute or chronic pain. Observe physical appearance for acute pain behaviors such as crying, moaning, or grimacing. Observe for chronic pain behaviors such as irritability or depression.

#### ADMINISTRATION IN ALTERNATE SETTINGS

Should be administered in short-term care settings where the client can be closely monitored. May be administered in other clinical settings under the supervision of a physician. Not recommended for home administration.

### EVALUATION: OUTCOMES OF DRUG THERAPY

#### EXPECTED OUTCOMES

PHYSICAL ASSESSMENT. Vital signs are within client's baseline with no tachycardia; bradycardia; slow, shallow respirations; or gasping. Clients with acute pain are without complaints of severe discomfort. Clients with chronic pain are without complaints of severe pain or mental cloudiness. No nausea, vomiting, or diarrhea. Skin warm, pink, and dry. Client shows no writhing, grimacing, or unnatural stillness.

LABORATORY. Elevated partial thromboplastin time (PTT) (occasional).

**NEGATIVE OUTCOMES**

Vital signs are more than 15% higher or lower than client's baseline. Clients with acute pain verbalize severe discomfort. Clients with chronic pain complain of severe pain. Clients complain of nausea, vomiting, or diarrhea. Skin pale and diaphoretic. Clients may show runny noses, "goose" flesh, excitement, irritability, or increased yawning.

## PENTAZOCINE

*Trade Name:* Talwin
*Canadian Availability:* Talwin
*Pregnancy Risk:* Category C
*pH:* 4–5
*Storage/Stability:* Store below 40° C. Protect from light.

**ASSESSMENT: DRUG CHARACTERISTICS**

**ACTION**

An opioid agonist-antagonist analgesic that binds to specific receptor sites in the CNS and alters perceptions and emotional responses to pain. Appears to bind to kappa- and sigma-receptor sites, and fails to bind to mu receptors widely found in the CNS. May antagonize mu-receptor agonists. May precipitate withdrawal symptoms in clients who are physically dependent on opioid substances. Has lower incidence of physical dependence than other opioid substances. Has lower analgesic effect than morphine or meperidine. Pain relief begins promptly and lasts about 2 hours.

**INDICATIONS**

Used to treat moderate to severe pain. Used also as an adjunct to anesthesia.

**CAUTIONS**

ADVERSE EFFECTS. Allergic response with difficulty breathing, histamine release, tachycardia or bradycardia or palpitations, hypertension, antidiuretic effect, dizziness, blurred vision, constipation, light-headedness, drowsiness, dry mouth, euphoria, malaise, headache, hypotension, restlessness, nausea, vomiting, nightmares, fatigue, or painful urination.

CONTRAINDICATIONS. Diarrhea associated with use of cephalosporins, lincomycins, penicillins, or other poisoning until all toxic material has been eliminated from the GI tract; respiratory depression, asthma, chronic respiratory diseases, inflammatory bowel diseases, biliary disease, hypertension, or head injury. Should be used with caution in clients ▼

with myocardial infarction, since pentazocine may increase cardiac workload.

**POTENTIAL DRUG/FOOD INTERACTIONS**

Incompatible with aminophylline and glycopyrrolate. May interact with alcohol or other CNS depressants such as hypnotics and sedatives to increase CNS depression. May potentiate the constipating effects of anticholinergics and antidiarrheals if given at the same time. May inhibit the GI effects of metoclopramide if given at the same time. May potentiate the effects of antihypertensives and MAO inhibitors if given at the same time. Neuromuscular blocking agents may potentiate the respiratory depression caused by pentazocine. Naloxone reverses the respiratory depression caused by pentazocine. Pentazocine may antagonize other opioid agonist substances, potentiate side effects, or cause withdrawal symptoms in clients who are physically dependent.

**INTERVENTIONS: ADMINISTRATION**

Does not require dilution if given by IV push, but it is preferable to dilute each 5 mg with at least 1 mL of sterile water.

**MODE/RATE OF ADMINISTRATION**

Given by IV push at 5 mg/min.

INTRAVENOUS USE (WITH NORMAL RENAL FUNCTION)

**Adults:** For pain the usual dose is 5–30 mg q3–4h as needed. The maximum daily dose should not exceed 360 mg.

**Children:** Dose not established.

**Infants/Neonates:** Dose not established.

**Geriatrics:** Elderly clients are more likely to experience respiratory depression and urinary retention and to have age-related decreases in hepatic and renal functioning that decrease the rate of drug metabolism. Older clients may require dose adjustment and lower doses.

INTRATHECAL USE OR OTHER INFUSION ROUTES AS INDICATED. Not recommended.

**POTENTIAL PROBLEMS IN ADMINISTRATION**

May cause pain and redness at IV infusion site.

**INDEPENDENT NURSING ACTIONS**

Assess client frequently for acute or chronic pain. Monitor vital signs. Monitor for changes in level of consciousness, irritability, or restlessness. Observe physical appearance for acute pain behaviors such as crying, moaning, or grimacing. Observe for chronic pain behaviors such as irritability or depression.

**ADMINISTRATION IN ALTERNATE SETTINGS**

May be given in a variety of clinical settings and in the home by a qualified infusion therapy nurse.

**EVALUATION: OUTCOMES OF DRUG THERAPY**

**EXPECTED OUTCOMES**

PHYSICAL ASSESSMENT. Vital signs are within client's base line with no tachycardia, hypertension, or tachypnea. Clients with acute pain verbalize less discomfort and are able to move without complaints of severe discomfort. Clients with chronic pain are able to carry out desired activities without complaints of severe pain or mental cloudiness. No nausea, vomiting, or diarrhea. Skin warm, pink, and dry. Client shows no writhing, grimacing, or unnatural stillness.

LABORATORY. No significant laboratory studies.

**NEGATIVE OUTCOMES**

Vital signs are more than 15% higher or lower than client's baseline. Clients may have tachycardia, hypertension, tachypnea, or gasping. Clients with acute pain verbalize severe discomfort and are unable to move without complaints of severe discomfort. Clients with chronic pain are unable to carry out desired activities without complaints of severe pain or mental cloudiness. Clients may complain of nausea, vomiting, or diarrhea. Skin pale and diaphoretic. Client shows writhing, grimacing, or sedation.

## ANTICONVULSANTS

### THERAPEUTIC EFFECTS

Anticonvulsants may act to control seizures by a variety of mechanisms. Some anticonvulsants such as phenobarbital act by inhibiting sensory conduction in the reticular formation and preventing transmission of impulses to the cortex. Others such as magnesium sulfate act by depressing the CNS and by reducing the release of acetylcholine at the myoneural junction. Still other anticonvulsants such as phenytoin sodium appear to act by stabilizing the neuronal membrane and damping the seizure spike.

### PHARMACOKINETICS

**Distribution.** Anticonvulsants are widely distributed throughout body tissues when administered intravenously. Drugs such as phenytoin accumulate in the brain tissue. Diazepam is extremely rapid acting.

**Metabolism/Elimination.** Anticonvulsants are metabolized by the liver and may accelerate the metabolism of other drugs. Most anticonvulsants are excreted via the kidneys.

### CAUTIONS

**Side/Adverse Effects.** Anticonvulsants may cause allergic reactions, CNS depression or paradoxical excitement, hepatic damage, or depression of white blood cell production.

#### Contraindications

***Pregnancy and Lactation.*** Studies have linked an increased incidence of birth defects to the use of anticonvulsants, but a causal relationship has not been established. Anticonvulsants should not be discontinued during pregnancy in women who are using anticonvulsants to control major seizure activity. Phenobarbital crosses the placental barrier, and many of the anticonvulsants may be passed in breast milk.

***Pediatrics.*** Children using anticonvulsants have been known to have an increased incidence of behavioral and cognitive impairments. Those impairments range from drowsiness to hyperactivity and from impaired task performance to impaired attending and short-term memory.

***Geriatrics.*** The elderly tend to metabolize anticonvulsants slowly. Serum levels of the anticonvulsant should be monitored to prevent overdoses from occurring.

## TOXICITY

See Table 21–3.

## POTENTIAL DRUG/FOOD INTERACTIONS

Anticonvulsants such as phenobarbital and phenytoin may interact with adrenocorticoids, alcohol or other CNS depressants, amiodarone, antacids, calcium, carbamazepine, chloramphenicol, cimetidine, diazoxide, disulfiram, estrogen-containing contraceptives, fluconazole, isoniazid, lidocaine, methadone, phenacemide, phenbutazone, propranolol, sulfonamides, streptozocin, xanthines, warfarin-based anticoagulants, or valproic acid. Magnesium sulfate has no known significant food or drug interactions.

# MAGNESIUM SULFATE

*Trade Name:* None specified
*Canadian Availability:* Magnesium sulfate
*Pregnancy Risk:* Category B
*pH:* 5.5–7
*Storage/Stability:* Store below 40° C. Protect from freezing.

### ASSESSMENT: DRUG CHARACTERISTICS

#### ACTION

An anticonvulsant, uterine relaxant, electrolyte replenisher, and antidysrhythmic that acts by depressing the CNS and by reducing the release of acetylcholine at the myoneural junction. Has a mild diuretic effect.

#### INDICATIONS

Used to treat seizures, cerebral edema, hypomagnesemia, and uterine tetany. Also added to total parenteral nutrition (TPN) solutions.

#### CAUTIONS

ADVERSE EFFECTS. Severe respiratory depression, circulatory collapse, diaphoresis, dysreflexia, hypotension, hypotonia, bradycardia, flushing, increased PR interval, prolonged ST interval, and increased QRS complex.

▼

**TABLE 21–3**
**Anticonvulsant Toxicities**

| Body System | Side/Toxic Effects | Physical Assessment Indicators | Laboratory Indicators | Nursing Interventions |
|---|---|---|---|---|
| Neurologic | Central nervous system toxicity | Cognitive impairments, mental depression or paradoxical excitement, hallucinations, confusion, drowsiness, slurred speech, poor judgment, "hangover" effect | N/A | Monitor client's cognitive and motor activity; report positive findings; provide for client safety. |
| | Hypotonia | Weakness, flaccidity, dysreflexia, peripheral neuropathy | | |
| Cardiovascular | Agranulocytosis or leukopenia | Fever, chills | Erythrocyte count > 4.4 $10^6/mm^3$, reticulocyte count > $25,000/mm^3$, Leukocyte count < $4500/mm^3$ | Use strict aseptic techniques with client; counsel client to avoid crowds, people with known infections. |
| | Circulatory collapse | Hypotension, hypotonia, and bradycardia | | |
| Respiratory | Respiratory depression | Slow respiratory rate | N/A | Encourage frequent position changes, coughing, and deep breathing |
| Renal/genitourinary | Peyronie's disease | Curvature of penis, pain on erection | N/A | Report client complaints of painful erection. |
| Gastrointestinal | Hepatic damage | Jaundice, fever, chills, enlarged liver | AST > 27 U/L, ALT >21 U/L | Monitor for jaundice; report immediately. |
| | | Gingival hyperplasia | N/A | Counsel client on safe techniques for oral care to avoid gingival infections. |
| Other | Allergic reactions | Skin rash, urticaria, wheezing | N/A | Auscultate lungs frequently; report immediately any evidence of allergic reaction; anticonvulsant drugs cannot be stopped without provision for client safety in the event of seizures. |

ALT = alanine aminotransferase, AST = aspartate aminotransferase, N/A = not applicable.

CONTRAINDICATIONS. Heart block, myocardial damage, or renal impairment or failure.

**POTENTIAL DRUG/FOOD INTERACTIONS**

No significant food interactions. Incompatible with alcohol alkalies, calcium preparations, clindamycin, dobutamine, hydrocortisone, IV fat emulsion 10% solution, phosphates, tobramycin, and vitamin B complex.

**INTERVENTIONS: ADMINISTRATION**

Does not require dilution to be given IV push. May be added to IV fluid for a minimum 20% solution.

**MODE/RATE OF ADMINISTRATION**

May be given IV push at a rate not to exceed 1.5 mL of 10% solution per minute or by continuous IV infusion over 3h, not to exceed 3 mL/min. Administered by infusion control device to ensure accuracy.

INTRAVENOUS USE (WITH NORMAL RENAL AND HEPATIC FUNCTION)

**Adults:** For seizures the usual dose is 1–4 g as a 10%–20% solution by IV push or 4 g in 250 mL of 0.9% NSS as an IV infusion at a rate not to exceed 3 mL/min.

For electrolyte imbalance the usual dose is 5 g in 1 L of 0.9% NSS over 3h or 8–24 mEq/24h in TPN solution.

Maximum daily dose should not exceed 40 g/d.

**Children 12 years:** Follow adult dosing schedule.

**Infants/Neonates:** For seizures the usual dose is 20–40 mg/kg of body weight as a 20% solution. For TPN, give 2–10 mEq/24 h.

**Geriatrics:** Elderly clients are more likely to have age-related decreases in hepatic and renal functioning that decrease the rate of drug metabolism. Elderly clients may require dose adjustment and lower doses.

INTRATHECAL USE OR OTHER INFUSION ROUTES AS INDICATED. Not recommended.

**POTENTIAL PROBLEMS IN ADMINISTRATION**

May cause toxic serum levels if administered too rapidly. Potentiates neuromuscular blocking agents.

**INDEPENDENT NURSING ACTIONS**

Assess client frequently for seizure activity. Monitor vital signs, especially blood pressure, respirations, and pulse rate and rhythm. Monitor for changes in level of consciousness, irritability, or restlessness. Check patellar reflex frequently; if absent, discontinue drug. Maintain a minimum of 100 mL of urine q4h.

**ADMINISTRATION IN ALTERNATE SETTINGS**

IV administration for electrolyte replacement may be done in a variety of clinical settings. IV administration for seizure therapy should be done in clinical settings where the client can be closely monitored. IV administration for electrolyte replacement may be done in home settings.

### EVALUATION: OUTCOMES OF DRUG THERAPY

#### EXPECTED OUTCOMES

PHYSICAL ASSESSMENT. No seizure activity. Vital signs within 15% of client's baseline. Client alert, calm, and able to carry out activities of daily living (ADLs) without hesitation.

LABORATORY. Complete blood count shows red blood cells (RBCs) between 4.4 and 5.5 $10^6/mm^3$, reticulocyte count between 25,000 and 75,000/$mm^3$, platelets between 150,000 and 450,000/$mm^3$, hemoglobin (Hgb) between 13.0 and 16.5 g/dL, hematocrit (Hct) between 40% and 50%. Aspartate aminotransferase (AST) between 7 and 27 U/L. Alanine aminotransferase (ALT) between 1 and 21 U/L. Blood urea nitrogen (BUN) between 8 and 25 mg/dL.

#### NEGATIVE OUTCOMES

Seizure activity. Pulse 15% less than baseline. Respirations are less than 16/min. Client drowsy, restless, irritable, and unable to carry out ADLs without hesitation.

## PHENOBARBITAL SODIUM

*Trade Name:* Luminal
*Canadian Availability:* Phenobarbital
*Pregnancy Risk:* Category D
*pH:* 9.2–10.2
*Storage/Stability:* Store below 40° C. Protect from freezing. Do not use if a precipitate is present or if solution is not clear. Should be used within 30 minutes after being reconstituted.

### ASSESSMENT: DRUG CHARACTERISTICS

#### ACTION

A sedative-hypnotic and anticonvulsant that depresses the sensory cortex, diminishes motor activity, and produces drowsiness and sedation. Appears to inhibit sensory conduction in the reticular formation and prevents transmission of impulses to the cortex. Onset of action is prompt; effects last 6 to 10 hours.

#### INDICATIONS

Used as an adjunct to anesthesia, to treat epilepsy, and to manage convulsions associated with tetanus, eclampsia, and meningitis.

#### CAUTIONS

ADVERSE EFFECTS. Allergic reactions, mental depression or paradoxical excitement, agranulocytosis, hallucinations, confusion, drowsiness, fever, hypothermia, slurred speech, hepatic damage, poor judgment, or "hangover" effect.

CONTRAINDICATIONS. Porphyria or a history of allergy to phenobarbital, substance abuse, hepatic impairment, pain, or depressed respiratory functioning.

▼

**POTENTIAL DRUG/FOOD INTERACTIONS**

May inhibit the action of adrenocorticoids and may decrease the action of warfarin-based anticoagulants. May increase the excretion rate and thus decrease the effectiveness of carbamazepine. May decrease the reliability of estrogen-containing contraceptives. May potentiate the CNS depressant effects of alcohol or other CNS depressants. May decrease the excretion rate and thus increase the effects of valproic acid and the incidence of hepatotoxicity. Incompatible with aminophylline, calcium chloride, cephalothin, chlorpromazine, cimetidine, clindamycin, hydralazine, insulin, meperidine, magnesium sulfate, morphine, pentazocine, phenytoin, vancomycin, and many other CNS depressants.

**INTERVENTIONS: ADMINISTRATION**

Add 3 mL of sterile water to a 120-mg vial; add 10 mL of sterile water to larger vials. May take up to 5 min to dissolve. Do not use if not completely clear after shaking and waiting 5 min.

**MODE-RATE OF ADMINISTRATION**

Given by IV push at a rate of not more than 65 mg/min. Not given as a continuous infusion.

INTRAVENOUS USE (WITH NORMAL RENAL FUNCTION)

**Adults:** For preanesthesia sedation the usual dose is 130–200 mg 1–1½h before surgery.

For hypnotic effect the usual dose is 100–325 mg.

For anticonvulsant effect the usual dose is 100–320 mg, repeated in 6h as necessary to a maximum daily dose of 600 mg.

For status epilepticus the usual dose is 10–20 mg/kg of body weight given slowly and repeated if necessary.

**Children >12 years:** Follow adult dosing schedule.

**Infants/Neonates:** For preanesthesia sedation and hypnotic effects the dose is individualized to the client.

For anticonvulsant effect the usual dose is 10–20 mg/kg of body weight initially, followed by 1–6 mg/kg/d.

For status epilepticus the usual dose is 15–20 mg/kg of body weight given over 15 min, not to exceed 40 mg/kg/24 h.

**Geriatrics:** Elderly clients are more likely to experience excitement, depression, confusion, and hypothermia and to have age-related decreases in hepatic and renal functioning that decrease the rate of drug metabolism. Older clients may require dose adjustment and lower doses.

INTRATHECAL USE OR OTHER INFUSION ROUTES AS INDICATED. Not recommended.

**POTENTIAL PROBLEMS IN ADMINISTRATION**

Maximal effect may not be reached until 15 min after IV administration. Caution should be exercised to give the lowest dose possible to avoid overdosing the client. Phenobarbital is highly alkaline. Avoid extravasation, which may cause severe irritation or tissue necrosis. If extravasation does occur, the area may be injected with 0.5% procaine solution.

**INDEPENDENT NURSING ACTIONS**

Assess client frequently for seizure activity. Monitor vital signs, especially blood pressure, respirations, and pulse rate and rhythm. Monitor for changes in level of consciousness, irritability, or restlessness.

**ADMINISTRATION IN ALTERNATE SETTINGS**

IV administration should be done in clinical settings where the client can be closely monitored and emergency resuscitation equipment is immediately available.

**EVALUATION: OUTCOMES OF DRUG THERAPY**

**EXPECTED OUTCOMES**

PHYSICAL ASSESSMENT. No seizure activity. Vital signs within 15% of client's baseline. Client alert, calm, and able to carry out ADLs without hesitation.

LABORATORY. Complete blood count shows RBCs between 4.4 and $5.5 \times 10^6/mm^3$, reticulocyte count between 25,000 and 75,000/$mm^3$, platelets between 150,000 and 450,000/$mm^3$, Hgb between 13.0 and 16.5 g/dL, Hct between 40% and 50%. AST between 7 and 27 U/L. ALT between 1 and 21 U/L. BUN between 8 and 25 mg/dL.

**NEGATIVE OUTCOMES**

Seizure activity. Pulse 15% less than baseline. Respiration less than 16/min. Client drowsy, restless, irritable, and unable to carry out ADLs without hestiation.

## PHENYTOIN SODIUM

*Trade Name:* Dilantin
*Canadian Availability:* Dilantin
*Pregnancy Risk:* Category C
*pH:* 12
*Storage/Stability:* Store between 15° and 30° C. Protect from freezing. Should not be used if darker than light yellow. If refrigerated, may form a preciptate that redissolves at room temperature.

**ASSESSMENT: DRUG CHARACTERISTICS**

**ACTION**

An anticonvulsant that appears to act by stabilizing the neuronal membrane and damping the seizure spike. Also acts as an antiarrhythmic by regulating sodium and calcium ion movement in the Purkinje fibers. Also has some antineuralgic and skeletal muscle relaxant activity. Onset of action is prompt.

**INDICATIONS**

Used to control epilepsy, status epilepticus, and neurosurgically induced seizures. Also may be used in treatment of supraventricular and ventricular dysrhythmias.

**CAUTIONS**

ADVERSE EFFECTS. CNS toxic activity such as ataxia, drowsiness, confusion, tremors, and visual disturbances; gingival hyperplasia; agranulocytosis; leukopenia, hepatitis; cognitive impairments; Peyronie's disease; or peripheral polyneuropathy; respiratory or cardiac arrest, hypotension, or skin rash.

CONTRAINDICATIONS. Heart block, blood dyscrasias, hepatic or renal impairment, porphyria, or allergy to phenytoin.

**POTENTIAL DRUG/FOOD INTERACTIONS**

May interact with adrenocorticotropins or estrogen-containing contraceptives to decrease the effectiveness of these agents. Alcohol, other CNS depressants, or diazoxide may decrease the effectiveness of phenytoin. May increase the incidence of toxicity if used with amiodarone. Antacids or calcium may decrease the uptake of phenytoin. Use with warfarin, chloramphenicol, cimetidine, disulfiram, isoniazid, phenbutazone, sulfonamides, or fluconazole may increase serum levels of phenytoin. May have an additive cardiac depressant effect if used with lidocaine or propranolol. May increase methadone metabolism and require dose adjustment. May inhibit streptozocin. May potentiate phenacemide. Valproic acid may block uptake of phenytoin. When used with xanthines, may facilitate hepatic metabolism of both agents.

**INTERVENTIONS: ADMINISTRATION**

Add 2.2 mL of diluent to a 100-mg vial or 5.2 mL to a 250-mg vial (1 mL = 50 mg). Shake to dissolve. May immerse in warm water to dissolve powder.

**MODE/RATE OF ADMINISTRATION**

May be given by IV push at a rate not to exceed 50 mg/min as an anticonvulsant; 25 mg/min as an antidysrhythmic. May be given by intermittent IV infusion over 1 h.

INTRAVENOUS USE (WITH NORMAL RENAL FUNCTION)

**Adults:** For seizures the usual dose is 15–20 mg/kg of body weight or 100–250 mg initially, then 100–150 mg in 30 min. May be repeated q4h. For dysrhythmias, dosage is 50–100 mg q10–15min, not to exceed total dose of 15 mg/kg.

**Children ≥ 12 years:** Follow adult dosing schedule.

**Children < 12 years:** The usual dose is 250 mg/m$^2$ or 10–15 mg/kg in divided doses of 5–10 mg/kg of body weight.

**Infants/Neonates:** For seizures the usual dose is

15–20 mg/kg of body weight at a rate not to exceed 50 mg/min.

**Geriatrics:** Elderly clients are more likely to have age-related decreases in hepatic and renal functioning that decrease the rate of drug metabolism. Older clients may require dose adjustment and lower doses. They also may require phenytoin at a slower rate.

INTRATHECAL USE OR OTHER INFUSION ROUTES AS INDICATED. Contraindicated.

#### POTENTIAL PROBLEMS IN ADMINISTRATION

Phenytoin is highly alkaline. Avoid extravasation, which may cause severe irritation. Follow each injection with saline flush.

#### INDEPENDENT NURSING ACTIONS

Assess client frequently for seizure activity. Monitor vital signs, especially blood pressure, respirations, and pulse rate and rhythm. Monitor for changes in level of consciousness, irritability, or restlessness.

#### ADMINISTRATION IN ALTERNATE SETTINGS

IV administration should be done in clinical settings where the client can be closely monitored. IV administration not recommended for home settings.

#### EVALUATION: OUTCOMES OF DRUG THERAPY

#### EXPECTED OUTCOMES

PHYSICAL ASSESSMENT. No seizure activity. Vital signs within 15% of client's baseline. Client alert, calm, and able to carry out ADLs without hesitation.

LABORATORY. Complete blood count shows RBCs between 4.4 and 5.5 × $10^6$/$mm^3$, reticulocyte count between 25,000 and 75,000/$mm^3$, platelets between 150,000 and 450,000/$mm^3$, Hgb between 13 and 16.5 g/dL, Hct between 40% and 50%. AST between 7 and 27 U/L. ALT between 1 and 21 U/L. BUN between 8 and 25 mg/dL.

#### NEGATIVE OUTCOMES

Seizure activity. Pulse 15% less than baseline. Respirations less than 16/min. Client drowsy, restless, irritable, and unable to carry out ADLs without hesitation.

## ANXIOLYTICS, SEDATIVES, AND HYPNOTICS

### THERAPEUTIC EFFECTS

Anxiolytic agents decrease anxiety and may also have antiemetic, antivertigo, amnestic, anticonvulsant, antipanic, and skeletal muscle relaxant effects, or sedative-hypnotic action. The benzodiazepines such as diazepam, lorazepam, and midazolam depress the CNS by facilitating the inhibitory neurotransmitter GABA. Promethazine acts as an antihistaminic by competing for $H_1$-receptor sites, thus blocking histamine effects rather than blocking histamine release. Pro-methazine also acts as an antivertigo and antiemetic agent by decreasing vestibular stimulation and depressing the CTZ.

## PHARMACOKINETICS

**Distribution.** Anxiolytic agents are widely distributed throughout the body when administered intravenously. Onset of action is rapid.

**Metabolism/Elimination.** Benzodiazepines and promethazine are metabolized by the liver and excreted in urine and feces. Slow-acting benzodiazepines, such as diazepam, have a prolonged half-life and therefore are slowly excreted.

## CAUTIONS

**Side/Adverse Effects.** Anxiolytic agents may cause allergic reactions, blood dyscrasias, CNS symptoms, and hepatic dysfunction. Seizure activity may result if anxiolytics are abruptly started or stopped in clients with epilepsy. Promethazine may cause anticholinergic effects.

### Contraindications

***Pregnancy and Lactation.*** The benzodiazepines have been associated with an increased incidence of congenital malformations when used in the first trimester. Benzodiazepines are secreted in breast milk and may cause sedation in the infant. Promethazine's safety for use in pregnancy has not been determined. It is not clear whether promethazine is passed in breast milk.

***Pediatrics.*** Benzodiazepines have an increased risk of causing CNS symptoms in children. Promethazine may cause dystonias in children, especially in children who are dehydrated. Promethazine may also cause a marked drowsiness in children.

***Geriatrics.*** Elderly clients are more likely to fall and suffer injury while taking benzodiazepines. They are more likely to have an increased incidence of CNS symptoms. The elderly are more likely to have conditions for which promethazine is contraindicated, such as cardiac and respiratory disease, prostatic hypertrophy, or narrow-angle glaucoma.

## TOXICITY

See Table 21–4.

## POTENTIAL DRUG/FOOD INTERACTIONS

Anxiolytics may interact with alcohol or other CNS depressants to enhance CNS depression. Anticholinergics, antithyroid agents, carbamazepine, cimetidine, epinephrine, erythromycin, levodopa, metrizamide, MAO inhibitors, probenecid, or zidovudine may alter the duration of action of anxiolytics, or anxiolytics may alter the effects of these drugs by interfering with hepatic metabolism.

**TABLE 21–4**
**Anxiolytic, Sedative, and Hypnotic Toxicities**

| Body System | Side/Toxic Effects | Physical Assessment Indicators | Laboratory Indicators | Nursing Interventions |
|---|---|---|---|---|
| Neurologic | Central nervous system symptoms | Confusion, memory impairment, extrapyramidal symptoms, ataxia, excitement, seizure activity, weakness, emergence delirium, hallucinations | N/A | Monitor client's cognitive and motor activity; report positive findings; provide for client safety. |
| Cardiovascular | Blood dyscrasias<br>Macrocytic anemia<br>Leukopenia<br>Thrombocytopenia<br>Agranulocytosis | Bruising, bleeding from gums, pink-tinged urine | Erythrocyte count $< 4.2$ $10^6/mm^3$, leukocyte count $< 4300/mm^3$ | Use strict aseptic technique with client; report positive findings promptly; counsel client to avoid crowds and people with known infections. |
| | Cardiac dysrhythmias | Tachycardia, irregular heartbeat | | |
| | Hypotension | Blood pressure more than 15% less than client's baseline | | |
| Respiratory | Respiratory depression | Slow respiratory rate, hyperventilation | N/A | Encourage frequent position changes, deep breathing, and coughing. |
| Gastrointestinal | Hepatic dysfunction<br>Anticholinergic effects | Nausea, vomiting, gastric distress,<br>Anorexia, dry mouth, constipation, diarrhea, | Serum cholesterol $> 220$ mg/dL, HDLs elevated | Provide comfort measures such as mouth care; report positive findings promptly. |
| Special senses | | Blurred vision, nystagmus, diplopia, tinnitus, vertigo | N/A | Provide for client safety; counsel client to avoid hazardous equipment and activities requiring sharp motor skills; monitor motor skills for falls, especially in the elderly. |
| Other | Allergic reactions | Skin rashes, hives, itching, or difficulty breathing | N/A | Auscultate lung sounds; report positive findings promptly; be prepared to administer emergency drugs for allergic reactions. |

## Diazepam

*Trade Name:* T-Quil, Valium, Zetran
*Canadian Availability:* Valium
*Pregnancy Risk:* Category D
*pH:* 6.2–6.9
*Storage/Stability:* Store below 40° C. Protect from freezing and from light. Should not be diluted with any medication or fluid because solution will be unstable.

### ASSESSMENT: DRUG CHARACTERISTICS

#### ACTION

An antianxiety agent (long-acting benzodiazepine) that also has sedative-hypnotic, amnestic, anticonvulsant, antipanic, and skeletal muscle relaxant effects. Acts as a CNS depressant by facilitating the inhibitory neurotransmitter GABA. Is very slowly excreted from the body.

#### INDICATIONS

May be used to treat anxiety, acute alcohol withdrawal, moderate to severe psychoneuroses, insomnia, seizures, various forms of epilepsy (especially acute status epilepticus), and skeletal muscle spasms. May also be used to induce amnesia related to traumatic procedures such as cardioversion and as an anesthesia adjunct.

#### CAUTIONS

ADVERSE EFFECTS. Respiratory depression, especially apnea, dyspnea, or hyperventilation; allergic reactions; blood dyscrasias; CNS symptoms such as ataxia, blurred vision, drowsiness, headache, or memory impairment; extrapyramidal symptoms such as tremors; hepatic dysfunction; weakness; or excitement. Seizure activity may result if diazepam is abruptly started or stopped in clients with epilepsy.

CONTRAINDICATIONS. Narrow-angle glaucoma, myasthenia gravis, or severe pulmonary obstructive disease; history of sensitivity to diazepam; shock or coma.

#### POTENTIAL DRUG-FOOD INTERACTIONS

May interact with alcohol or other CNS depressants to increase the CNS depression. Drugs such as erythromycin, cimetidine, carbamazepine, or zidovudine may prolong drug action by slowing hepatic metabolism. Incompatible with any drug in same syringe, as precipitation of drug will occur.

### INTERVENTIONS: ADMINISTRATION

Do not dilute before using and do not add to IV solution.

#### MODE/RATE OF ADMINISTRATION

Given by IV push at a rate not to exceed 5 mg/min. For children, administer total dose over a minimum of 3 min.

INTRAVENOUS USE (WITH NORMAL RENAL FUNCTION)

**Adults:** For alcohol withdrawal the usual initial dose is 10 mg, followed by 2–10

For amnesic effect the usual dose is 5–20 mg before the traumatic procedure.

For anticonvulsant effect the usual initial dose is 5–10 mg, followed by 5–10 mg q10–15min as necessary up to 30 mg. Dose may be repeated in 2–4h if needed.

For preoperative antianxiety or before cardioversion the usual dose is 5–15 mg.

For skeletal muscle relaxation the usual dosage is 5–10 mg q3–4h. If given for tetanus or endoscopic procedure, the dose may be larger.

**Children 5 years:** For status epilepticus, give 0.5–2 mg q2–5min up to 10 mg.

**Children 5–12 years:** For anticonvulsant effect the usual initial dosage is 1 mg q2–5min as necessary up to 10 mg. Dose may be repeated in 2–4h if needed.

For skeletal muscle relaxant effect the usual initial dose is 5–10 mg slowly. Dose may be repeated in 3–4h if needed.

**Children 12 years:** Follow adult dosing schedule.

**Neonates and newborns 30 days:** Dose not established.

**Infants and Children 30 days–5 years:** For anticonvulsant effect the usual initial dosage is 200–500 mcg (0.2–0.5 mg) slowly q3–5min as necessary up to 5 mg. Dose may be repeated in 2–4h if needed.

For skeletal muscle relaxant effect the usual initial dose is 1–2 mg slowly. Dose may be repeated in 3–4h if needed.

**Geriatrics:** Should not be given to the elderly client.

INTRATHECAL USE OR OTHER INFUSION ROUTES AS INDICATED. Not recommended.

#### POTENTIAL PROBLEMS IN ADMINISTRATION

Diazepam is quite irritating to veins and can cause thrombophlebitis. Small veins on back of hands should not be used. Care should be exercised not to cause extravasation. May cause laryngospasm if used as an adjunct to peroral endoscopic procedures.

#### INDEPENDENT NURSING ACTIONS

Observe for CNS effects such as dizziness, drowsiness, motor impairment, or sensory-perceptual dysfunction. Evaluate anxiety. Evaluate muscle strength and seizure activity. Document duration, loction, and intensity of seizure activity. Teach clients to seek assistance with ambulation and to avoid operating hazardous equipment. Teach clients to avoid alcohol and other CNS depressants. Bed rest is required for at least 3h after drug administration.

#### ADMINISTRATION IN ALTERNATE SETTINGS

Not recommended.

#### EVALUATION: OUTCOMES OF DRUG THERAPY

#### EXPECTED OUTCOMES

PHYSICAL ASSESSMENT. Client reports diminished anxiety, ability to rest quietly, no memory of traumatic procedures, no seizures, or no skeletal muscle spasms.

▼

LABORATORY. Complete blood count within client's baseline. ALT between 7 and 27 U/L. AST between 1 and 21 U/L.

**NEGATIVE OUTCOMES**

Client demonstrates CNS symptoms such as confusion or memory impairment, extrapyramidal symptoms, or excitement. Client demonstrates muscle weakness, skeletal muscle spasm, or seizure activity or experiences respiratory depression.

---

## LORAZEPAM

*Trade Name:* Ativan
*Canadian Availability:* Ativan
*Pregnancy Risk:* Category D
*pH:* Unknown
*Storage/Stability:* Store between 2° and 8° C. Protect from freezing and from light. Do not use if not clear or there is a precipitate present.

**ASSESSMENT: DRUG CHARACTERISTICS**

**ACTION**

An antianxiety, anticonvulsant, antiemetic, antipanic, amnestic, sedative-hypnotic, and skeletal muscle relaxant. Acts as a CNS depressant (long-acting benzodiazepine) by facilitating the inhibitory neurotransmitter GABA. Is slowly excreted via the urine.

**INDICATIONS**

May be used to treat anxiety and nausea and vomiting associated with chemotherapy. Is also commonly used as an anesthesia adjunct.

**CAUTIONS**

ADVERSE EFFECTS. Allergic reactions, blood dyscrasias, CNS symptoms such as confusion or memory impairment, extrapyramidal symptoms, hepatic dysfunction, weakness, or excitement.

CONTRAINDICATIONS. Narrow-angle glaucoma, myasthenia gravis, psychoses, severe pulmonary obstructive disease, or history of sensitivity to lorazepam.

**POTENTIAL DRUG/FOOD INTERACTIONS**

May interact with alcohol or other CNS depressants such as opioid analgesia and phenothiazines to increase the CNS depression. Drugs such as erythromycin, cimetidine, carbamazepine, probenecid, or zidovudine may prolong drug action by slowing hepatic metabolism. Potentiates MAO inhibitors and tricyclic antidepressants.

**INTERVENTIONS: ADMINISTRATION**

Dilute with an equal volume of sterile water, 0.9% NSS, or D5W solution immediately before use.

**MODE/RATE OF ADMINISTRATION**

Given by IV push at a rate of 2 mg/min.

INTRAVENOUS USE (WITH NORMAL RENAL FUNCTION)

**Adults** For antianxiety or amnesic effect the usual initial dose is 44 mcg (0.044 mg)/kg of body weight up to a maximum of 2 mg, given 15–20 min prior to the procedure.

For anticonvulsant effect the usual initial dose is 0.5 mg/kg of body weight to a total of 4 mg, followed by 0.5 mg/kg of body weight in 10–15 min as necessary. Dose may be repeated in another 10–15 min if needed. If seizures are still present after the third course, other measures should be instituted to control the seizures.

For antiemetic effect the usual dose is 2 mg 30 min before chemotherapy and 2 mg q4h as needed following chemotherapy.

Maximum dose should not exceed 8 mg in 12 h.

**Children:** Dose not established.

**Infants/Neonates:** Dose not established.

**Geriatrics:** Elderly clients are more sensitive to the effects of benzodiazepines such as lorazepam. Clients with diminished liver function are also more likely to demonstrate adverse reactions. If necessary, no more than 2 mg should be given.

INTRATHECAL USE OR OTHER INFUSION ROUTES AS INDICATED. Not recommended.

**POTENTIAL PROBLEMS IN ADMINISTRATION**

Lorazepam is quite irritating to veins. Small veins on back of hands should not be used. Care should be exercised not to cause extravasation. May cause laryngospasm if used as an adjunct to peroral endoscopic procedures.

**INDEPENDENT NURSING ACTIONS**

Observe for CNS effects such as dizziness, drowsiness, motor impairment, or sensory-perceptual dysfunction. Evaluate anxiety, muscle strength, and seizure activity. Document duration, location, and intensity of seizure activity. Teach clients to seek assistance with ambulation and to avoid operating hazardous equipment.

**ADMINISTRATION ALTERNATE SETTINGS**

Not recommended.

**EVALUATION: OUTCOMES OF DRUG THERAPY**

**EXPECTED OUTCOMES**

PHYSICAL ASSESSMENT. Client reports diminished anxiety, ability to rest quietly, no memory of traumatic procedures, no seizures, or no skeletal muscle spasms.

LABORATORY. Complete blood count within client's baseline. AST between 7 and 27 U/L. ALT between 1 and 21 U/L.

**NEGATIVE OUTCOMES**

Client demonstrates CNS symptoms such as confusion or memory impairment, extrapyramidal symptoms, or excitement. Client demonstrates muscle weakness, skeletal muscle spasm, or seizure activity.

## MIDAZOLAM HYDROCHLORIDE

*Trade Name:* Versed
*Canadian Availability:* Versed
*Pregnancy Risk:* Category D
*pH:* 3
*Storage/Stability:* Store between 15° and 30° C. Protect from freezing. Do not use if discolored or if precipitate is present. Stable for 24 hours if diluted with D5W or 0.9% NSS. Stable for 4 hours if diluted with Ringer's lactate.

### ASSESSMENT: DRUG CHARACTERISTICS

#### ACTION

An anesthetic, sedative-hypnotic (conscious sedation), and anesthesia adjunct agent that acts as a CNS depressant by facilitating the inhibitory neurotransmitter GABA. May cause a decrease in cerebrospinal fluid pressure and intraocular pressure and may cause respiratory depression.

#### INDICATIONS

Used to produce sedation and amnesia; also used as an anesthesia adjunct during induction and as an antianxiety agent.

#### CAUTIONS

ADVERSE EFFECTS. Respiratory depression, muscle tremors, excitement, and emergence delirium including confusion, hallucinations, or anxiety; hyperventilation; bradycardia, cardiac dysrhythmias; cardiac arrest; hypotension; ataxia; blurred vision; or allergic responses such as skin rashes, hives, itching, or difficulty breathing. Increased cough reflex and laryngospasm may occur, therefore, topical anesthetic is used with midazolam during peroral endoscopy.

CONTRAINDICATIONS. Myasthenia gravis, acute or chronic glaucoma, or severe pulmonary obstructive disease; history of sensitivity to midazolam; shock, coma, or acute alcohol intoxication.

#### POTENTIAL DRUG/FOOD INTERACTIONS

May interact with alcohol or other CNS depressants to increase the CNS depression. May be potentiated by antihistamines, opioids, and antidepressants.

### INTERVENTIONS: ADMINISTRATION

Dilute with NSS or D5W to allow slow titration, such as 1 mg/4 mL concentration.

#### MODE/RATE OF ADMINISTRATION

Given by IV push at a rate not to exceed 1 mg/min.

INTRAVENOUS USE (WITH NORMAL RENAL AND HEPATIC FUNCTION)

**Adults:** For conscious sedation in healthy adults younger than 60 years, the usual dose is 1–2.5 mg administered immediately before the procedure. Doses may be given q2min or more to achieve desired effects. Total dose should not exceed 5 mg.

As an anesthesia adjunct the usual dose is 150–350 mcg (0.15–0.35 mg)/kg of body weight over 20–30 s.

**Children 12 years:** Follow adult dosing schedule.

**Infants/Neonates:** For anesthesia adjunct, the usual dose is 50–200 mcg (0.05–0.2 mg)/kg of body weight.

**Geriatrics:** Elderly clients are more sensitive to the effects of benzodiazepines such as midazolam. Clients with diminished liver function are also more likely to demonstrate adverse reactions.

For conscious sedation in adults older than 60 years, the usual dose is 0.5–1.5 mg immediately before the procedure. Doses may be given q2min or more to achieve desired effects. Total dose should not exceed 3.5 mg.

As an anesthesia adjunct the usual dose is 150 mcg–350 mcg (0.15–0.35 mg)/kg of body weight over 20–30 s.

INTRATHECAL USE OR OTHER INFUSION ROUTES AS INDICATED. Not recommended.

#### POTENTIAL PROBLEMS IN ADMINISTRATION

Midazolam is very irritating to veins. Small veins on back of hands should not be used. Care should be exercised not to cause extravasation. May cause severe respiratory depression or cardiac dysrhythmias if given by bolus injection.

#### INDEPENDENT NURSING ACTIONS

Observe for CNS effects such as dizziness, drowsiness, motor impairment, or sensory-perceptual dysfunction. Monitor vital signs and ECG carefully. Evaluate anxiety. Teach clients to seek assistance with ambulation and to avoid operating hazardous equipment.

#### ADMINISTRATION IN ALTERNATE SETTINGS

Should only be given in settings where clients can be closely monitored and where emergency cardiac and respirtory support is available.

#### EVALUATION: OUTCOMES OF DRUG THERAPY

#### EXPECTED OUTCOMES

PHYSICAL ASSESSMENT. Pulse, respirations, and blood pressure remain within 15% of baseline. Client does not demonstrate confusion, delirium, motor impairment, or sensory-perceptual dysfunction. Client has no memory of traumatic procedure or anxiety.

LABORATORY. Complete blood count within client's baseline.

#### NEGATIVE OUTCOMES

Client demonstrates respiratory depression; hyperventilation; tachycardia; cardiac dysrhythmias; muscle tremors; emergence delirium including confusion, hallucinations, or anxiety; or allergic responses such as skin rashes, hives, or itching.

## PROMETHAZINE HYDROCHLORIDE

*Trade Name:* Phenergan, Phenazine, Prometh-50, Prothazine
*Canadian Availability:* Histantil, Phenergan, PMS Promethazine
*Pregnancy Risk:* Category C
*pH:* 4–5.5

▼

*Storage/Stability:* Store below 40° C. Refrigerate multidose vials or diluted solutions. Protect from freezing and from light. Do not use if discolored or if a precipitate is present.

## ASSESSMENT: DRUG CHARACTERISTICS

### ACTION

A potent antihistamine that also has antiemetic, antivertigo, and sedative-hypnotic effects. Acts as an antihistaminic by competing for $H_1$-receptor sites, thus blocking histamine effects rather than blocking histamine release. Acts as an antivertigo and antiemetic agent by decreasing vestibular stimulation and depressing the chemoreceptor trigger zone (CTZ). Is readily absorbed and excreted in the urine.

### INDICATIONS

Used to treat pruritus, rhinitis, sneezing, urticaria, angioedema, and conjunctivitis associated with allergies. Also used to treat motion sickness and the nausea and vomiting associated with motion sickness. May also be used as an anesthesia adjunct for sedation and as an antianxiety adjunct for clients experiencing pain.

### CAUTIONS

ADVERSE EFFECTS. Blood dyscrasias, respiratory depression, anticholinergic effects, CNS depression or excitation, extrapyramidal symptoms, hypotension, drowsiness, blurred vision, tinnitus, tachycardia, or cardiac or respiratory arrest.

CONTRAINDICATIONS. Urinary retention associated with bladder neck obstructions or benign prostatic hypertrophy, coma, glaucoma, or jaundice.

### POTENTIAL DRUG/FOOD INTERACTIONS

May interact with alcohol, other CNS depressants, anticholinergics, or MAO inhibitors to potentiate the effects of these medications. May increase the risk of agranulocytosis if used with antithyroid agents. May block the α-adrenergic effects of epinephrine or the antiparkinsonian effects of levodopa. If used with intrathecal metrizamide, may cause seizures. Should not be given with thiazide diuretics, epinephrine, or quinidine.

## INTERVENTIONS: ADMINISTRATION

Should be diluted, usually 25–50 mg in 9 mL NSS.

### MODE/RATE OF ADMINISTRATION

May be given IV push at a rate not to exceed 25 mg in 2 min.

INTRAVENOUS USE (WITH NORMAL RENAL FUNCTION)

**Adults:** For antiemetic effect the usual dosage is 12.5–25 mg q4h as needed.

For antihistaminic effect the usual dosage is 25 mg q2h if necessary.

For sedative-hypnotic effect the usual dose is 25–50 mg.

Maximum daily dose should not exceed 150 mg.

**Children:** IV injection usually not for children.

**Children 12 years:** Follow adult dosing schedule.

**Infants/Neonates:** Not recommended for infants younger than 2 years.

**Geriatrics:** Follow the adult dosing schedule but use caution.

INTRATHECAL USE OR OTHER INFUSION ROUTES AS INDICATED. Not recommended.

#### POTENTIAL PROBLEMS IN ADMINISTRATION

May cause severe arterial spasm if given by intraarterial injection. Promethazine is very irritating and extravasation should be avoided.

#### INDEPENDENT NURSING ACTIONS

Monitor vital signs, especially blood pressure and pulse. Observe for CNS depression or excitation, extrapyramidal symptoms, or drowsiness. Monitor for complaints of dry mouth, blurred vision, or tinnitus.

#### ADMINISTRATION IN ALTERNATE SETTINGS

May be given in most clinical settings. IV administration not generally recommended for the home setting.

#### EVALUATION: OUTCOMES OF DRUG THERAPY

#### EXPECTED OUTCOMES

PHYSICAL ASSESSMENT. Vital signs, especially blood pressure and pulse, remain with 15% of client's baseline. Client is calm and demonstrates CNS depression or excitation, extrapyramidal symptoms, or drowsiness. Client does not complain of dry mouth, blurred vision, or tinnitus.

LABORATORY. Complete blood count within client's baseline.

#### NEGATIVE OUTCOMES

Client complains of anticholinergic effects such as CNS depression or excitation, drowsiness, blurred vision, or tinnitus. Client demonstrates extrapyramidal symptoms, hypotension, or tachycardia.

## TRANQUILIZERS

### THERAPEUTIC EFFECTS

Tranquilizers such as the phenothiazines may act as antipsychotics, antiemetics, or antidyskinetics. Antipsychotic action is created by blocking postsynaptic dopaminergic receptors in the brain. Tranquilizers may also have an α-adrenergic blocking effect and may decrease hormone release from the hypothalamus and hypophysis. Antiemetic action is created by blocking dopamine receptors in the CTZ in the medulla and by blocking vagus stimulation in the GI tract.

### PHARMACOKINETICS

**Distribution**. Tranquilizers are widely distributed when administered intravenously. Peak effect may not be achieved for 4 to 7 days.

**Metabolism/Elimination**. Tranquilizers are metabolized by the liver and excreted in urine and bile.

## CAUTIONS

**Side/Adverse Effects**. Tranquilizers may cause akathisias (motor restlessness and an inability to sit still), extrapyramidal symptoms, tardive dyskinesia (continual chewing movements and darting movements of the tongue), anticholinergic effects, or skin rashes.

### Contraindications

***Pregnancy and Lactation.*** Tranquilizers may cause a decreased production of sperm in men. The effects of tranquilizers have not been well studied. The agents may be passed in breast milk and may cause tardive dyskinesia in infants.

***Pediatrics.*** Maternal use of phenothiazines may cause prolonged jaundice or extrapyramidal symptoms in neonates. Children are more likely to experience extrapyramidal symptoms.

***Geriatrics.*** The elderly are more sensitive to the anticholinergic and orthostatic hypotensive effects of phenothiazines.

## TOXICITY

See Table 21–5.

## POTENTIAL DRUG/FOOD INTERACTIONS

May interact with alcohol, other CNS depressants, tricyclic antidepressants, maprotiline, or MAO inhibitors, antithyroid agents, other hypotension-producing drugs, epineprhine, levodopa, lithium, and metrizamide.

---

## CHLORPROMAZINE HYDROCHLORIDE

*Trade Names:* Ormazine, Thorazine
*Canadian Availability:* Largactil
*Pregnancy Risk:* Category C
*pH:* 4–4.3
*Storage/Stability:* Store below 40° C. Protect from freezing and from light. Do not use if darker than very light yellow or if vial has a precipitate.

### ASSESSMENT: DRUG CHARACTERISTICS

### ACTION

An antipsychotic, antiemetic, and antidyskinetic. Acts as an antipsychotic by blocking postsynaptic dopaminergic receptors in the brain. May also have an α-adrenergic blocking effect and may decrease hormone release from the hypothalamus and hypophysis. Acts as an antiemetic by blocking dopamine receptors in the CTZ in the medulla and by blocking vagus stimulation in the GI tract.

### INDICATIONS

Used to treat psychotic disorders, nausea and vomiting, tetanus, acute and chronic porphyria, and hiccups. The IV route is used primarily to treat hiccups and tetanus and during surgery.

▼

**TABLE 21–5**
**Tranquilizer Toxicities**

| Body System | Side/Toxic Effects | Physical Assessment Indicators | Laboratory Indicators | Nursing Interventions |
|---|---|---|---|---|
| Neurologic | Dystonia | Akathisia, inability to move eyes, twitching, twisting movements, hypotension, Parkinsonian extrapyramidal symptoms such as shuffling gait, trembling of fingers, tardive dyskinesia such as lip smacking | N/A | Monitor client behavior; report evidence of motion difficulties; be prepared to administer agents such as cogentin to decrease symptoms of motion difficulties. |
| Cardiovascular | Agranulocytosis | High fever, chills, ulceration of mucous membrane | Leukocyte count $< 4{,}300/mm^3$ | Monitor vital signs, especially temperature; report elevations promptly. |
| | Orthostatic hypotension | Sudden decrease in blood pressure with position change to standing. | | Counsel clients to change position slowly. |
| Renal | | Difficulty urinating | N/A | Measure and record intake and output; report client difficulty with urination. |
| Sensory | Vision | Blurred vision | N/A | Provide for client safety. |
| Integumentary | | Skin rash, skin photosensitivity | N/A | Provide comfort measures; council client to avoid direct sunlight by wearing protective covering. |
| Gastrointestinal | Anticholinergic effects | Dry mouth, decreased sweating, dizziness, and drowsiness | N/A | Provide comfort measures such as frequent mouth care. |

**CAUTIONS**

ADVERSE EFFECTS. Akathesia, blurred vision, hypotension, agranulocytosis, skin rash, skin photosensitivity, difficulty urinating, dystonic extrapyramidal symptoms (e.g., inability to move eyes, muscle spasms of face, head, and neck, and twisting body movements), parkinsonian-like extrapyramidal symptoms (e.g., shuffling gait, trembling of fingers, difficulty swallowing, and masklike face), tardive dyskinesia (e.g., lip smacking, chewing motions or uncontrolled wormlike movements of arms and legs), and anticholinergic effects (e.g., dry mouth, decreased sweating, dizziness, and drowsiness).

CONTRAINDICATIONS. Severe cardiovascular disease, CNS depression, or coma. Should be given with caution to clients who are alcoholic or who have blood dyscrasias, hepatic dysfunction, or Reye's syndrome.

**POTENTIAL DRUG/FOOD INTERACTIONS**

May interact with alcohol or other CNS depressants to increase respiratory depression and liver toxicity. May potentiate the sedative and hypnotic effects of tricyclic antidepressants, maprotiline, or MAO inhibitors. May increase the incidence of agranulocytosis if used with antithyroid agents. Concurrent use with other extrapyramidal symptoms–producing agents or with other hypotension producing agents increases the incidence of those symptoms. Blocks the α-adrenergic effects of epinephrine and the antiparkinsonian activity of levodopa. Lithium may block intestinal absorption of chlorpromazine. If used with metrizamide, may lower the seizure threshold.

**INTERVENTIONS: ADMINISTRATION**

Dilute on 0.9% NSS, 1 mg/1 mL for a 1:1 concentration.

**MODE/RATE OF ADMINISTRATION**

May be given IV push at a rate not to exceed 1 mg/min. May be given by continuous IV infusion, using an infusion pump.

INTRAVENOUS USE (WITH NORMAL RENAL FUNCTION)

**Adults:** For nausea and vomiting during surgery the usual dose is up to 25 mg in 25 mL of 0.9% NSS at a rate not exceeding 2 mg q2min.

For hiccups the usual dose is 25–50 mg diluted in 500–1000 mL of 0.9% NSS at 1 mg/min.

For tetanus the usual dose is 25–50 mg diluted 1:1 with 0.9% NSS, given at not more than 1 mg/min.

Maximum daily dose should not exceed 1 g.

**Chidlren 5–12 years:** Maximum daily dosage should not exceed 75 mg/d.

**Children 12 years:** Follow adult dosing schedule.

**Infants 6 months:** Dose not established.

**Infants and Children 6 months–5 years:** For nausea and vomiting during surgery the usual dose is 275 mcg (0.275 mg)/kg of body weight diluted 1:1 with 0.9% NSS at a rate of 1 mg q2min.

For tetanus the usual dose is 550 mcg (0.55 mg)/kg of body weight diluted 1 : 1 with 0.9% NSS at a rate of 1 mg q2min.

Maximum daily dosage should not exceed 40 mg/d.

**Geriatrics:** Elderly clients are more likely to experience hypotension, orthostatic hypotension, and extrapyramidal effects when given chlorpromazine. They are also more sensitive to the anticholinergic effects of the agent. Elderly clients should initially be given half the recommended adult dose and monitored carefully.

INTRATHECAL USE OR OTHER INFUSION ROUTES AS INDICATED. Not recommended.

#### POTENTIAL PROBLEMS IN ADMINISTRATION

IV administration may cause severe hypotension. Clients should be in recumbent position when chlorpromazine is administered. May cause a contact dermatitis if skin contacts liquid during preparation.

#### INDEPENDENT NURSING ACTIONS

Monitor vital signs, especially blood pressure. Observe client carefully for extrapyramidal symptoms. Monitor intake and output. Teach client to change positions slowly to avoid orthostatic hypotension. Teach client to avoid exposure to sunlight and alcohol or other CNS depressants.

#### ADMINISTRATION IN ALTERNATE SETTINGS

Not recommended.

#### EVALUATION: OUTCOMES OF DRUG THERAPY

#### EXPECTED OUTCOMES

PHYSICAL ASSESSMENT. No nausea or vomiting. Decreased pychotic manifestations. Blood pressure within 15% of client's baseline. Intake and output within normal range for age. No extrapyramidal symptoms, no tardive dyskinesia, no skin rashes. Client does not complain of dry mouth or blurred vision.

LABORATORY. Complete blood cell count and liver function studies remain within client's baseline.

#### NEGATIVE OUTCOMES

Blood pressure more than 15% below client's baseline. Client experiences orthostatic hypotension or dizziness when changing position. Extrapyramidal symptoms or skin rashes observed. Client complains of difficulty urinating, blurred vision, or dry mouth.

---

## DROPERIDOL

*Trade Name:* Inapsine
*Canadian Availability:* Inapsine
*Pregnancy Risk:* Category C
*pH:* 3–8

*Storage/Stability:* Store between 15° and 30° C. Protect from freezing and from light. Stable for up to 10 days in concentrations of 1 mg/50 mL.

▼

**ASSESSMENT: DRUG CHARACTERISTICS**

**ACTION**

A tranquilizer and antianxiety agent that acts like the phenothiazines and haloperidol. Acts at the subcortical level to create a strong sedative effect. Inhibits α-adrenergic receptor binding sites in large doses. By inhibiting α-adrenergic receptor binding sites, may cause peripheral vasodilation, decreased vascular resistance, and marked hypotension. Has an antiemetic effect.

**INDICATIONS**

Used to create a calming effect to reduce nausea and vomiting during diagnostic and surgical procedures. Also used in conjunction with general anesthesia or with fentanyl (Innovar) for neuroleptanalgesia. Used to control nausea and vomiting resulting from chemotherapy, especially cisplatin, or resulting from surgery.

**CAUTIONS**

ADVERSE EFFECTS. Hypotension, tachycardia, cardiac dysrhythmias, dystonic reactions, akinesia, restlessness, hyperactivity, dizziness, chills, tremors, acute psychosis, depression, or severe respiratory depression. Respiratory depression is more likely to occur when droperidol is used with fentanyl (Innovar).

CONTRAINDICATIONS. Severe hypotension, severe cardiovascular disease, CNS depression, or coma. Should be given with caution to clients who are alcoholic or who have blood dyscrasias, hepatic or renal dysfunction, or Reye's syndrome.

**POTENTIAL DRUG/FOOD INTERACTIONS**

May interact with alcohol or other CNS depressants to increase respiratory depression and liver toxicity. May potentiate the sedative and hypnotic effects of tricyclic antidepressants, maprotiline, or MAO inhibitors. May increase the incidence of agranulocytosis if used with antithryoid agents. Concurrent use with other extrapyramidal symptom–producing agents or with other hypotension-producing agents increases the incidence of those symptoms. Blocks the α-adrenergic effects of epinephrine and the antiparkinsonian activity of levodopa. Lithium may block intestinal absorption of droperidol. Incompatible with epinephrine.

**INTERVENTIONS: ADMINISTRATION**

Can be given undiluted or mixed in D5W or 0.9% NSS to desired concentration. Available in 2.5 mg/mL-vials of 2-, 5-, and 10-mL ampules.

**MODE/RATE OF ADMINISTRATION**

May be given IV push at a rate of 1 mg/min. May be given by continuous IV infusion, usually by an anesthesiologist or nurse anesthetist.

INTRAVENOUS USE (WITH NORMAL RENAL FUNCTION)

**Adults:** For premedication the usual dose is 2.5–10 mg, given 30–60 min before surgery.

For anesthesia induction the usual dose is 0.22–0.275 mg/kg of body weight or 2.5 mg for q10–12kg of body weight.

For use during diagnostic procedures the usual dose includes the premedication dose plus additional doses of 1.25–2.5 mg as ordered by the physician.

For antiemetic purposes the usual dose is 0.5 mg q4h.

**Children 2–12 years:** Usual dose is 0.088–0.165 mg/kg of body weight, or 1–1.5 mg for q10–12kg of body weight.

**Children 12 years:** Follow adult dosing schedule.

**Infants/Neonates:** Do not give to infants younger than 2 years.

**Geriatrics:** Elderly clients may be more likely to have age-related decreases in renal or hepatic functioning that would require lower doses. Orthostatic hypotension frequently occurs in elderly clients receiving droperidol.

INTRATHECAL USE OF OTHER INFUSION ROUTES AS INDICATED. Not recommended.

**POTENTIAL PROBLEMS IN ADMINISTRATION**

Hypovolemia may increase the hypotensive effects of droperidol. Clients should receive adequate hydration during administration of this agent.

**INDEPENDENT NURSING ACTIONS**

Monitor vital signs, especially blood pressure and heart rate and rhythm. Observe client carefully for extrapyramidal symptoms. Measure and record intake and output. Position client in recumbent position to avoid orthostatic hypotension. Teach client to avoid alcohol or other CNS depressants.

**ADMINISTRATION IN ALTERNATE SETTINGS**

Should be administered in clinical settings where emergency resuscitation equipment is immediately available.

**EVALUATON: OUTCOMES OF DRUG THERAPY**

**EXPECTED OUTCOMES**

PHYSICAL ASSESSMENT. No nausea or vomiting; decreased anxiety. Vital signs, especially blood pressure and heart rate and rhythm, remain within 15% of client's baseline. Client does not exhibit extrapyramidal symptoms or anxiety. Intake and output are adequate to maintain a urine output of more than 50 mL/h.

LABORATORY. Complete blood cell count and renal and liver function studies remain within client's baseline.

**NEGATIVE OUTCOMES**

Vital signs, especially blood pressure and heart rate and rhythm, are more than 15% higher or lower than client's baseline. Client exhibits extrapyramidal symptoms or anxiety. Urine output less than 50 mL/h.

## PERPHENAZINE

*Trade Names:* Trilafon
*Canadian Availability:* Trilafon
*Pregnancy Risk:* Category Unknown
*pH:* 4.2–5.6
*Storage/Stability:* Store below 40° C. Protect from freezing and from light. Do not use if darker than very light yellow or if vial has a precipitate.

### ASSESSMENT: DRUG CHARACTERISTICS

#### ACTION

An antipsychotic, antianxiety, and antiemetic agent. Acts as an antipsychotic by blocking postsynaptic dopaminergic receptors in the brain. May also have an α-adrenergic blocking effect and may decrease hormone release from the hypothalamus and hypophysis. Acts as an antiemetic by blocking dopamine receptors in the CTZ in the medulla and by blocking vagus stimulation in the GI tract. Six times more potent than chlorpromazine.

#### INDICATIONS

Used to treat psychotic disorders, intractable hiccups, and severe nausea and vomiting.

#### CAUTIONS

ADVERSE EFFECTS. Akathesia, blurred vision, hypotension, agranulocytosis, skin rash, skin photosensitivity, difficulty urinating, dystonic extrapyramidal symptoms (e.g., inability to move eyes, muscle spasms of face, head, and neck, and twisting body movements), parkinsonian-like extrapyramidal symptoms (e.g., shuffling gait, trembling of fingers, difficulty swallowing, and mask-like face), tardive dyskinesia (e.g., lip smacking, chewing motions or uncontrolled wormlike movements of arms and legs), and anticholinergic effects (e.g., dry mouth, decreased sweating, dizziness, and drowsiness).

CONTRAINDICATIONS. Severe cardiovascular disease, CNS depression, or coma. Should be given with caution to clients who are alcoholic or who have blood dyscrasias, hepatic dysfunction, or Reye's syndrome.

#### POTENTIAL DRUG/FOOD INTERACTIONS

May interact with alcohol or other CNS depressants to increase respiratory depression and liver toxicity. May potentiate the sedative and hypnotic effects of tricyclic antidepressants, maprotiline, or MAO inhibitors. May increase the incidence of agranulocytosis if used with antithyroid agents. Concurrent use with othe extrapyramidal symptom–producing agents or with other hypotension-producing agents increases the incidence of those symptoms. Blocks the α-adrenergic effects of epinephrine and the antiparkinsonian activity of levodopa. Lithium may block intestinal absorption of perphenazine. If used with metrizamide, may lower the seizure threshold.

#### INTERVENTIONS: ADMINISTRATION

Dilute with NSS to a concentration of 0.5 mg/mL or less (or dilute each 5 mg [1 mL] with 9 mL NSS). May be further diluted for intermittent infusion.

#### MODE/RATE OF ADMINISTRATION

May be given IV push, only as absolutely necessary, at a rate not to exceed 1 mg q1–2min. May be given by intermittent IV infusion at a rate not to exceed 1 mg/min.

##### INTRAVENOUS USE (WITH NORMAL RENAL FUNCTION)

**Adults:** For nausea and vomiting the usual dose is up to 1–5 mg per dose.

Maximum dose should not exceed 5 mg. Allow 2–3 min between doses.

**Children 12 years:** Follow adult dosing schedule.

**Infants/Neonates:** Dose not established.

**Geriatrics:** Elderly clients are more likely to experience hypotension, orthostatic hypotension, and extrapyramidal effects when given perphenazine. They are also more sensitive to the anticholinergic effects of perphenazine. Elderly clients should initially be given half the recommended adult dose and monitored carefully.

INTRATHECAL USE OR OTHER INFUSION ROUTES AS INDICATED. Not recommended.

#### POTENTIAL PROBLEMS IN ADMINISTRATION

IV administration may cause severe hypotension. Clients should be in a recumbent position when perphenazine is administered.

#### INDEPENDENT NURSING ACTIONS

Monitor vital signs, especially blood pressure. Observe client carefully for extrapyramidal symptoms. Monitor intake and output. Teach client to change positions slowly to avoid orthostatic hypotension. Teach client to avoid exposure to sunlight and alcohol or other CNS depressants. Handle drug carefully to avoid contact dermatitis.

#### ADMINISTRATION IN ALTERNATE SETTINGS

Not recommended.

#### EVALUATION: OUTCOMES OF DRUG THERAPY

##### EXPECTED OUTCOMES

PHYSICAL ASSESSMENT. No nausea or vomiting; decreased anxiety and psychotic manifestations. Blood pressure within 15% of client's baseline. Intake and output within normal range for age. No extrapyramidal symptoms, no tardive dyskinesia, no skin rashes. Client does not complain of dry mouth or blurred vision.

LABORATORY. Complete blood cell count and liver function studies remain within client's baseline.

##### NEGATIVE OUTCOMES

Blood pressure more than 15% lower than client's baseline. Client experiences orthostatic hypotension or dizziness when changing position. Extrapyramidal symptoms or skin rashes observed.

## PROCHLORPERAZINE EDISYLATE

*Trade Names:* Compa-Z, Compazine, Utrazine-10
*Canadian Availability:* Prorazin, Stemetil
*Pregnancy Risk:* Category Unknown
*pH:* 4.2–6.2
*Storage/Stability:* Store below 40° C. Protect from freezing and light. Do not use if darker than light yellow or vial has a precipitate.

### ASSESSMENT: DRUG CHARACTERISTICS

#### ACTION

An antipsychotic and antiemetic. Acts as an antipsychotic by blocking postsynaptic dopaminergic receptors in the brain. May also have an α-adrenergic blocking effect and may decrease hormone release from the hypothalamus and hypophysis. Acts as an antiemetic by blocking dopamine receptors in the CTZ in the medulla and by blocking vagus stimulation in GI tract.

#### INDICATIONS

Psychotic disorders and nausea and vomiting

#### CAUTIONS

ADVERSE EFFECTS: Akathesia, blurred vision, hypotension, agranulocytosis, skin rash, skin photosensitivity, difficulty urinating, dystonic extrapyramidal symptoms (e.g., inability to move eyes, muscle spasms of face, head, and neck, and twisting body movements), parkinsonian-like extrapyramidal symptoms (e.g., shuffling gait, trembling of fingers, difficulty swallowing, and mask-like face), tardive dyskinesia (e.g., lip smacking, chewing motions or uncontrolled wormlike movements of arms and legs), and anticholinergic effects (e.g., dry mouth, decreased sweating, dizziness, and drowsiness).

CONTRAINDICATIONS. Severe cardiovascular disease, CNS depression, or coma. Should be given with caution to alcoholics or those with blood dyscrasias, hepatic dysfunction, or Reye's syndrome. Do not mix in syringe with another drug or solution.

#### POTENTIAL DRUG/FOOD INTERACTIONS

May interact with alcohol or other CNS depressants to increase respiratory depression and liver toxicity. May potentiate the sedative and hypnotic effects of tricyclic antidepressants, maprotiline, or MAO inhibitors. May increase the incidence of agranulocytosis if used with antithyroid agents. Concurrent use with other extrapyramidal symptom–producing agents or with other hypotension-producing agents increases the incidence of those symptoms. Blocks the α-adrenergic effects of epinephrine and the antiparkinsonian activity of levodopa. Lithium may block intestinal absorption of prochlorperazine. If used with metrizamide, may lower the seizure threshold. Incompatible with aminophylline, calcium gluconate, aminoglycosides, methicillin, prednisolone, phenytoin, and dexamethasone.

#### INTERVENTIONS: ADMINISTRATION

Dilute 5 mg with 9 mL NSS (1 mg = 1 mL); add 10–20 mg to 1 L of isotonic IV solution.

#### MODE/RATE OF ADMINISTRATION

May be given IV push at a rate not to exceed 5 mg/min or by continuous IV infusion, using an infusion pump.

##### INTRAVENOUS USE (WITH NORMAL RENAL FUNCTION)

**Adults:** For nausea and vomiting the usual adult dose is 5–10 mg at a rate not to exceed 5 mg/min. Maximum daily dose should not exceed 40 mg. For anxiety the usual dose is 2.5–1 mg at a rate not to exceed 5 mg/min. Maximum daily dosage should not exceed 40 mg/d.

**Children 12 years:** IV administration is unusual in children younger than 12.

**Children 12 years:** Follow adult dosing schedule.

**Infants/Neonates:** Dose not established for infants up to 2 years of age. IV administration is unusual in infants.

**Geriatrics:** Elderly clients are more likely to experience hypotension, orthostatic hypotension, and extrapyramidal effects from prochlorperazine. They are more sensitive to anticholinergic effects of prochlorperazine. They should initially be given half the recommended adult dose and monitored carefully.

INTRATHECAL USE OR OTHER INFUSION ROUTES AS INDICATED. Not recommended.

#### POTENTIAL PROBLEMS IN ADMINISTRATION

IV administration may cause severe hypotension. Clients should be in a recumbent position when prochlorperazine is administered. May cause a contact dermatitis if skin contacts liquid during preparation.

#### INDEPENDENT NURSING ACTIONS

Monitor vital signs, especially blood pressure. Observe client carefully for extrapyramidal symptoms. Monitor intake and output. Teach client to change positions slowly to avoid orthostatic hypotension and to avoid sunlight and alcohol or other CNS depressants.

#### ADMINISTRATION IN ALTERNATE SETTINGS

Not recommended.

#### EVALUATION: OUTCOMES OF DRUG THERAPY

#### EXPECTED OUTCOMES

PHYSICAL ASSESSMENT. No nausea or vomiting. Decreased anxiety. Blood pressure within 15% of client's baseline. Intake and output within normal range for age. No extrapyramidal symptoms, no tardive dyskinesia, no skin rashes. Client does not complain of dry mouth or blurred vision.

LABORATORY. CBC and liver function studies remain within client's baseline.

#### NEGATIVE OUTCOMES

Blood pressure more than 15% lower than client's baseline. Client experiences orthostatic hypotension or dizziness when changing position, also extrapyramidal symptoms or skin rashes.

## Promazine Hydrochloride

*Trade Names:* Primazine, Prozine-50, Sparine
*Canadian Availability:* Promazine hydrochloride
*Pregnancy Risk:* Category C
*pH:* 4–5.5
*Storage/Stability:* Store below 40° C. Protect from freezing and light. Do not use if darker than light yellow or if vial has a precipitate.

### ASSESSMENT: DRUG CHARACTERISTICS

#### ACTION

An antipsychotic, antianxiety, and antiemetic agent that acts by blocking postsynaptic dopaminergic receptors in the brain. May also have an α-adrenergic blocking effect and decrease hormone release from the hypothalamus and hypophysis.

#### INDICATIONS

Psychotic disorders and to control nausea and vomiting.

#### CAUTIONS

ADVERSE EFFECTS. Akathesia, blurred vision, hypotension, agranulocytosis, skin rash, skin photosensitivity, difficulty urinating, dystonic extrapyramidal symptoms (e.g., inability to move eyes, muscle spasms of face, head, and neck, and twisting body movements), parkinsonian-like extrapyramidal symptoms (e.g., shuffling gait, trembling of fingers, difficulty swallowing, and mask-like face), tardive dyskinesia (e.g., lip smacking, chewing motions or uncontrolled wormlike movements of arms and legs), and anticholinergic effects (e.g., dry mouth, decreased sweating, dizziness, and drowsiness).

CONTRAINDICATIONS. Severe cardiovascular disease, CNS depression, or coma. Given with caution to clients who are alcoholic or who have blood dyscrasias, hepatic dysfunction, or Reye's syndrome. May mask brain tumor, drug intoxication, or intestinal obstruction.

#### POTENTIAL DRUG/FOOD INTERACTIONS

Contraindicated for clients receiving quinidine, thiazide diuretics, or epinephrine. May interact with alcohol or other CNS depressants to increase respiratory depression and liver toxicity. May potentiate the sedative and hypnotic effects of tricyclic antidepressants, maprotiline, or MAO inhibitors. May increase the incidence of agranulocytosis if used with antithyroid agents. Concurrent use with ther extrapyramidal symptom–producing agents or with other hypotension-producing agents increases the incidence of those symptoms. Blocks the α-adrenergic effects of epinephrine and the antiparkinsonian activity of levodopa. Lithium may block intestinal absorption of promazine. If used with metrizamide, may lower the seizure threshold.

### INTERVENTIONS: ADMINISTRATION

May be diluted with NSS to a concentration 25 mg/mL or less. May be given undiluted in concentrations of 25 mg/mL or less.

**MODE/RATE OF ADMINISTRATION**

May be given IV push at a rate not to exceed 25 mg/min.

INTRAVENOUS USE (WITH NORMAL RENAL FUNCTION)

**Adults:** For psychotic disorder the usual dose is 25–50 mg, repeated in 4–6h if needed. Maximum daily dose should not exceed 1 g.

**Children:** IV administration unusual.

**Infants/Neonates:** Dose not established.

**Geriatrics:** Elderly clients are more likely to experience hypotension, orthostatic hypotension, and extrapyramidal effects when given promazine. They are also more sensitive to the anticholinergic effects of promazine. Elderly clients initially be given half the recommended adult dose and monitored carefully.

INTRATHECAL USE OR OTHER INFUSION ROUTES AS INDICATED. Not recommended.

**POTENTIAL PROBLEMS IN ADMINISTRATION**

IV administration may cause severe hypotension. Clients should be in a recumbent position when promazine is administered. May cause a contact dermatitis if skin contacts liquid during preparation.

**INDEPENDENT NURSING ACTIONS**

Monitor vital signs, especially blood pressure. Observe client carefully for extrapyramidal symptoms. Monitor intake and output. Teach client to change positions slowly to avoid orthostatic hypotension and to avoid sunlight and alcohol or other CNS depressants.

**ADMINISTRATION IN ALTERNATE SETTINGS**

Not recommended.

**EVALUATION: OUTCOMES OF DRUG THERAPY**

**EXPECTED OUTCOMES**

PHYSICAL ASSESSMENT. No nausea or vomiting. Decreased anxiety and psychotic manifestations. Blood pressure within 15% of client's baseline. Intake and output within normal range for age. No extrapyramidal symptoms, no tardive dyskinesia, no skin rashes. No dry mouth or blurred vision.

LABORATORY. CBC and liver function studies remain within client's baseline.

**NEGATIVE OUTCOMES**

Blood pressure more than 15% lower than client's baseline. Client experiences orthostatic hypotension or dizziness when changing position, also extrapyramidal symptoms or skin rashes.

# CHAPTER 22
# Fluid and Electrolyte Agents

*Elaine Kennedy*

**Caloric Agents**
- Amino Acid Injections
- Dextrose
- Fat Emulsions
- Invert Sugar

**Diuretic Agents**
- Acetazolamide Sodium
- Bumetanide
- Furosemide
- Mannitol
- Torsemide

**Replacement Agents**
- Calcium Chloride
- Calcium Gluconate
- Dextran 40
- Hetastarch
- Potassium Chloride
- Sodium Bicarbonate

Clients may be unable to secure, ingest, and metabolize sufficient nutrients for a variety of reasons such as surgery, severe trauma, gastrointestinal pathology, or other disease states. In addition, some drug therapies such as diuretic therapy may excessively deplete the body of needed substances such as potassium. Parenteral replacement of fluids, nutrients, and electrolytes provides the client with the necessary calories and structural elements to respond to stress, maintain structural mass, and heal the effects of trauma, surgery, or other depleting processes.

## CLASSIFICATION

### CALORIC AGENTS

Caloric agents provide various levels of carbohydrates, finely emulsified fat, and free fatty acids or varying amounts of all the essential amino acids. Amino acids conserve lean body mass or structural protein and promote wound healing. Dextrose provides a source of nonprotein calories so that lean body mass is not catabolized for energy. Fats emulsions are used to provide a source of nonprotein calories for energy and to prevent or reverse essential fatty acid deficiency (EFAD).

### DIURETIC AGENTS

Diuretic agents are usually carbonic anhydrase inhibitors, loop (high-ceiling) diuretics, or osmotic diuretics. Cabronic anhydrase inhibitors act by producing a systemic metabolic acidosis with resultant diuretic effect. Loop diuretics act by preventing the reabsorption of sodium and water in the ascending loop of Henle, thus increasing water loss. Osmotic diuretics act by increasing intravascular osmolality, thus drawing fluid into the vascular compartment. Further, osmotic diuretics are not reabsorbed by the kidney tubule, and they inhibit the reabsorption of water plus sodium, chloride, and other electrolytes.

### REPLACEMENT AGENTS

Replacement agents are used to supplement or increase electrolytes or other substances needed by the body to maintain homeostasis. Parenteral calcium is needed to raise serum calcium levels quickly to relieve the symptoms of tetany resulting from severe hypocalcemia. Potassium is needed primarily for cellular membrane functioning and electric excitability. Other replacement agents are used in emergencies as substitutes for missing substances.

Fluid and electrolyte infusion agents are grouped by subclassifications in Table 22–1.

## CALORIC AGENTS

### THERAPEUTIC EFFECTS

Caloric agents provide various levels of carbohydrates, finely emulsified fat, and free fatty acids or varying amounts

**TABLE 22–1**
**Fluid and Electrolyte Infusion Agents Grouped by Subclassifications**

| **Caloric Agents** | **Replacement Agents** |
|---|---|
| Amino acids | Calcium acetate* |
| Dextrose | Calcium chloride |
| Fat emulsions | Calcium gluceptate* |
| Invert sugar | Calcium gluconate |
| **Diuretic Agents** | Dextran 40 |
| Acetazolamide sodium | Dextran 70/75* |
| Bumetanide | Hetastarch |
| Chlorothiazide sodium* | Potassium acetate* |
| Ethacrynate sodium* | Potassium chloride |
| Furosemide | Potassium phosphate* |
| Mannitol | Sodium bicarbonate |
| Torsemide | Sodium chloride* |
| Urea* | |

*Not discussed in this Chapter.

of all the essential amino acids for energy, protein conservation, and synthesis.

## PHARMACOKINETICS

**Distribution.** Caloric agents are rapidly and widely distributed throughout the body when given intravenously.

**Metabolism/Elimination.** Caloric agents are metabolized as sugar, protein, and fat and are excreted via feces and urine.

## CAUTIONS

**Side/Adverse Effects.** Dextrose preparations may cause hyperglycemia and osmotic diuresis. Lipids may cause hyperlipidemia or allergic reactions. Amino acid preparations may cause hyperglycemic hyperosmolar nonketotic syndrome (HHNS) coma from the hypertonic solution.

### Contraindications

***Pregnancy and Lactation.*** There are no specific contraindications to using caloric agents during pregnancy or lactation.

***Pediatrics.*** Lipids have been known to cause death in preterm infants.

***Geriatrics.*** There are no specific contraindications to using caloric agents in the elderly.

## TOXICITY

See Table 22–2 for caloric agent toxicities.

## POTENTIAL DRUG/FOOD INTERACTIONS

Dextrose, invert sugar, or amino acid injections may increase the requirement for insulin. No significant interactions with lipids have been reported.

*Trade Name:* None specified

# AMINO ACID INJECTIONS

*Trade Names:* Aminosyn, Fre-Amine III, Travasol, Novamine

*Canadian Availability:* Not specified

*Pregnancy Risk:* Category C

*pH:* 5.0–7.0

*Storage/Stability:* Store below 40° C. Protect from freezing.

## ASSESSMENT: DRUG CHARACTERISTICS

### ACTION

A caloric agent used as part of parenteral therapy to prevent the loss of nitrogen when clients are unable to maintain adequate nutrition by any other means. The amino acids included in the ▼

**TABLE 22–2**
**Caloric Agent Toxicities**

| Body System | Side/Toxic Effects | Physical Assessment Indicators | Laboratory Indicators | Nursing Interventions |
|---|---|---|---|---|
| Cardiovascular | | Hypercoagulability, anemia, venous thrombosis, chest or back pain | N/A | Observe the client for phlebitis or complaints of chest pain; report symptoms promptly. |
| Renal | | Glycosuria, osmotic diuresis, water intoxication | Urine positive for sugar | Measure and record intake and output; observe client for evidence of dehydration; provide fluids. |
| Gastrointestinal | | Diarrhea, nausea or vomiting, jaundice, hyperglycemia | Serum glucose > 800 mg/dL<br>Serum bilirubin > 0.4 mg/dL | Monitor laboratory reports and observe for evidence of gastrointestinal disturbance; report promptly. |
| Endocrine | Hyperglycemic, hyperosmolar nonketotic syndrome | Dry mucous membranes, weight loss, weakness, fatigue | Serum glucose > 800 mg/dL<br>Serum osmolality > 350 mOsm/kg | Measure and record evidence of dehydration. |
| Other | Anaphylactic reactions<br>Infection | Urticaria, wheezing, rash<br>Local irritation | N/A | Monitor vital signs; be prepared to give medication for anaphylactic reactions. |

N/A = not applicable.

products provide varying amounts of all the essential amino acids for protein production in the body.

#### INDICATIONS

Used to prevent the loss of lean body mass and to promote wound healing.

#### CAUTIONS

ADVERSE EFFECTS. May cause HHNS from the hypertonic solution.

CONTRAINDICATIONS. Should be given with caution to clients with impaired renal or hepatic function, since nitrogenous waste products may cause severe elevations in blood urea nitrogen (BUN) or hepatic coma.

#### POTENTIAL DRUG/FOOD INTERACTIONS

May increase the requirement for insulin.

#### INTERVENTIONS: ADMINISTRATION

Solutions containing more than 4% amino acids should be given through a central venous catheter. Solutions containing less than 4% amino acids may be given peripherally.

#### MODE/RATE OF ADMINISTRATION

Given by continuous intravenous (IV) infusion, using an infusion pump.

INTRAVENOUS USE (WITH NORMAL RENAL AND HEPATIC FUNCTION)

**Adults:** Usual dosage of amino acids is based on 0.9 g/kg/d for the healthy adult. Clients with significant trauma such as burns, malnutrition. or infection require individual doses in excess of that amount.

**Children:** Usual dosage of amino acids is based on 1.4–2.2 g/kg/d for the healthy child. Clients with significant trauma such as burns, malnutrition, or infection require individual doses in excess of that amount.

**Infants/Neonates:** Follow children's dosing schedule.

**Geriatrics:** Elderly clients are more likely to have age-related decreases in renal function that may require lowered doses.

INTRATHECAL USE OR OTHER INFUSION ROUTES AS INDICATED. Not recommended.

#### POTENTIAL PROBLEMS IN ADMINISTRATION

Solutions containing amino acids are excellent media for bacterial growth. Care should be exercised to maintain strict aseptic technique when handling containers and equipment and at the injection site.

#### INDEPENDENT NURSING ACTIONS

Monitor vital signs, especially temperature and heart rate. Monitor for signs of infection such as temperature elevation, redness or swelling at the injection site, complaints of weakness, nausea, vomiting, or malaise. Monitor for symptoms of HHNS such as dehydration, confusion, glycosuria, and hypernatremia. Monitor BUN and creatinine levels.

#### ADMINISTRATION IN ALTERNATE SETTINGS

May be given in a variety of settings, including long-term care and the home.

**EVALUATION: OUTCOMES OF DRUG THERAPY**

**EXPECTED OUTCOMES**

PHYSICAL ASSESSMENT. Vital signs, especially temperature and heart rate, remain within 15% of client's baseline. Client has no temperature elevation, redness or swelling at the injection site, complaints of weakness, nausea, vomiting, or malaise. Client exhibits no signs of dehydration, confusion, glycosuria, or hypernatremia. Client has no restlessness, irritability, anxiety, or cool, clammy skin.

LABORATORY. Serum glucose between 80 and 120 mg/dL. BUN between 10 and 20 mg/dL. Creatinine between 0.7 and 1.4 mg/dL. Total protein between 6 and 8 g/dL. Serum sodium between 135 and 145 mEq/L. Serum albumin between 3.5 and 5 g/dL.

**NEGATIVE OUTCOMES**

Vital signs, especially temperature and heart rate, are more than 15% above client's baseline. Client has a temperature elevation, redness or swelling at the injection site, complaints of weakness, nausea, vomiting, or malaise. Client is dehydrated and confused and has glycosuria or hypernatremia. Client has restlessness, irritability, anxiety, and cool, clammy skin.

## DEXTROSE (GLUCOSE)

*Canadian Availability:* Dextrose (glucose)
*Pregnancy Risk:* Category C
*pH:* 3.5–6.5
*Storage/Stability:* Store below 40° C.

**ASSESSMENT: DRUG CHARACTERISTICS**

**ACTION**

A caloric agent that provides various levels of carbohydrate for energy and for protein conservation and synthesis. Hypertonic solutions (20% to 50%) act as diuretics. Excreted by the kidneys.

**INDICATIONS**

Used to prevent the loss of lean body mass and to promote wound healing by providing nonprotein calories as part of partial or total parenteral nutrition (PPN or TPN). Used to treat hypoglycemia (50% solution), shock (10% to 70% solution), hypercalcemia (20% solution), and diuresis (20% to 50% solution) and as a diluent for IV medications (2.5% to 10% solution).

**CAUTIONS**

ADVERSE EFFECTS. Hyperglycemia, glycosuria, osmotic diuresis, water intoxication (fluid overload), infection, venous thrombosis, or local irritation.

CONTRAINDICATIONS. High-dextrose concentrations should be given with caution to clients with a history of glucose intolerance, diabetes mellitus, or central or peripheral edema.

▼

**POTENTIAL DRUG/FOOD INTERACTIONS**

May increase the requirement for insulin. Incompatible with whole blood and blood products, kanamycin, and sodium bicarbonate.

**INTERVENTIONS: ADMINISTRATION**

May be given in various concentrations and may be found in combination with sodium chloride in varying concentrations.

**MODE/RATE OF ADMINISTRATION**

May be given IV push or by intermittent or continuous peripheral or central venous infusion. Hypertonic solutions with dextrose concentrations higher than 12.5% are given by central venous infusion. Avoid extravasation.

INTRAVENOUS USE (WITH NORMAL RENAL FUNCTION)

**Adults:** For caloric replacement, the usual dosage is 0.5 g/kg/h. The maximum dosage generally should not exceed 0.8 g/kg/h. Clients with significant trauma such as burns, malnutrition, or infection require individualized doses. For example, 10% dextrose provides 340 kcal/L. For intermittent use, give 500 mL of 20% solution over 30–60 min. For continuous infusion, give 10% solution at 1000 mL over 3 h. At a rate of 0.5 g/kg/h, a 30%–70% solution does not cause glycosuria. At 0.8 g/kg/h, 95% solution is retained, and glycosuria will occur.

For hypoglycemia the usual dose is 20–50 mL of 50% dextrose at a rate of 3 mL/min IV push.

**Children:** For caloric replacement the dose is based on age, weight, clinical condition, fluid and electrolyte and acid-base balance. The usual dosage is 0.5 g/kg/h. The maximum dosage generally should not exceed 0.8 g/kg/h. Clients with significant trauma such as burns, malnutrition, or infection require individualized doses.

For hypoglycemia the usual dose is 20–50 mL of 50% dextrose at a rate of 3 mL/min IV push.

**Infants/Neonates:** For hypoglycemia the usual dose is 2 mL/kg of 10%–25% dextrose at a rate of 3 mL/min IV push.

**Geriatrics:** Follow adult dosing schedule.

INTRATHECAL USE OR OTHER INFUSION ROUTES AS INDICATED. Low-concentration solutions may be given by hypodermoclysis (subcutaneous infusion), although not common.

**POTENTIAL PROBLEMS IN ADMINISTRATION**

Abrupt termination of TPN may cause rebound hypoglycemia with symptoms such as weakness, faintness, shakiness, sweating, confusion, and rapid heart rate. If next container of TPN is not immediately available, administer 10% dextrose to avoid rebound hypoglycemia. Solutions containing high concentrations of dextrose are excellent media for bacterial growth. Care should be exercised to maintain strict aseptic technique when handling containers and equipment and at the injection site. Do not administer dextrose with blood products.

**INDEPENDENT NURSING ACTIONS**

Monitor vital signs, especially temperature and heart rate. Monitor for signs of infection such as temperature elevation, redness or swelling at the injection site, complaints of weakness, nausea, vomiting, or malaise. Monitor for symptoms of HHNK coma such as dehyration, confusion, glycosuria, and hypernatremia. For clients receiving parenteral nutrition, monitor blood sugar frequently, check urine for ketones, and monitor weight and intake and output.

**ADMINISTRATION IN ALTERNATE SETTINGS**

May be given in a variety of settings, including the home.

**EVALUATION: OUTCOMES OF DRUG THERAPY**

**EXPECTED OUTCOMES**

PHYSICAL ASSESSMENT. Vital signs, especially temperature and heart rate, remain within 15% of client's baseline. Client has no temperature elevation, redness or swelling at the injection site, complaints of weakness, nausea, vomiting, or malaise. Client has no dehydration, confusion, glycosuria, or hypernatremia. Client has no restlessness, irritability, anxiety, or cool, clammy skin. For use as PPN or TPN, client remains in or achieves positive nitrogen balance, as enough dextrose is available for energy requirements.

LABORATORY. Serum glucose between 80 and 120 mg/dL. BUN between 10 and 20 mg/dL. Creatinine between 0.7 and 1.4 mg/dL. Total protein between 6 and 8 g/dL. Serum sodium between 135 and 145 mEq/L.

**NEGATIVE OUTCOMES**

Vital signs, especially temperature and heart rate, are more than 15% above client's baseline. Client has a temperature elevation, redness or swelling at the injection site, complaints of weakness, nausea, vomiting, or malaise. Client is dehydrated and confused and has glycosuria or hypernatremia. Client has restlessness, irritability, anxiety, and cool, clammy skin.

## FAT EMULSIONS

*Trade Names:* Intralipid, Liposyn, Liposyn II, Travamulsion (10% and 20% solutions)
*Canadian Availability:* Intralipid, Liposyn II
*Pregnancy Risk:* Category C
*pH:* 6–8.9
*Storage/Stability:* Store below 40° C. Protect from freezing.

**ASSESSMENT: DRUG CHARACTERISTICS**

**ACTION**

A caloric agent that provides finely emulsified fat

and free fatty acids that are metabolized and used for energy.

#### INDICATIONS

Used to treat nutritional deficiencies, to correct EFAD, and to provide calories for energy. Has an osmolality of 280 mOsm/L. Intralipid has a caloric value of 1.1 kcal/mL for a 10% solution.

#### CAUTIONS

ADVERSE EFFECTS. Hyperlipidemia, allergic reactions, infection, anemia, hypercoagulability, jaundice, chest or back pain, dyspnea, seizures, diarrhea, nausea, or vomiting. Has been known to cause death in preterm infants.

CONTRAINDICATIONS. Should be given with caution to clients with known hypersensitivity or with conditions that include abnormal fat metabolism such as diabetes mellitus, renal and hepatic impairment, or pancreatitis. Not given to clients with severe egg allergy or to those with history of fat embolism.

#### POTENTIAL DRUG/FOOD INTERACTIONS

Check with infusion pharmacist before adding any medications to container.

#### INTERVENTIONS: ADMINISTRATION

May be given separately or with both high-concentration dextrose and amino acid solutions as in three-in-one TPN or total nutrient admixture (TNA).

#### MODE/RATE OF ADMINISTRATION

May be given by intermittent or continuous peripheral or central venous infusion, using an infusion pump. Use of an in-line filter is contraindicated because some of the lipid molecules are larger than most filters tolerate. Rate is 0.5 mL/min of 20% fat solution or 1 mL/min of 10% fat solution for the first 15–30 min, then increased to a rate that infuses not more than 500 mL of 10% fat solution or 250 mL of 20% fat solution in 4–6 h.

INTRAVENOUS USE (WITH NORMAL RENAL FUNCTION)

**Adults:** The usual initial dosage for TPN is 250 mL of 20% fat solution or 500 mL of 10% fat solution q4–6h, then can be increased. The maximum dose should not exceed 3 g/kg/d. For EFAD, provide 8%–10% of total caloric intake per day with fat solution.

**Children 12 years:** Follow adult dosing schedule.

**Children <12 years:** 2–4 g/kg/d.

**Infants/Neonates:** The usual dose is 0.1 mL/min of 10% or 20% fat solution for 15–30 min, then not more than 100 mL/h of 10% fat solution or 50 mL/h of 20% fat solution. For TPN, up to 1 g/kg, then increase gradually. The maximum daily dose should not exceed 4 g/kg of body weight.

**Geriatrics:** Follow adult dosing schedule.

INTRATHECAL USE OR OTHER INFUSION ROUTES AS INDICATED. Not recommended.

**POTENTIAL PROBLEMS IN ADMINISTRATION**

Care should be exercised to maintain strict aseptic technique when handling containers and equipment and at the injection site. Use caution in administration of emulsion to neonates, as intravascular fat accumulation in lungs may occur.

**INDEPENDENT NURSING ACTIONS**

Monitor vital signs, especially temperature and heart rate. Monitor for signs of infection such as temperature elevation, redness or swelling at the injection site, complaints of weakness, nausea, vomiting, or malaise. Monitor for symptoms of HHNS such as dehydration, confusion, glycosuria, and hypernatremia. Monitor for fat embolism syndrome (dyspnea, chest pain, rash).

**ADMINISTRATION IN ALTERNATE SETTINGS**

May be given in a variety of settings, including the home.

**EVALUATION: OUTCOMES OF DRUG THERAPY**

**EXPECTED OUTCOMES**

PHYSICAL ASSESSMENT. Vital signs, especially temperature and heart rate, remain within 15% of client's baseline. Client has no temperature elevation, redness or swelling at the injection site, complaints of weakness, nausea, vomiting, or malaise. Client has no dehydration, confusion, glycosuria, or hypernatremia. Client has no restlessness, irritability, anxiety, or cool, clammy skin. Client maintains or gains weight.

LABORATORY. Serum glucose between 80 and 120 mg/dL. BUN between 10 and 20 mg/dL. Creatinine between 0.7 and 1.4 mg/dL. Total protein between 6 and 8 g/dL. Serum sodium between 135 and 145 mEq/L.

**NEGATIVE OUTCOMES**

Vital signs, especially temperature and heart rate, are more than 15% above client's baseline. Client has a temperature elevation, redness or swelling at the injection site, complaints of weakness, nausea, vomiting, or malaise. Client is dehydrated and confused and has glycosuria or hypernatremia. Client has restlessness, irritability, anxiety, and cool, clammy skin. Client loses weight.

## INVERT SUGAR

*Trade Name:* Travert
*Canadian Availability:* Not specified
*Pregnancy Risk:* Category Unknown
*pH:* 3.7–4
*Storage/Stability:* Store below 40° C.

**ASSESSMENT: DRUG CHARACTERISTICS**

**ACTION**

A caloric carbohydrate mix that provides various concentrations of combined dextrose and fructose for energy and for protein conservation and synthesis.

▼

#### INDICATIONS

Used as a source of calories and water for hydration.

#### CAUTIONS

ADVERSE EFFECTS. Hyperglycemia, glycosuria, osmotic diuresis, water intoxication, infection, venous thrombosis, or local irritation.

CONTRAINDICATIONS. Invert sugar solutions should be given with caution to clients with a history of glucose intolerance, diabetes mellitus, or with central or peripheral edema.

#### POTENTIAL DRUG/FOOD INTERACTIONS

May increase the requirement for insulin.

#### INTERVENTIONS: ADMINISTRATION

May be given in various concentrations and may be found in combination with sodium chloride in varying concentrations.

#### MODE/RATE OF ADMINISTRATION

May be given by intermittent or continuous, peripheral or central venous infusion.

INTRAVENOUS USE (WITH NORMAL RENAL FUNCTION)

**Adults:** For caloric replacement, the usual dose is 1–3 L of a 10% solution per day.

**Children:** For caloric replacement, the dose is based on age, weight, clinical condition, and fluid, electrolyte, and acid/base balance. The usual dose is 1–3 L of a 10% solution per day.

**Infants/Neonates:** For caloric replacement the dose is based on age, weight, clinical condition, and fluid, electrolyte, and acid/base balance. Dose is individualized.

**Geriatrics:** Follow adult dosing schedule.

INTRATHECAL USE OR OTHER INFUSION ROUTES AS INDICATED. Low concentration solutions may be given by hypodermoclysis.

#### POTENTIAL PROBLEMS IN ADMINISTRATION

Abrupt termination of invert sugar may cause rebound hypoglycemia with such symptoms as weakness, faintness, shakiness, sweating, confusion, and rapid heart rate. Solutions containing high concentrations of invert sugar are excellent media for bacterial growth. Care should be exercised to maintain strict aseptic technique when handling containers and equipment and at the injection site.

#### INDEPENDENT NURSING ACTIONS

Monitor vital signs, especially temperature and heart rate. Monitor for signs of infection, such as temperature elevation, redness or swelling at the injection site, complaints of weakness, nausea, vomiting, or malaise. Monitor for symptoms of HHNS, such as dehydration, confusion, glycosuria, and hypernatremia. Monitor for symptoms of hypoglycemia, such as restlnessness, irritability, anxiety, and cool, clammy skin.

**ADMINISTRATION IN ALTERNATE SETTINGS**

May be given in a variety of settings including the home.

**EVALUATION: OUTCOMES OF DRUG THERAPY**

**EXPECTED OUTCOMES**

PHYSICAL ASSESSMENT. Client's vital signs, especially temperature and heart rate, remain within 15% of baseline. Client has no temperature elevation, redness, or swelling at the injection site, or complaints of weakness, nausea, vomiting, or malaise. Client has no dehydration, confusion, glycosuria, or hypernatremia. Client has no restlessness, irritability, anxiety, or cool, clammy skin. Client gains weight.

LABORATORY. Serum glucose between 80 and 120 mg/dL. BUN between 10 and 20 mg/dL. Creatinine between 0.7 and 1.4 mg/dL. Total protein between 6 and 8 g/dL. Serum sodium between 135 and 145 mEq/L.

**NEGATIVE OUTCOMES**

Client's vital signs, especially temperature and heart rate, are more than 15% above baseline. Client has a temperature elevation, redness or swelling at the injection site, complaints of weakness, nausea, vomiting, or malaise. Client is dehydrated or confused or has glycosuria or hypernatremia. Client is restless, irritable, or anxious, or has cool, clammy skin. Client loses weight.

---

# DIURETIC AGENTS

## THERAPEUTIC EFFECTS

Acetazolamide sodium is a carbonic anhydrase inhibitor and acts by producing a systemic metabolic acidosis with resultant diuretic effect. Bumetanide and furosemide are loop diuretics that act by preventing the reabsorption of sodium and water in the ascending loop of Henle, thus increasing water loss. Mannitol and urea are osmotic diuretics that act by increasing intravascular osmolality, thus drawing fluid into the vascular compartment. Further, osmotic diuretics are not reabsorbed by the kidney tubule. The increased osmolality of the filtrate inhibits the reabsorption of water plus sodium, chloride, and other electrolytes.

## PHARMACOKINETICS

**Distribution.** Diuretic agents are widely distributed when administered intravenously.

**Excretion.** Carbonic anhydrase inhibitors, loop diuretics, and osmotic diuretics are excreted mainly in the urine.

## CAUTIONS

**Side/Adverse Effects.** Carbonic anhydrase inhibitors may cause gastrointestinal symptoms. Loop diuretics may cause electrolyte or acid-base imbalances. Osmotic diuretics may cause electrolyte imbalances or cardiovascular symptoms.

### Contraindications

***Pregnancy and Lactation.*** Carbonic anhydrase inhibitors such as acetazolamide sodium may be teratogenic, and use during pregnancy (especially the first trimester) is not recommended. Loop diuretics such as bumetanide and furosemide may cross the placental barrier. Studies have not documented adverse effects. Both carbonic anhydrase inhibitors and loop diuretics may be passed in breast milk. Osmotic diuretics such as mannitol and urea have not been studied sufficiently to determine fetal effects. Studies have not determined if they are passed in breast milk.

***Pediatrics.*** The effects of carbonic anhydrase inhibitors and osmotic diuretics on children have not been sufficiently studied to determine effects. Loop diuretics have a prolonged half-life in infants and should be used with caution.

***Geriatrics.*** The elderly are more likely to have age-related diminished renal function and may require lower doses of all types of diuretics. The elderly are especially prone to electrolyte disturbances, hypotension, and thromboembolic episodes when loop diuretics are used.

## TOXICITY

See Table 22–3 for diuretic toxicities.

## POTENTIAL DRUG/FOOD INTERACTIONS

Carbonic anhydrase inhibitors may interact with amphetamines, anticholinergics, methenamine, or quinidine. Loop diuretics may interact with amphotericin B, other nephrotoxic agents, anticoagulants, thrombolytic agents, other hypokalemia-producing agents, or lithium. Osmotic diuretics may interact with glycosides.

---

# ACETAZOLAMIDE SODIUM

*Trade Name:* Diamox
*Canadian Availability:* Diamox
*Pregnancy Risk:* Category C
*pH:* 9.2
*Storage/Stability:* Store below 40° C. May be stored for up to 1 week if refrigerated, after reconstituting with 5 mL of sterile water for injection.

#### ASSESSMENT: DRUG CHARACTERISTICS

#### ACTION

A carbonic anhydrase inhibitor diuretic that has antiglaucoma, anticonvulsant, and antiurolithic effects. Carbonic anhydrase inhibitors produce a systemic metabolic acidosis with resultant diuretic effects. As an anti-

▼

## TABLE 22–3
### Diuretic Toxicities

| Body System | Side/Toxic Effects | Physical Assessment Indicators | Laboratory Indicators | Nursing Interventions |
|---|---|---|---|---|
| Neurologic | Central nervous system effects | Headache, possible subarachnoid or epidural hemorrhage, depression, or drowsiness | N/A | Monitor LOC; report complaints of severe head pain or change in LOC promptly. |
| Cardiovascular | Hypovolemia | Orthostatic hypotension, chest pain, tachycardia, angina, peripheral edema | N/A | Measure and record vital signs, especially heart rate, rhythm, and blood pressure frequently; inspect intravenous site frequently; rotate sites frequently; auscultate lungs; encourage frequent position change, cough, and deep breathing. |
| | Thrombophlebitis | Redness, pain, heat at the injection site | | |
| Respiratory | | Pulmonary congestion, fever, chills | Leukocyte count $> 10{,}000/mm^3$ | |
| Renal | Electrolyte imbalance | Hyponatremia | Serum sodium $< 135$ mEq/L | Increase sodium, potassium, or chloride intake where possible. |
| | | Hypokalemia | Potassium $< 3.5$ mEq/L | |
| | | Hypochloremia | Chloride $< 100$ mEq/L | |
| | Acid-base imbalance | Alkalosis | $HCO_3 > 24$ mEq/L | |
| | Intrarenal damage | Crystalluria, renal calculi, renal failure | BUN $> 50$ mg/dL | Measure and record intake, output, and daily weight. Report depressed function; provide fluids to assure adequate urine flow to prevent crystalluria. |
| Gastrointestinal | Gastrointestinal disturbance | Loss of appetite, a metallic taste in the mouth, dry mouth, thirst, stomach cramps, nausea, vomiting, diarrhea | Serum potassium $< 3.5$ mEq/L | Observe client for vomiting or diarrhea; assess for complaints of nausea or stomach cramps; report promptly; provide comfort measures such as mouth care. |
| Sensory | Visual | Blurred vision | N/A | Provide for client safety. |
| Other | | Excessive fatigue<br>Premature ejaculation or difficulty keeping an erection | N/A | Assess male clients for possible concerns about changes in sexual performance. |

BUN = blood urea nitrogen, LOC = level of consciousness, N/A = not applicable.

glaucoma agent, reduces intraocular pressure by reducing production of aqueous humor by as much as 60%. The mechanism of action is not fully known. Anticonvulsant properties are not clearly understood but are believed to associated with retarded transmission of nerve impulses.

#### INDICATIONS

Used to treat glaucoma, congestive heart failure, and epilepsy. May also be used to treat elevated intracranial pressure, drug-induced edema, and drug overdose (aspirin and phenobarbital).

#### CAUTIONS

ADVERSE EFFECTS. Diarrhea, excessive fatigue, loss of appetite, metallic taste in the mouth, crystalluria, renal calculi, depression, drowsiness, fever, and bone marrow depression.

CONTRAINDICATIONS. Adrenal insufficiency, hyperchloremia, hypokalemia, respiratory acidosis, renal or hepatic dysfunction, renal calculi, or allergy to acetazolamide.

#### POTENTIAL DRUG/FOOD INTERACTIONS

May interact with amphetamines, anticholinergics, or quinidine to prolong the effects of those drugs. May inhibit the effectiveness of methenamine.

#### INTERVENTIONS: ADMINISTRATION

May be reconstituted (500 mg in 5 mL for a concentration of 100 mg/mL).

#### MODE/RATE OF ADMINISTRATION

May be given by IV push over 1–5 min (500 mg or less), by intermittent IV infusion over 4–8 h, or by continuous infusion. Filter may be used.

INTRAVENOUS USE (WITH NORMAL RENAL FUNCTION)

**Adults:** For antiglaucoma effect the usual dose is 500 mg. Dose may be repeated in 2–4 h. Client is usually switched to oral therapy.

For diuretic effect the usual dose is 5 mg/kg of body weight. Dose may be adjusted to maintain desired output.

For antiepilepsy effect the usual dose ranges from 8–30 mg/kg body weight over 24 hours in divided doses.

**Children:** For antiglaucoma effect the usual dosage is 5–10 mg/kg of body weight q6h.

For diuretic effect the usual dosage is 5 mg/kg of body weight q.d. for 1–2 d, followed by a drug-free day. Cycle may be repeated.

**Infants/Neonates:** Not commonly used.

**Geriatrics:** Elderly clients are more likely to have age-related decreases in renal function and are more sensitive to orthostatic hypotension. Lower doses may be required.

INTRATHECAL USE OR OTHER INFUSION ROUTES AS INDICATED. Not recommended.

#### POTENTIAL PROBLEMS IN ADMINISTRATION

Clients should maintain a high fluid intake to avoid renal complications such as calculi. Toxicity may occur with digitalis.

**INDEPENDENT NURSING ACTIONS**

Monitor vital signs, especially pulse and blood pressure. Monitor laboratory values for serum sodium, potassium, chlorides, and acid-base status. Evaluate client for complaints of blurred vision, chest pain, diarrhea, headache, anorexia, stomach cramps, or excessive fatigue.

**ADMINISTRATION IN ALTERNATE SETTINGS**

May be used for home administration or other clinical settings with careful monitoring.

**EVALUATION: OUTCOMES OF DRUG THERAPY**

**EXPECTED OUTCOMES**

PHYSICAL ASSESSMENT. Vital signs, especially pulse and blood pressure, remain within 15% of client's baseline. Client has no complaints of blurred vision, eye pain, diarrhea, headache, anorexia, stomach cramps, or excessive fatigue. Client does not show evidence of orthostatic hypotension.

LABORATORY. Serum sodium between 135 and 145 mEq/L. Serum potassium between 3.5 and 5 mEq/L. Serum chlorides between 100 and 106 mEq/L. Arterial pH between 7.35 and 7.5 BUN between 8 and 25 mg/dL or not more than 5 mg/dL above client's baseline.

**NEGATIVE OUTCOMES**

Vital signs, especially pulse and blood pressure, are more than 15% below client's baseline. Client complains of blurred vision, eye pain, diarrhea, headache, anorexia, stomach cramps, or excessive fatigue. Client shows evidence of orthostatic hypotension.

## BUMETANIDE

*Trade Name:* Bumex
*Canadian Availability:* Not specified.
*Pregnancy Risk:* Category C
*pH:* 7
*Storage/Stability:* Store below 40° C. Protect from freezing and from light. Diluted solutions should be used within 24 hours.

**ASSESSMENT: DRUG CHARACTERISTICS**

**ACTION**

A loop diuretic with antihypertensive and antihypercalcemic effects. Prevents the reabsorption of sodium and water in the ascending loop of Henle, thus increasing water loss. Antihypertensive effects can be attributed to the decrease in plasma and extracellular fluid volume.

**INDICATIONS**

Used to treat edema associated with congestive heart failure, acute pulmonary edema, liver and renal dysfunction, and hypertension.

▼

**CAUTIONS**

ADVERSE EFFECTS. Hyponatremia, hypokalemia, alkalosis, hypochloremia, orthostatic hypotension, premature ejaculation or difficulty keeping an erection, blurred vision, chest pain, diarrhea, headache, anorexia, stomach cramps, pruritus, thrombosis, or circulatory collapse.

CONTRAINDICATIONS. Anuria, renal dysfunction, or advanced cirrhosis.

**POTENTIAL DRUG/FOOD INTERACTIONS**

May interact with amphotericin B or other nephrotoxic agents to increase the risk of ototoxicity and nephrotoxicity. May increase blood glucose and precipitate diabetes mellitus. Anticoagulants or thrombolytic agents may be less effective if used with this agent. May produce severe hypokalemia if used with other hypokalemia-producing agents. May cause lithium toxicity if used with lithium. Incompatible with dobutamine.

**INTERVENTIONS: ADMINISTRATION**

May be diluted in 5% dextrose (D5W) or specified solution or given undiluted (0.25 mg/mL).

**MODE/RATE OF ADMINISTRATION**

Given by IV push over 1–2 min.

INTRAVENOUS USE (WITH NORMAL RENAL FUNCTION)

**Adults:** For diuresis the usual dose is 500 mcg (0.5 mg)–1 mg. Dose may be repeated q2–3h if needed. Maximum daily dose is 10 mg.

**Children:** Dose not established.

**Infants/Neonates:** Dose not established.

**Geriatrics:** Elderly clients are more likely to have age-related decreases in renal function and are more sensitive to orthostatic hypotension. Lower dose may be required.

INTRATHECAL USE OR OTHER INFUSION ROUTES AS INDICATED. Not recommended.

**POTENTIAL PROBLEMS IN ADMINISTRATION**

Clients should be sitting or in a recumbent position when bumetanide is given.

**INDEPENDENT NURSING ACTIONS**

Monitor vital signs, especially pulse and blood pressure. Monitor laboratory values for serum sodium, potassium, chlorides, and acid-base status. Evaluate client for complaints of burred vision, chest pain, diarrhea, headache, anorexia, stomach cramps, or premature ejaculation or difficulty keeping an erection. Weigh client daily; monitor intake and output.

**ADMINISTRATION IN ALTERNATE SETTINGS**

Not recommended for home administration or clinical settings other than short-term care.

**EVALUATION: OUTCOMES OF DRUG THERAPY**

**EXPECTED OUTCOMES**

PHYSICAL ASSESSMENT. Vital signs, especially pulse and blood pressure, remain within 15% of client's baseline. Client has no complaints of blurred vision, chest pain, diarrhea, headache, anorexia, stomach cramps, or premature ejaculation or difficulty keeping an erection. Client does not show evidence of othostatic hypotension. Client has increased urinary output and decreased fluid retention.

LABORATORY. Serum sodium between 135 and 145 mEq/L. Serum potassium between 3.5 and 5 mEq/L. Serum chlorides between 100 and 106 mEq/L. Arterial pH between 7.35 and 7.5 BUN between 8 and 25 mg/dL or not more than 5 mg/dL over client's baseline.

**NEGATIVE OUTCOMES**

Vital signs, especially pulse and blood presure, are more than 15% below client's baseline. Client complains of blurred vision, chest pain, diarrhea, headache, anorexia, stomach cramps, or premature ejaculation or difficulty keeping an erection. Client shows evidence of orthostatic hypotension.

## FUROSEMIDE

*Trade Name:* Lasix
*Canadian Availability:* Lasix
*Pregnancy Risk:* Category C
*pH:* 8.8–9.5
*Storage/Stability:* Store below 40° C. Protect from freezing and from light. Diluted solutions should be used within 24 hours. Do not use if yellow.

### ASSESSMENT: DRUG CHARACTERISTICS

**ACTION**

A loop diuretic with antihypertensive and antihypercalcemic effects. Prevents the reabsorption of sodium and water in the ascending loop of Henle, thus increasing water loss. Antihypertensive effects can be attributed to the decrease in plasma and extracellular fluid volume.

**INDICATIONS**

Used to treat edema associated with congestive heart failure, liver and renal dysfunction, and hypertension. May also be used as a diagnostic aid with renal disease. Used to treat hypercalcemia and nephrotic syndrome.

**CAUTIONS**

ADVERSE EFFECTS. Hyponatremia, hypokalemia, alkalosis, hypochloremia, orthostatic hypotension, blurred vision, diarrhea, headache, photosensitivity, anorexia, stomach cramps, confusion, leg cramps, tinnitus, hyperglycemia, and hyperuricemia.

CONTRAINDICATIONS. Anuria or renal dysfunction.

**POTENTIAL DRUG/FOOD INTERACTIONS**

May interact with amphotericin B or other nephrotoxic agents to increase the risk of ototoxicity and nephrotoxicity. Anticoagu-

▼

lants or thrombolytic agents may be less effective if used with this agent. May produce severe hypokalemia if used with other hypokalemia-producing agents. May cause lithium toxicity if used with lithium. Incompatible with corticosteroids, dobutamine, meperidine, tetracyclines, and any drug in the same syringe.

**INTERVENTIONS: ADMINISTRATION**

May be given undiluted or diluted in D5W or specified solution.

**MODE/RATE OF ADMINISTRATION**

May be given by IV push at a rate of 20 mg/min. May be given as a continuous infusion at a rate not to exceed 4 mg/min.

INTRAVENOUS USE (WITH NORMAL RENAL FUNCTION)

**Adults:** For diuresis the usual dose is 20–40 mg. Dose may be increased by 20 mg and given in 1–2 h if needed. Further doses may be increased by 20 mg until desired results are achieved. Maximum dose is 600 mg/ 24 h.

For antihypertensive effect the usual dose is 40–80 mg.

For hypertensive crisis with pulmonary edema the usual dose is 100–200 mg.

**Children 12 years:** Follow adult dosing schedule.

**Infants/Neonates:** For diuresis the usual initial dose is 1 mg/kg of body weight. The dose may be increased by 1 mg/kg of body weight and given in 2 h. Further doses may be increased by 1 mg/kg of body weight until desired results are achieved, not to exceed 5 mg/kg.

**Geriatrics:** Elderly clients are more likely to have age-related decreases in renal function and are more sensitive to orthostatic hypotension. Lower doses may be required.

INTRATHECAL USE OR OTHER INFUSION ROUTES AS INDICATED. Not recommended.

**POTENTIAL PROBLEMS IN ADMINISTRATION**

Clients should be sitting or in a recumbent position when furosemide is given.

**INDEPENDENT NURSING ACTIONS**

Monitor vital signs, especially pulse and blood pressure. Monitor laboratory values for serum sodium, potassium, chlorides, and acid-base status. Evaluate client for complaints of blurred vision, chest pain, diarrhea, headache, anorexia, stomach cramps, or premature ejaculation or difficulty keeping an erection. Monitor intake and output; weigh daily.

**ADMINISTRATION IN ALTERNATE SETTINGS**

Recommended for home administration or clinical settings other than short-term care if caregivers have been instructed in the proper monitoring of the client.

**EVALUATION: OUTCOMES OF DRUG THERAPY**

**EXPECTED OUTCOMES**

PHYSICAL ASSESSMENT. Client has increased urinary output and decreased fluid retention. Vital signs, especially pulse and blood pressure, remain within 15% of client's baseline. Client has no complaints of blurred vision, chest pain, diarrhea, headache, anorexia, stomach cramps, or premature ejaculation or difficulty keeping an erection. Client does not show evidence of orthostatic hypotension.

LABORATORY. Serum sodium between 135 and 145 mEq/L. Serum potassium between 3.5 and 5 mEq/L. Serum chloride between 100 and 106 mEq/L. Arterial pH between 7.35 and 7.5. BUN between 8 and 25 mg/dL or not more than 5 mg/dL over client's baseline.

**NEGATIVE OUTCOMES**

Vital signs, especially pulse and blood pressure, are more than 15% below client's baseline. Client complains of blurred vision, chest pain, diarrhea, headache, anorexia, stomach cramps, or premature ejaculation or difficulty keeping an erection. Client shows evidence of orthostatic hypotension.

## MANNITOL

*Trade Name:* Osmitrol
*Canadian Availability:* Osmitrol
*Pregnancy Risk:* Category C
*pH:* 4.5–7
*Storage/Stability:* Store below 40° C. Protect from freezing. Do not use if crystals are present and cannot be dissolved. Use immediately and discard unused portions.

### ASSESSMENT: DRUG CHARACTERISTICS

**ACTION**

An osmotic diuretic and anti-glaucoma agent that acts by increasing intravascular osmolality, thus drawing fluid into the vascular compartment. Is not reabsorbed by the kidney tubule. Increases the osmolality of the filtrate, thereby inhibiting the reabsorption of water plus sodium, chloride, and other electrolytes. Minimizes hemolysis when used as an irrigant during transurethral resections. May also be used as a diagnostic aid for renal disease.

**INDICATIONS**

Used to treat edema, especially cerebral edema. Also used to treat intraocular pressure from glaucoma and to prevent toxicity from overdoses of lithium, salicylates, or barbiturates. Used in the oliguric phase of acute renal failure.

**CAUTIONS**

ADVERSE EFFECTS. Electrolyte imbalances, tachycardia, angina, fever or chills, pulmonary congestion, renal failure, peripheral edema, thrombophlebitis at the injection site, dry mouth, headache, dizziness, convulsions, thirst, nausea, or vomiting.

▼

CONTRAINDICATIONS. Anuria, dehydration, intracranial bleeding, pulmonary edema, cardiac dysfunction, or significant renal dysfunction.

**POTENTIAL DRUG/FOOD INTERACTIONS**

May increase the risk of hypokalemia and subsequent toxicity if taken with digitalis glycosides.

**INTERVENTIONS: ADMINISTRATION**

Given undiluted.

**MODE/RATE OF ADMINISTRATION**

May be given by intermittent IV infusion or continuous infusion, using an infusion pump.

INTRAVENOUS USE (WITH NORMAL RENAL FUNCTION)

**Adults:** For diuresis the usual dose is 50–100 g of a 5%–25% solution given at a rate to maintain a urinary output of 30–50 mL/h. For intraocular pressure the usual dose is 0.25–2 g/kg of body weight of a 15%–25% solution over 30–60 min.

For toxicity the usual dose is 50–200 g as a 5%–25% solution given at a rate to maintain a urinary output of 100–500 mL/h.

Maximum daily dose should not exceed 6 g/kg of body weight.

**Children 12 years:** Follow adult dosing schedule.

**Infants/Neonates:** For diuresis the usual dose is 0.25–2 g/kg of body weight over 2–6 h.

For cerebral edema or intraocular pressure the usual dose is 1–2 g/kg of body weight of a 15% to 20% solution over 30–60 min.

For toxicity the usual dose is up to 2 g/kg of body weight of a 5%–10% solution.

**Geriatrics:** Elderly clients are more likely to have age-related decreases in renal function that may require lower doses.

INTRATHECAL USE OR OTHER INFUSION ROUTES AS INDICATED. Contraindicated.

**POTENTIAL PROBLEMS IN ADMINISTRATION**

Clients should be sitting or in a recumbent position when mannitol is given. Mannitol is very irritating. Extravasation should be avoided.

**INDEPENDENT NURSING ACTIONS**

Monitor vital signs, especially pulse and blood pressure. Monitor laboratory values for serum sodium, potassium, chlorides, and acid-base status. Evaluate client for complaints of blurred vision, eye pain, chest pain, diarrhea, headache, changes in neurologic status, anorexia, or stomach cramps. Weigh daily. Monitor intake and output.

**ADMINISTRATION IN ALTERNATE SETTINGS**

Not recommended for home administration or clinical settings other than short-term care.

**EVALUATION: OUTCOMES OF DRUG THERAPY**

**EXPECTED OUTCOMES**

PHYSICAL ASSESSMENT. Vital signs, especially pulse and

blood pressure, remain within 15% of client's baseline. Urinary output is equal to or more than 30 to 50 mL/h. Client has no complaints of blurred vision, eye pain, chest pain, diarrhea, headache, anorexia, or stomach cramps. Client does not show evidence of orthostatic hypotension. Client has increased urinary output, and there is improvement in neurologic symptoms.

LABORATORY. Serum sodium between 135 and 145 mEq/L. Serum potassium between 3.5 and 5 mEq/L. Serum chlorides between 100 and 106 mEq/L. Arterial pH between 7.35 and 7.5. BUN between 8 and 25 mg/dL or not more than 5 mg/dL over client's baseline.

**NEGATIVE OUTCOMES**

Vital signs, especially pulse and blood pressure, are more than 15% below client's baseline. Urinary output is less than 30 to 50 mL/h. Client complains of blurred vison, eye pain, chest pain, diarrhea, headache, anorexia, or stomach cramps. Client shows evidence of orthostatic hypotension or changes in level of consciousness, pupil changes, or deteriorating neurologic status.

## TORSEMIDE

*Trade Name:* Demadex
*Canadian Availability:* Not specified
*Pregnancy Risk:* Category C
*Storage/Stability:* Store below 40° C. Protect from freezing and from light. Diluted solutions should be used within 24 hours. Solution should be clear.

**ASSESSMENT: DRUG CHARACTERISTICS**

**ACTION**

A loop diuretic that prevents the reabsorption of sodium and water in the ascending loop of Henle. This causes an increase in water loss. The resulting decrease in plasma and extracellular fluid volume provides the antihypertensive effect.

**INDICATIONS**

Used to treat edema associated with congestive heart failure, renal disease, or hepatic disease. Used either alone or in combination with other drugs to treat hypertension.

**CAUTIONS**

ADVERSE EFFECTS. Headache, dizziness, nausea, vomiting, and hyperglycemia. These side effects are usually transient. Use cautiously with clients who have hepatic disease marked by cirrhosis and ascites, as sudden changes in fluid and electrolyte balance may cause hepatic coma. There is increased risk of hypokalemia and metabolic alkalosis. An ▼

aldosterone antagonist or another potassium-sparing diuretic should be given along with torsemide. Excessive diuresis may cause dehydration, hypovolemia, and possibly thrombosis and embolism, especially in elderly clients.

CONTRAINDICATIONS. Known hypersensitivity to torsemide or other sulfonylureas or anuria.

**POTENTIAL DRUG/FOOD INTERACTIONS**

Clients taking high doses of salicylates may experience salicylate toxicity if they also take torsemide. Probenecid decreases the diuretic effect of torsemide.

**INTERVENTIONS: ADMINISTRATION**

May be given undiluted.

**MODE/RATE OF ADMINISTRATION**

May be given by slow IV push over 2 min of a single dose, which should not exceed 200 mg.

INTRAVENOUS USE (WITH NORMAL RENAL AND HEPATIC FUNCTION)

**Adults:** For congestive heart failure the recommended initial dose is 10–20 mg q.d.

For chronic renal failure the recommended initial dose is 20 mg q.d.

For hepatic cirrhosis the recommended intial dose is 5–10 mg q.d.

If the diuretic response is inadequate, the dose should be titrated upward by approximately double until the desired result is achieved. Single doses should not exceed 200 mg for congestive heart failure or chronic renal failure or 40 mg for hepatic cirrhosis.

**Children 12 years:** Follow adult dosing schedule.

**Infants/Neonates:** Safety and effectiveness in infants and neonates has not been established.

**Geriatrics:** Elderly clients are more likely to have age-related decreases in renal function and are more sensitive to orthostatic hypotension, hypovolemia, and possibly thrombosis and embolism. Lower doses may be required.

INTRATHECAL USE OR OTHER INFUSION ROUTES AS INDICATED. Not recommended.

**POTENTIAL PROBLEMS IN ADMINISTRATION**

Clients should be sitting in a recumbent position during administration.

**INDEPENDENT NURSING ACTIONS**

Monitor vital signs, especially orthostatic pulse and blood pressure. Monitor laboratory values for serum sodium, potassium, chlorides, and acid-base status. Evaluate client for complaints of blurred vision and chest pain. Weigh client daily and monitor intake and output.

**ADMINISTRATION IN ALTERNATE SETTINGS**

Recommended for home administration or clinical settings other than short-term care if caregivers have been instructed in the proper monitoring of the client.

**EVALUATION: OUTCOMES OF DRUG THERAPY**

**EXPECTED OUTCOMES**

PHYSICAL ASSESSMENT. Client has increased urinary output and decreased fluid retention. Vital signs, especially pulse and blood pressure, remain within 15% of client's baseline. Client has no complaints of blurred vision or chest pain. Client does not experience orthostatic hypotension.

LABORATORY. Serum sodium between 135 and 145 mEq/L. Serum potassium between 3.5 and 5 mEq/L. Serum chloride between 100 and 106. Arterial pH between 7.35 and 7.5. BUN remains between 8 and 25 mg/dL or not more than 5 mg/dL over client's baseline.

**NEGATIVE OUTCOMES**

Vital signs, especially pulse and blood pressure, are more than 15% below client's baseline. Client complains of blurred vision and chest pain. Client complains of dizziness and light-headedness when changing from lying to sitting position.

---

# REPLACEMENT AGENTS

## THERAPEUTIC EFFECTS

Replacement agents are used to supplement or increase electrolytes or other substances required by the body to maintain homeostasis. Calcium is required for structural integrity and nervous system activity. Potassium is required for cellular membrane functioning; nerve activity in brain, heart, and skeletal muscle; renal function; and acid-base balance. Other agents such as hetastarch are used in emergencies as substitutes for missing substances such as albumin, which is required to provide colloidal oncotic pressure.

## PHARMACOKINETICS

**Distribution.** Calcium and potassium are widely and rapidly distributed throughout the plasma and body tissues when given intravenously. Hetastarch is distributed in plasma intravascularly.

**Excretion.** Calcium is excreted primarily in feces. Potassium is excreted primarily in the urine, with greater amounts (up to 40 and 50 mEq) being excreted by clients under stress. Hetastarch is excreted through the kidneys, with nearly 40% being excreted within 24 hours in clients with normal renal function.

## CAUTIONS

**Side/Adverse Effects.** Calcium may cause nausea, vomiting, flushing or sensation of warmth, sweating, paresthesias, drowsiness, headache, confusion, irritability, depression, or weakness. Potassium may cause symptoms of hyperkalemia.

Hetastarch may cause flulike symptoms or anaphylactoid reactions.

### Contraindications

***Pregnancy and Lactation.*** Calcium may be passed in breast milk but has not been documented to cause problems. Hetastarch should not be used in pregnant women unless the risk to the fetus is outweighed by benefits to the mother.

***Pediatrics.*** IV calcium may cause tissue necrosis and sloughing, and its use in children may be limited because of small veins. The effects of hetastarch on children has not been well studied.

***Geriatrics.*** The elderly are more likely to have hyperkalemia and clinical conditions such as stroke, congestive heart failure, or renal failure for which hetastarch is contraindicated.

## TOXICITY

See Table 22–4 for replacement agent toxicities.

## POTENTIAL DRUG/FOOD INTERACTIONS

Calcium may interact with calcium-containing medications to create hypercalcemia. If used with digitalis preparations, calcium may increase the risk of dysrhythmias. Calcium blocks the effectiveness of magnesium sulfate and gallium nitrate and decreases the effectiveness of cellulose sodium phosphate. Calcium prevents the absorption of etidronate. If used with angiotensin converting enzyme (ACE) inhibitors, nonsteroidal antiinflammatory drugs (NSAIDs), β-adrenergic blocking agents, old banked blood, or potassium-sparing diuretics, potassium may cause hyperkalemia. Potassium used with anticholinergics may cause intestinal lesions. Hetastarch has no reported interactions.

# CALCIUM CHLORIDE

*Trade Name:* None specified
*Canadian Availability:* Calciject
*Pregnancy Risk:* Category C
*pH:* 6–8.2
*Storage/Stability:* Store below 40° C. Protect from freezing.

## ASSESSMENT: DRUG CHARACTERISTICS

### ACTION

An antihypocalcemic agent that also has electrolyte replenishing, cardiotonic, antihyperkalemic, and antihypermagnesemic activity. Essential for structural integrity and nervous system activity. Replacement of a severely deficient supply of calcium is essential for life.

### INDICATIONS

Used to treat hypocalcemia and electrolyte imbalances and as an adjunct to treatment of cardiac arrest.

▼

**TABLE 22–4**
**Replacement Agent Toxicities**

| Body System | Side/Toxic Effects | Physical Assessment Indicators | Laboratory Indicators | Nursing Interventions |
|---|---|---|---|---|
| Neurologic | Central nervous system disturbance | Drowsiness, headache, confusion, irritability, depression, or weakness | Serum calcium $< 8.5$ mg/dL or $> 10.5$ mg/dL | Protect the client from injury; monitor and report changes in client's LOC; assist with ADLs as needed. |
| | Peripheral | Paresthesias | Serum potassium $< 3.5$ mEq/L or $> 5$ mEq/L | |
| Cardiovascular | Myocardial | Cardiac dysrhythmias, hypotension | Serum potassium $< 3.5$ mEq/L or $> 5$ mEq/L | Monitor vital signs, especially pulse and blood pressure; monitor laboratory values for potassium and calcium; report changes promptly. |
| Gastrointestinal | Gastrointestinal disturbance | Nausea, vomiting, diarrhea, abdominal cramps | Serum potassium $< 3.5$ mEq/L or $> 5$ mEq/L | Observe client for gastrointestinal disturbance; be prepared to give antiemetic or antidiarrheal agents. |
| Integumentary | | Flushing, sweating, sensation of warmth | Serum calcium $> 10.5$ mg/dL | |
| Other | | Weakness, fatigue | Serum potassium $< 3.5$ mEq/L | Observe client for evidence of reaction to agent; report promptly; be prepared to discontinue intravenous administration. |
| | Flulike symptoms* | Vomiting, mild temperature elevations, chills, itching, headache, muscle aches | | |
| | Anaphylactoid reaction* | Urticaria or wheezing | | |

*Hetastarch
ADL = activities of daily living, LOC = level of consciousness.

**CAUTIONS**

ADVERSE EFFECTS. In parenteral form, hypotension, cardiac dysrhythmias (bradycardia), nausea, vomiting, flushing or sensation of warmth, sweating, or paresthesias. Symptoms of hypercalcemia such as drowsiness, headache, confusion, irritability, depression, or weakness.

CONTRAINDICATIONS. Hypercalcemia, renal calculi, sarcoidosis, hypoparathyroidism, renal insufficiency, cardiac dysfunction, ventricular fibrillation during cardiac arrest, or digitalis toxicity.

**POTENTIAL DRUG/FOOD INTERACTIONS**

May interact with calcium-containing medications to create hypercalcemia. Use with digitalis preparations increases the risk of dysrhythmias. Blocks the effectiveness of magnesium sulfate and gallium nitrate. Decreases the effectiveness of cellulose sodium phosphate. Prevents the absorption of etidronate. Incompatible with amphotericin B, sodium bicarbonate, tetracyclines, phosphates, and sulfates.

**INTERVENTIONS: ADMINISTRATION**

May be given undiluted as a 10% solution. Vials of 100 mg/mL may be mixed with an equal amount of 0.9% normal saline solution (NSS) for a 5% solution.

**MODE/RATE OF ADMINISTRATION**

Given by IV push at a rate of 0.5–1 mL of 100-mg/mL solution per minute. For nutritional support may be given as a continuous IV infusion, using an infusion pump.

INTRAVENOUS USE (WITH NORMAL RENAL FUNCTION)

**Adults:** For antihypocalcemic effect the usual dosage is 500 mg–1 g (5–10 mL) q1–3d.

For antihyperkalemic and antihypermagnesemic effect the usual dose is titrated according to laboratory values. Initially, a dose of 500 mg (5 mL) is given, and further doses depend on client response.

For cardiotonic effect the usual dosage is 500 mg–1 gram q1–3d. An intraventricular dose of 200–800 mg may be given as a single dose.

**Children 12 years:** Follow adult dosing schedule.

**Infants/Neonates:** For antihypocalcemic effect the usual dose is 20–25 mg/kg of body weight.

**Geriatrics:** Elderly clients may have greater deficiency and may need higher doses.

INTRATHECAL USE OR OTHER INFUSION ROUTES AS INDICATED. Contraindicated.

**POTENTIAL PROBLEMS IN ADMINISTRATION**

Calcium is very irritating and may cause necrosis, tissue sloughing, or abscess formation if it extravasates.

**INDEPENDENT NURSING ACTIONS**

Monitor vital signs, especially pulse and blood pressure. Observe for flushing, drowsiness, confusion, irritability, depression, weakness, or sweating. Monitor client complaints of headache, nausea, vomiting, sensation of warmth, or paresthesias. Monitor for tetany.

**ADMINISTRATION IN ALTERNATE SETTINGS**

Except as a nutritional supplement, parenteral forms not recommended for settings other than short-term care.

**EVALUATION: OUTCOMES OF DRUG THERAPY**

**EXPECTED OUTCOMES**

PHYSICAL ASSESSMENT. Vital signs, especially pulse and blood pressure, remain within 15% of client's baseline. Client does not demonstrate flushing, drowsiness, confusion, irritability, depression, weakness, or sweating. Client does not complain of headache, nausea, vomiting, sensation of warmth, or paresthesias.

LABORATORY. Serum calcium between 8.5 and 10.5 mg/dL. Serum potassium between 3.5 and 5 mEq/L. Serum magnesium between 1.5 and 2 mEq/L.

**NEGATIVE OUTCOMES**

Vital signs more than 15% higher or lower than client's baseline. Pulse irregular. Blood pressure more than 15% less than client's baseline. Client demonstrates flushing, drowsiness, confusion, irritability, depression, weakness, or sweating. Client complains of headache, nausea, vomiting, sensation of warmth, or paresthesias.

## CALCIUM GLUCONATE

*Trade Name:* Kalcinate
*Canadian Availability:* Not specified
*Pregnancy Risk:* Category C
*pH:* 6–8.2
*Storage/Stability:* Store below 40° C. Protect from freezing. Precipitates may be dissolved by warming. Do not use if warming does not eliminate precipitates or if solution is discolored.

**ASSESSMENT: DRUG CHARACTERISTICS**

**ACTION**

An antihypocalcemic agent that also has electrolyte-replenishing, cardiotonic, antihyperkalemic, and antihypermagnesemic activity. Essential for structural integrity and nervous system activity. Replacement of a severely deficient supply of calcium is essential for life.

**INDICATIONS**

Used to treat hypocalcemia and electrolyte imbalances.

**CAUTIONS**

ADVERSE EFFECTS. In parenteral form, hypotension, cardiac dysrhythmias (bradycardia), nausea, vomiting, flushing or sensation of warmth, sweating, or paresthesias. Symptoms of hypercalcemia such

▼

as drowsiness, headache, confusion, irritability, depression, or weakness.

CONTRAINDICATIONS. Hypercalcemia, renal calculi, sarcoidosis, hypoparathyroidism, renal insufficiency, cardiac dysfunction, ventricular fibrillation during cardiac arrest, or digitalis toxicity.

**POTENTIAL DRUG/FOOD INTERACTIONS**

May interact with calcium-containing medications to create hypercalcemia. Use with digitalis preparations increases the risk of dysrhythmias. Blocks the effectiveness of magnesium sulfate and gallium nitrate. Decreases the effectiveness of cellulose sodium phosphate. Prevents the absorption of etidronate. Incompatible with amphotericin B, promethazine, cephalosporins, phosphates, sulfates, and carbonates.

**INTERVENTIONS: ADMINISTRATION**

May be given undiluted as a 10% solution. Vials of 97 mg/mL solution may be mixed with an equal amount of 0.9% NSS for a 5% solution.

**MODE/RATE OF ADMINISTRATION**

Given by IV push at a rate of 0.5 mL of 97 mg/mL solution per minute. For nutritional support may be given as a continuous IV infusion, using an infusion pump.

INTRAVENOUS USE (WITH NORMAL RENAL FUNCTION)

**Adults:** For antihypocalcemic or electrolyte replenishing effect the usual dose is 970 mg. Dose may be repeated if necessary for tetany.

For antihyperkalemic or antihypermagnesemic effect the usual dose is 1–2 g. Maximum daily dose should not exceed 15 g.

**Children 12 years:** Follow adult dosing schedule.

**Infants/Neonates:** For antihypocalcemic effect the usual dose is 200–500 mg.

For exchange transfusions, 97 mg is given after each 100 mL of citrated blood has been exchanged.

**Geriatrics:** Elderly clients may have greater deficiency and may need higher doses.

INTRATHECAL USE OR OTHER INFUSION ROUTES AS INDICATED. Contraindicated.

**POTENTIAL PROBLEMS IN ADMINISTRATION**

Calcium is very irritating and may cause necrosis, tissue sloughing, or abscess formation if it extravasates.

**INDEPENDENT NURSING ACTIONS**

Monitor vital signs, especially pulse and blood pressure. Observe for flushing, drowsiness, confusion, irritability, depression, weakness, or sweating. Monitor client complaints of headache, nausea, vomiting, sensation of warmth, or paresthesias. Monitor for tetany.

**ADMINISTRATION IN ALTERNATE SETTINGS**

Except as a nutritional supplement, parenteral forms not recommended for settings other than short-term care.

#### EVALUATION: OUTCOMES OF DRUG THERAPY

##### EXPECTED OUTCOMES

PHYSICAL ASSESSMENT. Vital signs, especially pulse and blood pressure, remain within 15% of client's baseline. Client does not demonstrate flushing, drowsiness, confusion, irritability, depression, weakness, or sweating. Client does not complain of headache, nausea, vomiting, sensation of warmth, or paresthesias.

LABORATORY. Serum calcium between 8.5 and 10.5 mg/dL. Serum potassium between 3.5 and 5.0 mEq/L. Serum magnesium between 1.5 and 2.0 mEq/L.

##### NEGATIVE OUTCOMES

Vital signs are more than 15% higher or lower than client's baseline. Pulse irregular. Blood pressure more than 15% less than client's baseline. Client demonstrates flushing, drowsiness, confusion, irritability, depression, weakness, or sweating. Client complains of headache, nausea, vomiting, sensation of warmth, or paresthesias.

---

## DEXTRAN 40

*Trade Names:* Gentran 40, Rheomacrodex
*Canadian Availability:* Hyskon, Macrodex, Rheomacrodex
*Pregnancy Risk:* Category C
*pH:* 3–7
*Storage/Stability:* Store below 25° C. Solution should not be used if not clear. Flakes may develop if refrigeration is uneven. Flakes may be dissolved by heating solution in a water bath at 100° C until clear.

#### ASSESSMENT: DRUG CHARACTERISTICS

##### ACTION

A plasma volume expander and low molecular weight polymer of glucose. Increases plasma colloidal osmotic pressure and acts by drawing fluid into the vascular space. Increases the plasma volume by once or twice its own volume.

##### INDICATIONS

Used for early fluid replacement and treatment of certain types of shock when blood or blood products are not available or when the urgency of the situation makes blood typing and crossmatching procedures too time consuming. May be used to treat shock from burns, surgery, hemorrhage, or trauma that causes hypovolemia. Does not replace other treatments for hypovolemia; it is supplemental. May also be used prophylactically for clients predisposed to thromboembolic complications.

▼

**CAUTIONS**

ADVERSE EFFECTS. Mild to severe allergic reactions, including anaphylactic shock; marked increases in viscosity and specific gravity of urine; renal tubular stasis or necrosis; impact on hepatic function, including elevating serum aspartate aminotransferase (AST) and alanine aminotransferase (ALT).

CONTRAINDICATIONS. Known hypersensitivity to dextran. Should be given with caution to clients with clinical dehydration, head trauma, congestive heart failure, pulmonary edema, renal failure, prolonged or known clotting disorders.

**POTENTIAL DRUG/FOOD INTERACTIONS**

No recorded interactions.

**INTERVENTIONS: ADMINISTRATION**

Solution is available in containers with D5W or D10W injection. Since solution has no preservatives, discard open but unused solution promptly. A 1.2-$\mu$m filter may be used.

**MODE/RATE OF ADMINISTRATION**

Given by IV infusion, using an infusion pump.

INTRAVENOUS USE (WITH NORMAL RENAL FUNCTION)

**Adults:** For treatment of shock the usual dose is calibrated on fluid loss and hemoconcentration. After a period of slow administration and careful observation to detect any hypersensitivity, clients may receive 1 g/kg of body weight (10 mL/kg) as rapidly as the solution can be administered. Clients should not receive more than 2 g/kg of body weight (20 mL/kg) of 10% solution in 24 h.

For priming fluid in extracorporeal pumps the usual dose is 2 g/kg of body weight (20 mL/kg).

For prophylactic treatment of thrombophlebitis after surgery the usual dose is 1 g/kg of body weight (10 mL/kg) the first day. Succeeding days may halve that amount.

**Children:** For treatment of shock, follow adult guidelines after adjusting dose to body weight. Children should not receive more than 2 g/kg of body weight (20 mL/kg) in 24 h.

For priming fluid in extracorporeal pumps the usual dose is adjusted to body weight. Children should not receive more than 2 g/kg of body weight (20 mL/kg).

**Infants/Neonates:** Follow dosing schedule for children.

**Geriatrics:** Follow adult dosing schedule.

INTRATHECAL USE OR OTHER INFUSION ROUTES AS INDICATED. Not recommended.

**POTENTIAL PROBLEMS IN ADMINISTRATION**

Clients should receive adequate hydration while they receive dextran.

**INDEPENDENT NURSING ACTIONS**

Monitor all vital signs carefully. Measure and

record intake and output frequently. If available, monitor central venous pressure. Observe for any allergic reactions or thrombophlebitis.

**ADMINISTRATION IN ALTERNATE SETTINGS**

Should be administered in clinical settings where emergency equipment is immediately available.

**EVALUATION: OUTCOMES OF DRUG THERAPY**

**EXPECTED OUTCOMES**

PHYSICAL ASSESSMENT. Heart rate, rhythm, and blood pressure remain within 15% of client's baseline. Breath sounds clear. Skin color pink. Urine output equal to or greater than 50 mL/h. Central venous pressure between 5 and 10 cm $H_2O$. Client does not have any wheezing, urticaria, nausea, or vomiting. Client does not complain of calf pain or have reddened tender areas in the calves.

LABORATORY. Hematocrit (Hct) between 37 and 54 mL/dL. AST between 10 and 30 Ux/L. ALT between 5 and 30 U/L. Urine specific gravity less than 1.035.

**NEGATIVE OUTCOMES**

Heart rate, rhythm, and blood pressure more than 15% below client's baseline. Breath sounds include crackles or wheezes. Skin color pale and skin cold and clammy. Urine output less than 50 mL/h. Central venous pressure less than 5 or greater than 12. Client has wheezing, urticaria, nausea, or vomiting. Client complains of calf pain or has reddened tender areas in the calves.

## HETASTARCH

*Trade Names:* HES, Hespan
*Canadian Availability:* Not specified
*Pregnancy Risk:* Category C
*pH:* 5.5
*Storage/Stability:* Store below 40° C. Protect from freezing. Do not use if discolored or if a precipitate is present.

**ASSESSMENT: DRUG CHARACTERISTICS**

**ACTION**

A plasma volume expander that acts by providing an osmotic effect similar to plasma albumin. Osmolality is 310 mOsm/L.

**INDICATIONS**

Used to treat early shock resulting from fluid volume deficit when blood or suitable blood products are not available or when time for typing and crossmatching is not available. Should not be used for non–volume deficit shock. Also used in leukapheresis to improve granulocyte harvesting.

**CAUTIONS**

ADVERSE EFFECTS. Flulike symptoms, vomiting, mild temperature elevations, chills, itching, headache, muscle aches, or anaphylactoid reactions such as urticaria or wheezing.

CONTRAINDICATIONS. Thrombocytopenia, severe bleeding disorders, congestive heart failure, closed head trauma, impaired renal or hepatic function, or history of allergy to hetastarch.

**POTENTIAL DRUG/FOOD INTERACTIONS**

No reported interactions.

**INTERVENTIONS: ADMINISTRATION**

Given undiluted as a 6% solution in 500 mL from manufacturer.

**MODE/RATE OF ADMINISTRATION**

Given as a continuous infusion using an infusion pump at a rate that should not exceed 1.2 g (20 mL)/kg/h.

INTRAVENOUS USE (WITH NORMAL RENAL FUNCTION)

**Adults:** For serum protein replacement as a shock therapy adjunct the usual dose is 30–60 g (500–1000 mL).

Maximum daily dose should not exceed 90 g (1500 mL). For leukapheresis 250–700 mL in continuous centrifuge procedures.

**Children 12 years:** Follow adult dosing schedule.

**Infants/Neonates:** Dose not established.

**Geriatrics:** Follow adult dosing schedule.

INTRATHECAL USE OR OTHER INFUSION ROUTES AS INDICATED. Not recommended.

**POTENTIAL PROBLEMS IN ADMINISTRATION**

Unknown.

**INDEPENDENT NURSING ACTIONS**

Monitor vital signs, intake and output, and bowel sounds. Observe for changes in level of consciousness, skin changes such as pallor, temperature, diaphoresis.

**ADMINISTRATION IN ALTERNATE SETTINGS**

Should be given in short-term care settings where the client can be closely monitored.

**EVALUATION: OUTCOMES OF DRUG THERAPY**

**EXPECTED OUTCOMES**

PHYSICAL ASSESSMENT. Vital signs remain within 15% of client's baseline. Urinary output more than 45 mL/h. Intake 1800 to 2200 mL/d. Bowel sounds present. Client alert, calm, and able to interact appropriately. Skin warm, pink, and dry.

LABORATORY. Complete blood count and serum electrolytes within client's baseline. Indirect bilirubin, hemoglobin, and erythrocyte sedimentation rate may be increased. Platelet count may be decreased.

**NEGATIVE OUTCOMES**

Vital signs more than 15% below client's baseline. Urinary output less than 45 mL/h. Intake is less than 1800 mL/d. Bowel sounds absent. Client somnolent or lethargic, restless, and unable to interact appropriately. Skin cool, pale, and clammy.

## Potassium Chloride

*Trade Name:* None specified
*Canadian Availability:* Potassium chloride
*Pregnancy Risk:* Category C
*pH:* 4–8
*Storage/Stability:* Store below 40° C. Protect from freezing.

### ASSESSMENT: DRUG CHARACTERISTICS

#### ACTION

An antihypokalemic agent that also has electrolyte-replenishing activity. Essential for cellular membrane functioning; nerve activity in brain, heart, and skeletal muscle; renal function; and acid-base balance. Replacement of a severely deficient supply of potassium is essential for life.

#### INDICATIONS

Used to treat hypokalemia and electrolyte imbalances.

#### CAUTIONS

ADVERSE EFFECTS. Symptoms of hyperkalemia (confusion, bradycardia, dysrhythmias, numbness and tingling around the lips or hands or feet, weakness, fatigue, abdominal cramps, diarrhea, or vomiting) may result from improper replacement.

CONTRAINDICATIONS. Diarrhea, gastric or intestinal obstruction, peptic ulcers, heart block, hyperkalemia, or conditions known to cause hyperkalemia such as renal failure or metabolic acidosis.

#### POTENTIAL DRUG/FOOD INTERACTIONS

Use of ACE inhibitors, NSAIDs, β-adrenergic blocking agents, old banked blood, or potassium-sparing diuretics with potassium may lead to hyperkalemia. Anticholinergics used with potassium may cause intestinal lesions. Thiazide diuretics may increase the risk of hypokalemia if unsupplemented with potassium. Incompatible with amikacin, amphotericin B, dobutamine, IV fat emulsion, mannitol, and penicillin G potassium.

### INTERVENTIONS: ADMINISTRATION

Vials of 1.5-to-2 mEq/mL solution **MUST** be diluted in 500–1000 mL of 0.9% NSS, D5W, combinations of dextrose and sodium chloride, or Ringer's lactate solution. Concentration should not exceed 80 mEq/L for peripheral infusions or 240 mEq in 250 mL for central infusion. **ONLY** vials of 0.1–0.4 mEq/mL may be given undiluted, using a calibrated infusion device.

#### MODE/RATE OF ADMINISTRATION

Given by continuous infusion at a rate not to exceed 10 mEq/h. Should **NEVER** be given IV push without dilution.

INTRAVENOUS USE (WITH NORMAL RENAL FUNCTION)

**Adults:** For antihypokalemic or electrolyte-replenishing effect the usual dosage is up to 400 mEq/d.

**Children 12 years:** Follow adult dosing schedule.

**Infants/Neonates:** For antihypokalemic effect the usual dosage is up to 3 mEq/kg/d.

**Geriatrics:** Elderly clients may have age-related renal changes that put them more at risk for hyperkalemia.

INTRATHECAL USE OR OTHER INFUSION ROUTES AS INDICATED. Contraindicated.

#### POTENTIAL PROBLEMS IN ADMINISTRATION

Potassium is highly irritating. Avoid extravasation. May require frequent IV site changes.

#### INDEPENDENT NURSING ACTIONS

Monitor vital signs, especially pulse and blood pressure. Observe for confusion, irritability, weakness, diarrhea, or vomiting. Monitor client complaints of nausea, fatigue, abdominal cramps, sensation of warmth, or numbness and tingling around the lips or hands or feet.

#### ADMINISTRATION IN ALTERNATE SETTINGS

Except for hydration, parenteral forms not recommended for settings other than short-term care. Dose should not exceed 20–40 mEq/L.

#### EVALUATION: OUTCOMES OF DRUG THERAPY

#### EXPECTED OUTCOMES

PHYSICAL ASSESSMENT. Vital signs, especially pulse and blood pressure, within 15% of client's baseline. Client alert and calm. Client does not complain of weakness, nausea, abdominal cramps, fatigue, or numbness and tingling around the lips or hands or feet. Client does not demonstrate diarrhea or vomiting.

LABORATORY. Serum potassium between 3.5 and 5.0 mEq/L. Serum sodium between 135 and 145 mEq/L. Serum chloride between 100 and 106 mEq/L.

#### NEGATIVE OUTCOMES

Pulse less than 60 beats per minute (bpm) or irregular. Client demonstrates confusion, diarrhea, or vomiting. Client complains of weakness, fatigue, abdominal cramps, or numbness and tingling around the lips or hands or feet.

## SODIUM BICARBONATE INJECTION

*Trade Name:* None specified
*Canadian Availability:* Sodium bicarbonate injection
*Pregnancy Risk:* Category C
*pH:* 7–8
*Storage/Stability:* Store below 40° C. Protect from freezing. May be stored up to 45 days at room temperature in a 7.5% solution. Do not use if there is a precipitate.

#### ASSESSMENT: DRUG CHARACTERISTICS

#### ACTION

An alkalizing agent with antacid action. Increases the

bicarbonate concentration in plasma and raises serum pH, reversing acidosis. Increases the free bicarbonate ion concentration in excreted urine, thereby raising urine pH. Reacts directly with hydrochloric acid to neutralize stomach pH.

**INDICATIONS**

Used to treat metabolic acidosis in renal disease or cardiac arrest, prevent renal calculi, treat gastric hyperacidity, replace bicarbonate loss from severe diarrhea, neutralize certain toxic substances such as barbiturates or salicylates, and keep urine alkaline to prevent crystalluria when clients are also taking sulfonamides. May be used to treat hyponatremia and diabetic ketoacidosis.

**CAUTIONS**

ADVERSE EFFECTS. Hypokalemia, metabolic alkalosis, peripheral edema, hypercalcemia, thirst, respiratory depression, headaches, hyperexcitability, or abdominal cramps.

CONTRAINDICATIONS. Metabolic or respiratory alkalosis, anuria or oliguria, hypochloremia from gastric suctioning or vomiting, hypocalcemia, hypertension, or sodium-retention states such as congestive heart failure.

**POTENTIAL DRUG/FOOD INTERACTIONS**

May interfere with the absorption of ketoconazole and tetracycline if given within 2 hours. Prolongs the effect of mecamylamine. Potentiates the action of amphetamines, ephedrine, and quinidine.

**INTERVENTIONS: ADMINISTRATION**

May be given diluted to a 1.5% (isotonic) solution up to a 8.5% (hypertonic) solution, depending on client condition and circumstances.

**MODE/RATE OF ADMINISTRATION**

May be given IV push at a rate of 1 mEq/kg of body weight over 1–3 min (in a cardiac arrest). May be given by continuous infusion.

INTRAVENOUS USE (WITH NORMAL RENAL FUNCTION)

**Adults:** As an alkalizing agent during cardiac arrest the usual adult dose is 1 mEq/kg of body weight. Additional dosages of 0.5 mEq/kg of body weight may be given q10min if needed during an arrest.

For metabolic acidosis the usual dose is 2–5 mEq/kg of body weight over 4–8 h, not to exceed 50 mEq/h.

As an antacid the usual dose is 2–5 mEq/kg of body weight over 4–8 h.

**Children:** As an alkalizing agent during cardiac arrest the usual dose is 1 mEq/kg of body weight. Additional dosages of 0.5 mEq/kg of body weight may be given q10min if needed during an arrest.

For metabolic acidosis, follow the adult dosing schedule.

As an antacid, follow the adult dosing schedule.

▼

**Infants/Neonates:** Rapid injection of 10 mL of hypertonic sodium bicarbonate may cause intracranial hemorrhage in neonates and infants younger than 2 years. Maximum dose is 8 mL of not more than 4.2% solution of sodium bicarbonate.

**Geriatrics:** Elderly clients are more likely to have age-related decreases in renal function that require lower doses.

INTRATHECAL USE OR OTHER INFUSION ROUTES AS INDICATED. Not recommended.

#### POTENTIAL PROBLEMS IN ADMINISTRATION

May cause hypokalemia and cardiac dysrhythmias if over administered. May cause severe alkalosis, hyperirritability, and tetany if given too rapidly.

#### INDEPENDENT NURSING ACTIONS

Monitor vital signs, especially heart rate, rhythm, and respiratory rate. Monitor laboratory values for potassium, chlorides, and calcium. Provide for adequate ventilation to assist in maintaining arterial pH.

#### ADMINISTRATION IN ALTERNATE SETTINGS

IV sodium bicarbonate should be given in short-term care settings and is not recommended for the home setting.

### EVALUATION: OUTCOMES OF DRUG THERAPY

#### EXPECTED OUTCOMES

PHYSICAL ASSESSMENT. Vital signs within 15% of client's baseline. Heart rate regular. Client does not complain of burning pain in esophagus or abdomen.

LABORATORY. Serum calcium between 8.5 and 10.5 mg/dL. Serum chlorides between 100 and 106 mEq/L. Arterial pH between 7.35 and 7.45. Bicarbonate between 22 and 24 mEq/L. Serum potassium between 3.5 and 5 mEq/L.

#### NEGATIVE OUTCOMES

Vital signs more than 15% above client's baseline. Heart rate rapid and irregular. Client complains of burning pain in esophagus or abdomen.

# CHAPTER 23

# Gastrointestinal Agents

*Elaine Kennedy*

**Antiemetic Drugs**
- Dimenhydrinate
- Ondansetron Hydrochloride

**Antiulcer/Antigastric Stasis Drugs**
- Cimetidine
- Famotidine
- Metoclopramide Hydrochloride
- Ranitidine

Gastrointestinal (GI) infusion agents are administered primarily to relieve nausea and vomiting. Some drugs are used to treat ulcers or problems associated with gastric stasis.

## CLASSIFICATION

GI infusion agents can be classified as antiemetic drugs and antiulcer or antigastric stasis drugs. The antiemetic drugs are given to control vomiting and to control the nausea that often precedes vomiting.

### ANTIEMETIC DRUGS

Antiemetic drugs control vomiting by controlling neural stimulation of the vomiting centers in the medulla. The neural stimulation can come from three different pathways. The first pathway is through higher central nervous system (CNS) functions and is triggered by events such as emotions, pain, or motion sickness. The second pathway involves the peripheral nervous system and is triggered by disease or injury to body tissue, especially in the GI tract. The third pathway is the chemoreceptor trigger zone (CTZ), also in the medullary center, which is sensitive to circulating toxins and drugs.

### ANTIULCER/ANTIGASTRIC STASIS DRUGS

The antiulcer drugs aid ulcer healing or prevent ulcer formation by blocking the action of histamine ($H_2$) on the $H_2$ receptors of parietal cells of the stomach, causing a decrease in gastric acid. Antigastric stasis drugs affect GI smooth muscle

**TABLE 23–1**
**Gastrointestinal Infusion Agents Grouped by Subclassifications**

| Antiemetic Agents | Antiulcer/Antigastric Stasis Agents |
|---|---|
| Benzquinamide* | Cimetidine |
| Diphenidol* | Famotidine |
| Dimenhydrinate | Metoclopramide hydrochloride |
| Ondansetron hydrochloride | Ranitidine |
| Prochlorperazine (see under Tranquilizers in Chapter 21) | |

*Not discussed in this chapter.

so that muscle tone is increased and gastric emptying time is decreased.

The infusion agents are grouped by subclassifications inTable 23–1.

## ANTIEMETIC AGENTS

### THERAPEUTIC EFFECTS

Antiemetic drugs are used to treat nausea and vomiting associated with anesthesia and surgery, antineoplastic drug therapy and radiation therapy, and vertigo associated with motion sickness and Meniere's disease.

### PHARMACOKINETICS

**Distribution**. Antiemetic drugs are widely distributed throughout the body and appear in high concentrations in the liver and kidneys. Onset of action is usually within 15 minutes after administration. Duration is 3 to 4 hours.

**Metabolism/Elimination**. Antiemetic drugs are metabolized by the liver and excreted in the urine in clients with normal kidney function.

### CAUTIONS

**Side/Adverse Effects**. The most common side effect is drowsiness. Clients may also have insomnia, headaches, excitement, dry mouth, blurred vision, flushing, dizziness, vertigo. Some drugs such as prochlorperazine may cause extrapyramidal effects, including dystonia, torticollis, (wryneck), oculogyric crisis, akathisia, (inability to sit still, restlessness), or gait disturbances.

**Contraindications**. Antiemetics should not be used to control nausea and vomiting if the source of the problem has not been fully determined. Antiemetics may mask the symptoms of toxic overdose or intestinal obstruction. Clients who must operate hazardous equipment should be cautioned not to use antiemetics.

***Pregnancy and Lactation.*** Antiemetics are probably teratogenic and may be passed in breast milk. Clients should be instructed in appropriate birth control measures. If the client is breast-feeding, antiemetic drugs should not be used.

***Pediatrics.*** In general antiemetics should not be used in children younger than 12 years. They should also not be used if Reye's syndrome is suspected. Antiemetic drugs may be hepatotoxic.

***Geriatrics.*** Elderly clients may be more prone to confusional episodes.

## TOXICITY

For antiemetic agent toxicities see Table 23–2.

## POTENTIAL DRUG/FOOD INTERACTIONS

Antiemetic drugs may potentiate the effects of other CNS depressants and anticholinergics. Antiemetics may mask symptoms of ototoxicity if given with ototoxic drugs.

**TABLE 23–2**
**Antiemetic Agent Toxicities**

| Body System | Side/ Toxic Effects | Physical Assessment Indicators | Laboratory Indicators | Nursing Interventions |
|---|---|---|---|---|
| Neurologic | CNS Depression | Restlessness, excitement, nervousness, euphoria, lethargy, seizures, hallucinations | N/A | Monitor LOC, institute safety precautions; keep environment quiet; be prepared to treat seizures with diazepam. |
| Gastrointestinal | | Dysphagia, anorexia, vomiting | N/A | Report continuing vomiting. |
| Cardiovascular | Blood pressure changes | Elevated blood pressure | N/A | Monitor blood pressure. |
| Genitourinary | Urinary retention | Palpable bladder, decreased urinary output | N/A | Monitor urinary output. |

*LOC = level of consciousness, N/A = not applicable.

## DIMENHYDRINATE

*Trade Names:* Dramamine, Dramanate, Dramocen
*Canadian Availability:* Gravol
*Pregnancy Risk:* Category B
*pH:* 6.4–7.2
*Storage/Stability:* Store below 40° C. Protect from freezing.

### ASSESSMENT: DRUG CHARACTERISTICS

#### ACTION

An antihistamine ($H_1$ receptor). Competes with histamine for receptor sites. Antagonizes the action of histamine rather than preventing its release. Seems to affect the CTZ and the labyrinthine functions to decrease sensitivity. Is also a CNS depressant.

#### INDICATIONS

Used to treat nausea and vomiting, motion sickness, and vertigo, especially associated with Meniere's disease.

#### CAUTIONS

ADVERSE EFFECTS. Blood dyscrasias, cardiac dysrhythmias, CNS depression (especially drowsiness), hypotension, cholinergic symptoms (flushed face and dry mouth), fever, CNS stimulation, or rarely blurred vision, confusion, difficulty with urination, or tachycardia.

CONTRAINDICATIONS. Impaired hepatic function, urinary tract obstruction, cardiac dysrhythmias, asthma, or glaucoma.

#### POTENTIAL DRUG/FOOD INTERACTIONS

May interact with alcohol, other CNS depressants such as phenothiazines, or monoamine oxidase (MAO) inhibitors to potentiate CNS depression. May interact with erythromycin or ketoconazole to increase the risk of cardiotoxicity. May mask the symptoms of ototoxicity if used with ototoxic drugs. Incompatible with corticosteroids, hydroxyzine, aminophylline, heparin, and phenytoin.

### INTERVENTIONS: ADMINISTRATION

Each 50 mg must be diluted in 10 mL of 0.9% normal saline solution (NSS) for injection.

#### MODE/RATE OF ADMINISTRATION

Given by rapid intravenous (IV) injection over at least 2 min.

INTRAVENOUS USE (WITH NORMAL RENAL AND HEPATIC FUNCTION)

**Adults:** Usual dose is 50–100 mg. May be repeated q4h if needed.

**Children:** Usual dose is 1.25 mg/kg of body weight. May be repeated q6h if needed. Maximum dosage should not exceed 300 mg/d.

**Infants/Neonates:** Dose not established.

**Geriatrics:** Elderly clients may be more sensitive to the effects of dimenhydrinate. Follow adult dosing schedule.

INTRATHECAL USE OR OTHER INFUSION ROUTES AS INDICATED. Not recommended.

#### POTENTIAL PROBLEMS IN ADMINISTRATION

May lower opioid requirement by as much as 50% if used preoperatively or post partum. May cause orthostatic hypotension and should be given with the client in a recumbent position.

#### INDEPENDENT NURSING ACTIONS

Monitor blood pressure and pulse. Instruct the client not to operate hazardous equipment if drowsy or experiencing visual changes.

#### ADMINISTRATION IN ALTERNATE SETTINGS

May be given in the home setting by a qualified infusion therapy nurse.

### EVALUATION: OUTCOMES OF DRUG THERAPY

#### EXPECTED OUTCOMES

PHYSICAL ASSESSMENT. Client states relief of nausea, vomiting, or vertigo. Client is alert. Blood pressure and pulse are within 15% of client's baseline.

LABORATORY. Complete blood count remains within baseline.

#### NEGATIVE OUTCOMES

Client experiences no relief of nausea, vomiting, or vertigo. Client is drowsy or restless and irritable. Blood pressure is more than 15% lower than client's baseline and pulse is greater than 100 beats per minute (bpm).

## ONDANSETRON HYDROCHLORIDE

*Trade Name:* Zofran
*Canadian Availability:* Not available
*Pregnancy Risk:* Category B
*pH:* 3.3–4
*Storage/Stability:* Store below 40° C. Protect from light. Diluted solutions may be stored for up to 48 hours.

### ASSESSMENT: DRUG CHARACTERISTICS

#### ACTION

A serotonin (5-$HT_3$) receptor antagonist. These receptors are located in the CTZ and on the vagus nerve of the peripheral nervous system.

#### INDICATIONS

Used to treat the nausea and vomiting associated with cancer chemotherapy or radiation therapy or surgery.

#### CAUTIONS

ADVERSE EFFECTS. Mild to moderate headache, transient diarrhea or constipation, fever, rash, blurred vision, or transient rises in liver enzymes (aspartate aminotransferase [AST] and alanine aminotransferase [ALT]).

CONTRAINDICATIONS. Pregnancy, breast-feeding, impaired hepatic function, or allergy to ondansetron.

▼

**POTENTIAL DRUG/FOOD INTERACTIONS**

May interact with corticosteroids to increase the antiemetic effects of ondansetron. Drugs that alter hepatic metabolism, such as phenobarbital or cimetidine, may affect the actions of ondansetron.

**INTERVENTIONS: ADMINISTRATION**

Should be diluted in at least 50 mL of solution. May use 5% dextrose in water (D5W), 0.9% NSS, or Ringer's lactate solution.

**MODE/RATE OF ADMINISTRATION**

Intermittent or continuous infusion. Intermittent infusion should take 15 min.

INTRAVENOUS USE (WITH NORMAL RENAL AND HEPATIC FUNCTION)

**Adults:** For high-risk emetogenic chemotherapy treatment the usual dose is 0.15 mg/kg of body weight given over 15 min at least 30 min before the beginning of chemotherapy. After chemotherapy, two more doses of 0.15 mg/kg of body weight should be given at 4 and 8 h. Oral therapy may then be ordered.

An alternative regimen is one 32-mg dose given over 15 min at least 30 min before the beginning of chemotherapy, with no doses given after chemotherapy.

For less emetogenic chemotherapy the usual dose is 0.15 mg/kg of body weight given over 15 min at least 30 minbefore beginning of chemotherapy.

**Children 4–18 years:** Follow adult dosing schedule.

**Children 1–4 years:** The usual dose is 3–5 mg/m$^2$ of body surface area (BSA) given over 15 min at least 30 min before the beginning of chemotherapy.

**Infants/Neonates:** Dose not established.

**Geriatrics:** Follow adult dosing schedule. Decreased drug clearance and prolonged half-life reported in clients over 75 years, but no safety risk.

INTRATHECAL USE OR OTHERINFUSION ROUTES AS INDICATED. Not recommended.

**POTENTIAL PROBLEMS IN ADMINISTRATION**

No specific problems identified.

**INDEPENDENT NURSING ACTIONS**

Obtain baseline liver function studies, including AST and ALT. Monitor for allergic response. Monitor client complaints of nausea, vomiting, or headache.

**ADMINISTRATION IN ALTERNATE SETTINGS**

May be given intravenously in outpatient settings by a qualified nurse.

**EVALUATION: OUTCOMES OF DRUG THERAPY**

**EXPECTED OUTCOMES**

PHYSICAL ASSESSMENT. Client does not experience nausea or vomiting. Client does not report headache.

LABORATORY. Hepatic function studies remain within client's baseline.

**NEGATIVE OUTCOMES**

Client experiences nausea or vomiting. Client reports headache or rash.

## ANTIULCER/ANTIGASTRIC STASIS AGENTS

### THERAPEUTIC EFFECTS

Antiulcer drugs are used to treat acute duodenal ulcers, gastric ulcers, gastroesophageal reflux disease (GERD), and pathologic hypersecretory conditions such as Zollinger-Ellison syndrome and to prevent stress-induced GI tract bleeding in critically ill clients (stress ulcers). Antigastric stasis drugs are used to treat gastric stasis and GERD and to prevent antineoplastic agent-induced emesis or postoperative nausea.

### PHARMACOKINETICS

**Distribution.** Antiulcer or antigastric stasis drugs are widely distributed throughout the body. Onset of action is about 1 hour after IV administration.

**Metabolism/Elimination.** Antiulcer or antigastric stasis drugs are metabolized by the liver and excreted through the urine. In clients with normal kidney function the plasma half-life averages between 2 and 4 hours.

### CAUTIONS

**Side/Adverse Effects.** Mild transient diarrhea, dizziness, rashes, urticaria, somnolence, headache, and restlessness are the most reported side effects.

**Contraindications.** Known hypersensitivity, renal impairment, mental depression especially suicidal tendencies, hepatic dysfunction, or required operation of hazardous equipment.

***Pregnancy and Lactation.*** Antiulcer or antigastric stasis drugs are passed through breast milk but are not known to be mutagenic or teratogenic. The agents should be used cautiously, if at all, with women who are breast-feeding.

***Pediatrics.*** Antiulcer or antigastric stasis drugs should not be given to children younger than 12 years.

***Infants/Neonates.*** Antiulcer or antigastric stasis drugs should not be given to children younger than 12 years.

***Geriatrics.*** Elderly clients may be more prone to psychotic disturbances.

### TOXICITY

For antiulcer or antigastric stasis agent toxicities see Table 23–3.

### POTENTIAL DRUG/FOOD INTERACTIONS

Antiulcer or antigastric stasis drugs may decrease hepatic activity and thus reduce absorption and metabolism of some drugs suchas aspirin, warfarin, phenytoin, propranolol, and some benzodiazepines. They may also potentiate CNS depressants or the myelosuppressive effects of alkylating agents. Some antacids may inhibit absorption of antiulcer or antigastric stasis drugs, thus delaying onset of action.

**TABLE 23–3**
**Antiulcer/Antigastric Stasis Drug Toxicities**

| Body System | Side/Toxic Effects | Physical Assessment Indicators | Laboratory Indicators | Nursing Interventions |
|---|---|---|---|---|
| Neurologic | CNS depression | Depression, headache, dizziness, fatigue, lethargy, seizures, hallucinations | N/A | Monitor LOC; institute safety precautions; keep environment quiet; discontinue medication. |
| Gastrointestinal | Peristaltic changes | Constipation, diarrhea, nausea, vomiting, flatulence, anorexia | N/A | Report continued vomiting, diarrhea, or constipation. |
| Cardiovascular | Changes in vital signs | Hypotension, dysrhythmias, sinus bradycardia | ECG changes | Monitor pulse and blood pressure. |
| Genitourinary | Nephrotoxicity | | Elevated BUN, serum creatinine | Monitor laboratory values; report elevations. |
| Hepatic | Hepatotoxicity | Jaundice | Elevated AST, ALT, total serum bilirubin | Monitor laboratory values; report elevations. |
| Hematopoietic | Leukocytosis, leukopenia, neutropenia, pancytopenia, eosinophilia, thrombocytopenia | Fever, chills | Elevated ESR, decreased WBC, platelets | Monitor temperature and laboratory values; report any decreases in WBC, platelets; institute bleeding precautions in the presence of thrombocytopenia. |
| Dermatologic | Skin lesions | Acne, pruritus, urticaria, dry skin, rash | N/A | Keep skin clean and dry; lubricate with mild emollients; keep fingernails short and smooth. |
| Other | Hypersensitivity, anaphylaxis, angioedema, bronchospasm | Facial edema, dyspnea, wheezing, swelling of extremities | N/A | Discontinue drug immediately; initiate emergency care for anaphylactic shock or severe respiratory distress. |

ALT = alanine aminotransferase, AST = aspartate aminotransferase, BUN = blood urea nitrogen, ECG = electrocardiogram, ESR = erythrocyte sedimentation rate, LOC = level of consciousness, N/A = not applicable, WBC = white blood cell count.

## CIMETIDINE

*Trade Name:* Tagamet
*Canadian Availability:* Tagamet
*Pregnancy Risk:* Category B
*pH:* 3.8–6
*Storage/Stability:* Store between 15° and 30° C. Protect from light and freezing. May be stored at room temperature for 48 hours. Cold temperatures may cause solution to look cloudy but do not affect cimetidine's action. Do not use if discolored or if there is a precipitate present.

### ASSESSMENT: DRUG CHARACTERISTICS

#### ACTION

An $H_2$-receptor antagonist that inhibits gastric acid secretion by competing with histamine for the $H_2$-receptor sites of the parietal cells. Inhibits stimulation of gastric acid secretion by food, caffeine, insulin, and vagal reflex. May also be used to treat urticaria because its action on the $H_2$-receptor sites blocks the inflammatory response of cutaneous blood vessels. May enhance healing of stress-induced gastric mucosa from acid ulceration by promoting the production of gastric mucus and the secretion of bicarbonate and stimulating gastric mucosal blood flow. Not used as commonly as newer $H_2$-receptor drugs, such as ranitidine.

#### INDICATIONS

Used to treat gastric and duodenal ulcers, gastric hypersecretory states, Zollinger-Ellison syndrome, multiple endocrine adenomas, gastroesophageal reflux, and upper gastrointestinal tract bleeding and to relieve GI distress from nonsteroidal antiinflammatory drugs (NSAIDs) used for arthritis therapy on a short-term basis. Also used to treat stress-induced GI tract bleeding.

#### CAUTIONS

ADVERSE EFFECTS. Allergic reaction, decreased libido, joint or muscle pain, or alopecia; cardiac dysrhythmias, hypotension, or death (rare) as IV push.

CONTRAINDICATIONS. Impaired renal or hepatic function or sensitivity to cimetidine.

#### POTENTIAL DRUG/FOOD INTERACTIONS

May reduce the absorption of ketoconazole. May interact with alcohol, tricyclic antidepressants, calcium channel blockers, metoprolol, phenytoin, propranolol, or xanthines to delay the elimination of these drugs and prolong their effects.

### INTERVENTIONS: ADMINISTRATION

May be reconstituted as 300 mg in 20 mL of NSS for IV push. Must be diluted in at least 50 mL of a compatible solution before giving as an intermittent infusion. May use D5W or D10W, NSS, combination of D5W and NSS, Ringer's lactate, or 5% sodium bicarbonate solutions.

**MODE/RATE OF ADMINISTRATION**

May be given by IV push over not less than 2 min (300 mg) or as an intermittent infusion of 300 mg in a 50- to 100-mL infusate over 15–20 min.

INTRAVENOUS USE (WITH NORMAL RENAL AND HEPATIC FUNCTION)

**Adults:** For acute ulcer states the usual dosage is 300 mg q6–8h by rapid IV or intermittent IV infusion. For continuous infusion the dosage is 37.5 mg/h to a maximum of 900 mg/d. For prevention of stress-related ulcers the usual dosage is 50 mg/h by continuous infusion for up to 7 d. If renal function is impaired, the dosage is reduced to 300 mg q12h. Maximum adult dose is 2.4 g/d.

**Children:** For acute ulcer states the usual dosage is 5–10 mg/kg q6–8h by rapid IV orintermittent IV infusion. Dose should be reduced if there is renal impairment.

**Infants/Neonates:** Dose not established.

**Geriatrics:** Follow adult dosing schedule. Elderly clients are more likely to have diminished renal function and may require a lower dose. Elderly clients are more at risk for confusion.

INTRATHECAL USE OR OTHER INFUSION ROUTES AS INDICATED. Not recommended.

**POTENTIAL PROBLEMS IN ADMINISTRATION**

Rapid bolus IV injection is not recommended because there is an increased risk of cardiac dysrhythmias and hypotension.

**INDEPENDENT NURSING ACTIONS**

Monitor client for nausea, vomiting, or complaints of abdominal pain. Monitor stool for character, amount, and color. Monitor vital signs, especially heart rate and blood pressure. Monitor laboratory values, especially for changes in hepatic function and elevations in serum creatinine. Monitor mental status, especially in the elderly.

**ADMINISTRATION IN ALTERNATE SETTINGS**

May be given in a wide variety of settings, including the home, by a qualified infusion therapy nurse.

**EVALUATION: OUTCOMES OF DRUG THERAPY**

**EXPECTED OUTCOMES**

PHYSICAL ASSESSMENT. Client has no complaints of nausea, vomiting, abdominal pain, GI tract bleeding, or diarrhea. Heart rate remains between 60 and 100 bpm and regular.

LABORATORY. Liver function studies and serum creatinine levels remain within client's baseline.

**NEGATIVE OUTCOMES**

Client continues to complain of nausea, vomiting, or abdominal pain. Client experiences GI tract bleeding, diarrhea, and confusion. Heart rate is irregular.

# FAMOTIDINE

*Trade Name:* Pepcid IV
*Canadian Availability:* Pepcid IV
*Pregnancy Risk:* Category B
*pH:* 5–5.6
*Storage/Stability:* Store between 15° and 30° C. Protect from light and freezing. May be stored at room temperature for 48 hours. Do not use if discolored or if there is a precipitate present.

## ASSESSMENT: DRUG CHARACTERISTICS

### ACTION

An $H_2$-receptor antagonist that inhibits gastric acid secretion by competing with histamine for the $H_2$-receptor sites of the parietal cells. Inhibits stimulation of gastric acid secretion by food, caffeine, insulin, and vagal reflex. May enhance healing of stress-induced acid ulceration by promoting the production of gastric mucus and the secretion of bicarbonate and by stimulating gastric mucosal blood flow.

### INDICATIONS

Used on a short-term basis to treat gastric and duodenal-ulcers, gastric hypersecretory states, Zollinger-Ellison syndrome, multiple endocrine adenomas, GERD, and upper GI tract bleeding and to relieve gastrointestinal distress from NSAIDs used for arthritis therapy. Also used to treat stress-induced GI tract bleeding.

### CAUTIONS

ADVERSE EFFECTS. Confusion, hallucinations, decreased libido, breast tenderness, drowsiness, dry mouth, joint or muscle pain, anorexia, alopecia, nausea or vomiting, tinnitus, skin rash, constipation or diarrhea, dizziness, fever, thrombocytopenia, or headache.

CONTRAINDICATIONS. Impaired renal or hepatic function or sensitivity to famotidine; not given to children.

### POTENTIAL DRUG/FOOD INTERACTIONS

May reduce the absorption of ketoconazole.

## INTERVENTIONS: ADMINISTRATION

Must be diluted before administration. For rapid injection famotidine 20 mg in 2 mL should be added to at least 10 mL of a compatible solution before administration. For intermittent infusion famotidine 20 mg in 2 mL should be added to at least 100 mL of a compatible solution. May use D5W or D10W, 0.9% NSS for injection, combinations of D5W and NSS, Ringer's lactate, or 5% sodium bicarbonate solutions.

### MODE/RATE OF ADMINISTRATION

May be given by IV push, 20 mg over not less than 2 min or by intermittent infusion over 15–30 min. Filter may be used.

INTRAVENOUS USE (WITH NORMAL RENAL AND HEPATIC FUNCTION)

**Adults:** For acute ulcer states the usual dosage is ▼

20 mg q12h by IV push or intermittent IV infusion.

**Children:** Dose not established.

**Infants/Neonates:** Dose not established.

**Geriatrics:** Follow adult dosing schedule. Clients are more likely to have diminished renal function and may require a lower dose. Drug half-life may be more than 20 h if creatinine clearance is less than 10 mL/min. Elderly clients are also more at risk for confusion.

INTRATHECAL USE OR OTHERINFUSION ROUTES AS INDICATED. Not recommended.

**POTENTIAL PROBLEMS IN ADMINISTRATION**

Rapid bolus IV injection is not recommended because there is an increased risk of cardiac arrhythmias and hypotension.

**INDEPENDENT NURSING ACTIONS**

Monitor client for nausea, vomiting, or complaints of abdominal pain. Monitor stool for character, amount, and color. Monitor vital signs, especially heart rate and regularity. Monitor laboratory values, especially for changes in hepatic function and elevations in serum creatinine. Monitor mental status, especially in the elderly.

**ADMINISTRATION IN ALTERNATE SETTINGS**

May be given in a wide variety of settings, including the home, by a qualified infusion therapy nurse.

**EVALUATION: OUTCOMES OF DRUG THERAPY**

**EXPECTED OUTCOMES**

PHYSICAL ASSESSMENT. Client has no complaints of nausea, vomiting, abdominal pain, GI tract bleeding, or diarrhea. Heart rate remains between 60 and 100 bpm and regular.

LABORATORY. Liver function studies and serum creatinine levels remain within client's baseline. Thrombocyte countremains within normal limits.

**NEGATIVE OUTCOMES**

Client continues to complain of nausea, vomiting, or abdominal pain. Client experiences GI tract bleeding, diarrhea, and confusion. Heart rate is irregular.

## METOCLOPRAMIDE HYDROCHLORIDE

*Trade Names:* Octamide, Reglan
*Canadian Availability:* Maxeran, Reglan
*Pregnancy Risk:* Category B
*pH:* 3–5
*Storage/Stability:* Store between 15° and 30° C. Protect from light. Diluted solutions may be stored up to 48 hours if protected from light. If diluted with 0.9% NSS, solutions may be stored frozen for up to 4 weeks.

**ASSESSMENT: DRUG CHARACTERISTICS**

**ACTION**

A dopaminergic blocking agent (antagonist) and antiemetic. Promotes gastric muscle contractions, relaxes lower esophageal and pyloric sphincters, and promotes gastric emptying into the duodenum. Increases duodenal and jejunal peristalsis to prevent paralytic ileus after surgery. Decreases chemoreceptor trigger zone (CTZ) response to afferent visceral nerves.

**INDICATIONS**

Used during GI tract (small bowel) intubation and for treatment of GERD and nausea and vomiting caused by diabetic gastroparesis, chemotherapy, or surgery.

**CAUTIONS**

ADVERSE EFFECTS. Agranulocytosis; hypotension or hypertension; tachycardia; drowsiness; extrapyramidal symptoms; parkinsonian-like symptoms or tardive dyskinesia symptoms (lip-smacking and chewing motions, uncontrolled movement of arms or legs), agitation, confusion, drowsiness, or diarrhea.

CONTRAINDICATIONS. Epilepsy, severe renal impairment, or conditions where GI stimulation is not indicated such as hemorrhage or mechancial obstruction.

**POTENTIAL DRUG/FOOD INTERACTIONS**

May increase the CNS depressant effects of alcohol or other CNS depressant drugs. May increase the risk of extrapyramidal symptoms if used with other drugs that cause extrapyramidal symptoms. Incompatible with calcium gluconate, cephalothin, cisplatin, erythromycin, methotrexate, and tetracycline.

**INTERVENTIONS: ADMINISTRATION**

Mix doses of more than 10 mg in 50 mL of NSS, D5W, D5W and 0.45% NSS, Ringer's lactate, or Ringer's lactate injection.

**MODE/RATE OF ADMINISTRATION**

May be given by IV push over 2 min. May be given by intermittent infusion over at least 15 min. Not recommended for long-term continuous infusion; may use filter.

INTRAVENOUS USE (WITH NORMAL RENAL AND HEPATIC FUNCTION)

**Adults:** For stimulating peristalsis the usual dose is 10 mg as a single dose. For postoperative nausea, the dose can be repeated q3–4h as needed. For antiemetic effect the usual dose is 2 mg/kg of body weight over 15 min given 30 min before chemotherapy. Dose may be repeated q2–3h as needed. Alternately, the dose may be 3 mg/kg of body weight by continuous infusion given 30 min before chemotherapy and 0.5 mg/kg/h for 8 h.

**Children:** The usual dose is 1 mg/kg of body weight as a single dose. The dose ▼

may be repeated once in 1 h. Maximum dose should not exceed 2 mg/kg of body weight.

**Infants/Neonates:** Dose not established.

**Geriatrics:** Elderly clients are more likely to show extrapyramidal, parkinsonian, and tardive dyskinesia symptoms.

INTRATHECAL USE OR OTHER INFUSION ROUTES AS INDICATED. Not recommended.

#### POTENTIAL PROBLEMS IN ADMINISTRATION

If given too rapidly by IV push, the client may experience brief, intense anxiety and restlessness, followed by drowsiness.

#### INDEPENDENT NURSING ACTIONS

Monitor client for nausea, vomiting, or complaints of abdominal pain. Monitor stool for character, amount, and color. Monitor vital signs, especially heart rate and regularity. Monitor laboratory values, especially for elevations in serum creatinine. Monitor mental status, especially in the elderly. Monitor for evidence of extrapyramidal, parkinsonian, or tardive dyskinesia symptoms.

#### ADMINISTRATION IN ALTERNATE SETTINGS

May be given in a wide variety of settings, including the home, by a qualified infusion therapy nurse.

#### EVALUATION: OUTCOMES OF DRUG THERAPY

#### EXPECTED OUTCOMES

PHYSICAL ASSESSMENT. Client has no complaints of nausea, vomiting, abdominal pain, GI tract bleeding, or diarrhea. Heart rate remains between 60 and 100 bpm and regular.

LABORATORY. Serum creatinine levels remain within client's baseline.

#### NEGATIVE OUTCOMES

Client continues to complain of nausea, vomiting, or abdominal pain. Client experiences GI tract bleeding, diarrhea, confusion, extrapyramidal, parkinsonian, or tardive dyskinesia symptoms. Heart rate is irregular.

---

## RANITIDINE

*Trade Name:* Zantac
*Canadian Availability:* Zantac
*Pregnancy Risk:* Category B
*pH:* 6.7–7.3
*Storage/Stability:* Store below 30° C. Protect from light and freezing. May be stored for 48 hours at room temperature. Store premixed solutions at 25° C. Do not use if discolored or if there is a precipitate present.

#### ASSESSMENT: DRUG CHARACTERISTICS

#### ACTION

An $H_2$-receptor antagonist that inhibits gastric acid secretion by competing with histamine for the $H_2$-receptor sites of the parietal cells. Inhibits stimulation of gastric acid secretion by food, caffeine, insulin, and vagal reflex. May also be used to treat urticaria because its action on the $H_2$-receptor sites blocks the inflammatory response of cutaneous blood vessels. May enhance healing of stress-induced acid ulceration by promoting the production of gastric mucus and the secretion of bicarbonate and stimulating gastric mucosal blood flow.

#### INDICATIONS

Used on a short-term basis to treat gastric and duodenal ulcers, gastric hypersecretory states, Zollinger-Ellison syndrome, multiple endocrine adenomas, GERD, and upper GI tract bleeding, and to relieve GI distress from NSAIDs used for arthritis therapy. Also used to treat stress-induced GI tract bleeding and to prevent stress ulcers associated with trauma or surgery.

#### CAUTIONS

ADVERSE EFFECTS. Allergic reactions, decreased libido, breast tenderness, joint or muscle pain, or loss of hair.

CONTRAINDICATIONS. Impaired renal or hepatic function or sensitivity to ranitidine.

#### POTENTIAL DRUG/FOOD INTERACTIONS

May reduce the absorption of ketoconazole. May inhibit the metabolism of warfarin, requiring careful monitoring of prothrombin time for warfarin dose adjustment. May interfere with the renal elimination of procainamide, causing an increase in blood concentrations of procainamide. May be incompatible with aminophylline, amphotericin B, and most cephalosporins.

#### INTERVENTIONS: ADMINISTRATION

Each 50 mg must be diluted in at least 20 mL of NSS before administration. May use D5Wor D10W, 0.9% NSS, combinations of D5W and NSS, Ringer's lactate, or 5% sodium bicarbonate solutions for intermittent infusion.

#### MODE/RATE OF ADMINISTRATION

Most commonly given by intermittent infusion over 15–20 min or by continuous infusion. May also be administered by IV push over 5 min.

INTRAVENOUS USE (WITH NORMAL RENAL AND HEPATIC FUNCTION)

**Adults:** Usual dosage is 50 mg q6–8h by intermittent IV infusion. For continuous infusion (not common) the dosage is 6.75 mg/h to a maximum of 900 mg/d. For IV push, give 50 mg over 5 min. If renal function is impaired, the dosage is reduced to 50 mg q18–24h. Lower doses may be required if there is impaired hepatic function.

**Children:** For acute ulcer states the usual dosage is 2–4 mg/kg/d by intermittent IV infusion. Dose should be reduced if there is renal impairment.

▼

**Infants/Neonates:** Dose not established.

**Geriatrics:** Follow adult dosing schedule. Elderly clients are more likely to have diminished renal function and may require a lower dose. Elderly clients are more at risk for confusion.

INTRATHECAL USE OR OTHER INFUSION ROUTES AS INDICATED. Not recommended.

#### POTENTIAL PROBLEMS IN ADMINISTRATION

Rapid bolus IV injection is not recommended because there is an increased risk of cardiac arrhythmias and hypotension.

#### INDEPENDENT NURSING ACTIONS

Monitor client for nausea, vomiting, or complaints of abdominal pain. Monitor stool for character, amount, and color. Monitor vital signs, especially heart rate and regularity. Monitor laboratory values, especially for changes in hepatic function and elevations in serum creatinine. Monitor mental status, especially in the elderly.

#### ADMINISTRATION IN ALTERNATE SETTINGS

May be given in a wide variety of settings, including the home, by a qualified IV nurse.

#### EVALUATION: OUTCOMES OF DRUG THERAPY

#### EXPECTED OUTCOMES

PHYSICAL ASSESSMENT. Client has no complaints of nausea, vomiting, abdominal pain, GI tract bleeding, or diarrhea. Heart rate remains between 60 and 100 bpm and regular.

LABORATORY. Liver function studies and serum creatinine levels remain within client's baseline.

#### NEGATIVE OUTCOMES

Client continues to complain of nausea, vomiting, or abdominal pain. Client experiences GI tract bleeding, diarrhea, and confusion. Heart rate is irregular.

CHAPTER 24

# Miscellaneous Infusion Agents

*Elaine Kennedy*

**Antidotes**
- Digoxin Immune Fab
- Edetate Disodium
- Flumazenil
- Leucovorin Calcium
- Mesna

**Antihistamines**
- Diphenhydramine

**Hormones**
- Desmopressin Acetate
- Dexamethasone Sodium Phosphate
- Diethylstilbestrol Diphosphate Sodium
- Glucagon Hydrochloride
- Hydrocortisone Sodium Succinate
- Insulin
- Levothyroxine Sodium
- Methylprednisolone Sodium Succinate
- Oxytocin
- Vasopressin

**Vitamins**
- Ascorbic Acid
- Multivitamin Infusion (MVI)
- Phytonadione
- Thiamine Hydrochloride

**Other Infusion Agents**
- $Alpha_1$ Proteinase Inhibitor
- Aminophylline (79% Theophylline)
- Cyclosporine
- Immune Globulin IV
- Tacrolimus

Miscellaneous infusion agents covered in this chapter include antidotes, antihistamines, hormones, vitamins, and other infusion agents. Some agents act as antidotes to other agents and counter the negative effects of these agents in a variety of ways. For example, leucovorin counters the inhibited folic acid production caused by methotrexate. Some agents absorb and bind other drugs for safe elimination from the body. An example is the way in which edetate sodium binds calcium, which is then eliminated in the urine. The calcium loss acts as an antagonist to digitalis glycosides when toxic levels of those glycosides have been reached.

Antihistamines act to minimize the effects of the release of histamine by the body in response to an allergen. In the presence of an allergen, the mast cells release histamine, which affects the body's vascular and bronchial smooth muscle. Histamine's effects on these muscles are manifested as hypersensitivity and allergic reactions.

Hormones secreted by the endocrine system may need to be replaced if the endocrine gland does not secrete sufficient quantities of the hormone or if the gland is surgically removed.

Vitamins are naturally occurring organic compounds required for growth and health, usually in small amounts. Clients frequently require supplements of vitamins during periods of intense stress caused by ill health or in the presence of malnutrition.

Some miscellaneous agents affect the immune system. Some agents, such as cyclosporine, may suppress the immune system, or other agents, such as immune globulin IV, provide passive immunity. Finally, some agents, such as theophylline, act as a stimulant.

Miscellaneous infusion agents are grouped by classifications in Table 24–1.

---

### TABLE 24–1
### Miscellaneous Infusion Agents Grouped by Classification

**Antidotes**
Digoxin immune fab
Edetate calcium disodium*
Edetate disodium
Flumazenil
Leucovorin calcium
Mesna
Pamidronate disodium*
Pralidoxime*
Protamine sulfate (see Chapter 19)
Sodium nitrite*
Sodium thiosulfate*

**Vitamins**
Ascorbic acid
Dexpanthenol*
Folic acid*
Menadiol sodium*
Multivitamin infusion (MVI)
Niacin*
Phytonadione
Pyridoxine hydrochloride*
Thiamine hydrochloride

**Other Infusion Agents**
Alpha₁ proteinase inhibitor
Aminophylline (79% Theophylline)
Cyclosporine
Immune globulin IV
Tacrolimus

**Antihistamines**
Brompheniramine*
Chlorpheniramine*
Diphenhydramine

**Hormones**
Alprostadil*
Betamethasone*
Calcitonin human*
Calcitonin salmon*
Conjugated estrogens*
Cosyntropin*
Corticotropin*
Desmopressin acetate
Dexamethasone sodium phosphate
Diethylstilbestrol diphosphate sodium
Gonadorelin acetate*
Gonadorelin hydrochloride*
Glucagon hydrochloride
Hydrocortisone sodium succinate
Insulin
Levothyroxine sodium
Liothyronine sodium*
Methylprednisolone sodium succinate
Prednisolone sodium phosphate*
Oxytocin
Vasopressin

* Not discussed in this chapter.

# Antidotes

## DIGOXIN IMMUNE FAB

*Trade Name:* Digibind
*Canadian Availability:* None specified
*Pregnancy Risk:* Category C
*pH:* 6–8
*Storage/Stability:* Refrigerate vials. Reconstituted drug stable for up to 4 hours if refrigerated after reconstitution.

### ASSESSMENT: DRUG CHARACTERISTICS

#### ACTION

Antibodies produced in sheep bind with molecules of digoxin or digitoxin to make them unavailable for binding at their site of action in the body.

#### INDICATIONS

Used to treat life-threatening digoxin or digitoxin toxicity.

#### CAUTIONS

ADVERSE EFFECTS. Rapid development of hypokalemia with associated muscle cramping, nausea, vomiting, hypoactive bowel sounds, abdominal distention, dyspnea, and postural hypotension; congestive heart failure (CHF); anaphylaxis or death in clients sensitive to ovine proteins or in clients who have previously received digoxin immune fab; large doses given rapidly may cause febrile reactions.

CONTRAINDICATIONS. None if given for specific indications; for clients with hypersensitivity, pretreat with corticosteroids and diphenhydramine; prepare to treat anaphylaxis as necessary.

#### POTENTIAL DRUG/FOOD INTERACTIONS

Initially a rise in serum digoxin levels; however, this will be bound to the fab fragments. Accurate serum digoxin levels are elusive until all the fab fragments are excreted. Catecholamines may aggravate arrhythmias caused by digitalis.

### INTERVENTIONS: ADMINISTRATION

Dosing is dependent on the amount of digoxin or digitoxin ingested. Each 40-mg vial will bind 0.6 mg of digoxin. If the ingested dose is unknown, administer 20 vials (800 mg). Dilute each vial of 40 mg with 4 mL of sterile water for injection for a final concentration of 10 mg/mL. May be further diluted with any amount of 0.9% normal saline solution (NSS), but be aware of potential for fluid overload with further dilution.

#### MODE/RATE OF ADMINISTRATION

Administer as an infusion through a 0.22-$\mu$m filter over 30 min. Use intravenous (IV) push if cardiac arrest is imminent.

▼

INTRAVENOUS USE (WITH NORMAL RENAL FUNCTION)

**Adults and Children:** When amount of digoxin or digitoxin is unknown, administer 800 mg IV or serum digoxin concentration × weight in kg divided by 100 = digoxin immune fab dose.

When amount of digoxin or digitoxin is known, calculate the total dose or total body load (TBL) in milligrams of digoxin or digitoxin. If digoxin tablets or elixir is ingested orally, multiply the amount ingested by 0.8. Dose of digoxin immune fab in milligrams = TBL × 66.7.

For toxicity during long-term digoxin or digitoxin therapy, administer 240 mg for adults and 40 mg for children.

**Geratrics:** Follow adult dosing schedule.

INTRATHECAL USE OR OTHER INFUSION ROUTES AS INDICATED. Contraindicated.

**POTENTIAL PROBLEMS IN ADMINISTRATION**

Large doses of digoxin immune fab act more quickly but increase the likelihood of febrile or allergic reactions than do small doses. Patients allergic to ovine proteins should be tested for sensitivity to digoxin immune fab before administration unless cardiac arrest is imminent. In case of shock, support blood pressure with dopamine. Clients with atrial fibrillation may develop a rapid ventricular response due to the binding of the digoxin or digitoxin.

**INDEPENDENT NURSING ACTIONS**

Use cardiac monitor and monitor vital signs, especially pulse rate and rhythm and temperature, prior to and during treatment. Assess for signs of CHF. Monitor laboratory electrolytes.

**ADMINISTRATION IN ALTERNATE SETTINGS**

Not recommended for administration in home settings or clinical settings where the client cannot be closely monitored.

**EVALUATION: OUTCOMES OF DRUG THERAPY**

**EXPECTED OUTCOMES**

PHYSICAL ASSESSMENT. Vital signs, especially pulse rate and rhythm and temperature remain within 15% of client's baseline. Client does not experience CHF. Serum digoxin levels slowly return to therapeutic range.

LABORATORY. Serum digoxin or digitoxin levels are not valid for 5 to 7 days after treatment.

**NEGATIVE OUTCOMES**

Vital signs, especially pulse rate and rhythm and temperature, are more than 15% higher or lower than client's baseline. Client demonstrates CHF with weight gain, dyspnea, peripheral edema, rales, or crackles in lungs.

# Edetate Disodium

*Trade Names:* Disotate, Endrate
*Canadian Availability:* None specified
*Pregnancy Risk:* Category C
*pH:* 6.5–7.5
*Storage/Stability:* Store below 40° C. Protect from freezing.

## ASSESSMENT: DRUG CHARACTERISTICS

### ACTION

A calcium-chelating agent that forms soluble complexes with calcium that are then filtered through the kidneys. The hypocalcemic effect acts as a temporary antagonist to the chronotropic and inotropic effects of digitalis glycosides. Also forms soluble complexes with other metals such as magnesium and zinc or other trace minerals.

### INDICATIONS

Used to treat hypercalcemia and dysrhythmias caused by digitalis toxicity. Also used to treat acute and chronic lead poisoning.

### CAUTIONS

ADVERSE EFFECTS. Thrombophlebitis at injection site, anemia, dermatitis, fever, gout, nephrotoxicity, hypokalemia, hypomagnesemia, hypocalcemia, cardiac dysrhythmias, abdominal pain, headache, anaphylaxis, or death.

CONTRAINDICATIONS. Hypocalcemia, renal dysfunction, heart disease, or seizures.

### POTENTIAL DRUG/FOOD INTERACTIONS

May antagonize the effects of digitalis glycosides. Magnesium deficiency may occur with prolonged use. Incompatible with any metal. Calcium gluconate is the antidote.

## INTERVENTIONS: ADMINISTRATION

Dilute the calculated dose in 500 mL of 5% dextrose in water (D5W) or 0.9% NSS.

### MODE/RATE OF ADMINISTRATION

Should not be given by IV push. Give by intermittent IV infusion over at least 1–3 h or by continuous infusion.

#### INTRAVENOUS USE (WITH NORMAL RENAL FUNCTION)

**Adults:** For hypercalcemia or digitalis toxicity the usual dosage is 50 mg/kg of body weight in 24 h. Dose may be repeated for 4 more days with at least 2 drug-free days before repeating the regimen. Regimen may be repeated for a total of 15 doses.

Maximum daily dose should not exceed 3 g.

**Children:** For hypercalcemia or digitalis toxicity the usual dosage is 35–40 mg/kg of body weight in 24 h. Dose may go as high as 70 mg/kg of body weight in 24 h.

**Infants/Neonates:** Follow children's dosing schedule.

▼

**Geriatrics:** Follow adult dosing schedule.

INTRATHECAL USE OR OTHER INFUSION ROUTES AS INDICATED. Contraindicated.

#### POTENTIAL PROBLEMS IN ADMINISTRATION

Agent is highly irritating. Too rapid infusion may cause a sudden decrease in serum calcium with subsequent cardiac or respiratory arrest, tetany, or convulsions.

#### INDEPENDENT NURSING ACTIONS

Monitor vital signs, especially pulse rate, rhythm, and temperature. Observe for dermatitis, thrombophlebitis, or gout. Monitor urinary output. Evaluate client for complaints of abdominal pain or headache. Monitor laboratory electrolytes.

#### ADMINISTRATION IN ALTERNATE SETTINGS

Not recommended for administration in home settings or clinical settings where the client cannot be closely monitored.

### EVALUATION: OUTCOMES OF DRUG THERAPY

#### EXPECTED OUTCOMES

PHYSICAL ASSESSMENT. Vital signs, especially pulse rate, rhythm, and temperature, remain within 15% of client's baseline. Client has no dermatitis, thrombophlebitis, or gout. Urinary output is more than 50 mL/h. Client has no complaints of abdominal pain or headache.

LABORATORY. Serum calcium is 8.5 to 10.5 mg/dL. Serum potassium is 3.5 to 5 mEq/L. Serum magnesium is 1.5 to 2 mEq/L. Serum digoxin levels are in therapeutic range.

#### NEGATIVE OUTCOMES

Vital signs, especially pulse rate, rhythm, and temperature, are more than 15% higher or lower than client's baseline. Client demonstrates dermatitis, thrombophlebitis, or gout. Urinary output is less than 50 mL/h. Client complains of abdominal pain or headache.

## FLUMAZENIL

*Trade Name:* Mazicon
*Canadian Availability:* None specified
*Pregnancy Risk:* Category C
*pH:* 4
*Storage/Stability:* Store at room temperature. Discard after 24 hours any drug that has been drawn into syringe or has been mixed with any solutions or if particulate matter or discoloration is noted.

### ASSESSMENT: DRUG CHARACTERISTICS

#### ACTION

A benzodiazepine antagonist antidote. Used to reverse sedation, psychomotor impairment, and recall due to the activity of benzodiazepine on the central nervous system (CNS).

**INDICATIONS**

Used to treat benzodiazepine overdose. Provides complete or partial reversal of benzodiazepine's sedative effects when general anesthesia has been induced or maintained with benzodiazepine.

**CAUTIONS**

ADVERSE EFFECTS. Abnormal vision, agitation, anxiety, dizziness, dry mouth, dyspnea; emotional lability, fatigue, flushing, headache, hot flashes, insomnia, pain at injection site, palpitations, paresthesia, sweating, tremors, and vomiting; clients who have taken large doses may experience agitation, anxiety, seizures, hyperesthesia, and increased muscle tone.

CONTRAINDICATIONS. History of hypersensitivity to benzodiazepines, concurrent use of benzodiazepines for treatment of potentially life-threatening conditions such as control of intracranial pressure or status epilepticus, and signs of serious cyclic antidepressant overdose (motor abnormalities, arrythmias, anticholinergic signs, cardiovascular collapse).

**POTENTIAL DRUG/FOOD INTERACTIONS**

May produce seizures in clients who use benzodiazepines to control seizure disorders, in those clients who are physically dependent on large doses of benzodiazepines, or in overdose situations when large doses of other drugs may have been ingested. May alter cerebral blood flow in clients with head trauma.

**INTERVENTIONS: ADMINISTRATION**

May be given undiluted or diluted further with D5W, Ringer's lactate, or 0.9% NSS.

**MODE/RATE OF ADMINISTRATION**

May be given IV push through the side arm of a running IV in small pulse doses to allow for a controlled reversal of sedation without the client experiencing an abrupt awakening. This method of administration also minimizes the potential for side effects.

INTRAVENOUS USE (WITH NORMAL HEPATIC FUNCTION)

**Adults:** For reversal of conscious sedation in general anesthesia, initial dosage is 0.2 mg in 15 s, may repeat 0.2 mg dose in 45 s then at 60-s intervals until desired wakefulness established, but cumulative dose should not exceed 1 mg in a 20-min period. If resedation occurs, may repeat dose at 20-min intervals. Cumulative dose should not exceed 3 mg in a 60-min period.

For benzodiazepine overdose, initial dosage is 0.2 mg over 30 s, may repeat after 30 s with 0.3 mg over 30 s if desired level of consciousness is not achieved. Subsequent dosages of 0.5 mg over 30 s may be administered at 60-s intervals. Maximum dosage of 3 mg in 1 h.

**Children:** Dose not established.

▼

**Infants/Neonates:** Dose not established.

**Geriatrics:** Follow adult dosing schedule.

INTRATHECAL USE OR OTHER INFUSION ROUTES AS INDICATED. Not recommended.

**POTENTIAL PROBLEMS IN ADMINISTRATION**

Administer into a large vein through the side arm of a running IV to prevent pain and inflammation at IV site. If medication spills on skin, rinse with water immediately.

**INDEPENDENT NURSING ACTIONS**

Monitor the client's arterial blood gases before treatment and at 30-min intervals during treatment. Assess airway and prepare to intervene should reestablishment of airway and assistance with ventilation be necessary. Observe awakened client for resedation and respiratory depression, as flumazenil may wear off before benzodiazepines.

**ADMINISTRATION IN ALTERNATE SETTINGS**

Not recommended.

**EVALUATION: OUTCOMES OF DRUG THERAPY**

**EXPECTED OUTCOMES**

PHYSICAL ASSESSMENT. Client awakens without seizures or signs of respiratory depression. No complaints of dizziness, nausea, vomiting, headache, blurred vision, agitation, dry mouth, hyperventilation, or dyspnea.

LABORATORY. Arterial blood gases remain within normal limits for client.

**NEGATIVE OUTCOMES**

Client experiences seizures, anxiety, or respiratory depression. Client has recurring somnolence with respiratory depression.

## Leucovorin Calcium

*Trade Name:* Wellcovorin
*Canadian Availability:* Leucovorin calcium
*Pregnancy Risk:* Category C
*pH:* 6–8
*Storage/Stability:* Store below 40° C. Protect from freezing and light. Solutions containing leucovorin should be used within 24 hours if reconstituted with sterile water. If bacteriostatic water for injection is used, solution may be stored for up to 7 days if refrigerated.

**ASSESSMENT: DRUG CHARACTERISTICS**

**ACTION**

A folic acid antagonist antidote. Leucovorin is unaffected by the blockage of enzymes that inhibit folic acid production, hich may be caused by agents such as methotrexate. DNA, RNA, and protein synthesis can occur since leucovorin is a reduced form of folic acid.

**INDICATIONS**

Used to treat methotrexate, pyrimethamine, and trimethoprim toxicity. May be used to treat megaloblastic leukemia and as an adjunct to fluorouracil in the treatment of colorectal cancer.

**CAUTIONS**

ADVERSE EFFECTS. May cause an allergic reaction.

CONTRAINDICATIONS. Should not be used for clients with renal impairment or as the only antianemic agent for clients with pernicious anemia or vitamin $B_{12}$ deficiency.

**POTENTIAL DRUG/FOOD INTERACTIONS**

May inhibit the activity of barbiturate, hydantoin, or primidone antiseizure agents. May increase the effects of fluorouracil.

**INTERVENTIONS: ADMINISTRATION**

May be reconstituted to a 10–20 mg/mL concentration. May be given undiluted. May be used with sterile water (no preservatives) for all doses more than 10 mg/m$^2$.

**MODE/RATE OF ADMINISTRATION**

May be given IV push at a rate not to exceed 160 mg/min. May be given by intermittent or continuous IV infusion at ordered rate, but not to exceed 160 mg/min.

INTRAVENOUS USE (WITH NORMAL RENAL FUNCTION)

**Adults:** As an antidote the usual dosage is 10 mg/m$^2$ of body surface area (BSA) q6h until methotrexate blood levels fall to less than $5 \times 10^{-8}$ mol/L. If the serum methotrexate level exceeds the pretreatment level by 50% after 24 h, leucovorin should be increased to 100 mg/m$^2$ of BSA q3h until the serum methotrexate levels fall to the appropriate level.

For colorectal cancer therapy the usual dosage is 200 mg/m$^2$ of BSA over at least 3 min followed by fluorouracil 370 mg/m$^2$ of BSA q.d. for 5 d. The regimen may be repeated q4wk.

**Children:** As an antidote, follow adult dosing schedule. For colorectal cancer therapy, dose has not been established.

**Infants/Neonates:** Dose not established.

**Geriatrics:** Elderly clients are more likely to have age-related decreases in renal function that may require lower doses.

INTRATHECAL USE OR OTHER INFUSION ROUTES AS INDICATED. Not recommended.

**POTENTIAL PROBLEMS IN ADMINISTRATION**

Should be given intravenously when used to "rescue" clients from methotrexate toxicity because nausea and vomiting may interfere with absorption. Should be physically present if being used for "rescue." Should be given after methotrexate to prevent interfering with methotrexate's antineoplastic activity.

**INDEPENDENT NURSING ACTIONS**

Monitor the client for allergic reactions such as difficulty breathing, wheezing, urticaria, or hypotension. ▼

Monitor laboratory values, especially serum creatinine, methotrexate levels, urine pH, serum folate levels, hemoglobin, hematocrit, and reticulocyte counts.

**ADMINISTRATION IN ALTERNATE SETTINGS**

Not recommended.

**EVALUATION: OUTCOMES OF DRUG THERAPY**

**EXPECTED OUTCOMES**

PHYSICAL ASSESSMENT. Client has no evidence of anaphylactic shock.

LABORATORY. Serum creatinine is between 0.6 and 1.5 mg/dL. Serum methotrexate levels are less than $5 \times 10^8$. Urine pH is between 5 and 7. Serum folic level is more than 3.3 ng/mL. Hemoglobin is between 12 and 18 g/dL. Hematocrit is between 37% and 52%. Reticulocyte count is 0.5% to 2.5% red blood cell.

**NEGATIVE OUTCOMES**

Client has symptoms of an allergic response.

## MESNA

*Trade Name:* Mesnex
*Canadian Availability:* Uromitexan
*Pregnancy Risk:* Category B
*pH:* 6.5–8.5
*Storage/Stability:* Store at room temperature. Stable at room temperature for 24 hours after dilution. Recommended use within 6 hours. Discard any unused medications.

**ASSESSMENT: DRUG CHARACTERISTICS**

**ACTION**

In the kidney, mesna reacts with ifosfamide urotoxic metabolites to decrease hemorrhagic cystitis.

**INDICATIONS**

Used to decrease the incidence of ifosfamide-induced hemorrhagic cystitis. There is some indication that it may reduce hemorrhagic cystitis associated with cyclophosphamide.

**CAUTIONS**

ADVERSE EFFECTS. Bad taste in mouth; soft stools and with larger doses diarrhea, limb pain, headache, fatigue, nausea, hypotension, allergic reaction; in some instances, hematuria.

CONTRAINDICATIONS. Sensitivity to mesna or thiol (rubber) compounds.

**POTENTIAL DRUG/FOOD INTERACTIONS**

None noted.

**INTERVENTIONS: ADMINISTRATION**

Dilute each 100-mg vial with D5W or 0.9% NSS to make a final concentration of 20 mg/mL.

**MODE/RATE OF ADMINISTRATION**

As a single dose, administer over a minimum of 1 min if given alone. If given with ifosfamide, administer at same rate as ifosfamide is given.

INTRAVENOUS USE (WITH NORMAL RENAL FUNCTION)

**Adults:** Total daily dose of mesna equals 60% of daily ifosfamide dose. Mesna is given in a dosage equal to 20% of the ifosfamide dosage at the time of ifosfamide administration. This same dose of mesna is repeated at 4 and 8 h after initial dose. If hemorrhagic cystitis is not controlled with mesna at these doses, decreased doses of ifosfamide may be required.

**Children:** Dose not established.

**Infants/Neonates:** Dose not established.

**Geriatrics:** Follow adult dosing schedule.

INTRATHECAL USE OR OTHER INFUSION ROUTES AS INDICATED. Not recommended.

**POTENTIAL PROBLEMS IN ADMINISTRATION**

The effectiveness of mesna is greatest when the ifosfamide dose is less than 1.2 $gm^2$/24 h; less effective when ifosfamide dose is more than 2 $gm^2$/24 h.

**INDEPENDENT NURSING ACTIONS**

Instruct client of the potential for a bad taste in mouth. Monitor for nausea and amount and frequency of diarrhea. Observe client for postural hypotension. Examine first morning urine for blood. Instruct client to inform nurse or physician of headache or limb pain.

**ADMINISTRATION IN ALTERNATE SETTINGS**

Not recommended.

**EVALUATION: OUTCOMES OF DRUG THERAPY**

**EXPECTED OUTCOMES**

PHYSICAL ASSESSMENT. Stools are soft but not watery or frequent. Urine is clear and pale yellow. Client denies severe nausea, headache, or limb pain.

LABORATORY. Client's urine remains free of blood. Urine may test positive for ketones. There is no decrease in pretreatment hematocrit or hemoglobin.

**NEGATIVE OUTCOMES**

Client experiences severe diarrhea with associated signs and symptoms of hypotension. Client complains of severe headache, nausea, and limb pain. Urine is bloody.

## Antihistamines

### DIPHENHYDRAMINE

*Trade Names:* Bena-D, Benadryl, Benahist, Ben-Allergin, Benoject, Dihydrex, Diphenacen, Hyrexin, Nordryl, Wehdryl

*Canadian Availability:* Benadryl

*Pregnancy Risk:* Category B

*pH:* 5–6

*Storage/Stability:* Store at room temperature.

▼

## ASSESSMENT: DRUG CHARACTERISTICS

### ACTION

An antihistamine that blocks the effects of histamine at various receptor sites, either eliminating histamine's effects or reducing them.

### INDICATIONS

Relieve allergic responses caused by histamine release in the presence of an allergen. Useful as an antiemetic due to anticholinergic activity and for motion sickness. Indicated in the short-term treatment of parkinsonism. Used with epinephrine in the treatment of anaphylaxis. Useful as an antitussive and antipruritic. May be given as a pretreatment for blood product or amphotericin B administration.

### CAUTIONS

ADVERSE EFFECTS. Minimal when used in the treatment of anaphylaxis; drowsiness, dizziness, blurred vision, tinnitus, muscular weakness, dry mouth, urinary frequency, retention, dysuria, anorexia, palpitations, hypotension, tremors, seizures, constipation, diarrhea, epigastric distress, thickening of bronchial secretions, chest tightness, wheezing, tachycardia, photosensitivity.

The very young, the elderly, or debilitated may experience paradoxical excitation (insomnia, restlessness, euphoria, nervousness, or tremors).

Clients may exhibit signs and symptoms of allergic reaction.

CONTRAINDICATIONS. Hypersensitivity to antihistamines; pregnancy, lactation, concurrent use of monoamine oxidase (MAO) inhibitors, premature infants; narrow-angle glaucoma, stenosing peptic ulcers, prostatic hypertrophy, pyloroduodenal obstruction, bladder neck obstruction; acute asthmatic attacks; use with care in clients with liver disease.

### POTENTIAL DRUG/FOOD INTERACTIONS

Likely to cause additive CNS depression when used with other antihistamines, alcohol, opioids, sedatives, tranquilizers, or hypnotics. Potentiates the effectiveness of epinephrine. MAO inhibitors prolong anticholinergic effects. Effects of anticoagulants and corticosteroids may be reduced. Potentiates action of other anticholinergics and antihistamines.

## INTERVENTIONS: ADMINISTRATION

May be given undiluted.

### MODE/RATE OF ADMINISTRATION

In emergency situations, administer each 25 mg or fraction over 1 min. In nonemergency a longer administration is recommended.

INTRAVENOUS USE (WITH NORMAL RENAL FUNCTION)

**Adults:** 10–50 mg per dose. May require 100 mg per dose. Do not exceed 400 mg/d.

**Children:** 5 mg/kg/d in divided doses q6–8h. Do not exceed 300 mg/d.

**Infants/Neonates:** Not recommended.

**Geriatrics:** Lower doses are recommended.

INTRATHECAL USE OR OTHER INFUSION ROUTES AS INDICATED. Not recommended.

**POTENTIAL PROBLEMS IN ADMINISTRATION**

May have additive effect with other drugs associated with CNS depression.

**INDEPENDENT NURSING ACTIONS**

Monitor client for signs and symptoms of allergic response (urticaria, rashes, shortness of breath, [SOB], wheezing, hypotension). Assess client for nausea, vomiting, bowel sounds, etc. Instruct client to avoid concurrent use of alcohol, opioids, tranquilizers, sedatives, or hypnotics and to avoid activities that require alertness or motor skills. Monitor vital signs, including respiratory rate and depth and lung sounds. Assess children, the elderly, and debilitated clients for paradoxical reactions such as excitement. Offer frequent fluids and gum for clients with dryness of mouth and lips. Monitor closely for any untoward effects.

**CAUTIONS**

ADVERSE EFFECTS. Minimal when used in the treatment of anaphylaxis; drowsiness, dizziness, blurred vision, tinnitus, muscular weakness, dry mouth, urinary frequency, retention dysuria, anorexia, palpitations, hypotension, tremors, seizures, constipation, diarrhea, epigastric distress, thickening of bronchial secretions, chest tightness, wheezing, tachycardia, photosensitivity.

**ADMINISTRATION IN ALTERNATE SETTINGS**

May be given in a variety of clinical settings and in the home by a qualified infusion therapy nurse.

**EVALUATION: OUTCOMES OF DRUG THERAPY**

**EXPECTED OUTCOMES**

PHYSICAL ASSESSMENT. If given as treatment for allergic reaction, vital signs stabilize and respiratory status improves. Itching and rash resolve. Client may complain of sleepiness and dry mouth, throat, and lips. If used as pretreatment for blood products or amphotericin B administration, client does not experience febrile reaction or rigors. Children, the elderly, or debilitated clients do not experience paradoxical reactions or seizures. There is no nausea, vomiting, or dizziness.

LABORATORY. Clients who are undergoing intradermal sensitivity testing may have false-negative results if allergens are administered within 4 days of diphenhydramine.

**NEGATIVE OUTCOMES.**

No response when given as a treatment for allergic reaction. Client's reaction proceeds to anaphylaxis. When

▼

used as a pretreatment for blood product or amphotericin B administration, client experiences febrile reaction or rigors. Children, the elderly, or debilitated clients experience paradoxical excitation. Client complains of nausea, vomiting, or dizziness.

## Hormones

### DESMOPRESSIN ACETATE

*Trade Names:* DDAVP, Stimate, Vasopressin
*Canadian Availability:* DDAVP
*Pregnancy Risk:* Category B
*pH:* 3.5–4
*Storage/Stability:* Store at 4° C. Protect from freezing.

#### ASSESSMENT: DRUG CHARACTERISTICS

**ACTION**

An antidiuretic (synthetic analog of human antidiuretic hormone [ADH]) with antihemorrhagic effects. Acts by increasing water reabsorption from the collecting ducts. The antihemorrhagic action is unknown but thought to result from direct action on the vessel wall, as well as increasing clotting factor VIII and von Willebrand's factor.

**INDICATIONS**

Used to treat diabetes insipidus, hemophilia A, von Willebrand's hemophilia, and primary nocturnal enuresis.

**CAUTIONS**

ADVERSE EFFECTS. Hypertension, hypernatremia, abdominal cramps, flushing, headache, or nausea.

CONTRAINDICATIONS. Coronary artery disease or hypertension.

**POTENTIAL DRUG/FOOD INTERACTIONS**

Carbamazepine, chlorpropamide, clofibrate lithium, or norepinephrine may decrease the antidiuretic effect of desmopressin.

#### INTERVENTIONS: ADMINISTRATION

Does not need to be diluted. May be diluted with 0.9% NSS if needed.

**MODE/RATE OF ADMINISTRATION**

Given IV push over 1 min. May be given by intermittent IV infusion over 15–30 min to control hemorrhage.

INTRAVENOUS USE (WITH NORMAL RENAL FUNCTION)

**Adults:** For diabetes insipidus, the usual dosage is 2–4 mcg (0.002–0.004 mg)/d. Dose is divided; one half given in the morning, one half given in the evening.

For antihemorrhagic effect, the usual dose is 0.3 mcg (0.0003 mg)/kg of body weight in 50 mL of 0.9% NSS. Dose may be repeated if necessary.

**Children:** For children weighing more than 10 kg, for antihemorrhagic effect, the usual dose is 0.3 mcg (0.0003 mg)/kg of body weight diluted in 50 mL of 0.9% NSS.

For children weighing less than 10 kg, for antihemorrhagic effect, the usual dose is 0.3 mcg (0.0003 mg)/kg of body weight diluted in 10 mL of 0.9% NSS.

**Infants/Neonates:** Not recommended for infants under 3 mo.

**Geriatrics:** Elderly clients are sensitive to the effects of desmopressin and must be closely monitored for hypernatremia and water intoxication.

INTRATHECAL USE OR OTHER INFUSION ROUTES AS INDICATED. Not recommended.

**POTENTIAL PROBLEMS IN ADMINISTRATION**

May cause rapid decrease in effectiveness if given more often than q24–48h.

**INDEPENDENT NURSING ACTIONS**

Monitor vital signs, especially blood pressure. Monitor intake and output. Weigh the client daily. Monitor laboratory values, especially serum and urine osmolarity, hematocrit, and serum and urine sodium. Monitor for abdominal cramps, flushing, headache, or nausea.

**ADMINISTRATION IN ALTERNATE SETTINGS**

May be given in a variety of clinical settings and in the home by a qualified IV nurse.

**EVALUATION: OUTCOMES OF DRUG THERAPY**

**EXPECTED OUTCOMES**

PHYSICAL ASSESSMENT. Vital signs, especially blood pressure, remain within 15% of client's baseline. Intake and output are balanced and adequate for homeostasis. Daily weight fluctuations remain within 0.5 lb. Client does not complain of abdominal cramps, flushing, headache, or nausea. No evidence of bleeding.

LABORATORY. Serum osmolarity is between 280 and 295 mOsm/kg. Urine osmolarity is between 500 and 800 mOsm/L. Urine specific gravity is between 1.003 and 1.035. Hematocrit is between 44% and 52%. Serum sodium is between 135 and 145 mEq/L. Urine sodium is between 80 and 180 mEq/L.

**NEGATIVE OUTCOMES**

Vital signs, especially blood pressure, are more than 15% from client's baseline. Intake is less than output and is inadequate for homeostasis. Weight changes more than 0.5 lb daily. Client complains of abdominal cramps, flushing, headache, or nausea. Bleeding is excessive.

## Dexamethasone Sodium Phosphate

*Trade Names:* Dalalone, Decadron Phosphate, Decadrol
*Canadian Availability:* Decadron
*Pregnancy Risk:* Category C
*pH:* 7–8.5
*Storage/Stability:* Store below 40° C. Protect from freezing and from light.

### ASSESSMENT: DRUG CHARACTERISTICS

#### ACTION

A glucocorticoid with anti-inflammatory, immunosuppressant, and antiemetic effects. Replaces or supplements adrenal production of adrenocorticoids. Decreases inflammation by stabilizing the lysosomal membrane. Suppresses immune response by reducing T lymphocytes and decreasing immunoglobulin binding to receptor sites.

#### INDICATIONS

Used to treat adrenocortical insufficiency and to suppress inflammation. Also used to decrease cerebral edema. Used to treat cisplatin-induced vomiting, viral hepatitis, shock and thyroid crisis.

#### CAUTIONS

ADVERSE EFFECTS. Allergic reactions, sudden blindness, burning, numbness, weakness, delirium, hallucinations, manic-depressive episodes, depression, or paranoia; long-term effects include acne, avascular necrosis, hypokalemia, nausea, vomiting, muscle weakness, striae, or unusual bruising (Cushing's syndrome).

CONTRAINDICATIONS. Human immunodeficiency virus (HIV) infection, herpes simplex infections, cardiac disease, CHF, renal dysfunction, diabetes mellitus, fungal infections, myasthenia gravis, septic shock, or tuberculosis.

#### POTENTIAL DRUG/FOOD INTERACTIONS

May interact with amphotericin B, carbonic anhydrase inhibitors, or other diuretics to cause severe hypokalemia. Hypokalemia may increase the incidence of digitalis toxicity. Sodium-containing foods and medications used with dexamethasone may cause retention of fluid and edema. May increase blood glucose concentrations, and diabetic clients may require more insulin or other antidiabetic agents. May increase the potential of client's acquiring viral disease if client is given live virus vaccine. Incompatible with amikacin, doxorubicin, prochlorperazine, and vancomyin.

### INTERVENTIONS: ADMINISTRATION

May be given undiluted or added to D5W or 0.9% NSS; use diluted solutions within 24 h.

#### MODE/RATE OF ADMINISTRATION

Given by IV push over 1–2 min. May be given by

continuous IV infusion by electron flow control device.

INTRAVENOUS USE (WITH NORMAL RENAL FUNCTION)

**Adults:** For cerebral edema the usual initial dose is 10 mg followed by 4 mg doses q2–4h until symptoms decrease.

For shock the usual initial dose is 20 mg followed by 3 mg/kg of body weight in 24 h. Alternatively, may give 2–6 mg/kg of body weight as a single dose, or 40 mg as a single dose.

Maximum daily dose should not exceed 80 mg.

**Children:** IV route generally not used for children.

**Infants/Neonates:** IV route generally not used for infants and neonates.

**Geriatrics:** Older women are more likely to develop osteoporosis in long-term therapy.

INTRATHECAL USE OR OTHER INFUSION ROUTES AS INDICATED. May give intraarticularly, by intralesion route, or into soft tissue.

**POTENTIAL PROBLEMS IN ADMINISTRATION**

Read label carefully. Do not give dexamethasone acetate by IV route. Giving high doses of dexamethasone intravenously by IV push may cause anaphylactoid reactions, convulsions, and cardiac dysrhythmias.

**INDEPENDENT NURSING ACTIONS**

Monitor vital signs for hypertension or fever. Monitor intake and output. Observe client for evidence of delirium, hallucinations, manic-depressive episodes, depression, or paranoia. Observe for nausea, vomiting, muscle weakness, striae, unusual bruising, delayed healing, or allergic reactions.

**ADMINISTRATION IN ALTERNATE SETTINGS**

May be given in various clinical settings and in the home if client has been stabilized in an acute care setting first.

**EVALUATION: OUTCOMES OF DRUG THERAPY**

**EXPECTED OUTCOMES**

PHYSICAL ASSESSMENT. Vital signs remain within 15% of client's baseline. Client demonstrates no evidence of infection. Urinary output is more than 50 mL/h. Client has no delirium, hallucinations, manic-depressive episodes, depression, or paranoia. Client does not complain of nausea, vomiting, or muscle weakness. Client has no striae, unusual bruising, delayed healing, or allergic reactions. Symptoms of increased intracranial pressure (ICP) have abated.

LABORATORY. Serum potassium is between 3.5 and 5 mEq/L. Serum sodium is between 135 and 145 mEq/L.

**NEGATIVE OUTCOMES**

Client's blood pressure is more than 15% higher or lower than client's baseline, or temperature is more than 37.5° C. Client demonstrates evidence of infection. Urinary output is less than 50

▼

mL/h, or client shows evidence of edema. Client is delirious or has hallucinations, manic-depressive episodes, depression, or paranoia. Client complains of nausea, vomiting, or muscle weakness. Client has striae, unusual bruising, delayed healing, or allergic reactions. Symptoms of increased ICP remain unchanged.

## Diethylstilbestrol Diphosphate Sodium

*Trade Name:* Stilphostrol
*Canadian Availability:* Honvol
*Pregnancy Risk:* Category X
*pH:* 9–10.5
*Storage/Stability:* Store below 21° C. Protect from freezing.

### ASSESSMENT: DRUG CHARACTERISTICS

#### ACTION

An estrogen that acts as an antiprostatic cancer agent by decreasing the production of luteinizing hormone from the pituitary and by direct effect on the testes to decrease production of testosterone.

#### INDICATIONS

Used primarily as palliative treatment of prostatic cancer.

#### CAUTIONS

ADVERSE EFFECTS. Breast tenderness or pain, peripheral edema, gynecomastia, amenorrhea, menorrhagia, breakthrough vaginal bleeding, breast tumors, hepatitis, gallbladder obstruction, abdominal cramping, thrombophlebitis, nausea, vomiting, headache, dizziness, or anorexia.

CONTRAINDICATIONS. Most breast cancers, vaginal bleeding, hypercalcemia, or thrombophlebitis.

#### POTENTIAL DRUG/FOOD INTERACTIONS

May interact with bromocriptine to increase incidence of amenorrhea. May inhibit the effectiveness of cyclosporine. May increase the risk of hepatotoxicity if used with other hepatotoxic drugs. Incompatible with calcium gluconate.

### INTERVENTIONS: ADMINISTRATION

Mix 500 mg in 250 mL of 0.9% NSS or D5W solution.

#### MODE/RATE OF ADMINISTRATION

Given by intermittent IV infusion. Run at 1 mL/min for 10 min, then adjust rate to complete dose in 1 h.

INTRAVENOUS USE (WITH NORMAL RENAL FUNCTION)

**Adults:** For antineoplastic effect the usual initial dosage is 500 mg/d. Dose may be increased to 1 g/d for the next 5 or more days.

For maintenance the usual dose is 250–500 mg 1–2 times per week.

**Children:** Not given to children.

**Infants/Neonates:** Not given to infants or neonates.

**Geriatrics:** Follow adult dosing schedule.

INTRATHECAL USE OR OTHER INFUSION ROUTES AS INDICATED. Not recommended.

**POTENTIAL PROBLEMS IN ADMINISTRATION**

Client may complain of vaginal or perineal burning if agent administered too rapidly.

**INDEPENDENT NURSING ACTIONS**

Monitor vital signs. Monitor client for complaints of breast tenderness or pain, abdominal cramping, nausea, vomiting, headache, or anorexia. Monitor urinary output. Observe for peripheral edema, gynecomastia, amenorrhea, menorrhagia, break-through vaginal bleeding, breast tumors, hepatitis, gallbladder obstruction, or thrombophlebitis. Teach client to limit sodium intake.

**ADMINISTRATION IN ALTERNATE SETTINGS**

May be given in a variety of clinical settings and in the home by a qualified IV nurse.

**EVALUATION: OUTCOMES OF DRUG THERAPY**

**EXPECTED OUTCOMES**

PHYSICAL ASSESSMENT. Vital signs remain within 15% of client's baseline. Client has no complaints of breast tenderness or pain, abdominal cramping, nausea, vomiting, headache, or anorexia. Client does not have peripheral edema, gynecomastia, amenorrhea, menorrhagia, breakthrough vaginal bleeding, breast tumors, hepatitis, gallbladder obstruction, or thrombophlebitis.

LABORATORY. No significant laboratory values.

**NEGATIVE OUTCOMES**

Client's blood pressure is more than 15% above client's baseline. Client complains of breast tenderness or pain, abdominal cramping, nausea, vomiting, headache, or anorexia. Client has peripheral edema, gynecomastia, amenorrhea, menorrhagia, break-through vaginal bleeding, breast tumors, hepatitis, gallbladder obstruction, or thrombophlebitis.

## GLUCAGON HYDROCHLORIDE

*Trade Name:* Glucagon
*Canadian Availability:* Glucagon
*Pregnancy Risk:* Category B
*pH:* 2.5–3
*Storage/Stability:* Store between 15 and 30° C. After reconstituting with the diluent provided by the manufacturer, may be stored for 48 hours. Solution should be used immediately if reconstituted with sterile water for injection.

▼

## ASSESSMENT: DRUG CHARACTERISTICS

### ACTION

Antihypoglycemic and diagnostic agent that acts by stimulating the liver to convert glycogen to glucose (glycogenolysis) and to convert fats and protein to glucose (gluconeogenesis). Will not produce effects if liver stores of glycogen are depleted.

### INDICATIONS

Used to counter severe hypoglycemia and as a diagnostic aid to provide a hypotonic state in gastrointestinal radiography.

### CAUTIONS

ADVERSE EFFECTS. May cause allergic reactions, nausea, vomiting, or severe hypokalemia; but these effects are rare.

CONTRAINDICATIONS. Should not be given to clients with a history of allergic response to glucagon or as a diagnostic tool if client has a history of diabetes mellitus, insulinoma, or pheochromocytoma.

### POTENTIAL DRUG/FOOD INTERACTIONS

May increase the effects of warfarin anticoagulants.

## INTERVENTIONS: ADMINISTRATION

Given undiluted after reconstituting with manufacturer-provided diluent to a concentration of 1 USP unit per milliliter.

### MODE/RATE OF ADMINISTRATION

Given by IV push at a rate of 1 USP unit (1 mg) per minute.

INTRAVENOUS USE (WITH NORMAL RENAL FUNCTION)

**Adults and Children >12 Years:** For antihypoglycemic effect the usual dose is 0.5–1 USP unit (0.5–1 mg). Dose may be repeated in 10 min if needed.

As a diagnostic aid the usual dose is 0.25–1 USP unit (0.25–1 mg).

**Children <12 Years and Infants/Neonates:** For antihypoglycemic effect the usual dose is 0.025 USP unit (0.025 mg) per kilogram of body weight up to a maximum of 1 mg. Dose may be repeated in 10 min.

**Geriatrics:** Follow adult dosing schedule.

INTRATHECAL USE OR OTHER INFUSION ROUTES AS INDICATED. Not recommended.

### POTENTIAL PROBLEMS IN ADMINISTRATION

Client should show response within 5 minutes of IV injection. If client shows no response after second dose, further medical assistance is needed. Will probably cause nausea and vomiting.

### INDEPENDENT NURSING ACTIONS

Monitor vital signs. Monitor laboratory values, especially blood glucose and serum potassium levels. Observe for level of consciousness. Turn client to side to prevent aspiration of vomitus. Client should be able to ingest glucose within 15 to 20 minutes to prevent rebound hypoglycemia.

### ADMINISTRATION IN ALTERNATE SETTINGS

May be given in a variety

of clinical settings. Inappropriate for home setting.

**EVALUATION: OUTCOMES OF DRUG THERAPY**

**EXPECTED OUTCOMES**

PHYSICAL ASSESSMENT. Vital signs within 15% of client's baseline. Client alert and oriented. No complaints of nausea or vomiting. Able to ingest food.

LABORATORY. Blood glucose is between 80 and 120 mg/dL. Serum potassium is between 3.5 and 5 mEq/L.

**NEGATIVE OUTCOMES**

Vital signs more than 15% higher or lower than client's baseline. Client unresponsive. Client complains of nausea or is vomiting. Unable to ingest food.

## HYDROCORTISONE SODIUM SUCCINATE

*Trade Names:* Hydrocortone, Solu-Cortef
*Canadian Availability:* Solu-Cortef
*Pregnancy Risk:* Category C
*pH:* 7–8
*Storage/Stability:* Store below 40° C. Protect from freezing and from light.

**ASSESSMENT: DRUG CHARACTERISTICS**

**ACTION**

An adrenocorticoid with antiinflammatory, immunosuppressant, and antiemetic effects. Replaces or supplements adrenal production of adrenocorticoids. Decreases inflammation by stabilizing the lysosomal membrane. Suppresses immune response by reducing T lymphocytes and decreasing immunoglobulin binding to receptor sites.

**INDICATIONS**

Used to treat adrenocortical insufficiency and to suppress inflammation. Also used to treat shock.

**CAUTIONS**

ADVERSE EFFECTS. Allergic reactions, sudden blindness, burning, numbness, delirium, hallucinations, manic-depressive episodes, depression, or paranoia; long-term effects include acne, avascular necrosis, hypokalemia, nausea, vomiting, muscle weakness, striae, or unusual bruising.

CONTRAINDICATIONS. HIV infection, herpes simplex infections, cardiac disease, CHF, renal dysfunction, diabetes mellitus, fungal infections, myasthenia gravis, or tuberculosis.

**POTENTIAL DRUG/FOOD INTERACTIONS**

May interact with amphotericin B, carbonic anhydrase inhibitors, or other diuretics to cause severe hypokalemia. Hypokalemia may increase the incidence of digitalis toxicity. Sodium-containing foods and medications used with hydrocortisone may cause retention of fluid and edema. May in-

▼

crease blood glucose concentrations, and diabetic clients may require more insulin or other antidiabetic agents. May increase the potential of client's acquiring viral disease if client is given live virus vaccine. Incompatible with calcium gluconate, cephalosporins, erythromycin, kanamycin, methicillin, phenobarbital, prochlorperazine, promazine, tetracycline, vancomycin, and vitamin B complex with C.

**INTERVENTIONS: ADMINISTRATION**

May be given without diluting.

**MODE/RATE OF ADMINISTRATION**

May be given by IV push over 1–2 min or by continuous IV infusion.

INTRAVENOUS USE (WITH NORMAL RENAL/HEPATIC FUNCTION)

**Adults:** The usual dosage is 100–250 mg q2–6h. Total dose not to exceed 1g/24 h.

**Children:** 2–8 mg/kg body weight per 24 h. For acute adrenal insufficiency, give 1–2 mg/kg IV push, then 150–250 mg/kg in divided doses.

**Infants/Neonates:** Total dose not to exceed 150 mg/kg over 24 h in divided doses.

**Geriatrics:** Older women are more likely to develop osteoporosis in long-term therapy.

INTRATHECAL USE OR OTHER INFUSION ROUTES AS INDICATED. Read label carefully. Do not give hydrocortisone acetate by IV route. Giving high doses of hydrocortisone intravenously by IV push may cause anaphylactoid reactions, convulsions, and cardiac dysrhythmias.

**INDEPENDENT NURSING ACTIONS**

Monitor vital signs for hypertension or fever. Monitor intake and output. Observe client for evidence of delirium, hallucinations, manic-depressive episodes, depression, or paranoia. Observe for nausea, vomiting, muscle weakness, striae, unusual bruising, delayed healing, or allergic reactions.

**ADMINISTRATION IN ALTERNATE SETTINGS**

May be given in various clinical settings and in the home if client has been stabilized in an acute care setting first.

**EVALUATION: OUTCOMES OF DRUG THERAPY**

**EXPECTED OUTCOMES**

PHYSICAL ASSESSMENT. Vital signs remain within 15% of client's baseline. Client demonstrates no evidence of infection. Urinary output is more than 50 mL/h. Client has no delirium, hallucinations, manic-depressive episodes, depression, or paranoia. Client does not complain of nausea, vomiting, or muscle weakness. Client has no striae, unusual bruising, delayed healing, or allergic reactions.

LABORATORY. Serum potassium is between 3.5 and 5 mEq/L. Serum sodium is between 135 and 145 mEq/L.

**NEGATIVE OUTCOMES**

Client's blood pressure is more than 15% higher or

lower than client's baseline, or temperature is more than 37.5° C. Client demonstrates evidence of infection. Urinary output is less than 50 mL/h, or client shows evidence of edema. Client is delirious or has hallucinations, manic-depressive episodes, depression, or paranoia. Client complains of nausea, vomiting, or muscle weakness. Client has striae, unusual bruising, delayed healing, or allergic reactions.

## INSULIN

*Trade Names:* Iletin, Regular Insulin, Humulin R
*Canadian Availability:* Regular Iletin
*Pregnancy Risk:* Unknown
*pH:* 7.4
*Storage/Stability:* Store between 2° and 8° C. Do not use if discolored, cloudy, or thick.

### ASSESSMENT: DRUG CHARACTERISTICS

#### ACTION

An antidiabetic agent that controls fat, protein, and carbohydrate metabolism. Affects the storage and metabolism of fat, protein, and carbohydrates in liver, muscle, and adipose tissue.

#### INDICATIONS

Used to treat insulin-dependent diabetes mellitus and diabetic ketoacidosis. Also used in combination with glucose to treat hyperkalemia.

#### CAUTIONS

ADVERSE EFFECTS. Excessive doses may cause hypoglycemia, evidenced by anxiety, excessive hunger, nervousness, nausea, shakiness, tiredness, vision changes, or difficulty with concentration. Too little insulin may cause hyperglycemia, evidenced by drowsiness, flushed dry skin, anorexia, tiredness, thirst, increased urination, fruity breath odor, stomach cramps, nausea, or vomiting.

CONTRAINDICATIONS. Should not be given to clients who are unable to ingest food and who have no supplementary nutrition. Dose adjustment may be necessary for clients with infection, fever, surgery, diarrhea, renal or hepatic dysfunction, nausea, or vomiting.

#### POTENTIAL DRUG/FOOD INTERACTIONS

Drugs such as adrenocorticoids, amphetamines, furosemide, phenytoin, thyroid hormones, and diazide diuretics raise blood sugar levels and may decrease the effectiveness of insulin. Alcohol, disopyramide, MAO inhibitors, and salicylates may increase the hypoglycemic effects of insulin. β-Adrenergic blocking agents may cause either hyperglycemia or hypoglycemia.

### INTERVENTIONS: ADMINISTRATION

May be diluted with 0.9% or 0.45% NSS for continuous

▼

infusion. Can be given undiluted at 50 U over 1 min.

**MODE/RATE OF ADMINISTRATION**

Given by slow continuous infusion, using an electronic infusion device or IV push.

INTRAVENOUS USE (WITH NORMAL RENAL FUNCTION)

**Adults:** For diabetic ketoacidosis the usual dosage is 0.1 U/kg of body weight per hour. Rate should be decreased when blood glucose level reaches 250 mg/dL.

**Children:** For ketoacidosis, follow adult dosing schedule.

**Infants/Neonates:** For ketoacidosis, follow adult dosing schedule.

**Geriatrics:** Follow adult dosing schedule.

INTRATHECAL USE OR OTHER INFUSION ROUTES AS INDICATED. Not recommended.

**POTENTIAL PROBLEMS IN ADMINISTRATION**

*Only* regular or crystalline insulin may be given intravenously.

**INDEPENDENT NURSING ACTIONS**

Monitor vital signs and intake and output. Observe client for evidence of hypoglycemia and hyperglycemia. Monitor laboratory values, especially blood glucose levels. Note that regular or crystalline insulin is made from pork, beef, a combination of beef and pork, or genetically engineered (recombinant DNA) human insulin. Clients should not be switched from one type of crystalline insulin to another, since each product has some variability in absorption. In addition, there may be religious or cultural prohibitions to the use of a particular type of crystalline insulin.

**ADMINISTRATION IN ALTERNATE SETTINGS**

May be given in a variety of clinical settings and in the home setting by a qualified IV nurse.

**EVALUATION: OUTCOMES OF DRUG THERAPY**

**EXPECTED OUTCOMES**

PHYSICAL ASSESSMENT. Vital signs remain within 15% of client's baseline. Client does not demonstrate anxiety, excessive hunger, nervousness, nausea, shakiness, tiredness, vision changes, difficulty with concentration, drowsiness, flushed dry skin, anorexia, thirst, increased urination, fruity breath odor, stomach cramps, or vomiting.

LABORATORY. Serum glucose is between 80 and 120 mg/dL. Serum sodium is between 135 and 145 mEq/L. Serum potassium is between 3.5 and 5 mEq/L. Acetone negative. Hematocrit is 37% to 52%. Serum osmolality is between 280 and 296 mOsm/kg.

**NEGATIVE OUTCOMES**

Vital signs vary more than 15% higher or lower than client's baseline. Client demonstrates anxiety, excessive hunger, nervousness, nausea, shakiness, tiredness, vision changes, difficulty with concentration, drowsiness, flushed dry skin, anorexia, thirst, increased urination, fruity breath odor, stomach cramps, or vomiting.

## Levothyroxine Sodium

*Trade Names:* Levothroid, Synthroid
*Canadian Availability:* Synthroid
*Pregnancy Risk:* Category A
*pH:* Not specified
*Storage/Stability:* Store below 40° C. Protect from light. Solution should be used immediately after being reconstituted.

### ASSESSMENT: DRUG CHARACTERISTICS

#### ACTION

A thyroid hormone with antineoplastic effects. Contains $T_4$. Acts by stimulating cellular metabolism, growth, and development in all body tissues. Increases protein synthesis and the use and mobilization of glycogen.

#### INDICATIONS

Used to treat hypothyroidism, goiter, and thyroid carcinoma and as a diagnostic agent for thyroid function.

#### CAUTIONS

ADVERSE EFFECTS. Allergic response; symptoms of hyperthyroidism such as chest pain, diarrhea, tachycardia, hand tremors, or irritability; symptoms of hypothyroidism such as dry puffy skin, weight gain, listlessness, coldness, clumsiness, or changes in menstruation; severe headaches in children.

CONTRAINDICATIONS. Should not be given to clients with adrenocortical insufficiency, cardiovascular disease, history of hyperthyroidism, pituitary insufficiency, or history of hypersensitivity to levothyroxine. Should be given with caution to a client with a long history of untreated hypothyroidism because the client is likely to be more sensitive to levothyroxine.

#### POTENTIAL DRUG/FOOD INTERACTIONS

May increase the anticoagulant effects of warfarin anticoagulants. Cholestyramine or colestipol may decrease the effects of levothyroxine by binding the agent or preventing absorption. May increase the cardiovascular effects of sympathomimetic drugs and increase the risk of cardiac insufficiency.

### INTERVENTIONS: ADMINISTRATION

Reconstitute by adding 2 mL of NSS for injection to a 200-mcg (0.2-mg) vial for a concentration of 100 mcg (0.1 mg)/mL.

#### MODE/RATE OF ADMINISTRATION

Given IV push at a rate of 100 mcg (0.1 mg)/min.

#### INTRAVENOUS USE (WITH NORMAL RENAL FUNCTION)

**Adults:** For antihypothyroid effect the usual dosage is 50–100 mcg (0.05–0.1 mg) daily.

For myxedema coma the usual dosage is 200–500 mcg (0.2–0.5 mg) q.d. Dose may be increased an additional 100–300 mcg (0.1–0.3 mg) if no improvement is observed.

**Children $>$ 10 Years:** The usual dosage is 2–3 mcg

▼

(0.002–0.003 mg)/kg of body weight per day.

**Children 6–10 Years:** The usual dosage is 4–5 mcg (0.004–0.005 mg)/kg of body weight per day.

**Children 1–5 Years:** The usual dosage is 5–6 mcg (0.005–0.006 mg)/kg of body weight per day.

**Infants 6 Months–1 Year:** The usual dosage is 6–8 mcg (0.006–0.008 mg)/kg of body weight per day.

**Neonates and Infants 0–6 Months:** The usual dosage is 8–10 mcg (0.008–0.01 mg)/kg of body weight per day.

**Geriatrics:** Follow adult dosing schedule.

INTRATHECAL USE OR OTHER INFUSION ROUTES AS INDICATED. Not recommended.

#### POTENTIAL PROBLEMS IN ADMINISTRATION

Too large a dose given to clients with myxedema or cardiac disease may cause severe cardiac symptoms.

#### INDEPENDENT NURSING ACTIONS

Monitor vital signs, especially temperature, pulse rate and regularity, and blood pressure. Observe for evidence of hyperthyroidism or hypothyroidism. Monitor laboratory values, especially thyroid function studies.

#### ADMINISTRATION IN ALTERNATE SETTINGS

IV administration should be done in clinical settings where the client can be closely monitored.

### EVALUATION: OUTCOMES OF DRUG THERAPY

#### EXPECTED OUTCOMES

PHYSICAL ASSESSMENT. Vital signs remain within 15% of client's baseline. Client does not demonstrate symptoms of hyperthyroidism such as chest pain, diarrhea, tachycardia, hand tremors, or irritability. Client does not demonstrate symptoms of hypothyroidism such as dry puffy skin, weight gain, listlessness, coldness, clumsiness, or changes in menstruation. Client does not complain of headache.

LABORATORY. Total $T_4$ is between 4 and 12 mg/dL. Total $T_3$ is between 75 and 195 ng/dL.

#### NEGATIVE OUTCOMES

Vital signs are more than 15% higher or lower than client's baseline, with fever, tachycardia, or hypertension. Client demonstrates symptoms of hyperthyroidism such as chest pain, diarrhea, tachycardia, hand tremors, or irritability. Client demonstrates symptoms of hypothyroidism such as dry puffy skin, weight gain, listlessness, coldness, clumsiness, or changes in menstruation. Client complains of headache.

## Methylprednisolone Sodium Succinate

*Trade Name:* Solu-Medrol
*Canadian Availability:* Solu-Medrol
*Pregnancy Risk:* Category C
*pH:* 7–8
*Storage/Stability:* Store below 40° C. Use reconstituted solution within 48 hours. Do not use if solution is cloudy or if solution contains a precipitate.

### ASSESSMENT: DRUG CHARACTERISTICS

#### ACTION

An adrenocorticoid with antiinflammatory and immunosuppressant effects. Replaces or supplements adrenal production of adrenocorticoids. Decreases inflammation by stabilizing the lysosomal membrane. Suppresses immune response by reducing T lymphocytes and decreasing immunoglobulin binding to receptor sites. Less likely to cause electrolyte imbalances.

#### INDICATIONS

Used to treat adrenocortical insufficiency and to suppress inflammation. Also used in the treatment of hypersensitivity reactions, severe shock, ulcerative colitis, severe infections, esophageal burns, and multiple sclerosis.

#### CAUTIONS

ADVERSE EFFECTS. Allergic reactions, sudden blindness, burning, numbness, delirium, hallucinations, manic-depressive episodes, depression, paranoia, and hypertension; long-term effects include acne, avascular necrosis, hypokalemia, nausea, vomiting, muscle weakness, striae, or unusual bruising.

CONTRAINDICATIONS. HIV infection, herpes simplex infections, cardiac disease, CHF, renal dysfunction, diabetes mellitus, fungal infections, myasthenia gravis, or tuberculosis.

#### POTENTIAL DRUG/FOOD INTERACTIONS

May interact with amphotericin B, carbonic anhydrase inhibitors, or other diuretics to cause severe hypokalemia. Hypokalemia may increase the incidence of digitalis toxicity. Sodium-containing foods and medications used with methylprednisolone may cause retention of fluid and edema. May increase blood glucose concentrations, and diabetic clients may require more insulin or other antidiabetic agents. May increase the potential of client's acquiring viral disease if client is given live virus vaccine. Incompatible with aminophylline, calcium gluconate, insulin, nafcillin, tetracyclines, promethazine, and vitamin B complex.

### INTERVENTIONS: ADMINISTRATION

Diluted with diluent supplied in Mix-O-Vial only.

#### MODE/RATE OF ADMINISTRATION

Usually given IV push at a rate of 500 mg over 1–2 min.

▼

May be given as intermittent IV infusion over 30 min.

INTRAVENOUS USE (WITH NORMAL RENAL FUNCTION)

**Adults:** The usual dose is 10–40 mg, repeated as needed.

For "pulse" therapy the usual dose is 30 mg/kg of body weight over at least 30 min. Dose may be repeated q4–6h if needed.

For multiple sclerosis the usual dosage is 160 mg/d for 7 d, followed by 64 mg every other day for 1 mo.

**Children > 13 Years:** For adrenocortical insufficiency the usual dosage is 117 mcg (0.117 mg)/kg of body weight in three divided doses every third day or 39–58.5 mcg (0.039–0.585 mg)/kg of body weight per day. For acute spinal injury the usual dosage is 30 mg/kg of body weight over 15 min. After 15 min a continuous infusion of 5.4 mg/kg of body weight per hour for 23h.

**Children < 13 Years:** Dosage not established.

**Geriatrics:** Older women are more likely to develop osteoporosis in long-term therapy.

INTRATHECAL USE OR OTHER INFUSION ROUTES AS INDICATED. Not recommended.

**POTENTIAL PROBLEMS IN ADMINISTRATION**

Read label carefully. Do not give methylprednisolone acetate by IV route. Giving high doses of methylprednisolone by IV push may cause anaphylactoid reactions, convulsions, and cardiac dysrhythmias.

**INDEPENDENT NURSING ACTIONS**

Monitor vital signs for hypertension or fever. Monitor intake and output. Observe client for evidence of delirium, hallucinations, manic-depressive episodes, depression, or paranoia. Observe for nausea, vomiting, muscle weakness, striae, unusual bruising, delayed healing, or allergic reactions.

**ADMINISTRATION IN ALTERNATE SETTINGS**

May be given in various clinical settings and in the home if client has been stabilized in an acute care setting first.

**EVALUATION: OUTCOMES OF DRUG THERAPY**

**EXPECTED OUTCOMES**

PHYSICAL ASSESSMENT. Vital signs remain within 15% of client's baseline. Client demonstrates no evidence of infection. Urinary output is more than 50 mL/h. Client has no delirium, hallucinations, manic-depressive episodes, depression, or paranoia. Client does not complain of nausea, vomiting, or muscle weakness. Client has no striae, unusual bruising, delayed healing, or allergic reactions. Signs and symptoms of spinal cord trauma diminished.

LABORATORY. Serum potassium is between 3.5 and 5 mEq/L. Serum sodium is between 135 and 145 mEq/L.

#### NEGATIVE OUTCOMES

Blood pressure is more than 15% higher or lower than client's baseline, or temperature is more than 37.5° C. Client demonstrates evidence of infection. Urinary output is less than 50 mL/h, or client shows evidence of edema. Client is delirious, has hallucinations, manic-depressive episodes, depression, or paranoia. Client complains of nausea, vomiting, or muscle weakness. Client has striae, unusual bruising, delayed healing, or allergic reactions. Signs and symptoms of spinal cord trauma are not alleviated.

---

## OXYTOCIN

*Trade Names:* Pitocin, Syntocinon
*Canadian Availability:* Oxytocin
*Pregnancy Risk:* Category X
*pH:* 2.5–4.5
*Storage/Stability:* Store below 40° C. Protect from freezing.

### ASSESSMENT: DRUG CHARACTERISTICS

#### ACTION

A uterine stimulant that may be used to control postpartum bleeding or as a diagnostic aid. Acts by stimulating uterine smooth muscle contraction to simulate labor and slows uterine blood flow.

#### INDICATIONS

Used to induce or stimulate labor and in the management of incomplete or therapeutic abortions. May also be used to help control postpartum uterine hemorrhage.

#### CAUTIONS

ADVERSE EFFECTS. Nausea, vomiting, and maternal premature ventricular contractions; fetal bradycardia, postpartal hemorrhage, cardiac arrhythmias, psychotic reactions, seizures, or tachycardia.

CONTRAINDICATIONS. Should not be given to clients who are allergic to oxytocin. If given during labor, should not be given to clients with cephalopelvic disproportion, prolapsed cord, placenta previa, fetal distress, hypertonic uterine responses, obstetric emergencies requiring surgery, or prolonged use for uterine inertia or toxemia.

#### POTENTIAL DRUG/FOOD INTERACTIONS

May interact with hydrocarbon anesthetic agents to cause maternal hypotension. May increase the pressor effects of vasopressor agents. If used with other oxytocics, may cause marked uterine hypertonia or rupture. Incompatible with levarterenol, prochlorperazine, and warfarin.

▼

**INTERVENTIONS: ADMINISTRATION**

Must be diluted. For stimulation of labor, add 10 USP U to 1000 mL of 0.9% NSS to produce a concentration of 10 milliunits (0.01 U)/mL. To control postpartum hemorrhage, add 20–40 USP units to 1000 mL of 0.9% NSS to produce a concentration of 20–40 milliunits (0.02–0.04 U)/mL.

**MODE/RATE OF ADMINISTRATION**

Given by continuous IV infusion using an electronic flow device. Given through a side port to allow for rapid disconnection while maintaining a freely flowing IV infusion for emergency use.

INTRAVENOUS USE (WITH NORMAL RENAL FUNCTION)

**Adults:** To induce labor the usual initial dosage is 1–2 milliunits (0.001–0.002 U) of 10 U/1000 mL solution per minute. Dosage may be increased by 1–2 milliunits (0.001–0.002 U) q15–30min until contractions appear like normal labor. Maximum dosage is 20 milliunits (0.02 U)/min.

For incomplete or therapeutic abortion the usual dosage is 20–40 milliunits (0.02–0.04 U) of 20–40 U/1000 mL solution per minute.

For postpartal hemorrhage the usual dosage is 20–40 milliunits (0.02–0.04 U) of 20–40 U/1000 mL solution per minute.

**Children:** Inappropriate.

**Infants/Neonates:** Inappropriate.

**Geriatrics:** Inappropriate.

INTRATHECAL USE OR OTHER INFUSION ROUTES AS INDICATED. Not recommended.

**POTENTIAL PROBLEMS IN ADMINISTRATION**

Large doses given to clients with hypertonic response to oxytocin may cause uterine spasm, tetany, rupture, abruptio placentae, decreased uterine blood flow, amniotic fluid embolism, and fetal trauma. Large doses of oxytocin with high volumes of fluid may cause water intoxication. May retard placental expulsion. May cause hypotension, reflex hypertension, or tachycardia.

**INDEPENDENT NURSING ACTIONS**

Monitor maternal vital signs, especially pulse rate, regularity, and blood pressure. Monitor fetal heart rate constantly. Monitor for signs of fetal distress with contractions. Monitor contractions timing and strength q15min or as needed. Monitor intake and output and observe for evidence of fluid retention.

**ADMINISTRATION IN ALTERNATE SETTINGS**

Should be given in acute settings where client can be continuously monitored.

**EVALUATION: OUTCOMES OF DRUG THERAPY**

**EXPECTED OUTCOMES**

PHYSICAL ASSESSMENT. Maternal vital signs, especially pulse rate, regularity, and blood pressure, remain within 15% of client's baseline. Fetal heart rate remains constant with no signs of fetal heart deceleration or distress with contractions. Contractions continue at 3 to 4 minutes apart or less and moderate to strong. No evidence of fluid retention.

LABORATORY. Serum sodium is between 135 and 145 mEq/L.

**NEGATIVE OUTCOMES**

Maternal vital signs, especially pulse rate, regularity, and blood pressure, are more than 15% higher or lower than client's baseline. Client may be hypotensive or hypertensive. Client may have tachycardia or premature ventricular contractions. Fetal heart rate is irregular. Fetal distress is apparent with contractions. Contractions are hypertonic. Evidence of fluid retention.

## VASOPRESSIN

*Trade Name:* Pitressin
*Canadian Availability:* Pitressin, Pressyn
*Pregnancy Risk:* Category C
*pH:* 2.5–4.5
*Storage/Stability:* Store at 4° C. Protect from freezing.

**ASSESSMENT: DRUG CHARACTERISTICS**

**ACTION**

A posterior pituitary hormone with antidiuretic and antihemorrhagic effects. Acts by increasing water reabsorption from the collecting ducts. Also causes contraction of vascular and gastrointestinal smooth muscle and increases the secretion of corticotropin, follicle-stimulating hormone (FSH), and growth hormone.

**INDICATIONS**

Used to treat diabetes insipidus.

**CAUTIONS**

ADVERSE EFFECTS. Allergic response, chest pain or myocardial infarction, water intoxication with drowsiness, coma, confusion, headache, seizures, or weight gain; hypernatremia, abdominal cramps, flushing, diarrhea, nausea, or vomiting.

CONTRAINDICATIONS. Coronary artery disease, hypertension, or renal dysfunction.

**POTENTIAL DRUG/FOOD INTERACTIONS**

Carbamazepine, chlorpropamide, or clofibrate lithium may increase the antidiuretic effect of vasopressin. Norepinephrine may decrease the antidiuretic effect of vasopressin.

**INTERVENTIONS: ADMINISTRATION**

Add 1 vial of 20 USP posterior pituitary units per milliliter to an amount of 0.9% NSS to achieve a concentration of 0.1–1 U/mL.

**MODE/RATE OF ADMINISTRATION**

Given by continuous IV infusion, using an infusion pump.

▼

INTRAVENOUS USE (WITH NORMAL RENAL FUNCTION)

**Adults:** For diabetes insipidus the usual dosage is 0.2–0.4 U/min.

For antihemorrhagic effect the usual dosage is 0.2–0.4 U/min. Dosage is increased to a maximum of 0.9 U/min, depending on client response.

**Children:** Dose not established for IV administration.

**Infants/Neonates:** Dose not established for IV administration.

**Geriatrics:** Elderly clients are sensitive to effects of vasopressin and must be closely monitored for hypernatremia and water intoxication.

INTRATHECAL USE OR OTHER INFUSION ROUTES AS INDICATED. May be given intraarterially via the superior mesenteric artery, inferior mesenteric artery, or the splenic/celiac artery. Infusion catheter placement should be verified by angiography. Client response to vasopressor activity should be carefully evaluated by angiography within 20 to 30 minutes after infusion has begun.

**POTENTIAL PROBLEMS IN ADMINISTRATION**

Caution should be taken to avoid extravasation. May cause tissue necrosis.

**INDEPENDENT NURSING ACTIONS**

Monitor vital signs, especially blood pressure. Monitor intake and output. Weigh the client daily. Monitor laboratory values, especially serum and urine osmolarity, hematocrit, and serum and urine sodium. Client is alert and oriented. Observe for seizures, diarrhea, or vomiting. Monitor for abdominal cramps, flushing, headache, or nausea.

**ADMINISTRATION IN ALTERNATE SETTINGS**

May be given in a variety of clinical settings and in the home by a qualified IV nurse.

**EVALUATION: OUTCOMES OF DRUG THERAPY**

**EXPECTED OUTCOMES**

PHYSICAL ASSESSMENT. Vital signs, especially blood pressure, remain within 15% of client's baseline. Intake and output are balanced and adequate for homeostasis. Daily weight fluctuations remain within 0.5 lb. Client is alert and oriented. Client has no seizures, diarrhea, or vomiting. Client does not complain of chest pain, abdominal cramps, flushing, headache, or nausea.

LABORATORY. Serum osmolarity is between 280 and 295 mOsm/kg. Urine osmolarity is between 500 and 800 mOsm/L. Urine specific gravity is between 1.003 and 1.035. Hematocrit is between 44% and 52%. Serum sodium is between 135 and 145 mEq/L. Urine sodium is between 80 and 180 mEq/L.

**NEGATIVE OUTCOMES**

Vital signs, especially blood pressure, are more than 15% higher or lower than client's baseline. Intake is less than output and is in adequate for homeostasis. Weight changes more than 0.5 lb daily. Client is drowsy or confused. Client has seizures, diarrhea, or vomiting. Client complains of abdominal cramps, flushing, headache, or nausea.

## Vitamins

### ASCORBIC ACID

*Trade Names:* Cee-500, Cetane 500, Cenolate
*Canadian Availability:* Ascorbic acid
*Pregnancy Risk:* Category C
*pH:* 5.5–7
*Storage/Stability:* Store below 40° C. Protect from freezing and from light.

**ASSESSMENT: DRUG CHARACTERISTICS**

**ACTION**

A water-soluble vitamin that is essential for collagen and soft tissue formation and repair. Ascorbic acid is involved in carbohydrate metabolism, lipid synthesis, the metabolism of several amino acids, and protein synthesis and is necessary for blood vessel integrity.

**INDICATIONS**

Used to treat vitamin C deficiency and as a reducing agent for the in vitro labeling of red blood cells. May be used as a dietary supplement, especially for clients receiving total parenteral nutrition (TPN) for conditions such as severe burns or extensive trauma.

**CAUTIONS**

ADVERSE EFFECTS. Kidney stone, diarrhea with large doses; dizziness or faintness if injection is too rapid; headache, mild increase in urine output, nausea, vomiting, or abdominal cramps.

CONTRAINDICATIONS. Should be given with caution to clients with a history of renal stones or sensitivity to ascorbic acid. High doses of ascorbic acid may interfere with blood glucose level determination in diabetic clients or cause a crisis for clients with sickle cell anemia.

**POTENTIAL DRUG/FOOD INTERACTIONS**

May cause cardiac decompensation from increased iron toxicity if used with deferoxamine. May cause the destruction of vitamin $B_{12}$ if used in large doses.

**INTERVENTIONS: ADMINISTRATION**

May be given undiluted. May be diluted in most common IV solutions.

**MODE/RATE OF ADMINISTRATION**

Given IV push in doses of 100 mg or less over 1 min.

INTRAVENOUS USE (WITH NORMAL RENAL FUNCTION)

**Adults:** For dietary supplement the usual dosage is 100–250 mg 1–3 times q.d.

Maximum daily dose should not exceed 6 g.

▼

**Children:** Follow adult dosing schedule.

**Infants/Neonates:** For dietary supplement in infants the usual dose is 100–300 mg in divided doses over 24 h.

For nutritional supplement in premature infants the usual dose is 75–100 mg in divided doses over 24 h.

**Geriatrics:** Follow adult dosing schedule.

INTRATHECAL USE OR OTHER INFUSION ROUTES AS INDICATED. Not recommended.

#### POTENTIAL PROBLEMS IN ADMINISTRATION

None anticipated.

#### INDEPENDENT NURSING ACTIONS

Monitor client's vital signs. Monitor intake and output. Observe client for diarrhea or vomiting. Monitor client for dizziness, faintness, nausea, or stomach cramps. Monitor wound healing.

#### ADMINISTRATION IN ALTERNATE SETTINGS

May be given in a variety of clinical settings and in the home by a qualified IV nurse.

#### EVALUATION: OUTCOMES OF DRUG THERAPY

#### EXPECTED OUTCOMES

PHYSICAL ASSESSMENT. Vital signs remain within 15% of client's baseline. Intake and output are balanced. Client has no diarrhea or vomiting. Client has no complaints of dizziness, faintness, headache, nausea, or stomach cramps. Client exhibits wound closure or soft tissue repair.

LABORATORY. Urine pH is 4.5 to 8.

#### NEGATIVE OUTCOMES

Vital signs are more than 15% higher or lower than client's baseline. Output exceeds intake. Client has diarrhea or vomiting. Client complains of dizziness, faintness, headache, nausea, or stomach cramps. There is no evidence of wound closure or soft tissue repair.

---

## MULTIVITAMIN INFUSION (MVI)

*Trade Names:* MVC 9 + 3, MVI-12
*Canadian Availability:* None specified
*Pregnancy Risk:* Category A
*pH:* Not specified
*Storage/Stability:* Store between 15 and 30° C. Protect from light. Solution is bright yellow and will color solutions yellow. Infusions are stable for up to 24 hours.

#### ASSESSMENT: DRUG CHARACTERISTICS

#### ACTION

Water- and fat-soluble vitamins that serve to replace or increase naturally manufactured vitamins.

#### INDICATIONS

Used to treat vitamin deficiencies or to provide optimum levels of vitamins needed for tissue maintenance or repair after trauma, surgery, or burns.

**CAUTIONS**

ADVERSE EFFECTS. Allergic reaction, especially if client is sensitive to thiamine hydrochloride.

CONTRAINDICATIONS. Known allergic responses to MVI.

**POTENTIAL DRUG/FOOD INTERACTIONS**

Large amounts of pyridoxine ($B_6$) may inhibit action of levodopa.

**INTERVENTIONS: ADMINISTRATION**

Each 5- to 10-mL vial must be diluted with at least 500 mL of solution. May be diluted in 0.9% NSS, D5W, combinations of dextrose and normal saline, most other electrolyte replacement solutions, and protein amino acid solutions.

**MODE/RATE OF ADMINISTRATION**

Usually given by continuous IV infusion, using an infusion pump.

INTRAVENOUS USE (WITH NORMAL RENAL FUNCTION)

**Adults:** Usual dosage is 5–10 mL q24h.

**Children:** Follow adult dosing schedule.

**Infants/Neonates:** Dose not established.

**Geriatrics:** Follow adult dosing schedule.

INTRATHECAL USE OR OTHER INFUSION ROUTES AS INDICATED. Not recommended.

**POTENTIAL PROBLEMS IN ADMINISTRATION**

May cause allergic reactions.

**INDEPENDENT NURSING ACTIONS**

Monitor client's nutritional status, especially body weight and wound healing. Monitor laboratory values, especially total protein and albumin-globulin (A-G) ratio.

**ADMINISTRATION IN ALTERNATE SETTINGS**

May be given in a variety of clinical settings and in the home by a qualified IV nurse.

**EVALUATION: OUTCOMES OF DRUG THERAPY**

**EXPECTED OUTCOMES**

PHYSICAL ASSESSMENT. Client has no loss of body weight. Wound healing is not delayed.

LABORATORY. Total protein is 6 to 8.4 g/dL. A-G ratio is 1.5:1 to 2.5:1.

**NEGATIVE OUTCOMES**

Client has a loss of body weight more than 0.5 lb/wk. Wound healing is delayed.

## PHYTONADIONE

*Trade Names:* AquaMEPHYTON, Konakion, Vitamin K
*Canadian Availability:* Konakion
*Pregnancy Risk:* Unknown
*pH:* 3.5–7

*Storage/Stability:* Store below 40° C. Protect from freezing and light. Prepare solutions just prior to using and discard any unused solution promptly.

▼

### ASSESSMENT: DRUG CHARACTERISTICS

#### ACTION

A synthetic fat-soluble vitamin K that acts to promote hepatic formation of prothrombin and other essential factors for normal blood clotting. Excreted as metabolized in the urine.

#### INDICATIONS

Used to treat anticoagulant or treatment-induced prothrombin deficiencies, such as seen in warfarin overdose. Such deficiencies may result from gastrointestinal surgery, prolonged use of TPN, inflammatory diseases of the bowel, and various malabsorption syndromes. May also be used to treat hemorrhagic disease in newborns.

#### CAUTIONS

ADVERSE EFFECTS. Severe allergic reaction, flushing of the face, redness or pain at IV site, or complaints of a peculiar taste; cyanosis, diaphoresis, dyspnea, hypotension, tachycardia, or death.

CONTRAINDICATIONS. Hepatic dysfunction or known allergy to phytonadione.

#### POTENTIAL DRUG/FOOD INTERACTIONS

May decrease the effectiveness of warfarin or indandione-based anticoagulants. Use with antidiabetic agents, methyldopa, penicillin, quinidine, quinine, or sulfonamides may increase the hemolytic side effect of the drugs. Incompatible with ascorbic acid, dextran, phenobarbital, phenytoin, and vancomycin.

### INTERVENTIONS: ADMINISTRATION

Dilute with 0.9% NSS, D5W, or normal saline and dextrose combinations; add 10 mL of diluent.

#### MODE/RATE OF ADMINISTRATION

Given IV push at a rate not to exceed 1 mg/min.

INTRAVENOUS USE (WITH NORMAL RENAL FUNCTION)

**Adults:** For anticoagulant-induced hypoprothrombinemia the usual dose is 2.5–25 mg. Maximum dose should not exceed 50 mg.

For hypoprothrombinemia from other causes the usual dose is 2–25 mg.

For prolonged TPN the usual dosage is 5–10 mg/wk.

**Children:** For hypoprothrombinemia the usual dose is 5–10 mg.

For prolonged TPN the usual dosage is 2–5 mg/wk.

**Infants/Neonates:** Not usually given IV.

**Geriatrics:** Follow adult dosing schedule.

INTRATHECAL USE OR OTHER INFUSION ROUTES AS INDICATED. Not recommended.

#### POTENTIAL PROBLEMS IN ADMINISTRATION

May cause a severe allergic response if administered too rapidly.

#### INDEPENDENT NURSING ACTIONS

Monitor vital signs, especially blood pressure and pulse. Monitor client for evidence of bleeding such as bleeding from the gums, pink or red urine, or abnormal bruising. Monitor laboratory values, especially the prothrombin time.

**ADMINISTRATION IN ALTERNATE SETTINGS**

Not recommended.

**EVALUATION: OUTCOMES OF DRUG THERAPY**

**EXPECTED OUTCOMES**

PHYSICAL ASSESSMENT. Vital signs remain within 15% of client's baseline. Client demonstrates no evidence of bleeding or abnormal bruising.

LABORATORY. Prothrombin time deviates less than 2 seconds from control.

**NEGATIVE OUTCOMES**

Blood pressure is more than 15% less than client's baseline. Client's pulse is rapid, thready, or weak. Client is pale, restless, or confused, and client has bleeding gums, pink or red urine, or abnormal bruising on body.

## THIAMINE HYDROCHLORIDE

*Trade Names:* Betalin S, Biamine
*Canadian Availability:* Betaxin
*Pregnancy Risk:* Category A
*pH:* 2.5–4.5
*Storage/Stability:* Store below 40° C. Protect from freezing and from light.

**ASSESSMENT: DRUG CHARACTERISTICS**

**ACTION**

A water-soluble vitamin also known as vitamin $B_1$. Forms an essential coenzyme needed for carbohydrate metabolism.

**INDICATIONS**

Used to treat deficiency of vitamin $B_1$.

**CAUTIONS**

ADVERSE EFFECTS. Severe allergic response.

CONTRAINDICATIONS. History of sensitivity to thiamine.

**POTENTIAL DRUG/FOOD INTERACTIONS**

None reported.

**INTERVENTIONS: ADMINISTRATION**

Does not need to be diluted. May be diluted in most common IV solutions.

**MODE/RATE OF ADMINISTRATION**

Given by IV push over 5 min. May be given by intermittent or by continuous IV infusion.

INTRAVENOUS USE (WITH NORMAL RENAL FUNCTION)

**Adults:** For nutritional deficiency the usual dosage is 5–100 mg t.i.d.

**Children:** For nutritional deficiency the usual dosage is 10–25 mg/d.

**Infants/Neonates:** Follow children's dosing schedule.

**Geriatrics:** Follow adult dosing schedule.

INTRATHECAL USE OR OTHER INFUSION ROUTES AS INDICATED. Not recommended.

▼

**POTENTIAL PROBLEMS IN ADMINISTRATION**

IV administration should be done only if client is unable to take oral forms of thiamine. A test dose should be given intradermally prior to giving the first IV dose.

**INDEPENDENT NURSING ACTIONS**

Monitor client's vital signs. Monitor intake and output and body weight. Observe client for difficulty breathing, urticaria, swelling of face, or wheezing.

**ADMINISTRATION IN ALTERNATE SETTINGS**

Should be given intravenously in clinical settings where the client can be monitored. After establishing that client is not allergic, can be given by a qualified IV nurse in a variety of settings including the home.

**EVALUATION: OUTCOMES OF DRUG THERAPY**

**EXPECTED OUTCOMES**

PHYSICAL ASSESSMENT. Vital signs remain within 15% of client's baseline. Client has no urticaria, swelling of face, or wheezing. Client has no complaints of difficulty breathing. Client's body weight remains stable or increases, depending on goals of therapy.

LABORATORY. No significant laboratory values.

**NEGATIVE OUTCOMES**

Vital signs are more than 15% higher or lower than client's baseline. Client has urticaria, swelling of face, or wheezing. Client complains of difficulty breathing. Client's body weight decreases.

## Other Infusion Agents

### ALPHA$_1$ PROTEINASE INHIBITOR

*Trade Name:* Prolastin
*Canadian Availability:* Prolastin
*Pregnancy Risk:* Category C
*pH:* 6.6–7.4
*Storage/Stability:* Store in refrigerator. Do not refrigerate after reconstitution. Use within 3 hours and discard any unused portion.

**ASSESSMENT: DRUG CHARACTERISTICS**

**ACTION**

Replacement therapy for clients with alpha$_1$ antitrypsin deficiency. Restores balance between elastase (enzyme responsible for degradation of elastin tissue in lower respiratory tract) and alpha$_2$ proteinase inhibitor (inhibits neutrophil elastase).

**INDICATIONS**

Used as a treatment of the potentially fatal congenital alpha$_1$ antitrypsin deficiency and for long-term treatment of demonstrated panacinar emphysema associated with alpha$_1$ antitrypsin deficiency. Not appropriate for clients with irreversible destruction of lung tissue due to $alpha_1$ antitrypsin deficiency.

**CAUTIONS**

ADVERSE EFFECTS. Light-headedness, dizziness, transient leukocytosis a few hours after administration.

CONTRAINDICATIONS. Hypersensitivity to polyethylene glycol; $alpha_1$ antitrypsin deficiency when risk of panacinar emphysema is limited (phenotypes of PiMZ and PiMS); immunoglobulin A (IgA) deficiency with anti-IgA antibodies has an increased risk of hypersensitivity reactions.

**POTENTIAL DRUG/FOOD INTERACTIONS**

Sufficient information is unavailable. Do not mix with other drugs.

**INTERVENTIONS: ADMINISTRATION**

Bring bottles to room temperature. Using sterile water for injection provided by the manufacturer, reconstitute to yield a concentration of 20 mg/mL. If necessary, may dilute with 0.9% NSS.

**MODE/RATE OF ADMINISTRATION**

Administer by direct infusion at a rate of at least 0.8 mg/kg/min.

INTRAVENOUS USE (WITH NORMAL RENAL FUNCTION)

**Adults:** Usually 60 mg/kg/wk.

**Children:** Use not established.

**Infants/Neonates:** Use not established.

**Geriatrics:** Follow adult dosing schedule.

INTRATHECAL USE OR OTHER INFUSION ROUTES AS INDICATED. Not recommended.

**POTENTIAL PROBLEMS IN ADMINISTRATION**

$Alpha_1$ proteinase inhibitor is obtained from human plasma. Although each unit is tested and found nonreactive to HIV antibody and hepatitis B surface antigen, the possibility of contracting these viruses exists. Clients should be immunized against hepatitis B before beginning treatment.

**INDEPENDENT NURSING ACTIONS**

Inform client of risks and safety precautions observed in the manufacturing process. Assess lung sounds and character and rate of respirations before each treatment. Instruct client to report any changes in breathing patterns or sputum production. Caution against heavy smoking.

**ADMINISTRATION IN ALTERNATE SETTINGS**

Should be given intravenously in clinical settings where the client can be monitored. After establishing that client is not allergic, can be given by a qualified IV nurse in a variety of settings including the home.

**EVALUATION: OUTCOMES OF DRUG THERAPY**

**EXPECTED OUTCOMES**

PHYSICAL ASSESSMENT. Client does not exhibit any signs

▼

and symptoms of allergic reaction. Client may complain of dizziness or light-headedness. Lung sounds are clear. Respiratory effort diminishes.

LABORATORY. White blood cell count may rise within a few hours of administration. Count returns to normal within 8 hours.

**NEGATIVE OUTCOMES**

Client experiences signs and symptoms of acute allergic response. Client contracts HIV or hepatitis B virus. Lung sounds or respiratory effort does not improve.

## AMINOPHYLLINE (79% THEOPHYLLINE)

*Canadian Availability:* Elixophyllin
*Pregnancy Risk:* Category C
*pH:* 8.6–9
*Storage/Stability:* Store below 40° C. Protect from freezing. Do not use if not clear.

**ASSESSMENT: DRUG CHARACTERISTICS**

**ACTION**

A xanthine bronchodilator and respiratory stimulant. Acts by relaxing bronchial smooth muscle and the smooth muscle of pulmonary blood vessels to decrease bronchospasms. Also appears to stimulate the respiratory center in the medulla by making the center more responsive to carbon dioxide.

**INDICATIONS**

Used to treat bronchial asthma, bronchitis, and chronic obstructive pulmonary disease.

**CAUTIONS**

ADVERSE EFFECTS. Gastrointestinal distress such as gastroesophageal reflux or vomiting, allergic reactions, chest pain, hypotension, dizziness, tachypnea, palpitations, or symptoms of toxicity such as confusion, seizures, diarrhea, dizziness, cardiac dysrhythmias, headache, anorexia, stomach cramps, or weakness; may lead to cardiac arrest.

CONTRAINDICATIONS. Should not be given to clients with peptic ulcers or gastritis, cardiac dysrhythmias, hypertension, CHF, or cystic fibrosis. Should be given with caution to clients with liver dysfunction, alcoholism, or hyperthyroidism. Elimination of drug is prolonged in children younger than 1 year and in the elderly.

**POTENTIAL DRUG/FOOD INTERACTIONS**

May cause hypernatremia if given with adrenocorticoids. Phenytoin may increase hepatic clearance of theophylline. Cimetidine, erythromycin, ciprofloxacin, norfloxacin, or ranitidine may decrease hepatic clearance of theophylline and increase the incidence of toxicity. May block the effects of β-adrenergic blocking agents. Smoking may decrease the effectiveness of theophylline. Incompatible with most IV drugs.

**INTERVENTIONS: ADMINISTRATION**

May be given undiluted. May be further diluted if required.

**MODE/RATE OF ADMINISTRATION**

May be given IV push at a rate not to exceed 25 mg/min. Most often given by intermittent or continuous IV infusion, using an electronic infusion device.

INTRAVENOUS USE (WITH NORMAL RENAL FUNCTION)

**Adults:** For acute bronchial asthma, if the client is *not* currently receiving theophylline preparations, the usual loading dose is 5 mg/kg of body weight over 20 min.

For acute bronchial asthma, if the client is currently receiving theophylline preparations and the serum theophylline level is not available, the dosage is 2.5 mg/kg/d. If the serum theophylline level is available, the dose can be calculated, since each 0.5 mg of theophylline per kilogram of body weight will elevate the serum theophylline level 1 mcg/ml.

For maintenance for bronchial asthma the usual dosage is 700 mcg (0.7 mg)/kg of body weight per hour.

For clients with CHF or liver failure and in need of maintenance for bronchial asthma, the usual dosage is 200 mcg (0.2 mg)/kg of body weight per hour.

**Children ≤ 16 Years:** For acute bronchial asthma, if the client is *not* currently receiving theophylline preparations, the usual loading dose is 5 mg/kg of body weight over 20 min.

For acute bronchial asthma, if the client is currently receiving theophylline preparations and a serum the-ophylline level cannot be obtained, the usual dosage is 2.5 mg/kg/d. If the level has been obtained, the dose can be calculated, since 0.5 mg/kg of body weight of theophylline will elevate the serum theophylline level 1 mcg/mL.

**Children 12–15 Years:** If child does not smoke, the usual maintenance dosage is 500 mcg (0.5 mg)/kg of body weight per hour.

If child smokes, the usual maintenance dosage is 700 mcg (0.7 mg)/kg of body weight per hour.

**Children 9–11 Years:** The usual maintenance dosage is 700 mcg (0.7 mg)/kg of body weight per hour.

**Children 1–8 Years:** The usual maintenance dosage is 800 mcg (0.8 mg)/kg of body weight per hour.

**Infants < 1 Year:** The usual maintenance dose is calculated by the formula:

Dose in mg/kg of Body Weight = (0.008) (Age in Weeks) + 0.21

**Geriatrics:** For maintenance for bronchial asthma the usual dosage is 260 mcg

▼

(0.26 mg)/kg of body weight per hour. Used with caution in the elderly.

INTRATHECAL USE OR OTHER INFUSION ROUTES AS INDICATED. Not recommended.

**POTENTIAL PROBLEMS IN ADMINISTRATION**

Frequent serum theophylline levels must be drawn to calculate the appropriate dose.

**INDEPENDENT NURSING ACTIONS**

Monitor vital signs, especially respiratory rate, rhythm, and depth. Monitor client for hypotension, tachycardia, or dysrhythmias. Observe the client for vomiting, diarrhea, or seizures. Monitor client for gastrointestinal distress such as gastroesophageal reflux, chest pain, dizziness, or symptoms of toxicity such as confusion, dizziness, headache, anorexia, stomach cramps, or weakness.

**ADMINISTRATION IN ALTERNATE SETTINGS**

Should be given in clinical settings where the client can be monitored. Not recommended for home administration.

**EVALUATION: OUTCOMES OF DRUG THERAPY**

**EXPECTED OUTCOMES**

PHYSICAL ASSESSMENT. Vital signs remain within 15% of client's baseline. Client breathes without effort. Breath sounds clear. Client does not have vomiting, diarrhea, or seizures. Client does not complain of gastrointestinal distress such as gastroesophageal reflux, chest pain, dizziness, or symptoms of toxicity such as confusion, dizziness, headache, anorexia, stomach cramps, or weakness.

LABORATORY. Serum theophylline level is 10 to 20 mcg/mL.

**NEGATIVE OUTCOMES**

Vital signs are more than 15% higher than client's baseline. Client shows obvious respiratory effort. Breath sounds contain crackles or wheezes. Client has vomiting, diarrhea, or seizures. Client complains of gastrointestinal distress such as gastroesophageal reflux, chest pain, dizziness, or symptoms of toxicity such as confusion, dizziness, headache, anorexia, stomach cramps, or weakness.

## CYCLOSPORINE

*Trade Name:* Sandimmune
*Canadian Availability:* Sandimmune
*Pregnancy Risk:* Category C
*pH:* Not specified
*Storage/Stability:* Store below 40° C. Protect from freezing. Reconstituted solutions are stable for up to 24 hours in D5W. Solutions are stable for 6 hours if stored in polyvinyl chloride containers or up to 12 hours if stored in glass containers.

### ASSESSMENT: DRUG CHARACTERISTICS

#### ACTION

A potent immunosuppressant whose exact mechanism of action is unknown. Appears to inhibit interleukin-2. Does not cause significant myelosuppression. Excreted in bile and urine.

#### INDICATIONS

Used to treat transplant rejection and prophylactically to prevent organ transplant rejection.

#### CAUTIONS

ADVERSE EFFECTS. Nephrotoxicity, hypertension, or lymphomas; gingival hyperplasia, seizures, infection, allergic reactions, elevated potassium levels, pancreatitis, hand tremors, acne, headache, nausea, or vomiting; leukopenia (usually not severe).

CONTRAINDICATIONS. Should not be given to clients with active viral infections such as chicken pox or herpes zoster. Should be given cautiously to clients with hepatic or renal impairment or with an infection.

#### POTENTIAL DRUG/FOOD INTERACTIONS

May increase the hepatotoxic risk if used with androgens, cimetidine, danazol, diltiazem, erythromycin, estrogens, or miconazole. May cause elevated potassium levels if used with potassium-sparing diuretics, enalapril, lisinopril, or potassium supplements. May increase the incidence of infection if used with other immunosuppressants. May increase the risk of acute renal failure if used with lovastatin in cardiac transplantation. May markedly increase the risk of disease if clients receive live virus vaccine within 3 months to 1 year after receiving cyclosporine.

### INTERVENTIONS: ADMINISTRATION

Dilute each 50 mL of cyclosporine with 20–100 mL of D5W or 0.9% NSS immediately prior to use.

#### MODE/RATE OF ADMINISTRATION

Given by intermittent or continuous IV infusion over 2–6 h, using an infusion pump.

INTRAVENOUS USE (WITH NORMAL RENAL FUNCTION)

**Adults:** The usual dosage is 2–6 mg/kg of body weight per day beginning 4–12 h after surgery until the client can tolerate oral therapy.

**Children:** Follow adult dosing schedule. Doses may be higher or more frequent because of faster clearance.

**Infants/Neonates:** Dose not established.

**Geriatrics:** Elderly clients are more likely to have decreased renal function that would require lower doses.

INTRETHECAL USE OR OTHER INFUSION ROUTES AS INDICATED. Not recommended.

#### POTENTIAL PROBLEMS IN ADMINISTRATION

Rapid administration may cause nephrotoxicity. May cause a severe allergic reaction. Necessary equipment and medications should be on hand to combat anaphy-

▼

lactic shock before administering cyclosporine.

#### INDEPENDENT NURSING ACTIONS

Monitor for allergic reaction. Monitor for evidence of transplant rejection. Monitor vital signs, especially blood pressure and temperature. Observe for gingival hyperplasia, seizures, infection, hand tremors, acne, or vomiting. Monitor client for headache or nausea. Monitor laboratory values, especially for renal functioning, serum potassium, and serum amylase. Use glass container only.

#### ADMINISTRATION IN ALTERNATE SETTINGS

Not recommended.

#### EVALUATION: OUTCOMES OF DRUG THERAPY

#### EXPECTED OUTCOMES

PHYSICAL ASSESSMENT. Client has no evidence of an allergic reaction such as difficulty breathing, urticaria, or wheezing. Client has no symptoms of transplant rejection. Vital signs, especially blood pressure and temperature, remain within 15% of client's baseline. Client has no gingival hyperplasia, seizures, infection, hand tremors, acne, or vomiting. Client does not complain of headache or nausea.

LABORATORY. Blood urea nitrogen (BUN) is between 8 and 25 mg/dL. Creatinine is between 0.6 and 1.5 mg/dL. Serum potassium is between 3.5 and 5 mEq/L. Serum amylase is between 4 and 25 U/mL.

#### NEGATIVE OUTCOMES

Client has evidence of an allergic reaction such as difficulty breathing, urticaria, or wheezing. Client has symptoms of transplant rejection. Vital signs, especially blood pressure and temperature, are more than 15% higher or lower than client's baseline. Client has gingival hyperplasia, seizures, infection, hand tremors, acne, or vomiting. Client complains of headache or nausea.

## IMMUNE GLOBULIN IV

*Trade Names:* Gammagard, Gammar-IV, Sandoglobulin, Gamimune
*Canadian Availability:* IVgam
*Pregnancy Risk:* Category C
*pH:* 6.4–7.2
*Storage/Stability:* Store below 20° C. (Gamimune must be stored at 2° to 8° C.) Protect from freezing. Do not use if product has been frozen. Use immediately and discard any unused solution after 2 to 3 hours, depending on manufacturer's recommendations. Do not use if darker than straw colored or cloudy.

### ASSESSMENT: DRUG CHARACTERISTICS

#### ACTION

A passive immunizing agent that is made from

large pools of donor plasma. The antibody activities of the intravenous immune globin (IVIg) are representative of the donor plasma. The drug provides immediate antibody levels lasting for 3 weeks.

**INDICATIONS**

Used to treat primary immunodeficiencies such as congenital agammaglobulinemia and thrombocytopenic purpura and as a treatment adjunct for chronic lymphocytic leukemia to prevent infections.

**CAUTIONS**

ADVERSE EFFECTS. Hypotension and severe allergic reactions such as difficulty breathing, wheezing, urticaria, erythema, or tachycardia; backache, chills, chest tightness, flushing, headache, muscle aches, nausea, malaise, or fever within an hour after infusion.

CONTRAINDICATIONS. Allergic reactions to IVIg, known antibodies to IgA, or history of cardiac dysfunction. IVIg is obtained from human plasma. Although each unit has been tested and found nonreactive to HIV antibody and hepatitis B surface antigen, there is a possibility of contracting these viruses.

**POTENTIAL DRUG/FOOD INTERACTIONS**

May interfere with the body's response to live virus vaccines. Vaccines should be given 2 weeks prior to or 3 months after administration of IVIg.

**INTERVENTIONS: ADMINISTRATION**

May be diluted with manufacturer's suggested diluent only.

**MODE/RATE OF ADMINISTRATION**

Given by continuous IV infusion, using an electronic infusion device.

INTRAVENOUS USE (WITH NORMAL RENAL FUNCTION)

**Adults:** For immunodeficiency the usual initial dosage is 200–400 mg/kg/mo. Maintenance doses of at least 100 mg/kg of body weight are given monthly.

For idiopathic thrombocytopenic purpura the usual initial dose is 1 g/kg of body weight. If the client does not respond adequately, up to two more doses of 1 g/kg of body weight may be given every other day.

For bacterial infections with chronic lymphocytic leukemia the usual dose is 400 mg/kg of body weight a day for 4 d.

**Children:** Follow the adult dosing schedule.

**Infants/Neonates:** Follow the adult dosing schedule.

**Geriatrics:** Follow the adult dosing schedule.

INTRATHECAL USE OR OTHER INFUSION ROUTES AS INDICATED. Not recommended.

**POTENTIAL PROBLEMS IN ADMINISTRATION**

May cause a severe allergic reaction. Epinephrine should be available before giving IVIg.

▼

**INDEPENDENT NURSING ACTIONS**

Monitor vital signs, especially temperature, respirations, and blood pressure. Observe for dyspnea, wheezing, urticaria, or erythema. Monitor client for complaints of backache, chills, chest tightness, headache, muscle aches, nausea, or malaise. Inform client of risks and safety precautions observed in the manufacturing process.

**ADMINISTRATION IN ALTERNATE SETTINGS**

May be administered by a qualified IV nurse in a variety of clinical settings or in the home if the client can be carefully monitored.

**EVALUATION: OUTCOMES OF DRUG THERAPY**

**EXPECTED OUTCOMES**

PHYSICAL ASSESSMENT. Vital signs, especially temperature, respirations, and blood pressure, remain within 15% of client's baseline. Client does not have dyspnea, wheezing, urticaria, or erythema. Client does not complain of backache, chills, chest tightness, headache, muscle aches, nausea, or malaise.

LABORATORY. Serum IgG should be at or above 400 to 500 mg/dL after 4 weeks.

**NEGATIVE OUTCOMES**

Client's temperature is more than 37.5° C, respirations are more than 24 breaths per minute, and blood pressure is more than 15% higher than client's baseline. Client has dyspnea, wheezing, urticaria, or erythema. Client complains of backache, chills, chest tightness, headache, muscle aches, nausea, or malaise.

## TACROLIMUS

*Trade Name:* Prograf
*Canadian Availability:* None specified
*Pregnancy Risk:* Category C
*pH:* Not specified
*Storage/Stability:* Ampules may be stored at room temperature. Diluted IV infusions in polyethylene or glass containers may be stored at room temperature for 24 hours. Preparation should be discarded after 24 hours. Do not use polyvinyl chloride containers.

**ASSESSMENT: DRUG CHARACTERISTICS**

**ACTION**

A macrolide immunosuppressant that inhibits T-cell activation, thus delaying rejection of allografts. Survival of kidney, liver, heart, bone marrow, small bowel, skin, cornea, and lung has been prolonged in animal studies using the drug.

**INDICATIONS**

Used to prolong the survival of liver transplants by preventing organ rejection.

**CAUTIONS**

ADVERSE EFFECTS. Neurotoxicity including headache and tremors; nephrotoxicity, hyperkalemia, hyperglycemia, hypertension, nausea, vomiting, and diarrhea; increased incidence of infection; risk for skin malignancies and lymphomas. CONTRAINDICATIONS. Known sensitivity to tacrolimus or known hypersensitivity to hydrogenated castor oil.

**POTENTIAL DRUG/FOOD INTERACTIONS**

May potentiate the nephrotoxic effects of aminoglycosides, amphotericin B, cisplatin, or cyclosporine. Potassium-sparing diuretics should not be used because of the risk of hyperkalemia. May interact with other immunosuppressives to increase the incidence of infection. Should be started at least 24 hours after the last dose of cyclosporine. Calcium channel blockers, some antifungal agents, and other agents that inhibit liver enzymes may cause delayed metabolism of tacrolimus. Agents that induce liver enzyme activity, such as rifampin and rifabutin, and some anticonvulsants will cause accelerated metabolism of tacrolimus. May render vaccinations ineffective.

**INTERVENTIONS: ADMINISTRATION**

Dilute tacrolimus 5 mg/mL ampule with 0.9% NSS or D5W solution to a concentration of 4–20 g/mL (0.004–0.02 mg/mL).

**MODE/RATE OF ADMINISTRATION**

Each daily dose is infused continuously over 24 h.

INTRAVENOUS USE (WITH NORMAL RENAL FUNCTION)

**Adults:** Usual dose range is 50–100 mcg/kg (0.05–0.1 mg/kg)/d. Adults will usually respond to the lower range.

**Children:** Usual dosage is 100 mcg/kg (0.1 mg/kg)/d. Children will usually need the full amount, but dose may require adjustment.

**Infants/Neonates:** Dose not established.

**Geriatrics:** Elderly clients are more likely to have preexisting conditions that increase the likelihood of liver and renal dysfunction. Follow the adult dosing schedule and monitor.

INTRATHECAL USE OR OTHER INFUSION ROUTES AS INDICATED. Not recommended.

**POTENTIAL PROBLEMS IN ADMINISTRATION**

May cause anaphylactic shock when administered intravenously. Observe for 30 minutes after starting the infusion. If symptoms of an allergic response develop, stop the infusion immediately. Clients with allergic reactions may require epinephrine and oxygen.

**INDEPENDENT NURSING ACTIONS**

Monitor all vital signs carefully. Monitor laboratory reports carefully, especially those reflecting renal and liver function. Observe for any allergic reactions or evidence of transplant rejection.

▼

**ADMINISTRATION IN ALTERNATE SETTINGS**

Should be administered in clinical settings where emergency equipment is immediately available and the client can be continuously monitored.

**EVALUATION: OUTCOMES OF DRUG THERAPY**

**EXPECTED OUTCOMES**

PHYSICAL ASSESSMENT. Heart rate, rhythm, blood pressure, and weight remain within 15% of client's baseline. Breath sounds are clear. Client does not have abdominal pain, wheezing, urticaria, anorexia, nausea, vomiting, or night sweats. Client remains alert and oriented. Client has no symptoms of transplant rejection.

LABORATORY. Serum potassium is between 3.5 and 5.5 mEq/L. Fasting blood glucose is between 70 and 115 mg/dL. Aspartate aminotransferase (AST) is between 10 and 30 U/L. Alanine aminotransferase (ALT) is between 5 and 30 U/L. BUN is between 11 and 23 mg/dL. Total serum creatinine is between 15 and 25 mg/kg body weight per 24 hours.

**NEGATIVE OUTCOMES**

Heart rate, blood pressure, and weight are more than 15% higher or lower than client's baseline. Lungs have wheezes or crackles on auscultation. Client has urticaria or vomiting. Client complains of anorexia, nausea, or abdominal pain. Client demonstrates mental status changes such as irritability, somnolence, convulsions, or coma. Client has symptoms of transplant rejection.

# Bibliography

This list includes both cited works and other works the user might find helpful.

Alexander, W. J., & Peck, M. D. (1991). Future considerations for nutrition. In J. E. Fischer (Ed.), *Total parenteral nutrition* (p. 294). Boston: Little, Brown.

Almadrones, L., & Yerys, C. (1990). Problems associated with the administration of intraperitoneal therapy using the Port-A-Cath system. *Oncology Nursing Forum, 17*(1), 75–80.

American Red Cross, Council of Community Blood Centers, American Association of Blood Banks. (1991, December). *Circular of information for the use of human blood and blood components.* Author.

American Society of Parenteral and Enteral Nutrition (ASPEN). (1993). Section II: Rationale for adult nutrition support guidelines. *Journal of Parenteral and Enteral Nutrition, 17*(4), 5SA–6SA.

Bagan, M., Robson, J., & Soderstrom, R. (1971). Ethnic differences in skin fold thickness. *American Journal of Clinical Nutrition, 24,* 864–868.

Baird, S. B., McCorkle, R., & Grant, M. (Eds.). (1991). *Cancer nursing: A comprehensive textbook.* Philadelphia: W. B. Saunders.

Baranowski, L. (1992). Current trends in blood component therapy: The evolution of a safer, more effective product. *Journal of Intravenous Nursing, 15*(3), 135–151.

Beason, R., Bourguignon, J., Fowler, D., et al. (1992). Evaluation of a needle-free intravenous access system. *Journal of Intravenous Nursing, 15*(1), 11–16.

Bistrian, B. R., Blackburn, G. L., Sherman M., & Scrimshaw, N. S. (1975). Therapeutic index of nutritional depletion in hospitalized patients. *Surgical Gynecology and Obstetrics, 141,* 512–516.

Black, J. M., & Matassarin-Jacobs, E. (1993). *Luckmann and Sorensen's Medical surgical nursing: A psychophysiologic approach* (4th ed.). Philadelphia: W. B. Saunders.

Blackburn, G. L., & Bistrian, B. R. 1974, November. Protein status of general surgical patients. *Journal of the American Medical Association. 230*(6), 858–860.

Blackburn, G. L., & Bistrian, B. R. 1976, October. Nutritional care of the injured and/or septic patient. *Surgical Clinics of North America. 56*(5), 1195–1224.

Blanchard, J., Menk, E., Ramamurtky, S., & Hoffman, J. (1990). Subarachnoid and epidural calcitonin in patients with pain due to metastatic cancer. *Journal of Pain and Symptom Management, 5*(1), 42–45.

Bolander, V. B. (1994). *Sorensen and Luckmann's Basic nursing* (3rd ed.). Philadelphia: W. B. Saunders.

Bookman, M. A. (1989). Biologic therapy for ovarian cancer. *Current Opinions in Oncology, 1,* 112–118.

Borden, E. (1984). Progress toward therapeutic application in interferons. *Cancer, 54*(11), 2770–2776.

Brickman, K., Rega, P., & Guinnes, M. (1986). A comparative study of intraosseous, intravenous, and intra-arterial pH changes during hypoventilation in dogs. *Annals of Emergency Medicine, 16,* 487.

Brown, J. M. (1990). Peripherally inserted central catheters use in home care. *Journal of Intravenous Nursing, 12*(3), 144–147.

Camp-Sorrell, D., Fernandez, K., & Reardon, M. B. (1990). Teaching oncology nurses about epidural catheters. *Oncology Nursing Forum 17*(4), 683–689.

Carney-Gersten, P. J., Moore, M. D., & Giuffre, M. (1990). Intraperitoneal alpha interferon for ovarian cancer: A case report. *Oncology Nursing Forum, 17*(3), 403–407.

Carroll, H. J., & Oh, M. S. (1989). *Water, electrolyte and acid-base metabolism, diagnosis and management.* Philadelphia: J. B. Lippincott.

Clark-Christoff, N., Watters, V., Sparks, W., et al. (1992). Use of triple-lumen subclavian catheters for administration of total parenteral nutrition. *Journal of Parenteral and Enteral Nutrition, 16*(5), 402–407.

Collins, J., & Lutz, R. (1991). In vitro study of simultaneous infusion of incompatible drugs in multilumen catheters. *Heart and Lung, 20*(3), 271–277.

Coulter, K. (1992). Intravenous therapy for the elder patient: Implications for the intravenous nurse. *Journal of Intravenous Nursing, 15*(Suppl.), S18–A93.

Dedrick, R. L., Myers, C. E., Bungay, P. M., et al. (1978). Pharmacokinetic rationale for peritoneal drug administration in the treatment of ovarian cancer. *Cancer Treatment Report, 62*(1), 1–11.

DeWit, S. C. (1994). *Rambo's Nursing skills for clinical practice* (4th ed.). Philadelphia: W. B. Saunders.

Dick, M. J., Maree, S. M., Gray, J. (1992, June). How to boost the odds of a painless IV start. *American Journal of Nursing, 92,* 49–50.

Dodd, R. Y. (1992). The risk of transfusion-transmitted infection. *New England Journal of Medicine, 327*(6), 419–421.

Drigger, D. A., Johnson, R., Steiner, J., et al. (1991, March). Emergency resuscitation in children: The role of intraosseous infusion. *Postgraduate Medicine, 89*(4), 129–132.

Dunajcik, L. (1998, January). Controlling the dangers of epidural analgesia. *RN, 88,* 40–45.

Falchuk, K., Peterson, L., & McNeil, B. J. (1985). Microparticulate-induced phlebitis. *New England Journal of Medicine, 312,* 78–82.

Foley, K. M. (1985). Treatment of cancer pain. *New England Journal of Medicine, 313*(2), 84–95.

Foster, L. R., Hunsberger, M. M., Anderson, J. J T. (1989). *Family-centered nursing care of children.* Philadelphia: W. B. Saunders.

Frederick, V. (1991, December). Pediatric IV therapy: Soothing the patient. *RN, 91,* 39–42.

Gahart, B. L. (1995). Intravenous medications: *A handbook for nurses and allied health professionals* (11th ed.). St. Louis: Mosby–Year Book.

Gardner, C. (1989). IV specialization: Current issues. *Journal of Intravenous Nursing, 12*(Suppl.), S3–S9.

Gianino, M. S., Brunt, L. M., & Eisenberg, T. G. (1992). The impact of a nutritional support team on the cost and management of multilumen central venous catheters. *Journal of Intravenous Nursing, 15*(6), 327–331.

Giger, J. N., Davidhizar, R., & Cherry, B. (1991, April/May). Biological variations in the black patient. *NSNA/Imprint,* pp. 95–105.

Ginsberg, B., Grichnik, K., & Schobelock, M. (1993, May). Managing postoperative pain with epidural analgesia. *Pharmacy Times,* pp. 92–101.

Goode, C. J., Kleiber, C., Titler, M., et al. (1993). Improving practice through research: The case of heparin vs. saline for peripheral intermittent infusion devices. *Med Surg Nursing, 2,* 23–27.

Hadaway, L. C. (1989). Evaluation and use of advanced I.V. technology, Part 1: Central venous access devices. *Journal of Intravenous Nursing, 12*(2), 73–81.

Hampton, J. K. (1991). *The biology of human aging*. Dubuque, IA: Wm. C. Brown.

Handy, C. M. (1989) Vascular access devices hospital to home care. *Journal of Intravenous Nursing, 12*(1), S10–S18.

Hansberry, J., Bannick, K., & Durkan, M. (1990). Management of chronic pain with a permanent epidural catheter. *Nursing 90* pp. 53–55.

Hilton, E., Haslett, T., Borenstein, M., et al. (1988) Central catheter infections: Single versus triple-lumen catheters. Influence of guidewires on infection rates when used for replacement of catheter. *American Journal of Medicine 84*(4), 667–672.

Holcombe, V. J., Forloines-Lynn, S., & Garmhausen, L. W. (1992). Restoring patency of long-term central venous access devices. *Journal of Intravenous Nursing, 15*(1), 36–41.

Hutchinson, D. (1991, December). Pediatric IV therapy: Starting the line. *RN, 91,* 43–47.

Ignatavicius, D. D., Workman, M. L., & Mishler, M. A. (1995). *Medical-surgical nursing: A nursing process approach* (2nd ed.). Philadelphia: W. B. Saunders.

Intravenous Nurses Society. (1990). *Intravenous nursing standards of practice*. Philadelphia: J. B. Lippincott.

Intravenous Nurses Society. (1995). *Intravenous therapy: Clinical principles and practice*. Philadelphia: W. B. Saunders.

Isselbacher, K. J., Adams, R. D., Braunwald, E., et al. (1980). *Harrison's Principles of internal medicine* (9th ed.). New York: McGraw-Hill.

Kaufman, M. V. (1992). Intravenous therapy education in associate degree nursing programs. *Journal of Intravenous Nursing, 15,* 238–242.

Keeney, S. (1993). Nursing care of the postoperative patient receiving epidural analgesia. *MedSurg Nursing, 2*(3), 191–196.

Keys, A., Brogek, J., Henschel, A., et al. (1950). *The biology of human starvation* (Vols. 1–2). Minneapolis: University of Minnesota Press.

Kinney, J. M. (1991). Energy requirements for parenteral nutrition. In Fischer, J. E. (Ed.). *Total parenteral nutrition* (pp. 181–187). Boston: Little, Brown.

Kinney, M. R. (1981). *AACN's Clinical reference for critical-care nursing*. New York: McGraw-Hill.

Laffer U., Knusli, C., Hauder, F., et al. (1988). Intraperitoneal chemotherapy for gastrointestinal malignancies. *Antibiotic Chemotherapy, 40,* 26–34.

LaRocca, J. C., & Otto, S. E. (1993). *Pocket guide to intravenous therapy* (2nd ed.). St. Louis: Mosby–Year Book.

Leib, R. A., & Hurtig, J. B. (1985). Epidural and intrathecal narcotics for pain management. *Heart and Lung, 14,* 164–174.

Levenson, S. M. (1975). *Manual of surgical nutrition* (pp. 236–264). Philadelphia: W. B. Saunders.

Long, C. L. (1984). Energy and protein requirements in stress and trauma. In *Critical care nursing currents* (Vol. 2, No. 2, pp. 7– 12). Columbus, OH: Ross Laboratories.

Lotze M., Custer, M., & Rosenberg, S. (1986). Intraperitoneal administration of interleukin-2 in patients with cancer. *Archives of Surgery, 121,* 1373–1379.

Manley, L. (1988). Intraosseous infusion: A lifesaving technique that should be used more widely. *Journal of Intravenous Nursing, 12*(6), 367–368.

Manley, L, Halley, K., Dick, M. (1988). Intraosseous infusion: Rapid vascular access for critically ill or injured infants and children. *The Journal of Emergency Nursing, 14*(2), 63–68.

Markman, M. (1987). Intracavitary administration of biological agents. *Journal of Biological Response Modifiers, 6,* 404–411.

Markman, M., Hakes, T., Reichman, B., et al. (1991). Intraperitoneal cisplatin and cytarabine in the treatment of refractory or recurrent ovarian cancer. *Journal of Clinical Oncology, 9,* 204–210.

Masoorli, S., & Angeles, T. (1990, January). PICC lines: The latest home care challenge. *RN, 90,* 44–51.

McLaughlin-Hagan, M. (1990). Continuous subcutaneous infusion of narcotics. *Journal of Intravenous Nursing, 13,* 119–121.

Milliam, D. (1988). Are nurses prepared to perform I.V. therapy? *Nursing, 18*(3), 43.

Mosca, R., Curtas, S., Forbes B., et al. (1987). The benefits of isolator cultures in the management of suspected catheter sepsis. *Surgery, 102,* 718–723.

Moulin, D. E., Johnson, N. G., Murray-Parsons, N. et al. (1992, Mar. 15). Subcutaneous narcotic infusions for cancer pain: Treatment outcome and guidelines for use. *Canadian Medical Association Journal, 146*(6), 891–897.

Moulin, D. E., Kreeft, J. H., Murray-Parsons, N., et al. (1991, Feb. 23). Comparison of continuous subcutaneous and intravenous hydromorphone infusions for management of cancer pain. *Lancet, 337*(8739), 465–468

Mukau, L., Talamini, M. D., Sitzmann, J. V. et al. (1992). Long-term central venous access vs. other home therapies: Complications in patients with acquired immunodeficiency syndrome. *Journal of Parenteral and Enteral Nutrition, 16*(5), 455–459.

National Coordinating Committee on Large Volume Parenterals. (1979). Recommendations to pharmacists for solving problems with large-volume parenterals. *American Journal of Hospital Pharmacy 37,* 663–666.

Nentwich, P. F. (1990). *Intravenous therapy and medication administration.* Boston: Jones & Bartlett, 1990.

Neufeld, J. D. G., Light, A., & Marx, J. A. (1986). A comparison of peripheral, central, and intraosseous routes in resuscitation of hemorrhagic shock in pigs. *Annals of Emergency Medicine, 16,* 487.

Nitescu, P., Applegren, L., Linder, L.-E., et al. (1990). Epidural versus intrathecal morphine-bupivacaine: Assessment of consecutive treatments in advanced cancer pain. *Journal of Pain and Symptom Management, 5*(1), 18–26.

*Nutrition and your health: Dietary guidelines for Americans.* (1990, 3rd ed.). Hyattsville, MD: U. S. Department of Agriculture, U. S. Department of Health and Human Services.

Nutritional Assessment Kit. (1988). Columbus, OH: Ross Laboratories.

O'Toole, M. (Ed.). (1992). *Miller-Keane Encyclopedia and dictionary of medicine, nursing, and allied health* (5th ed.). Philadelphia: W. B. Saunders.

Ommaya, A. K. (1963, November 9). Subcutaneous reservoir and pump for sterile access to ventricular cerebrospinal fluid. *Lancet, 2,* 983–984.

Oncology Nursing Society. (1988). Cancer chemotherapy guidelines. Pittsburgh: Oncology Nursing Society.

Peterson, K. J. (1992). Nursing management of autologous blood transfusion. *Journal of Intravenous Nursing, 15*(3), 128–134.

Pharmacia, Inc. Port-A-Cath intraperitoneal system professional manual. Piscataway, NJ: Pharmacia, Inc.

Plumer, A. (1987). *Principles and practice of intravenous therapy* (4th ed.). Boston: Little, Brown.

Rahr, V. (1986). Giving intrathecal drugs. *American Journal of Nursing, 7,* 829–831.

Sazama, K. (1990). Reports of 355 transfusion-associated deaths: 1976 through 1985. *Transfusion, 30*(7), 583–590.

Scalley, R. D., Van, C. S. & Cochran, R. S. (1992). The impact of an I.V. team on the occurrence of intravenous-related phlebitis. *Journal of Intravenous Nursing, 15,* 100–107.

Shoor, P. M., Berryhill, R. E., & Benumof, J. L. (1972). Intraosseous infusions: Pressure flow relationship in pharmacokinetics. *Journal of Trauma, 19,* 772–774.

Silberman, H. (1989). *Parenteral and enteral nutrition.* Norwalk, CT: Appleton & Lange.

Solomon, E. P. (1992). *Introduction to human anatomy and physiology.* Philadelphia: W. B. Saunders.

Speer, E. W. (1990). Central venous catheterization: Issues associated with the use of single and multiple-lumen catheters. *Journal of Intravenous Nursing, 13*(1), 30–39.

Spivey, W. H. (1987). Intraosseous infusions. *The Journal of Pediatrics, 111*(5), 639–643.

Swenson, K., Erikson, J. (1986). Nursing management of intraperitoneal chemotherapy. *Oncology Nursing Forum, 12*(5), 33–39.

Uram, M. S. (1992, May). A new delivery system makes pain control easier. *RN, 92,* 46–51.

Vidal, R., Kisson, N., & Gayle, M. (1993, June). Compartment syndrome following intraosseous infusion. *Pediatrics, 91*(6), 1201–1202.

Warshawsky, K. Y. (1992). Intravenous fat emulsions in clinical practice. *Nutrition in Clinical Practice, 7*(4), 187–196.

Weinstein, S. M. (1993). *Plumer's principles and practice of intravenous therapy* (5th ed.). Philadelphia: J. B. Lippincott.

Wheeler, C. (1988). Pediatric intraosseous infusion: An old technique in modern health care technology. *Journal of Intravenous Nursing, 12*(6), 371–376.

Wild, L., & Coyne, C. (1992). The basics and beyond: Epidural analgesia. *American Journal of Nursing, 4,* 26–34.

Zook-Enck, D. (1990). Intraperitoneal therapy via the Tenckhoff catheter: prevention and management of complications. *Journal of Intravenous Nursing, 13*(6), 375–382.

# PART V

# APPENDIXES

# Appendix A

# The Occupational Safety and Health Administration's Occupational Exposure to Bloodborne Pathogens: Final Rule (1991)

In 1987 the Centers for Disease Control (CDC) published recommendations for blood and body fluid precautions to be used by all health care workers to prevent the spread of human immunodeficiency virus (HIV) and other bloodborne pathogens. These recommendations, referred to as universal blood and body fluid precautions or universal precautions, were adopted by most health care agencies.

In 1991 the Occupational Safety and Health Administration (OSHA), the federal agency responsible for the safety of the country's workers, published its *Occupational Exposure to Bloodborne Pathogens: Final Rule.* This document took the CDC's recommendations to a new level, making universal precautions fully enforceable under the law. In addition, OSHA outlined what inspectors will monitor in various agencies as it relates to compliance with these occupational safety rules.

Health care workers are continuously at risk for exposure to blood and body fluids that may contain pathogens that cause hepatitis B (HBV) and acquired immunodeficiency syndrome (AIDS [HIV]). According to OSHA, through a combination of engineering, work practice controls, barrier precautions, equipment, training, medical surveillance, hepatitis B vaccination, signs and labels, and other provisions, the health care worker's exposure can be minimized or eliminated.

The following is a list that summarizes some of the rules agencies must follow to be in compliance with the latest OSHA regulations.

**Hepatitis B Vaccine.** All employees who are at risk for exposure to blood and body fluids and consequently HBV must be offered the hepatitis B vaccine at no charge to the employee. The agency must offer the vaccine "at a reasonable time and place." New employees must be offered the vaccine "within 10 working days of initial assignment."

**Universal Precautions.** All health care workers are now legally bound to observe all human blood and certain human body fluids as though they were known to be infectious for HIV, HBV, and other bloodborne pathogens.

**Sharps and Waste Disposal.** All contaminated sharps and needles must be placed in puncture-resistant, leak-proof containers, which are labeled or color coded. These containers must be easily accessible, kept in an upright position, and routinely replaced.

**Protective Equipment.** Whenever there is the potential for the employee's clothes, skin, eyes, mouth, or other mucous membranes to be exposed to blood or other infectious materials, the agency must provide protective equipment to the employee. This includes but is not limited to gloves, gowns, protective eyewear, and shields.

**Gloves.** When hand contact with infectious materials can be anticipated, gloves must be worn. Disposable gloves may be washed or decontaminated for reuse, but they must be discarded if they are torn, punctured, or cracked. The agency must provide hypoallergenic gloves or a suitable alternative for employees who are allergic to the standard gloves used in the agency.

**Laundry.** Contaminated laundry must be handled with a minimum amount of agitation. When moving contaminated laundry, it must be in labeled or color-coded bags or containers. Leak-proof containers must be available for wet laundry. Laundry workers must wear gloves for protection.

**Communicating Hazards.** Containers holding regulated waste and refrigerators or freezers used to store infectious materials must be marked with orange-red or fluorescent signs, which include the official "BIOHAZARD" legend.

In addition, health care workers are responsible for using good infection control practices to protect themselves and their clients. Some of these practices include the following.

**Handwashing.** Hands should be washed before applying gloves, and immediately after removing them. Gloves should either be washed or replaced when moving from client to client. Hands and other skin surfaces should be washed immediately and thoroughly if contaminated with blood or other body secretions.

**Protection Against Injury.** The nurse should take precautions to prevent injury when handling any sharps (needles, scalpels, etc.) during procedures, when cleaning used instruments, and during disposal of used needles. Used needles are *never* recapped. Any used disposable sharp is dropped into a puncture-proof container. Reusable sharps should be placed in a separate puncture-proof container to transport to the processing area.

Appendix B

# Continuous Ambulatory Drug Delivery Pumps (CADD Pumps)

## STARTING THE PUMP

Press and HOLD the Stop/Start key until three dashes on the display screen DISAPPEAR. The pump will scroll through the program and the word "STOP" will disappear from the display screen.

## STOPPING THE PUMP

Press and HOLD the Stop/Start key until three dashes APPEAR on the display screen. "STOP" will appear on the display screen.

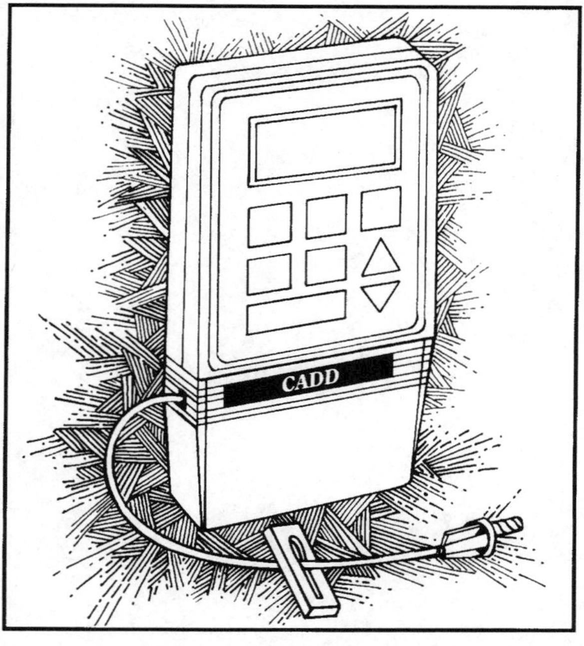


CADD pump.

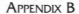

## CHANGING THE CASSETTE

When your cassette is almost empty with 5 mL or less remaining, the "RESVOL" display will flash and a variable tone alarm will sound. At this point, you may change the medication cassette. When the display reads "000," the pump stops pumping and "STOP" will appear on the display screen. The pump will alarm twice each second. The medication cassette *must* be changed at this time.

## SUPPLIES

- Medication cassette system
- Alcohol preps
- Key or coin (dependent on type of pump)

Always: ☑

- ☐ Take the medication cassette system out of the refrigerator _______ minutes before your infusion.
- ☐ Check the label on the medication cassette system for medication name, expiration date, and patient name.
- ☐ Clean the work area with soap and water.
- ☐ Wash your hands.

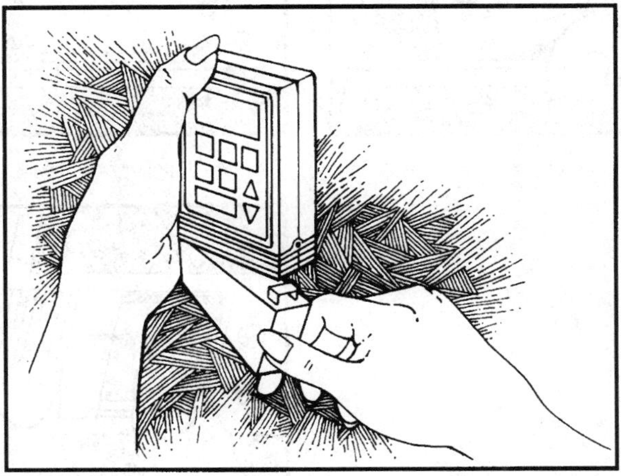

Changing the medication reservoir.

## CHANGING THE BATTERY

When changing the battery, use a fresh, 9V alkaline or lithium battery.

Procedure:

1. Slide open the battery compartment cover and remove the used battery.
2. Install the new battery, flat end first. Match the polarity markings (+ and −) with those on the battery compartment. If you put the battery in backward, the screen will remain blank and you will not hear a beeping sound.
3. Press the battery down into the compartment with your thumb and replace the compartment cover by pressing it down directly over the battery and sliding the cover forward toward the polarity markings.
4. Remember to restart the pump.

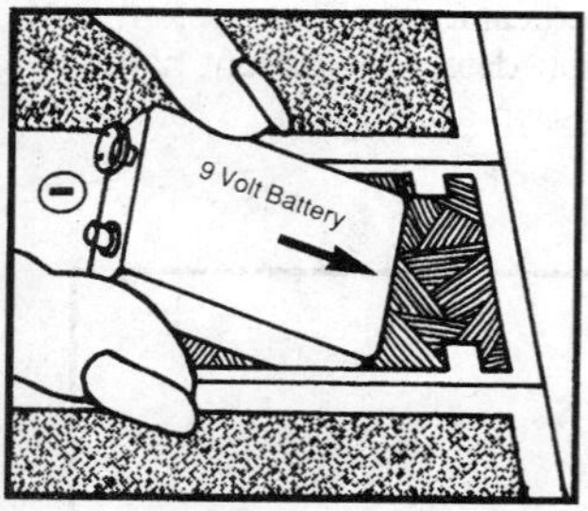


Insert battery flat end first.

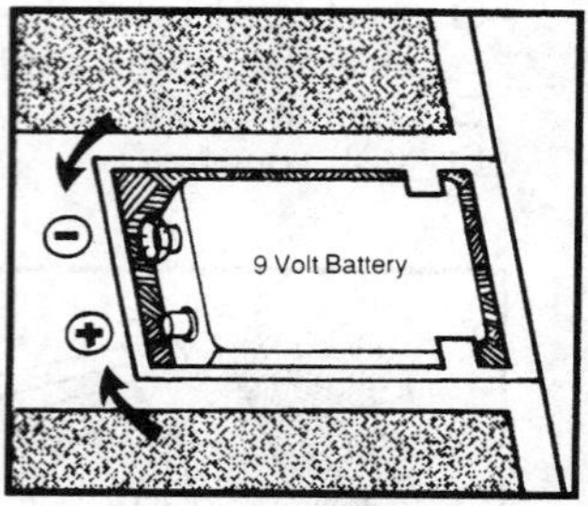


Match polarity markings.

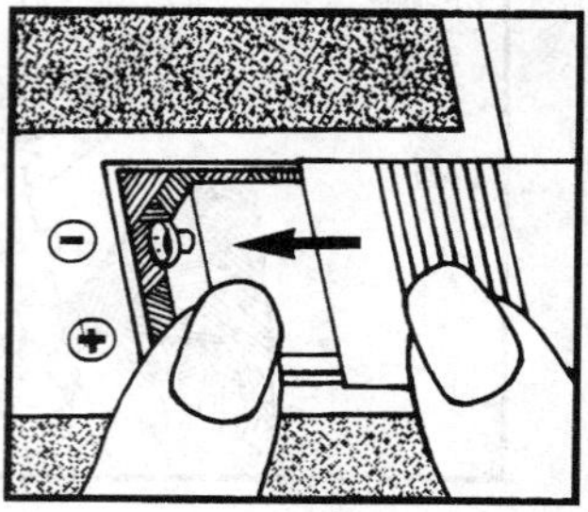

Install battery, relace cover.

**Procedure:**

1. Stop the pump.
2. Disconnect the medication tubing from your access device.
3. Unlock the used medication cassette from the pump by inserting a coin or key into the locking button and turning it one-quarter turn clockwise. The locking button will pop out and release the medication cassette.
4. Remove the medication cassette from the pump by sliding the cassette reservoir hooks from the pump hinge pins.
5. Attach the new medication cassette to the pump by inserting the cassette hooks into the hinge pins on the pump.
6. Place the pump with the medication cassette attached in an upright position on a firm, flat surface and press down on the pump to ensure that the medication cassette fits tightly against the pump.
7. Lock the medication cassette to the pump by inserting a coin or key into the locking button and turning it one-quarter turn counterclockwise.
8. Open all clamps on the medication cassette system tubing. If necessary, prime the tubing by pressing and holding the prime key until "PPP" appears. Release the prime key and quickly press the key again and HOLD until fluid fills the tubing.
9. Press the Set/Clear key to automatically reset the residual volume (RESVOL) to ______________.
10. Connect the medication cassette system tubing to the access device and secure.
11. Turn on the pump.

## Troubleshooting Guidelines • Continuous Ambulatory Drug Delivery Pumps • (CADD Pumps)

| Problem | Corrective Action |
|---|---|
| Three beeps sound every 5 minutes.<br>"LO BAT" blinks on the display. | The battery power is low but the pump is operable. Change the battery soon. |
| A continuous variable-tone alarm sounds.<br>"LO BAT" remains on the display. | The battery power is too low to operate the pump; the pump operation stops. Change the battery immediately. Be sure to restart the pump. |
| A continuous variable-tone alarm sounds, "HI P" appears on the display. | The high pressure alarm may be the result of a blockage or kink in the tubing or a blockage in the access device. Try to locate and correct the cause of the blockage or kink in the tubing. After correcting, the alarm will cease and the pump will resume operation. If you suspect that the blockage is in the access device, contact your nurse. |
| A continuous variable-tone alarm and the letter "E" and two numbers appear on the display or "OFF" appears on the display. | There may be a problem with the pump. The pump operation stops.<br>Clamp the tubing and call your nurse. |
| Three beeps sound every 5 minutes and "STOP" blinks on the display. | The pump has stopped. Start the pump as necessary. |
| Wetness near the IV site or access device cap. | Wash your hands.<br>Tighten any loose connections.<br>Dry the area.<br>If wetness returns, stop your infusion and call your nurse. |

**Troubleshooting Guidelines Continued**
**• Continuous Ambulatory Drug Delivery Pumps**
**• (CADD Pumps)**

| Problem | Corrective Action |
|---|---|
| Resistance met when access device is being flushed or cannot be flushed | Do not try to force the flush solution through the access device. Check that the clamp is open on the access device. If unsuccessful, call your nurse. |
| Redness, swelling, or soreness at access device site | Do not infuse medication. Call your nurse. |
| Itching skin, tingling lips, rash and or hives | Do not infuse medication. *Immediately* call your nurse. |
| Tightness in your chest, shortness of breath, difficulty breathing | *Stop medication. Call 911.* |

Name of Nurse: ______________________________

Telephone Number: (   ) ______________________________

APPENDIX C

# Basic Infusion Fluid Calculations

## Determining the Minute Volume (Milliliters per Minute)

$$\text{Minute volume} = \frac{\text{Hourly volume of fluid}}{60 \text{ min}}$$

EXAMPLE

The physician orders 1 L of IV fluid to run over 6 hours. How many milliliters per minute will be delivered?

In this example, first determine the hourly volume of IV fluid (flow rate), which is the total volume divided by the number of hours, or 1000 mL/6 h, which equals 167 mL/h (rounded hourly volume). Then use the formula above to calculate the minute volume: 167 mL/60 min, which equals 2.7 or approximately 3 mL/min.

## Determining the Drip Rate (Drops per Minute)

$$\begin{matrix}\text{Drip} \\ \text{rate}\end{matrix} = \frac{\text{Amount of solution infused (mL)}}{\text{Amount of time for infusion (min)}} \times \begin{matrix}\text{Drop factor} \\ \text{(gtt/mL)}\end{matrix}$$

EXAMPLE

The physician orders a continuous infusion to run at 150 mL/h. What is the drip rate? (Drop factor = 10.) (NOTE: Drop factor is found on infusion tubing package.)

In this example the amount of solution is 150 mL in 60 min: (150 mL/60 min) × 10 = 25 gtt/min.

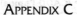

APPENDIX D

# Special Calculations for IV Drugs

## Determining Milliequivalents per Hour

EXAMPLE 1

The physician orders 1 L of IV solution with 80 mEq potassium chloride added to infuse over 10 hours. What amount of drug will the client receive per hour?

In this example the calculation is done by simply dividing the amount of medication by the total hours of infusion, or 80 mEq/10 h, which equals 8 mEq/h.

## Determining Infusion Flow Rate (mL/h) When Drug Dosage is Known

EXAMPLE 2

The physician orders a continuous heparin infusion of 1100 U/h. The solution from the pharmacy comes as 20,000 U of heparin diluted in 1000 mL of IV solution. What flow rate is need to deliver the prescribed amount of medication?

Using ratio and proportion, the calculation can be set up as:

$$\frac{1000 \text{ mL}}{x \text{ mL}} = \frac{20{,}000 \text{ U}}{1100 \text{ U}}$$

$$20{,}000x = 1{,}100{,}000$$

$$x = 55 \text{ mL/h}$$

## Determining IV Drug Concentration

EXAMPLE 3

The physician orders magnesium sulfate 10 g in 500 mL IV fluid. What is the concentration of the drug in solution?

This calculation is easier if the grams of drug are first converted to milligrams to eliminate working with decimals. Since 1 g is equal to 1000 mg, 10 g are equal to 10,000 mg (10 × 1000). Then, divide the amount of the drug in milligrams by the amount of solution to obtain the answer:

10,000 mg/500 mL = 20 mg/mL. For each milliliter of IV solution, there are 20 mg of magnesium sulfate.

## Determining the Flow Rate (mL/h) when the Drug Concentration Is Known

EXAMPLE 4

The physician orders terbutaline sulfate IV infusion to start at 10 mcg/min. The drug is mixed as 5 mcg/mL of solution. What flow rate is needed to deliver the prescribed amount of medication? This problem requires two steps. First, ratio and proportion or the formula (D/H) × Q ([desired amount/on hand amount of drug] × unit quantity) can be used. With this formula (10 mcg/5 mcg) ×1 mL = 2 mL. This value means that the desired amount of terbutaline (10 mcg) that must be infused is in 2 mL of solution. To find the flow rate per hour, multiply 2 mL × 60 min to get 120 mL/h.

## Determining Flow Rate for Drugs Prescribed in Micrograms per Kilogram per Minute

EXAMPLE 5

The physician orders lidocaine 20 mcg/kg/min for a 220-lb client. One gram of lidocaine is diluted in 500 mL of IV solution. What flow rate (milliliters per hour) is needed to deliver the prescribed amount?

This calculation requires several steps. First, the 220 lb must be converted to kilograms: divide 220 by 2.2 because there are 2.2 lb in 1 kg. The client weighs 100 kg.

In step 2, determine the amount of lidocaine that a 100-kg client requires. If 20 mcg/kg/min is ordered, then this client needs 20 mcg × 100 kg, or 2000 mcg/min. Since 1000 mcg is equivalent to 1 mg, the client needs 2 mg/min, or 120 mg/h (2 mg × 60 min).

Once the desired dose is calculated, the drug concentration that is available must be determined, as was calculated in Example 3 above. Convert 1 g to 1000 mg of lidocaine in 500 mL of solution; then divide the amount of drug in milligrams by the amount of solution to obtain the answer: 1000 mg/500 mL = 2 mg/mL of drug is on hand.

Finally, using ratio and proportion:

$$\frac{2 \text{ mg}}{1 \text{ mL}} = \frac{120 \text{ mg}}{x \text{ mL}}$$

$$2x = 120$$

$$x = 60$$

The flow rate required to deliver the prescribed dose of lidocaine is 60 mL/h.

## APPENDIX E

# Medication-Solution Compatibilities

| | | | | D5 + | | | | | |
|---|---|---|---|---|---|---|---|---|---|
| **Medications** | **D5W** | **D10W** | **NSS** | **0.25NSS** | **0.5NSS** | **NSS** | **R** | **D5R** | **RL** |
| acyclovir | C | | | | | C | | | |
| amikacin | C | C | C | C | C | C | | | C |
| amphotericin B | C | | | | | | | | |
| ampicillin | C | | | | C | C | | | C |
| ampicillin/ sulbactam | C | | C | | C | | | | C |
| aztreonam | C | C | C | C | C | C | C | | C |
| bretylium | C | | C | | C | C | | C | C |
| bumetanide | C | | C | | | | | | C |
| cefamandole | C | C | C | C | C | C | | C | |
| cefazolin | C | C | C | C | C | C | | C | C |
| cefonicid | C | C | C | C | C | C | C | C | C |
| ceforanide | C | C | C | C | C | | | C | C |
| cefotaxime | | | | C | C | C | | | |
| cefotetan | C | | C | | | | | | |
| cefoxitin | C | C | C | C | C | C | C | C | C |
| ceftazidime | C | C | C | C | C | C | C | C | C |
| ceftizoxime | C | C | C | C | C | C | | | C |
| ceftriaxone | C | C | C | | C | | | | C |
| cefuroxime | C | C | C | | C | C | C | | C |
| cephalothin | C | C | C | | | C | C | C | C |
| cephapirin* | C | C | C | C | C | C | | C | |
| chloramphenicol | C | C | C | C | C | C | | C | C |
| cimetidine | C | C | C | C | C | | C | C | C |
| ciprofloxacin | C | | C | | | | | | |
| corticotropin | C | | C | | | C | | | C |
| dobutamine† | C | | C | | C | C | | C | C |
| dopamine | C | | C | | C | C | | C | C |
| doxycycline | C | | C | | | | | C | C |
| erythromycin | C | | C | | | | | | C |
| esmolol† | C | | C | | C | C | C | C | C |
| ganciclovir‡ | C | | C | | | | C | C | C |
| gentamicin | C | | C | | | | C | | |
| heparin | C | | C | | C | | C | | |
| isoproterenol† | C | C | C | C | C | C | | C | C |
| imipenem- cilastatin | C | C | C | C | C | C | | | |

*Other: D20W
†Other: 0.45 NSS
‡Other: D5RL

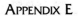

| Medications | D5W | D10W | NSS | D5 + 0.25NSS | D5 + 0.5NSS | D5 + NSS | R | D5R | RL |
|---|---|---|---|---|---|---|---|---|---|
| lidocaine* | C | | C | | C | C | | C | C |
| metaraminol | C | C | C | | | C | C | C | C |
| methicillin | C | C | C | | | C | C | | C |
| metoclopramid | C | | | | | C | | | |
| metronidazole | C | | C | | | | | | C |
| mezlocillin | C | C | C | C | C | C | C | | C |
| miconazole | C | | C | | | | | | |
| morphine* | C | C | C | | | | C | | C |
| moxalactam | C | C | C | | C | C | C | C | C |
| nafcillin | C | C | C | | C | C | C | C | C |
| naloxone | C | | C | | | | | | |
| netilmicin | C | C | C | | | C | C | C | C |
| nitroglycerin | C | C | C | | | | | | |
| nitroprusside | C | | | | | | | | |
| ofloxacin | C | C | C | | | C | | C | |
| ondansetron | C | | C | | C | C | | | |
| oxacillin | C | | C | | | C | | | C |
| oxytocin | C | C | C | | C | C | C | C | C |
| penicillin G | C | C | C | | C | C | C | C | C |
| pentamidine | C | | | | | | | | |
| piperacillin | C | | C | | | C | | | C |
| procainamide | C | | | | | | | | |
| rifampin | C | | C | | | | | | |
| ritodrine | C | | | | | | | | |
| theophylline | C | | | | | | | | |
| ticarcillin-clavulanate | C | | C | | | | C | | C |
| ticarcillin | C | | C | | | | C | | C |
| tobramycin | C | C | C | | | C | C | | C |
| vancomycin | C | C | C | | | | | | C |
| vasopressin | C | | C | | | | | | |
| vidarabine* | C | C | C | C | C | C | C | C | C |

*Other: 0.45 NSS

D5W, 5% dextrose in water; D10W, 10% dextrose in water; D20W, 20% dextrose in water; NSS, normal saline solution; D5 + 0.25 NSS, 5% dextrose in one-fourth strength normal saline solution; D5 + 0.5 NSS, 5% dextrose in half strength normal saline solution; D5 + NSS, 5% dextrose in normal saline solution; R, Ringer's solution; D5R, 5% dextrose in Ringer's solution; RL, lactated Ringer's solution; D5RL, 5% dextrose in lactated Ringer's solution.

APPENDIX F

# Medication-Medication Compatibilities

## Legend

| | |
|---|---|
| blank | Data either unavailable or sources inconsistent. |
| c | Found to be compatible when in contact in a syringe, at a Y site, or in an admixture. |
| cs | Found to be compatible when in contact in a syringe. |
| cy | Found to be compatible when in contact at a Y site. |
| ca | Found to be compatible when in contact in an admixture. |
| x | Found to be incompatible when in contact in a syringe, at a Y site, or in an admixture. |
| xs | Found to be incompatible when in contact in a syringe. |
| xy | Found to be incompatible when in contact at a Y site. |
| xa | Found to be incompatible when in contact in an admixture. |
| x* | Should be given 1 hour apart to avoid inactivation of either one or both medications. |
| ***XA**** | Manufacturer recommends that this medication not be admixed. |
| ~ | If medications administered concurrently, administer each at a separate site. |

| | Acyclovir | Amikacin ***XA**** | Aminophylline ***XA**** | Amphotericin-B | Ampicillin | Ampicillin and sulbactam | Ascorbic acid | Atracurium | Atropine | Aztreonam | Bleomycin | Carboplatin |
|---|---|---|---|---|---|---|---|---|---|---|---|---|
| Acyclovir | - | cy | | | cy | | | | | | | |
| Amikacin ***XA**** | cy | - | | | x* | x* | ca | | | | | |
| Aminophylline ***XA**** | | | - | | | | | cy | | | | |
| Amphotericin-B | | | | - | | | | | | | | |
| Ampicillin | cy | x* | | | - | | | | | | | |
| Ampicillin and sulbactam | | x* | | | | - | | | | | | |
| Ascorbic acid | | ca | | | | | - | | | | xa | |
| Atracurium | | | cy | | | | | - | | | | |
| Atropine | | | | | | | | | - | | | |
| Aztreonam | | | | | | | | | | - | | |
| Bleomycin | | | xa | | | | xa | | | | - | |
| Carboplatin | | | | | | | | | | | | - |
| Carmustine | | | | | | | | | | | | |
| Cefazolin | cy | ~ | | | | | xs | cy | | ca | xa | |
| Cefonicid | cy | ~ | | | | | | | | | | |
| Cefoperazone | cy | ~ | | | | | | | | | | |
| Cefotaxime | cy | ~ | | | | | | | | | | |
| Cefotetan | | ~ | cy | | cy | | | | cy | | | |
| Cefoxitin | cy | ~ | | | | | | | | | | |
| Ceftazidime | cy | ~ | | | | | | | | | | |
| Ceftriaxone ***XA**** | cy | ~ | | | | | | | | | | |
| Cefuroxime | cy | ~ | | | | | | cy | | | | |
| Chloramphenicol | cy | ca | | | cs | | ca | | | | | |
| Chlorpromazine | | | | xa | xa | | ca | | cs | | | |
| Cimetidine | cy | ca | cay | xa | | | | cy | cs | | | |
| Ciprofloxacin | | | | | | | | | | cay | | |
| Cisplatin | | | | | | | | | | | csy | csy |
| Clindamycin | cy | csa | | | ca | | | | | csa | | |
| Cyclophosphamide | | cy | | | cy | | | | | | csy | |
| Cytarabine | | | | | | | | | | | | |

| Carmustine | Cefazolin | Cefonicid | Cefoperazone | Cefotaxime | Cefotetan | Cefoxitin | Ceftazidime | Ceftriaxone ***XA**** | Cefuroxime | Chloramphenicol | Chlorpromazine | Cimetidine | Ciprofloxacin | Cisplatin | Clindamycin | Cyclophosphamide | Cytarabine |
|---|---|---|---|---|---|---|---|---|---|---|---|---|---|---|---|---|---|
| | cy | cy | cy | cy | | cy | cy | cy | cy | cy | | cy | | | cy | | |
| | ~ | ~ | ~ | ~ | ~ | ca | | | | ca | | ca | | | csa | cy | |
| | | | | | | | | | | | | cay | | | | | |
| | | | | | | | | | | | | xa | | | | | |
| | | | | | cy | | | | | cs | xa | | | | ca | cy | |
| | | | | | | | | | | | xa | | | | | | |
| | xs | | | | | | | | | ca | ca | | | | | | |
| | cy | | | | | | | | cy | | | cy | | | | | |
| | | | | | cy | | | | | | cs | cs | | | | | |
| | ca | | | | | | | | | | | | cay | | csa | | |
| | xa | | | | | | | | | | | | | csy | | csy | |
| | | | | | | | | | | | | | | csy | | | |
| - | | | | | | | | | | | | | | | | | |
| | - | | | | | | | | | | | xs | | | ca | cy | |
| | | - | | | | | | | | | | | | | ca | | |
| | | | - | | | | | | | | | ca | | | ca | cy | |
| | | | | - | | | | | | | | | | | ca | | |
| | | | | | - | | | | | | | cy | | | | | |
| | | | | | | - | | | | | | ca | | | ca | cy | |
| | | | | | | | - | | | | | | cay | | ca | | |
| | | | | | | | | - | | | | | | | | | |
| | | | | | | | | | - | | | | | | ca | cy | |
| | | | | | | | | | | - | xa | - | | | | cy | |
| | | | | | | | | | | xa | | xs | | | | | |
| | xs | | ca | | cy | ca | | | | | xs | - | | | ca | | |
| | | | | | | | cay | | | | | | - | | | | |
| | | | | | | | | | | | | | | - | | csy | |
| | ca | ca | ca | ca | | ca | ca | xa | ca | | | ca | | | - | cy | |
| | cy | | cy | cy | | cy | | | cy | cy | | | | csy | cy | - | |
| | | | | | | | | | | | | | | | | | |

| | Dacarbazine | Daunorubicin | Dexamethasone | Digoxin ***XA**** | Dimenhydrinate | Diphenhydramine | Dobutamine | Dopamine | Doxorubicin ***XA**** | Doxycycline | Droperidol |
|---|---|---|---|---|---|---|---|---|---|---|---|
| Acyclovir | | | cy | | cy | cy | xya | xya | | cy | |
| Amikacin ***XA**** | | | | | | ca | | | | | |
| Aminophylline ***XA**** | | | | | | xa | xy | xa | | | |
| Amphotericin-B | | | | | | | | | | | |
| Ampicillin | | | | | | | | xa | | | |
| Ampicillin and sulbactam | | | | | | | | | | | |
| Ascorbic acid | | | | | | ca | | | | | |
| Atracurium | | | | | | | cy | cy | | | |
| Atropine | | | | | cs | cs | | | | | cs |
| Aztreonam | | | | | | | | | | | |
| Bleomycin | | | | | | | | | csy | | |
| Carboplatin | | | | | | | | | | | |
| Carmustine | | | | | | | | | | | |
| Cefazolin | | | | | | | | | | | |
| Cefonicid | | | | | | | | | | | |
| Cefoperazone | | | | | | | | | | | |
| Cefotaxime | | | | | | | | | | | |
| Cefotetan | | | | cy | | | | cy | | xa | |
| Cefoxitin | | | | | | | | | | | |
| Ceftazidime | | | | | | | | | | | |
| Ceftriaxone ***XA**** | | | | | | | | | | | |
| Cefuroxime | | | | | | | | | | | |
| Chloramphenicol | | | | | ca | | | | | | |
| Chlorpromazine | | | | | xs | cs | | | | | cs |
| Cimetidine | | | ca | ca | | cs | | | | | cs |
| Ciprofloxacin | | | | | | | | | | | |
| Cisplatin | | | | | | | | | csy | | csy |
| Clindamycin | | | | | | | | | | | |
| Cyclophosphamide | | | | | | | | | csy | cy | csy |
| Cytarabine | cy | | | | | | | | | | |

| | Epinephrine | Etoposide | Famotidine | Filgrastim | Fluconazole ***XA**** | Fludarabine | Fluorouracil ***XA**** | Foscarnet | Furosemide | Ganciclovir | Gentamicin | Heparin | Hydrocortisone Na Suc | Idarubicin ***XA**** | Ifosfamide | Imipenem and cilastatin | Insulin regular | Isoproterenol | Leucovorin |
|---|---|---|---|---|---|---|---|---|---|---|---|---|---|---|---|---|---|---|---|
| | | | | | | | | x | | | cy | cy | cy | | | cy | | | |
| | ca | | | | | cy | | cy | cy | | | xsa | ca | | | | | | |
| | | | cy | | | cy | | | | | | | | | | | | | |
| | | | | | | | | xy | | | | | | | | | | | |
| | xy | | cy | | | cy | | | | | x* | cs | | | | | | | |
| | | | cy | | | cy | | | | | x* | | | | | | | | |
| | | | | | | | | | | | | ca | | | | | | | |
| | cy | | | | | | | | | | cy | cy | cy | | | | | cy | |
| | | | cy | | | | | | | | | csy | cy | | | | | | |
| | | | | | | cy | | cy | | | | | | | | | | | |
| | | | | | | cy | csy | | | | | csy | xa | | | | | | csy |
| | | | | | | cy | xa | | | | | | | | ca | | | | |
| | | | | | | cy | | | | | | | | | | | | | |
| | | | cy | | cy | cy | | cy | | | ~ | cs | | | | | cy | | |
| | | | | | | | | | | | ~ | | | | | | | | |
| | | | cy | | | cy | | cy | ca | | ~ | cs | | | | | | | |
| | | | | | xy | cy | | | | | ~ | | | | | | | | |
| | cy | | cy | | cy | cy | | | cy | | ~ | xa | | | | | cy | | |
| | | | cy | | cy | | | cy | | | ~ | cs | | | | | | | |
| | | | cy | | xy | cy | | cy | | | ~ | | | | | | | | |
| | | | | | xy | cy | | cy | | | ~ | | | | | | | | |
| | | | cy | | xy | cy | | cy | ca | | ~ | ca | | | | | | | |
| | | | | | xy | | | cy | xa | | | csa | ca | | | | | | |
| | | | | | cy | xy | | | | | | cy | cy | | | | | | |
| | | | | | cy | cy | | cy | ca | | ca | csy | | | | | | | |
| | | | | | | | | | | | | xy | | | | | | | |
| | | ca | | | | csy | csy | | csy | | | csy | | | ca | | | | c |
| | | | | | xy | cy | | cy | | | cs | csa | ca | | | | | | |
| | | | | | | cy | csy | | csy | | | csy | | | | | | | csy |
| | | | | | | cy | xay | | | | | xa | | | | | xa | | |

| | Lidocaine | Methotrexate | Methylprednisolone | Metoclopramide | Metronidazole **XA*** | Mezlocillin | Miconazole **XA*** | Mitomycin | Morphine sulfate | M.V.I. | Nafcillin | Netilmicin **XA*** |
|---|---|---|---|---|---|---|---|---|---|---|---|---|
| Acyclovir | | | cy | cy | cy | | | | cy | cy | cy | |
| Amikacin **XA*** | | | | | ca | x* | | | cy | | x* | |
| Aminophylline **XA*** | | | | | | | | | | | | cy |
| Amphotericin-B | | | | | | | | | | | | |
| Ampicillin | | | | | | | | | cy | | | x* |
| Ampicillin and sulbactam | | | | | | | | | cy | | | x* |
| Ascorbic acid | | | | | | | | | | | xa | |
| Atracurium | | | | | | | | | cy | | | |
| Atropine | | | | cs | | | | | cs | | cy | |
| Aztreonam | | | | | xa | | | | | | xa | |
| Bleomycin | | csy | | | | | | csy | | | xa | |
| Carboplatin | | | | | | | | | | | | |
| Carmustine | | | | | | | | | | | | |
| Cefazolin | cy | | | | ca | | | | cy | cy | | ~ |
| Cefonicid | | | | | | | | | | | | ~ |
| Cefoperazone | | | | | | | | | cy | | | ~ |
| Cefotaxime | | | | | | | | | | | | ~ |
| Cefotetan | | | | | | cy | | | cy | cy | | ~ |
| Cefoxitin | | | | | ca | | | | | ca | | ~ |
| Ceftazidime | | | | | ca | | | | | | | ~ |
| Ceftriaxone **XA*** | | | | | | | | | cy | | | ~ |
| Cefuroxime | | | | | ca | | | | cy | | | ~ |
| Chloramphenicol | ca | | ca | xs | ca | | | | cy | | ca | |
| Chlorpromazine | | | | cs | | | | | cs | | | ca |
| Cimetidine | | | ca | | | | | | cs | | cs | |
| Ciprofloxacin | | | | | ca | xya | | | | | | |
| Cisplatin | | csy | | csy | | | | csy | | | | |
| Clindamycin | | csy | ca | ca | cay | cy | | csy | cy | cy | cy | ca |
| Cyclophosphamide | cs | cy | | csy | cy | cy | | csy | | | cy | |
| Cytarabine | | ca | | cs | | | | | | | xa | |

| Nitroglycerin | Ondansetron | Oxacillin | Oxytocin | Penicillin G potassium | Perphenazine | Phenytoin ***XA**** | Phytonadione | Piperacillin | Potassium chloride | Prochlorperazine | Promethazine | Propranolol | Ranitidine | Sargramostim | Sodium bicarbonate | Theophylline | Ticarcillin | Ticarcillin and clavulanate |
|---|---|---|---|---|---|---|---|---|---|---|---|---|---|---|---|---|---|---|
| | xy | cy | | cy | cy | | | cy | cy | | | | cy | cy | cy | cy | cy | |
| | cy | x* | | x* | | | ca | | cy | | | | cy | | ca | | x* | x* |
| | xy | | | | | | | | cy | | | | cy | | | | | |
| | xy | | | | | | | | xa | | | | | | | | | xa |
| | xy | | | | | | | | cy | | | | | | | | | |
| | xy | | | | | | | | | | | | | | | | | |
| | | | | ca | | | | | | | | | | | xa | | | |
| cy | | | | | | | | | | | | | cy | | xs | | | |
| | | | | | cs | | | | cy | cs | cs | | cs | | xa | | | |
| | cy | | | | | | | | | | | | | | | | | |
| | | | | xa | | | | | | | | | | | | | | |
| | cy | | | | | | | | | | | | | cy | | | | |
| | cy | | | | | | | | | | | | | cy | xa | | | |
| | cy | | | | | | | | | | | | | cy | | | | |
| | | | | | | | | | | | | | | xy | | | | |
| | xy | | | | xy | | | | | | | | | xy | | | | |
| | | | | | | | | | | | | | | | | | | |
| | | | cy | cy | | | | cy | | | | | | cy | | | cy | |
| | cy | | | | cy | | | | | | | | | | | | | |
| | cy | | | | | | | | | | | | | xy | | | | |
| | | | | | | | | | | | | | | cy | | | | |
| | cy | | | | cy | | | | ca | | | | | cy | xa | | | |
| | | ca | | csa | cy | | | | ca | xa | xa | | ca | | ca | | | |
| | cy | | | xa | | | | | cy | | | | | xy | | | | |
| | cy | | | csa | cs | | | | ca | cs | cs | | | cy | | | | |
| | | | | | | | | cay | | | | | | | | | | |
| | csy | | | | | | | | | | | | | csy | xa | | | |
| | cy | cy | | ca | cy | | | ca | ca | | | | xa | cy | ca | | | |
| | cy | cy | | cy | | | cy | | | | | | | cy | | | cy | |
| | cy | xa | | xa | | | | | ca | | | | | cy | ca | | | |

| | Tobramycin | Trimethoprim-sulfa. ***XA**** | Vancomycin |
|---|---|---|---|
| Acyclovir | cy | cy | cy |
| Amikacin ***XA**** | | | ca |
| Aminophylline ***XA**** | | | |
| Amphotericin-B | | | |
| Ampicillin | x* | | |
| Ampicillin and sulbactam | x* | | |
| Ascorbic acid | | | |
| Atracurium | | cy | cy |
| Atropine | | | |
| Aztreonam | | | xy |
| Bleomycin | | | |
| Carboplatin | | | |
| Carmustine | | | |
| Cefazolin | ~ | | |
| Cefonicid | ~ | | |
| Cefoperazone | ~ | | |
| Cefotaxime | ~ | | |
| Cefotetan | ~ | | |
| Cefoxitin | ~ | | |
| Ceftazidime | ~ | | |
| Ceftriaxone ***XA**** | ~ | | xy |
| Cefuroxime | ~ | | |
| Chloramphenicol | | | xa |
| Chlorpromazine | | | |
| Cimetidine | | | ca |
| Ciprofloxacin | cay | | |
| Cisplatin | | | |
| Clindamycin | ca | | |
| Cyclophosphamide | cy | cy | cy |
| Cytarabine | | | |

| | Verapamil | Vinblastine | Vincristine | Zidovudine |
|---|---|---|---|---|
| Acyclovir | xy | | | cy |
| Amikacin ***XA**** | | | | |
| Aminophylline ***XA**** | | | | |
| Amphotericin-B | xa | | | cy |
| Ampicillin | ca | | | |
| Ampicillin and sulbactam | | | | |
| Ascorbic acid | | | | |
| Atracurium | | | | |
| Atropine | | | | |
| Aztreonam | | | | cy |
| Bleomycin | | csy | csy | |
| Carboplatin | | | | |
| Carmustine | | | | |
| Cefazolin | ca | | | |
| Cefonicid | | | | |
| Cefoperazone | | | | |
| Cefotaxime | | | | |
| Cefotetan | | | | |
| Cefoxitin | | | | |
| Ceftazidime | | | | cy |
| Ceftriaxone ***XA**** | | | | |
| Cefuroxime | | | | |
| Chloramphenicol | ca | | | |
| Chlorpromazine | | | | |
| Cimetidine | ca | | | cy |
| Ciprofloxacin | | | | |
| Cisplatin | | csy | csy | |
| Clindamycin | ca | | | cy |
| Cyclophosphamide | | csy | csy | |
| Cytarabine | | | ca | |

| | Acyclovir | Amikacin ***XA**** | Aminophylline ***XA**** | Amphotericin-B | Ampicillin | Ampicillin and sulbactam | Ascorbic acid | Atracurium | Atropine | Aztreonam | Bleomycin | Carboplatin |
|---|---|---|---|---|---|---|---|---|---|---|---|---|
| Dacarbazine | | | | | | | | | | | ca | |
| Daunorubicin | | | | | | | | | | | | |
| Dexamethasone | cy | | ca | | | | | | | | ca | |
| Digoxin ***XA**** | | | | | | | | | | | | |
| Dimenhydrinate | cy | ca | xy | | | | | | cs | | | |
| Diphenhydramine | cy | ca | ca | | | | ca | | cs | | ca | |
| Dobutamine | xya | | xya | | | | | cy | ca | | | |
| Dopamine | x | | ca | xa | xa | | | cy | | | | |
| Doxorubicin ***XA**** | | | | | | | | | | | csy | |
| Doxycycline | cy | | | | | | | | | | | |
| Droperidol | | | | | | | | | cs | | csy | |
| Epinephrine | | ca | | | xy | | | cy | | | | |
| Etoposide | | | | | | | | | | | | |
| Famotidine | | | cy | | cy | cy | | | cy | | | |
| Filgrastim | | | | | | | | | | | | |
| Fluconazole ***XA**** | cy | cy | cy | xy | xy | cy | | | | | cy | |
| Fludarabine | xy | cy | cy | xy | cy | cy | | | | cy | cy | cy |
| Fluorouracil ***XA**** | | | xa | xa | | | | | | | c | xa |
| Foscarnet | x | cy | xa | cy | | | | | | | | |
| Furosemide | | cay | ca | | ca | | | | ca | | csy | |
| Ganciclovir | | | xa | xa | | | | | | | | |
| Gentamicin | cy | | xa | xa | x* | x* | | cy | | ca | ca | |
| Heparin | cy | xsa | c | c | cs | ca | cay | cs | cs | c | csa | |
| Hydrocortisone Na Suc | cy | | ca | cy | | | cy | | | xa | | |
| Idarubicin ***XA**** | | | | | | | | | | | | ca |
| Ifosfamide | | | | | | | | | | | | |
| Imipenem and cilastatin | cy | xa | | xa | xa | xa | | | | xa | | |
| Insulin regular | | | xa | | cy | cy | | | | cy | | |
| Isoproterenol | | | xa | | | | | cy | | | | |
| Leucovorin | | | | | | | | | | | csy | |

| Carmustine | Cefazolin | Cefonicid | Cefoperazone | Cefotaxime | Cefotetan | Cefoxitin | Ceftazidime | Ceftriaxone ***XA**** | Cefuroxime | Chloramphenicol | Chlorpromazine | Cimetidine | Ciprofloxacin | Cisplatin | Clindamycin | Cyclophosphamide | Cytarabine |
|---|---|---|---|---|---|---|---|---|---|---|---|---|---|---|---|---|---|
| ca | | | | | | | | | | | | | | | | ca | ca |
| | | | | | | | | | | | | | | | | | |
| | | | | | | | | | | | | ca | | | | | |
| | | | | | | | | | | | | ca | | | | | |
| | | | | | | | | | | ca | xs | | | | | | |
| | | | | | | | | | | | csa | cs | | | | | |
| | | | | | | | | | | | | | | | | | |
| | | | | | | cy | | | | ca | | | | | | | |
| | | | | | | | | | | | | | | csy | | csy | |
| | | | | | | xa | | | | | | | | | | cy | |
| | | | | | | | | | | | cs | cs | | csy | | csy | |
| | | | | | | cy | | | | | | ca | | | | | |
| | | | | | | | | | | | | | | ca | | | |
| | cy | | cy | cy | cy | cy | cy | | cy | | | | | | | | |
| | | | | | | | | | | | | | | | | | |
| | cy | | | xy | cy | cy | xy | xy | xy | xy | cy | cy | | | xy | | |
| cy | cy | | cy | cy | cy | | cy | cy | cy | | xy | cy | | cy | cy | cy | cy |
| | | | | | | | | | | | | | | csy | | c | xa |
| | cy | | cy | | | cy | cy | cy | cy | cy | | ca | | xa | cy | | xa |
| | | | ca | | | | | | ca | | xa | ca | | csy | | csy | |
| | | | | | | | | | | | | | | | | | |
| | | ~ | ~ | ~ | ~ | ~ | ~ | ~ | ~ | | | ca | | | csa | cy | |
| cs | cs | cs | cs | cs | cs | cs | | | | csa | xsy | cs | cy | csa | | csy | xa |
| | | | | | | | | | ca | cy | | | | ca | | | |
| | | | | | | | | | | | | | | ca | | | |
| | | | | | | | | | | | | | | ca | | | |
| | xa | xa | xa | xa | xa | xa | xa | xa | xa | xa | | | xa | | xa | | |
| | cy | | | | cy | | | | | | | ca | | | | | xa |
| | | | | | | | | | | | | ca | | | | | |
| | | | | | | | | | | | | | | c | | csy | |

| | Dacarbazine | Daunorubicin | Dexamethasone | Digoxin ***XA**** | Dimenhydrinate | Diphenhydramine | Dobutamine | Dopamine | Doxorubicin ***XA**** | Doxycycline | Droperidol | Epinephrine |
|---|---|---|---|---|---|---|---|---|---|---|---|---|
| Dacarbazine | | | | | | | | | ca | | | |
| Daunorubicin | | | xa | | | | | | | | | |
| Dexamethasone | | xa | | | | | | | xa | | | |
| Digoxin ***XA**** | | | | | | | xa | | | | | |
| Dimenhydrinate | | | | | | | | | | | cs | |
| Diphenhydramine | | | | | | | | | | | cs | |
| Dobutamine | | | | xa | | | - | cay | | | | ca |
| Dopamine | | | | | | | cay | - | | | | |
| Doxorubicin ***XA**** | | | xa | | | | | | | | csy | |
| Doxycycline | | | | | | | | | | | | |
| Droperidol | | | | | | cs | cs | | csy | | | |
| Epinephrine | | | | | | | ca | | | | | |
| Etoposide | | | | | | | | | | | | |
| Famotidine | | | cy | cy | | | cy | cy | | | | cy |
| Filgrastim | | | | | | | | | | | | |
| Fluconazole ***XA**** | | | cy | | | cy | | | | | cy | |
| Fludarabine | cy | xy | cy | | | cy | | | cy | cy | cy | |
| Fluorouracil ***XA**** | | | | | | | | | csy | | xsy | |
| Foscarnet | | | | | | | | | | | | |
| Furosemide | | | ca | | | | xa | | xsy | | xsy | |
| Ganciclovir | | | | | | | | | | | | |
| Gentamicin | | | | | | | | | | | | |
| Heparin | | xsa | cy | cs | csa | cy | cs | c | xy | | xs | csy |
| Hydrocortisone Na Suc | | ca | | cy | xa | cy | | cay | xa | | cy | cy |
| Idarubicin ***XA**** | | | | | | | | | | | | |
| Ifosfamide | | | | | | | | | | | | |
| Imipenem and cilastatin | | | | | | | | | | xa | | |
| Insulin regular | | | | | | | cy | | | | | |
| Isoproterenol | | | | | | | ca | | | | | |
| Leucovorin | | | | | | | | | csy | | xsy | |

| Etoposide | Famotidine | Filgrastim | Fluconazole XA* | Fludarabine | Fluorouracil XA* | Foscarnet | Furosemide | Ganciclovir | Gentamicin | Heparin | Hydrocortisone Na Suc | Idarubicin XA* | Ifosfamide | Imipenem and cilastatin | Insulin regular | Isoproterenol | Leucovorin |
|---|---|---|---|---|---|---|---|---|---|---|---|---|---|---|---|---|---|
| | | | | cy | ca | | | | | | xa | | | | | | |
| | | | | xy | | | | | | xa | ca | | | | | | |
| | cy | | cy | cy | | cy | ca | | | | | | | | | | |
| | cy | | xs | | | xs | ca | | | cs | | | | | | | |
| | | | | | | | | | | csa | xy | | | | | | |
| | | | cy | cy | | xy | | | | cy | cy | | | | | | |
| | cy | | | | | xy | xa | | | cs | | | | | cy | ca | |
| | cy | | | | | cy | | | | c | cay | | | | | | |
| | | | | cy | csy | | xsy | | | xsy | xa | | | | | | csy |
| | | | | cy | | | | | | | | | | | | | |
| | | | cy | cy | xsy | xy | xsy | | | xs | cy | | | | | | xsy |
| | cy | | | | ca | | | | | csy | cy | | | | | | |
| | | | | cy | ca | | | | | | | | ca | | | | |
| | | | cy | cy | | | cy | | cy | cy | cy | | | cy | cy | cy | |
| | | | | | | | | | | | cy | | | xy | | | cy |
| | cy | | | cy | | cy | xy | cy | cy | cy | cy | | | xy | | | cy |
| cy | cy | | cy | | cy | | cy | xy | cy | cy | cy | | cy | cy | | | |
| ca | | | | cy | | | cy | | | csy | cy | | | | | | c |
| | | | | | | | | | | | | | | | | | |
| | cy | | xy | cy | csy | | | | xy | c | cy | | | | | | csy |
| | cy | | cy | xy | | xy | | | | | | | | | | | |
| | cy | | cy | cy | | cy | | | - | x | | | | | cy | | |
| | cy | | cy | cy | cs | csy | c | | x | - | | | | | cy | cay | csy |
| | | | | | cy | | cy | | | | - | | | | cy | cy | |
| | | | | | | | | | | xs | | | | | | | |
| ca | | | | cy | ca | | | | | | | | | | | | |
| | cy | | xy | | | cy | | | xa | | | | | | | | |
| | cy | | | | | | | | | cy | | | | cy | | | |
| | cy | | cy | | | | xa | | | cay | cy | | | | | - | |
| | | | | | c | xy | csy | | | csy | | | | | | | - |

| | Lidocaine | Methotrexate | Methylprednisolone | Metoclopramide | Metronidazole ***XA**** | Mezlocillin | Miconazole ***XA**** | Mitomycin | Morphine sulfate | M.V.I. | Nafcillin | Netilmicin ***XA**** |
|---|---|---|---|---|---|---|---|---|---|---|---|---|
| Dacarbazine | | ca | | | | | | | | | | |
| Daunorubicin | | | | | | | | | | | | |
| Dexamethasone | ca | | | cs | | | | | cy | | ca | ca |
| Digoxin ***XA**** | ca | | | | | | | | cy | | | |
| Dimenhydrinate | | | | cs | | | | | cs | | | |
| Diphenhydramine | ca | | | cs | | | | | cs | | ca | ca |
| Dobutamine | cay | | | | | | | | ca | | | |
| Dopamine | cay | | ca | | | | | | cy | | | |
| Doxorubicin ***XA**** | | csy | | csy | | | | csy | | | | |
| Doxycycline | | | | | | | | | cy | | xa | |
| Droperidol | | xsy | | csy | | | | csy | cs | | xy | |
| Epinephrine | | | | | | | | | | | | |
| Etoposide | | | | | | | | | | | | |
| Famotidine | cy | | cy | cy | | cy | | | cy | | cy | |
| Filgrastim | | | | | | | | | cy | | | |
| Fluconazole ***XA**** | | | | | cy | | | | cy | | cy | |
| Fludarabine | | cy | cy | cy | | cy | | | cy | cy | | cy |
| Fluorouracil ***XA**** | | c | | csy | | | | csy | | | | |
| Foscarnet | | | | | | | | | | | | |
| Furosemide | | csy | | x | | | | csy | xy | | | xya |
| Ganciclovir | | | | | | | | | | | | |
| Gentamicin | | | | | ca | | | | cy | cy | xa | |
| Heparin | csa | csy | ca | csy | | cs | | csy | xa | | csa | xs |
| Hydrocortisone Na Suc | cya | | | cs | ca | | | | cy | | xa | ca |
| Idarubicin ***XA**** | | | | | | | | | | | | |
| Ifosfamide | | | | | | | | | | | | |
| Imipenem and cilastatin | | | | | | xa | | | | | xa | xa |
| Insulin regular | ca | | xa | cs | | | | | cy | | | |
| Isoproterenol | xa | | | | | | | | | ca | | ca |
| Leucovorin | | csy | | csy | | | | csy | | | | |

| Nitroglycerin | Ondansetron | Oxacillin | Oxytocin | Penicillin G potassium | Perphenazine | Phenytoin ***XA**** | Phytonadione | Piperacillin | Potassium chloride | Prochlorperazine | Promethazine | Propranolol | Ranitidine | Sargramostim | Sodium bicarbonate | Theophylline | Ticarcillin | Ticarcillin and clavulanate |
|---|---|---|---|---|---|---|---|---|---|---|---|---|---|---|---|---|---|---|
| | cy | xa | | | | | | | | | | | | cy | | | | |
| | cy | | | | | | | | | | | | | | | | | |
| | cy | | | | | | | | cy | ca | | | cs | cy | | | | |
| | | | | | | | | | cy | | | | | | | | | |
| | | | | ca | cs | | | | ca | ca | xs | | cs | | | | | |
| | cy | | | ca | cs | | | | cy | cs | cs | | cs | | | | | |
| cay | | | | | | xa | xy | | cy | | | ca | c | | xa | | | |
| cay | | ca | | xa | | | | | cay | | | | c | | x | | | |
| | cy | | | | | | | | | | | | | | | | | |
| | cy | xa | | xa | cy | | | | | | | | cay | cy | | | | |
| | cy | | | | cs | | | | cy | cs | cs | | | cy | | | | |
| | | | | | | | cy | | cy | | | | | | xa | | | |
| | cy | | | | | | | | | | | | | cy | | | | |
| cy | cy | cy | | | cy | | cy | cy | cy | | | | | cy | cy | cy | cy | |
| | | | | ca | | | | | | | | | | | | | | |
| | cy | cy | | cy | | cy | | xy | | cy | cy | | | cy | | | xy | |
| | cy | | | | | | | | cy | | cy | | cy | | cy | | cy | |
| | | | | | | | | | cy | | | | | cy | | | | |
| | | | | | | | | | | | | | | | | | | |
| ca | xy | | | ca | | | | | cay | | | | | ca | cy | ca | | |
| | xy | | | | | | | | | | | | | xy | | | | |
| | cy | | | | cy | | | | | | | | ca | cy | | | xa | |
| | cy | cy | cy | csy | | xy | cy | cs | ca | | xas | | cay | cy | cay | | | |
| | cy | cy | cy | cay | | | cy | ca | ca | cy | xa | cy | | | cay | | | |
| | | | | | | | | | | | | | | xy | | | | |
| | cy | | | | | | | | | | | | | cy | | | | |
| | cy | xa | | xa | | | | xa | | | | | | xy | | | xa | xa |
| | | | cy | | | xa | | | cy | | | | | | cy | | cy | cy |
| | | | | | | | | | cay | | | | cs | | xa | | | |
| | | | | | | | | | | | | | | | | | | |

| | Tobramycin | Trimethoprim-sulfa. ***XA**** | Vancomycin |
|---|---|---|---|
| Dacarbazine | | | |
| Daunorubicin | | | |
| Dexamethasone | | | xa |
| Digoxin ***XA**** | | | |
| Dimenhydrinate | | | ca |
| Diphenhydramine | | | |
| Dobutamine | | | |
| Dopamine | | | |
| Doxorubicin ***XA**** | | | |
| Doxycycline | | | |
| Droperidol | | | |
| Epinephrine | | | |
| Etoposide | | | |
| Famotidine | | | |
| Filgrastim | | | |
| Fluconazole ***XA**** | cy | xy | cy |
| Fludarabine | cy | cy | |
| Fluorouracil ***XA**** | | | |
| Foscarnet | | | |
| Furosemide | cay | | |
| Ganciclovir | | | |
| Gentamicin | | | |
| Heparin | xsy | cs | xsy |
| Hydrocortisone Na Suc | | | ca |
| Idarubicin ***XA**** | | | |
| Ifosfamide | | | |
| Imipenem and cilastatin | xa | xa | xa |
| Insulin regular | cy | | cy |
| Isoproterenol | | | |
| Leucovorin | | | |

| | Verapamil | Vinblastine | Vincristine | Zidovudine |
|---|---|---|---|---|
| Dacarbazine | | ca | | |
| Daunorubicin | | | | |
| Dexamethasone | ca | | | cy |
| Digoxin ***XA**** | ca | | | |
| Dimenhydrinate | | | | |
| Diphenhydramine | | | | |
| Dobutamine | cy | | | cy |
| Dopamine | cay | | | cy |
| Doxorubicin ***XA**** | | cy | csy | xa |
| Doxycycline | | | | |
| Droperidol | | csy | csy | |
| Epinephrine | ca | | | |
| Etoposide | | | | |
| Famotidine | cy | | | |
| Filgrastim | | | | |
| Fluconazole ***XA**** | | | | cy |
| Fludarabine | cy | cy | cy | cy |
| Fluorouracil ***XA**** | | csy | csya | |
| Foscarnet | | | | |
| Furosemide | ca | | | |
| Ganciclovir | | | | |
| Gentamicin | ca | | | cy |
| Heparin | csa | cy | cy | cy |
| Hydrocortisone Na Suc | ca | | | |
| Idarubicin ***XA**** | | | | |
| Ifosfamide | | | | |
| Imipenem and cilastatin | | | | cy |
| Insulin regular | ca | | | |
| Isoproterenol | ca | | | |
| Leucovorin | | csy | csy | |

| | Acyclovir | Amikacin ***XA**** | Aminophylline ***XA**** | Amphotericin-B | Ampicillin | Ampicillin and sulbactam | Ascorbic acid | Atracurium | Atropine | Aztreonam | Bleomycin | Carboplatin |
|---|---|---|---|---|---|---|---|---|---|---|---|---|
| Lidocaine | | | ca | | | | | | | | | |
| Methotrexate | | | | | | | | | | | csy | |
| Methylprednisolone | cy | | | | | | | | | | | |
| Metoclopramide | cy | | cs | | xs | | cs | | cs | | csy | |
| Metronidazole ***XA**** | cy | ca | ca | | | | | | | xa | | |
| Mezlocillin | | x* | | | | | | | | | | |
| Miconazole ***XA**** | | | | | | | | | | | | |
| Mitomycin | | | | | | | | | | | csy | |
| Morphine sulfate | | cy | cy | | cy | cy | | cy | cs | | | |
| M.V.I. | cy | | | | cy | | | | | | xa | |
| Nafcillin | cy | | | | | | xa | | cy | xa | xa | |
| Netilmicin ***XA**** | | | cy | | ~ | ~ | | | ca | | | |
| Nitroglycerin | | | | | | | | | | | | |
| Ondansetron | xy | cy | xy | xy | xy | xy | | | | cy | cy | cy |
| Oxacillin | cy | | | | | | | | | | | |
| Oxytocin | | | | | | | | | | | | |
| Penicillin G potassium | cy | xa | xa | xa | | | ca | | | | | |
| Perphenazine | cy | cy | | | cy | | | | cs | | | |
| Phenytoin ***XA**** | | | | | | | | | | | | |
| Phytonadione | | ca | | | cy | | | | | | | |
| Piperacillin | cy | x* | | | | | | | | | | |
| Potassium chloride | cy | | cay | xa | cy | | | | cy | | | |
| Prochlorperazine | | ca | xya | xa | xa | | ca | | cs* | | | |
| Promethazine | | ca | xya | | | | ca | | cs | | | |
| Propranolol | | | | | | | | | | | | |
| Ranitidine | cy | ca | cay | xa | | | | cy | cs | | | |
| Sargramostim | xy | cy | cy | | xy | xy | | | | cy | cy | cy |
| Sodium bicarbonate | cy | ca | ca | ca | | | xa | | ca | | | xa |
| Theophylline | cy | | | | | | xa | | | | | |
| Ticarcillin | cy | x* | | | | | | | | | | |
| Ticarcillin and clavulanate | | x* | | | | | | | | | | |
| Tobramycin | cy | | | | x* | x* | | | | ca | ca | |
| Trimethoprim-sulfa. ***XA**** | cy | | | | | | | cy | | | | |
| Vancomycin | cy | ca | | | | | | cy | | xy | | |
| Verapamil | | | | | xy | | | | | | | |
| Vinblastine | | | | | | | | | | | csy | |
| Vincristine | | cy | | | | | | | | | csy | |
| Zidovudine | cy | cy | | cy | | | | | | cy | | |

| Carmustine | Cefazolin | Cefonicid | Cefoperazone | Cefotaxime | Cefotetan | Cefoxitin | Ceftazidime | Ceftriaxone ***XA**** | Cefuroxime | Chloramphenicol | Chlorpromazine | Cimetidine | Ciprofloxacin | Cisplatin | Clindamycin | Cyclophosphamide | Cytarabine |
|---|---|---|---|---|---|---|---|---|---|---|---|---|---|---|---|---|---|
| | cy | | | | | | | | | ca | | ca | | | | | |
| | | | | | | | | | | | | | | csy | | c | ca |
| | | | | | | | | | | ca | | ca | | | ca | | |
| | | | | | | | | | | xs | cs | | | csy | ca | csy | cs |
| | ca | | | ca | | | ca | | ca | ca | | | ca | | ca | cy | |
| | | | | | | | | | | | | | xa | | | cy | |
| | | | | | | | | | | | | | | | | | |
| | | | | | | | | | | | | | | csy | | csy | |
| | cy | | cy | cy | cy | cy | | cy | cy | cy | cs | cs | | | cy | | |
| | cy | | | | | ca | | | | | | | | | | | |
| | | | | | | | | | | ca | | cs | | | | cy | xa |
| | | | | | | | | | ca | | ca | | | | ca | | |
| | | | | | | | | | | | | | | | | | |
| cy | cy | | xy | cy | | cy | cy | | cy | | cy | cy | | cy | cy | cy | cy |
| | | | | | | | | | | ca | | | | | | cy | xa |
| | | | | | | | | | | ca | | | | | | | |
| | | | | | | | | | | | xa | ca | | | | cy | |
| | cy | | xy | cy | | cy | | | cy | cy | | cs | | | cy | | |
| | | | | | | | | | | | | | | | | | |
| | | | | | | | | | | ca | | ca | | | | | |
| | | | | | | | | | | | | | cay | | ca | cy | |
| | | | | | | | | | | ca | cy | ca | | | ca | | ca |
| | | | | | | | | | | xya | | cs* | | | | | |
| | | | xy | | | | | | | xya | | cs | | | | | |
| | | | | | | | | | | | | | | | | | |
| | | | | | | | | | | ca | | | | | xa | | |
| cy | cy | | xy | cy | cy | | xy | cy | cy | | xy | cy | | cy | cy | cy | cy |
| xa | | | | xa | | ca | | | | ca | | ca | | xa | ca | | ca |
| | | | | | | | | | | | xa | | | | | | |
| | | | | | | | | | | | | | | | | cy | |
| | | | | | | | | | | | | | | | | cy | |
| | | | | | ca | | | | | | | cay | | ca | cy | | |
| | | | | | | | | | | | | | | | cy | | |
| | | | | | | | | | xa | | ca | | | | cy | | |
| | | | | | | | | | | | | | | | | | |
| | | | | | | | | | | | | | csy | | csy | | |
| | | | | | | | | | | | | | csy | | csy | | |
| | | | | | | cy | cy | | | | cy | | | cy | | | |

| | Dacarbazine | Daunorubicin | Dexamethasone | Digoxin ***XA**** | Dimenhydrinate | Diphenhydramine | Dobutamine | Dopamine | Doxorubicin ***XA**** | Doxycycline | Droperidol | Epinephrine |
|---|---|---|---|---|---|---|---|---|---|---|---|---|
| Lidocaine | | | ca | | | ca | cay | ca | | | | |
| Methotrexate | | | | | | | | | csy | | xsy | |
| Methylprednisolone | | | | | | | | ca | | | | |
| Metoclopramide | | | cs | | cs | cs | | | csy | | csy | |
| Metronidazole ***XA**** | | | | | | | | xa | | | | |
| Mezlocillin | | | | | | | | | | | | |
| Miconazole ***XA**** | | | | | | | | | | | | |
| Mitomycin | | | | | | | | | csy | | csy | |
| Morphine sulfate | | | cy | cy | cs | cs | ca | cy | | | cs | |
| M.V.I. | | | | | | | | | | | | |
| Nafcillin | | | ca | | | ca | | | | | xy | |
| Netilmicin ***XA**** | | | ca | | | ca | | | | | | |
| Nitroglycerin | | | | | | | | | | | | |
| Ondansetron | cy | cy | cy | | | cy | | | cy | cy | cy | |
| Oxacillin | | | | | | | | | | | | |
| Oxytocin | | | | | | | | | | | | |
| Penicillin G potassium | | | | | ca | ca | | xa | | | | |
| Perphenazine | | | | | cs | cs | | | | cy | cs | |
| Phenytoin ***XA**** | | | | | | | | | | | | |
| Phytonadione | | | | | | | xy | | | | | cy |
| Piperacillin | | | | | | | | | | | | |
| Potassium chloride | | | cy | cy | ca | cy | cy | cy | | | cy | cy |
| Prochlorperazine | | | ca | | ca | cs* | | | | | cs* | |
| Promethazine | | | | | xsy | cs | | | | | cs | |
| Propranolol | | | | | | | | | | | | |
| Ranitidine | | | cs | | cs | cs | cy | cy | | ca | | |
| Sargramostim | cy | | cy | | | cy | | | cy | cy | cy | |
| Sodium bicarbonate | | | | | | | xa | xa | | | | xa |
| Theophylline | | | | | xa | | | | | | | |
| Ticarcillin | | | | | | | | | | | | |
| Ticarcillin and clavulanate | | | | | | | | | | | | |
| Tobramycin | | | | | | | | | | | | |
| Trimethoprim-sulfa. ***XA**** | | | | | | | | | | | | |
| Vancomycin | | | xa | | ca | | | | | | | |
| Verapamil | | | | | | | cy | cy | | | | |
| Vinblastine | | | | | | | | | cy | | csy | |
| Vincristine | | | | | | | | | csy | | csy | |
| Zidovudine | | | cy | | | | cy | cy | | | | |

| | Etoposide | Famotidine | Filgrastim | Fluconazole ***XA**** | Fludarabine | Fluorouracil ***XA**** | Foscarnet | Furosemide | Ganciclovir | Gentamicin | Heparin | Hydrocortisone Na Suc | Idarubicin ***XA**** | Ifosfamide | Imipenem and cilastatin | Insulin regular | Isoproterenol | Leucovorin |
|---|---|---|---|---|---|---|---|---|---|---|---|---|---|---|---|---|---|---|
| | | cy | | | | | | ca | | | ca | ca | | | | ca | | |
| | | | | | cy | c | | csy | | | cy | | | | | | | csy |
| | | cy | | | | | | | | | ca | | | | | xa | | |
| | | cy | | cy | cy | csy | cy | xsy | | | csy | cs | | | | cs | | csy |
| | | | | cy | | | cy | | | ca | ca | | | | | | | |
| | | cy | | | cy | | | | | x* | cs | | | | | | | |
| | | | | | xy | | cy | | | | | | | | | | | |
| | | | | | | csy | | csy | | | csy | | | | | | | csy |
| | | cy | | cy | cy | | cy | xy | | cy | cy | cy | | | | cy | | |
| | | | | | cy | | | | | cy | | | | | | | ca | |
| | | cy | | cy | | | cy | | | xa | csa | xa | | | | xy | | |
| | | | | | cy | | | xy | | | xy | ca | | | | | ca | |
| | | | | | | | | | | | | | | | | | | |
| | cy | cy | | cy | cy | | | xy | xy | cy | cy | cy | | cy | cy | | | |
| | | cy | | cy | | | cy | | | | cy | cy | | | | | | |
| | | | | | | | | | | | cy | cy | | | | cy | | |
| | | | | cy | | | cy | ca | | xa | cs | ca | | | | | | |
| | | cy | | | | | | | | cy | | | | | | | | |
| | | cy | | cy | | | cy | | | | | | | | | | | |
| | | cy | | | | | | | | | cy | cy | | | | | | |
| | | cy | | xy | cy | | cy | | | x* | cs | ca | | | | | | |
| | | cy | | | cy | cy | | cay | | | ca | ca | | | | cy | cy | |
| | | | | cy | cy | | xy | xa | | | | cy | | | | | | |
| | | | | cy | cy | | xy | | | | xsa | xya | | | | | | |
| | | | | | | | | | | | cy | cy | | | | | | |
| | | | | | cy | | cy | ca | | ca | cay | | | | | | cs | |
| | cy | cy | | | | cy | | cy | xy | cy | cy | xy | xy | cy | xy | | | |
| | | cy | | | cy | | | | | | ca | ca | | | xa | cy | xa | |
| | | cy | | | | | | | | | | | | | | | | |
| | | cy | | xy | cy | | | | | x* | | | | | | cy | | |
| | | cy | | cy | cy | | cy | | | x* | | | | | | cy | | |
| | | | | cy | cy | | cy | cay | | | xsy | | | | | cy | | |
| | | | | | cy | | xy | | | | cs | | | | | | | |
| | | | | cy | cy | | | | | | xs | ca | | | | cy | | |
| | | cy | | | | | | | | | cs | | | | | | | |
| | | | | | cy | csy | | xsy | | | cy | | | | | | | csy |
| | | | | | | csy | | xsy | | | csy | | | | | | | csy |
| | | | | cy | cy | | | | | cy | cy | | | | cy | | | |

| | Lidocaine | Methotrexate | Methylprednisolone | Metoclopramide | Metronidazole ***XA**** | Mezlocillin | Miconazole ***XA**** | Mitomycin | Morphine sulfate | M.V.I. | Nafcillin | Netilmicin ***XA**** |
|---|---|---|---|---|---|---|---|---|---|---|---|---|
| Lidocaine | - | | | | | | | | cy | | | |
| Methotrexate | | | | cy | | | | csy | | | | |
| Methylprednisolone | | | | cs | | | | | cy | | xa | |
| Metoclopramide | cs | cy | cs | | | | | csy | cs | ca | | |
| Metronidazole ***XA**** | | | | | | | | | cy | ca | | ca |
| Mezlocillin | | | | | | | | | cy | | | x* |
| Miconazole ***XA**** | | | | | | | | | | | | |
| Mitomycin | | csy | | csy | | | | | | | | |
| Morphine sulfate | cy | | cy | csy | cy | cy | | | | | cy | |
| M.V.I. | | | | ca | | | | | | | | ca |
| Nafcillin | | | xa | | | | | | cy | | | |
| Netilmicin ***XA**** | | | | | ca | | | | | ca | x* | |
| Nitroglycerin | | | | | | | | | | | | |
| Ondansetron | | cy | xy | cy | | xy | cy | cy | cy | | | |
| Oxacillin | | | | | | | | | cy | | | |
| Oxytocin | | | | | | | | | cy | | | ca |
| Penicillin G potassium | ca | | ca | xs | | | | | cy | | | xa |
| Perphenazine | | | | cs | cy | cy | | | cs | | cy | |
| Phenytoin ***XA**** | | | | | | | | | | | | |
| Phytonadione | | | | | | | | | | | | ca |
| Piperacillin | | | | | | | | | cy | | | x* |
| Potassium chloride | cay | | ca | ca | | | | | cy | | ca | ca |
| Prochlorperazine | ca | | | cs* | | | | | | | ca | |
| Promethazine | | | | cs | | | | | | | | ca |
| Propranolol | | | | | | | | | cy | | | |
| Ranitidine | ca | | | cs | | | | | csy | | | |
| Sargramostim | | cy | xy | cy | cy | cy | cy | xy | xy | | | cy |
| Sodium bicarbonate | ca | ca | | xs | | | | | cy | ca | ca | ca |
| Theophylline | | | ca | | | | | | | | | |
| Ticarcillin | | | | | | | | | cy | | | x* |
| Ticarcillin and clavulanate | | | | | | | | | cy | | | x* |
| Tobramycin | | | | | ca | | | | cy | | x* | |
| Trimethoprim-sulfa. ***XA**** | | | | | | | | | cy | | | |
| Vancomycin | | cy | | | | | | | cy | | | |
| Verapamil | | | | | | xy | | | | | xy | |
| Vinblastine | | csy | | csy | | | | csy | | | | |
| Vincristine | | csy | | csy | | | | csy | | | | |
| Zidovudine | | | | cy | | | | | cy | | cy | |

| Nitroglycerin | Ondansetron | Oxacillin | Oxytocin | Penicillin G potassium | Perphenazine | Phenytoin *XA** | Phytonadione | Piperacillin | Potassium chloride | Prochlorperazine | Promethazine | Propranolol | Ranitidine | Sargramostim | Sodium bicarbonate | Theophylline | Ticarcillin | Ticarcillin and clavulanate |
|---|---|---|---|---|---|---|---|---|---|---|---|---|---|---|---|---|---|---|
| | | | | ca | | xa | | | cay | ca | | | ca | | ca | | | |
| | cy | | | | | | | | | | | | xs | cy | ca | | | |
| | xy | | | ca | | | | | cy | | | | | xy | | | | |
| | cy | | | xs | cs | | | | ca | cs | cs | | cs | cy | xs | | | |
| | | | | | cy | | | | | | | | | cy | | | | |
| | xy | | | | cy | | | | | | | | | cy | | | | |
| | cy | | | | | | | | | | | | | cy | | | | |
| | cy | | | | | | | | | | | | | xy | | | | |
| | cy | cy | cy | cy | cs | xa | | cy | cy | | | cy | csy | xy | cy | | cy | cy |
| | | | | | | | | | | | | | | | ca | | | |
| | | | | | cy | | | | ca | ca | | | | | ca | | | |
| | | x* | ca | x* | | | ca | x* | ca | | ca | | | cy | | | x* | x* |
| | | | | | | | | | | | | | | | | | | |
| | | | | | | | | xy | cy | cy | | | cy | xy | xy | | cy | cy |
| | | - | | | cy | | | | cay | | | | | | ca | | | |
| | | | | | | | | | cy | | | | | | ca | | | |
| | | | | | cy | | | | cay | ca | xa | | | | | | | |
| | | cy | | cy | | | | cy | | | | | cs | | | | cy | cy |
| | | | | | | - | | | xy | | | | | | | | | |
| | | | | | | xy | | | cy | | | | | | ca | | | |
| | xy | | | | cy | | | | ca | | | | | xy | | | | |
| | cy | cay | cy | cay | | xy | cy | ca | | cy | | cy | ca | cy | cay | | | |
| | cy | | | xy | | xy | | | cy | | | | cs* | cy | ca | | | |
| | cy | | | xya | | xy | | | | | | | cs | cy | | | | |
| | | | | | | | | | cy | | | | | | | | | |
| cy | cy | | | ca | cs | | | | ca | cs | cs | | | cy | | | ca | |
| | xy | | | | | | | xy | cy | cy | cy | | cy | - | xy | | cy | cy |
| | | ca | ca | | | ca | ca | | cay | ca | | | | xy | | | | |
| | | | | xa | | xa | | | | xa | xa | | | | | | | |
| | cy | | | | cy | | | | | | | | ca | cy | | | | |
| | cy | | | | cy | | | | | | | | | cy | | | | |
| | | x* | | x* | cy | | | x* | | | | | ca | xy | | | x* | x* |
| | | | | | cy | | | | | | | | | cy | | | | |
| | cy | | | | cy | | | | ca | | | | ca | cy | | | | |
| | | xy | | cy | | | | cy | | | | | | | xy | | cy | |
| | cy | | | | | | | | | | | | | cy | | | | |
| | cy | | | | | | | | | | | | | cy | | | | |
| | cy | cy | | | | | | cy | cy | | | | cy | cy | | | | |

| | Tobramycin | Trimethoprim-sulfa. ***XA**** | Vancomycin | Verapamil | Vinblastine | Vincristine | Zidovudine |
|---|---|---|---|---|---|---|---|
| Lidocaine | | | | ca | | | |
| Methotrexate | | | cy | | csy | c | |
| Methylprednisolone | | | | ca | | | |
| Metoclopramide | | | | ca | csy | csy | cy |
| Metronidazole ***XA**** | ca | | | | | | |
| Mezlocillin | x* | | | xy | | | |
| Miconazole ***XA**** | | | | | | | |
| Mitomycin | | | | | csy | csy | |
| Morphine sulfate | cy | cy | cy | ca | | | cy |
| M.V.I. | | | | ca | | | |
| Nafcillin | | | | xy | | | cy |
| Netilmicin ***XA**** | | | | | | | |
| Nitroglycerin | | | | | | | |
| Ondansetron | | | cy | | cy | cy | cy |
| Oxacillin | | | | xy | | | cy |
| Oxytocin | | | | ca | | | |
| Penicillin G potassium | x | | | cay | | | |
| Perphenazine | cy | cy | | cy | | | |
| Phenytoin ***XA**** | | | | | | | |
| Phytonadione | | | | | | | |
| Piperacillin | x* | | | cay | | | cy |
| Potassium chloride | | | ca | ca | | | cy |
| Prochlorperazine | | | | | | | |
| Promethazine | | | | | | | |
| Propranolol | | | | ca | | | |
| Ranitidine | ca | | ca | ca | | | cy |
| Sargramostim | xy | cy | | cy | cy | cy | cy |
| Sodium bicarbonate | | | | | | | |
| Theophylline | | | xa | ca | | | |
| Ticarcillin | x* | | | cay | | | |
| Ticarcillin and clavulanate | x* | | | | | | |
| Tobramycin | - | | | ca | | | cy |
| Trimethoprim-sulfa. ***XA**** | | - | | xa | | | cy |
| Vancomycin | | | - | ca | | | cy |
| Verapamil | | | | - | | | |
| Vinblastine | | | | | - | csy | |
| Vincristine | | | | | csy | - | |
| Zidovudine | cy | cy | cy | | | | - |

APPENDIX G

# Food and Drug Administration Pregnancy Categories

The Food and Drug Administration (FDA) developed its list of pregnancy categories to alert and inform physicians, nurses, and pregnant women of the effects of certain drugs on the fetus. Most drugs are given a rating as a category A, B, C, D, or X. Category A drugs are the least dangerous to the fetus. These drugs have been tested in controlled studies and have been proven to cause no harm to the fetus even in the first trimester. In contrast, category X drugs are the most dangerous to the fetus. Category X drugs are known to cause harm in the human fetus, and there is no therapeutic benefit to be derived from these drugs that outweighs the risk to the fetus. The danger associated with categories B, C, and D fall between category A and category X drugs.

| Category | Description |
|---|---|
| A | Controlled studies have been completed in women. These studies have failed to show evidence of fetal harm. |
| B | Either (1) animal studies show no fetal risk, but studies have not been done in women *or* (2) animal studies indicate a risk of fetal harm, but studies in women show no risk. |
| C | Either (1) animal studies show a risk of fetal harm, but no studies have been done in women *or* (2) no studies have been done in women or animals. |
| D | Studies in women show proof of fetal damage. Use only if risk of untreated disease is greater than risk of drug use. The "warnings" section of the drug's label includes a statement of risk. |
| X | Studies in women or animals show definite risk of fetal abnormality. Risk outweighs any possible benefit. The "contraindications" section of the drug's label includes a statement of risk. |

APPENDIX H

# Recommendations for the Safe Handling and Disposal of Antineoplastic (Cytotoxic) Medications

Most antineoplastic or cytotoxic medications possess carcinogenic (ability to produce cancer), mutagenic (ability to induce a change in genetic material), or teratogenic (cause developmental anomalies in the embryo) attributes. In addition, many antineoplastics induce local irritation on direct contact with the skin, eyes, and mucous membranes or ulceration and necrosis of tissue. The toxicities associated with antineoplastic medications dictate that health care agencies develop and implement policies and procedures that minimize occupational exposure to these agents while assuring the maintenance of aseptic conditions during their preparation and administration.

Pharmacists, nurses, and housekeeping personnel are at risk for exposure to antineoplastic medications through the inhalation of aerosolized drug and direct skin contact. Exposure can occur during preparation, administration, or disposal of the medications or equipment used to prepare or administer the agents to the client. Education of all members of the health care team is the key to minimizing occupational risks. The National Institutes of Health (NIH) Division of Safety and the NIH Clinical Center Pharmacy Department and Cancer Nursing Service published "Recommendations for the Safe Handling of Antineoplastic (Cytotoxic) Drugs" (NIH Publication No. 92-2621) to assist health care workers in all settings minimize exposure to these agents.

## PERSONNEL CONSIDERATIONS

Only properly educated personnel should handle cytotoxic medications. It is recommended that new employees who risk exposure by virtue of their job responsibilities (pharmacists, technicians, nurses, aides, and housekeeping personnel) be offered training sessions that focus on reducing exposure and the safe handling of these agents and contaminants.

Employees should be informed that certain activities should not be performed in areas where cytotoxic agents are handled. Applying makeup near chemotherapeutic agents can prove hazardous. Inadvertent contamination of cosmetics may provide prolonged exposure. Eating, drinking, chewing gum, smoking, or storing food in areas where antineoplastic medications are stored or prepared should be prohibited. There is a risk of accidental ingestion with any of these activities. Periodic observation and monitoring of employees involved in any aspect of handling cytotoxic drugs is recommended to ensure compliance with procedures designed to reduce occupational exposure.

Employees who prepare cytotoxic agents should have periodic health examinations. Acute exposures should be documented, and the exposed employee referred for medical follow-up.

Because of the well-documented mutagenic, teratogenic, and abortifacient properties of certain cytotoxic agents, female employees who are pregnant or are attemping to conceive should exercise extreme caution when handling these medications. Although no studies to date address the possible risks associated with the occupational exposure to cytotoxic agents and their passage into breast milk, it is prudent for women who are breast-feeding to exercise caution when handling antineoplastic medications.

## PREPARATION OF ANTINEOPLASTIC AGENTS

All procedures involved in the preparation of parenteral cytotoxic medications should be performed by appropriately trained personnel in a class II type A or B laminar flow biologic safety cabinet. A class II type B safety cabinet is the cabinet of choice because it discharges exhaust to the outdoors. A class II type A safety cabinet discharges filtered exhaust into the room, but the installation of an exhaust canopy over the cabinet reroutes the exhaust to the outdoors. The safety cabinet should be inspected and certified at least annually by qualified personnel and anytime the cabinet is moved.

The safety cabinet's work surface should be cleaned with 70% alcohol before and after each use. Before preparing any cytotoxic medications, the safety cabinet's work surface should be covered with plastic-backed absorbent paper. This reduces the potential for dispersion of droplets and spills and facilitates clean up. This paper should be changed after any overt spills and at the end of the work shift.

The cabinet should be operated with the blower on 24 h/d, 7 d/wk unless it is used infrequently. If the cabinet is used for mixing only once or twice per week, it may be turned off after careful cleaning. Before beginning the next mixing session, the blower should be allowed to run for a minimum of 15 minutes. All materials necessary for preparing the medications should be placed in the cabinet before beginning the mixing session to avoid interruptions in cabinet air flow. Allow the cabinet blower to run for 2 to 3 minutes before beginning work so the unit can purge any airborne contaminants.

All cytotoxic drug preparation should take place with the view screen at the recommended access opening. The areas within 3 inches of the sides near the front opening are the least efficient areas of the cabinet in terms of product and personnel protection. All work should be performed in the cabinet away from these areas.

Personnel preparing the medications should wash their hands thoroughly before applying unpowdered latex surgical gloves and after removing them. A closed-front disposable or washable gown with elastic or knit ribbed cuffs is recommended. The cuffs should be pulled over the glove-covered wrists so that no skin is exposed. Gloves should be changed every 30 minutes when working continuously with cytotoxic agents. Protective clothing should not be worn outside of the drug preparation area. Any of this protective garb that becomes overtly contaminated or torn must be changed immediately.

In the event of skin contact with the antineoplastic agent, the affected area should be washed with soap and water, taking care not to abrade the area with excessive rubbing or a brush. If the eye is affected, flush immediately with copious amounts of water for 15 minutes while holding the eyelid open. The employee should then be evaluated by a physician.

The use of a venting device such as a 0.22-$\mu$m hydrophobic filter or chemotherapy dispensing pin reduces internal pressure and the probability of spraying and spillage when reconstituting vials of antineoplastic agents. Luer lock connections should be used for all equipment. A sterile alcohol prep should be wrapped around the needle when withdrawing it from the vial septum. This same technique should be used to control dripping and aerosol production when ejecting air or bubbles from a filled syringe.

The external surfaces of all syringes and drug solution containers (IV bags, bottles, cassettes, etc.) should be wiped with alcohol to remove any drug contamination before removal from the safety cabinet.

The procedure for opening glass ampules should include making certain that no drug is in the top of the ampule and wrapping the neck of the ampule with a sterile alcohol prep to contain aerosolized medication and protect fingers from laceration by glass shards. Withdraw the medication using a

5-$\mu$m filter needle or straw. Any excess drug should be placed in a closed collection vessel labeled as "Cytotoxic Waste," in the biologic safety cabinet, or in the original vial.

All cytotoxic products should be labeled with "Caution—Chemotherapy, Dispose of Properly." The prepared antineoplastic medication should be placed in a transparent plastic container and protected from leaking or breaking. The container should be labeled "Do Not Open if Contents Appear to be Broken."

After completion of the drug preparation, the interior of the safety cabinet should be wiped down with sterile water (appropriate for injection or irrigation) followed by 70% alcohol, using disposable towels. The towels and any contaminated preparation equipment, uncapped needles, filters, syringes, absorbent paper, gloves, disposable gowns, etc., should be disposed of intact in a puncture-resistant container. The container is then placed in a box that is sealed and labeled "Cytotoxic Waste Only." This box is disposed of according to federal, state, and local guidelines for regulated waste.

## ADMINISTRATION OF ANTINEOPLASTIC AGENTS

Only registered nurses with specialized training and knowledge may administer antineoplastic medications. Precautions similar to those used in the preparation of these medications are appropriate for nurses administering chemotherapeutic drugs. Unpowdered latex surgical gloves are put on after thorough handwashing. A closed-front disposable or washable gown with elastic or knit ribbed cuffs must be worn. Cuffs should be pulled over the glove-covered wrists to avoid skin exposure. Protective eye goggles may be worn.

All syringes and administration sets should have Luer lock connections to avoid drug leakage or spills. Special care must be taken when priming IV administration sets. Remove the distal tip or needle cover before priming. Prime the administration set into a sterile alcohol prep or a closed container such as the cytotoxic waste container. Do not prime sets or syringes into the sink or any open receptacle.

## DISPOSAL OF ANTINEOPLASTIC AGENTS

All contaminated supplies are disposed of intact to prevent aerosolization, leaks, and spills. All disposables used in the preparation and administration of the antineoplastic medications (including gloves and gowns) are placed in a large leak-proof, puncture-proof container labeled "Cytotoxic Waste." After securing the container cover, the container is placed in a box, taped, and labeled as indicated in agency policy and procedure. Some agencies use 4-mil polyethylene or 2-mil polypropylene bags instead of boxes. In either case the hazardous waste is labeled as such and disposed of according to federal, state, and local laws.

Nondisposable gowns or linens contaminated with body secretions of clients who received anitneoplastic medications within the previous 48 hours are placed in a laundry bag, which is placed in a special impervious bag marked with the appropriate labeling. Employees handling heavily soiled linens are instructed to wear two pairs of unpowdered surgical latex gloves, protective gowns, and possibly eye protection.

Spills must be attended to as soon as possible. Personnel should wear two pairs of unpowdered surgical latex gloves, gowns, and protective eyewear. Some agencies have spill kits for this purpose. Small amounts of liquid drug may be cleaned up with gauze pads. Larger spills require larger absorbent pads. After the drug is removed, the area is cleaned thoroughly three times with detergent. A final rinse with clean water completes the procedure.

## CLIENTS IN THE HOME SETTING

Clients who are receiving antineoplastic medications in the home and their caregivers should be instructed in the safe handling and disposal of the drug, supplies, and any linens, etc., contaminated with the medication or the client's body fluids. The client's home care nurse can provide this instruction. The pharmacy providing the drug will supply the client with a spill kit, gloves, a large puncture-proof, leak-proof container, labels, and gowns. The home care nurse can explain the use of each of these supplies. The pharmacy providing the medication is responsible for retrieving and disposing of any disposable hazardous waste according to federal, state, and local laws.

If the client receives the antineoplastic medication in the hospital or an outpatient clinic setting, it is the responsibility of the nurse to instruct the client and caregiver in the safe handling of any linens or surfaces that may become contaminated with the client's body fluids for a 48-hour period after the medication administration.

# Index

Note: Page numbers in *italics* refer to illustrations; page numbers followed by t refer to tables; drug names in *italics* refer to drugs not discussed in the text.

## C

## D

## I

## J



## K

## O